Total Fitness and Wellness

Canadian Edition

Total Fitness and Wellness
Canadian Edition

Scott K. Powers
University of Florida

Stephen L. Dodd
University of Florida

Angela M. Thompson
St. Francis Xavier University

Camie C. Condon
Wilfrid Laurier University

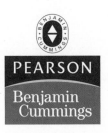

PEARSON

Benjamin
Cummings

Toronto

Library and Archives Canada Cataloguing in Publication

Total fitness and wellness/Scott K. Powers ... [et al.].—Canadian ed.

Includes index.

ISBN 0-205-44548-9

1. Physical fitness—Textbooks. 2. Health—Textbooks. I. Powers, Scott K. (Scott Kline), 1950–

RA781.T68 2006   613.7   C2005-904342-3

Vice President, Editorial Director: Michael J. Young

Editor-in-Chief: Gary Bennett

Acquisitions Editor: Kelly Torrance

Marketing Manager: Janet Piper

Developmental Editor: Madhu Ranadive

Production Editor: Marisa D'Andrea

Copy Editor: Kelli Howey

Proofreader: Jonathan Dore

Production Coordinator: Patricia Ciardullo

Literary Permissions Researcher: Lynn McIntyre

Photo Researcher: Amanda McCormick

Indexer: Nancy Mucklow

Page Layout: Joan M. Wilson

Art Director: Julia Hall

Interior and Cover Design: Miguel Acevedo

Cover Image: Getty Images/America 24-7/Jamie Squire

Statistics Canada information is used with the permission of the Minister of Industry, as Minister responsible for Statistics Canada. Information on the availability of the wide range of data from Statistics Canada can be obtained from Statistics Canada's Regional Offices, its World Wide Web site at http://www.statcan.ca, and its toll-free access number 1-800-263-1136. The Statistics Canada CANSIM II database can be accessed at http://cansim2.statcan.ca/.

10 11 12   15 14 13 12 11

Printed and bound in the United States.

PEARSON

Benjamin
Cummings

To my mother who encouraged me to pursue academic endeavours.   *Scott Powers*

To my family Haney, Will, Mom, and Dad. Your love and encouragement have always meant more than you will ever know.   *Stephen Dodd*

For all my previous, current, and future students who fuel my passion to be in the classroom. *Angie Thompson*

If this work is great, it is because I am supported by the broad shoulders of extraordinary colleagues, supportive family, and awe-inspiring students.   *Camie Condon*

Brief Contents

Contents

CHAPTER 3   General Principles of Exercise for Health and Fitness   67

CHAPTER 4   Exercise Prescription Principles: Cardiorespiratory Endurance   81

CHAPTER 8   Physical Activity, Dietary Intake, and Weight Maintenance   195

CHAPTER 9   Stress Management and Modifying Unhealthy Behaviour   227

CHAPTER 13   Prevention and Rehabilitation of Physical Activity–Related Injuries   291

CHAPTER 14   Prevention of Cardiovascular Disease   307

CHAPTER 15 Prevention of Cancer   325

Preface

Good health is our most precious possession. Although it is usually only in times of illness or injury that we really appreciate good health, more and more people are realizing that health is not simply the lack of disease. Indeed, there are degrees of health, or wellness, on which lifestyle can have a major impact.

Intended for an introductory post-secondary course in physical fitness and wellness, *Total Fitness and Wellness*, Canadian Edition, focuses on how lifestyle can be altered to achieve a high degree of physical fitness and wellness. Two major aspects of daily life that most affect our level of wellness are physical activity and dietary intake. Hence, the essential role of regular physical activity and good nutrition in achieving total fitness and wellness are major themes of the text.

Total Fitness and Wellness, Canadian Edition, is built on a strong foundation of exercise physiology and nutrition. The text provides clear and objective research-based information to post-secondary students during their first course in physical fitness and wellness. By offering a research-based text, we hope to dispel many myths associated with physical fitness, physical activity, nutrition, weight maintenance, and wellness. For the evaluation of various wellness components, such as physical fitness levels and nutritional status, a how-to approach is used. Ways to change your lifestyle that will improve wellness (e.g., designing a physical activity program and altering food choices) are described. Indeed, the title of the book—*Total Fitness and Wellness*—reflects our goals.

Numerous physical fitness and wellness texts are available today. Our motivation in writing this textbook was to create a unique *Canadian* physical fitness text, one that not only covers primary concepts of physical fitness and wellness but also addresses important issues, such as behaviour change, exercise-related injuries, physical activity and the environment, and physical activity for special populations.

Foundation in Exercise Physiology

We believe it is imperative that students develop an understanding of the basic physiological adaptations that occur in response to acute physical activity and regular training. Without this understanding, it is impossible to plan, modify, and properly execute a lifetime approach to physical activity and physical fitness.

Strong Emphasis on Nutrition

Because we feel so strongly about the important interaction between nutrition and physical activity, a nutritional theme is incorporated throughout the text. Each chapter includes Nutritional Links to Fitness boxes, which explain how nutrition affects health and wellness in areas such as cardiorespiratory endurance, muscular strength and endurance, and prevention of cardiovascular disease and cancer. We place major emphasis on and provide comprehensive coverage of basic nutrition and weight maintenance by dedicating separate chapters to each topic: Chapter 7, Nutrition, Health, and Physical Activity (includes the newly developed Dietary Reference Intakes [DRIs]) and Chapter 8, Physical Activity, Dietary Intake, and Weight Maintenance.

Coverage of the Latest Scientific Research on Physical Fitness, Nutrition, and Wellness

We firmly believe that post-secondary physical fitness and wellness texts should contain the latest scientific information and include references for scientific studies to support key information about physical activity, physical fitness, nutrition, and wellness. Our approach is to provide current scientific references that document the validity of presented facts. Accordingly, source information and suggested readings are placed at the end of each chapter.

The most current research in the arena of fitness and wellness is offered in *Total Fitness and Wellness*, Canadian Edition. For example, it is now clear that physical activity plays a role in reducing the risk of some cancers and can contribute to a longer life. While there has long been speculation about the health benefits of physical activity, evidence that supports this connection has only recently become available. In the area of nutrition, scientific data now suggest that vitamins may play a new role in preventing certain diseases and combating the aging process. In addition, while it is well accepted that fat in the diet increases our risk of heart disease, it has just lately been shown that dietary fat plays a greater role than other nutrients in weight gain.

With any attempt to present the most current information, there is always the danger of presenting ideas that are not fully substantiated by good research. We have made a concerted effort to avoid such a risk by using information from the most highly respected scientific journals and by consulting with experts in the field.

Each chapter of the Canadian edition has been revised to include the newest research developments in physical activity, physical fitness, wellness, and health-related nutrition. New and improved art and photos have been added to the text, as well as new and updated references in every chapter.

Layout and Features

While many topic and organization options have to be considered when developing a text, the best way to determine content and order is to ask instructors. Therefore, with input from instructors across the country, we have included the following coverage, layout, and features:

- Coverage: By design, *Total Fitness and Wellness,* Canadian Edition, contains more material than can be covered in a typical 15-week semester. The text is comprehensive in order to afford instructors a large degree of freedom in selecting concepts to be covered in their courses.

- Unique Topics: Several unique chapters are offered in the Canadian edition, which are not contained in other introductory fitness and wellness texts. For example, this book includes chapters on physical activity and the environment, physical activity for special populations, and prevention and rehabilitation of exercise-related injuries. Furthermore, in several chapters we have incorporated an elementary discussion of the physiology of exercise to improve students' knowledge of how the body operates and responds to regular physical activity.

- Informational Boxes: Each chapter contains informational A Closer Look boxes that offer extended coverage of concepts discussed in the body of the text with suggestions for practical application. Nutritional Links to Health and Fitness boxes emphasize the importance of nutrition to physical activity and physical fitness. Also included in this Canadian edition are boxed features called Ask an Expert, Fitness and Wellness for All, and Fitness–Wellness Consumer. Ask an Expert boxes provide the latest information from internationally known experts in the fields of resistance training, physical activity and nutrition, obesity, weight maintenance, physical activity and the environment, and the maintenance of a lifetime of physical activity. Fitness and Wellness for All boxes contain fitness, wellness, and nutritional information with respect to diversity. Fitness–Wellness Consumer boxes provide physical activity and wellness information related to consumer issues.

- Lab Exercises: Most chapters contain easy-to-follow, application-based lab exercises, such as fitness testing, nutritional evaluation, and cardiovascular risk assessment.

- Food Appendices: To assist students in tracking and modifying food intake, caloric and nutrient content of common foods and fast foods is offered in Appendices A and B.

- Pedagogical Aids: To stimulate students' interest and alert them to the significance of the material to be covered, Learning Objectives open each chapter. To emphasize and support understanding of material, important terms are boldfaced in the text, defined in a running glossary at the bottom of text pages, and compiled in the Glossary at the end of the text. Also, several features are offered at the end of each chapter to reinforce learning. For students' review, the Chapter Summary sections succinctly restate the most significant ideas

presented in the chapter. Study Questions encourage analysis of chapter discussions and prepare students for tests. Suggested Readings and References offer quality information sources for further study of fitness and wellness.

Instructor Supplements

A complete resource package accompanies *Total Fitness and Wellness,* Canadian Edition, to assist the instructor with classroom preparation and presentation.

- **Instructor's Resource CD-ROM (ISBN 0-205-48421-2)**

  The Instructor's Resource CD-ROM (IRCD) contains everything you need for efficient course preparation. All of the supplements on the IRCD have been revised to reflect changes made to the Canadian edition. The Instructor's CD-ROM contains the following:

  - **Instructor's Manual**

    The Instructor's Manual includes suggestions for class discussion, student activities, readings, lecture outlines, learning objectives, chapter summaries, web references, and media resources.

  - **Test Generator**

    The TestGen includes more than 1000 multiple-choice, true-or-false, short-answer, and matching questions in a format that allows instructors to incorporate these questions into their exams.

  - **PowerPoint® Lecture Slides**

    The PowerPoint Lecture Slides provide instructors with lecture notes to supplement their in-class discussions.

- **Companion Website (www.pearsoned.ca/powers)**

  This student resource site offers approximately 500 practice quiz questions, interactive activities, and web links to sites for further information.

Also Available—U.S. Instructor Supplements

Supplements from the U.S. edition are also available. Contact your Pearson Education Canada sales representative for more details.

- **Discovery Health Channel Health and Wellness Lecture Launcher Videos and CD-ROM (Volume I, 0-8053-5369-0; Volume II, 0-8053-6001-8, CD ROM, 0-8053-7830-8)**

  Created in partnership with Discovery Health Channel and Benjamin Cummings, these VHS tapes and CD-ROM feature a series of quick lecture launcher clips on topics from nutrition and stress management to substance abuse. There are 24 clips in all, each one between 5 and 10 minutes in length. This resource provides an excellent way to engage your students and enliven your lectures.

- **Benjamin Cummings Health Video Series**

  In addition to the Discovery Lecture Launcher series, additional videos are available to qualified adopters on a variety of topics. Contact your sales representative for a complete list of videos.

- **Films for the Humanities**

  More than 80 videos from respected sources are available to qualified adopters.

- **Transparency Acetates**

  More than 140 transparency acetates contain all figures, graphs, and tables from the main text. The transparencies are excellent for the presentation of information in a clear manner consistent with that of the textbook.

- **My HealthLab**

  My HealthLab features online access to a selection of print and media supplements to help motivate your students with personalized self-assessment, including activities, quizzes and tests, and other important study tools. The preloaded content on the interactive website includes an interactive e-book, self-assessment worksheets, Behavior Change Log Book and Wellness Journal, and links to e-themes from *The New York Times*, Research Navigator, and the Discovery Channel Lecture Launcher clips.

U.S. Student Supplements

- **Behavior Change Log Book and Wellness Journal**

  This assessment tool helps students track daily exercise and nutritional intake and create a long-term nutritional and fitness prescription plan. It also includes a behaviour change contract and topics for journal-based activities.

- **Stand-Alone EvaluEat Windows-Only CD-ROM**

  EvaluEat diet analysis software helps students track their eating habits and evaluate the nutritional content of their diets. This software features a database of more than 6200 food items and can report on dozens of different nutrients. Students can do a single- or multi-day diet analysis, create a variety of reports, and determine whether they are meeting the DRIs for various vitamins and minerals. This program also allows users to input their activity levels to create expenditure reports.

- **My HealthLab**

  My HealthLab features online access to a selection of print and media supplements for students and makes studying convenient and fun. The preloaded content on the interactive website includes an interactive e-book, self-assessment worksheets, Behavior Change Log Book and Wellness Journal, and links to e-themes from *The New York Times*, Research Navigator, and the Discovery Channel Lecture Launcher clips.

Acknowledgments

There are a lot of people to acknowledge for their contributions to this Canadian edition of *Total Fitness and Wellness*. Kelly Torrance, Senior Acquisitions Editor, was the driving force for bringing together the "Canadian" writing team of Angie Thompson and Camie Condon. Her positive encouragement, support, and guidance of our initial writing efforts are thoroughly appreciated. Tremendous gratitude also goes to Madhu Ranadive, Senior Developmental Editor, who provided significant support and guidance throughout the various stages of development of this Canadian edition. Dave Ward also deserves our gratitude for taking over the helm once the book was in the progress of revisions.

This book has also been greatly improved because of the significant contributions of Marisa D'Andrea, Editorial Coordinator; Patricia Ciardullo, Production Coordinator; Miguel Acevedo, Designer; Joan Wilson, Compositor; Kelli Howey, Copy Editor; and Jill Tracey, Technical Reviewer. Without their expert services, this book would not have the polished look that it does today.

A special thank you to Jonathan Bell and Lindsay Gosse who gave their time and energy to model for the photos showing the correct techniques for several cardiorespiratory fitness tests, strength and flexibility training, and body composition analysis.

It would be negligent if we did not also acknowledge the writers and various editors of the first through fourth U.S. editions of *Total Fitness and Wellness*. Clearly these authors and editors laid the groundwork that we quite simply followed, expanded, and updated for a first Canadian edition. We are indebted to you for providing a quality manuscript with which to work.

Finally, we acknowledge the many reviewers who provided substantive comments and suggestions for each stage of our revisions:

Ken Brooks, Conestoga College

Susan Brown, Centennial College

Kimberley Gammage, Brock University

Dan Kato, Grant MacEwan College

Robin Laking, Georgian College, Orillia Campus

Aletheia Mendes, Taylor University College

Ginette Michel, Laurentian University

Galen Plett, Briercrest College

Keith W. Russell, University of Saskatchewan

Bill Sheel, University of British Columbia

Patti Thorne, Memorial University

Melody Torcolacci, Queen's University

Jill Tracey, Wilfrid Laurier University

Darren Warburton, University of British Columbia

Gordon Wilcox, Algonquin College

Ilsa Wong, University of Lethbridge

A Great Way to Learn and Instruct Online

The Pearson Education Canada Companion Website is easy to navigate and is organized to correspond to the chapters in this textbook. Whether you are a student in the classroom or a distance learner you will discover helpful resources for in-depth study and research that empower you in your quest for greater knowledge and maximize your potential for success in the course.

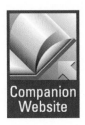
Companion Website

[www.pearsoned.ca/powers] Enter

PEARSON
Benjamin
Cummings

Jump to... http://www.pearsoned.ca/powers ⬍ Home Search Help Profile

Companion Website

Home >

Companion Website

Total Fitness and Wellness, Canadian Edition, by Powers, Dodd, Thompson, Condon

Total Fitness and Wellness
Canadian Edition

Student Resources

The modules in this section provide students with tools for learning course material. These modules include:

- Chapter Objectives
- Quizzes
- Weblinks
- Self Assessment
- Glossary and Flashcards
- Journal Topics

In the quiz modules students can send answers to the grader and receive instant feedback on their progress through the Results Reporter. Coaching comments and references to the textbook may be available to ensure that students take advantage of all available resources to enhance their learning experience.

Instructor Resources

The modules in this section provide instructors with additional teaching tools. Downloadable PowerPoint Presentations, Electronic Transparencies, and an Instructor's Manual are just some of the materials that may be available in this section. Where appropriate, this section will be password protected. To get a password, simply contact your Pearson Education Canada Representative or call Faculty Sales and Services at 1-800-850-5813.

CHAPTER 1

Understanding Health-Related Physical Activity and Wellness

1

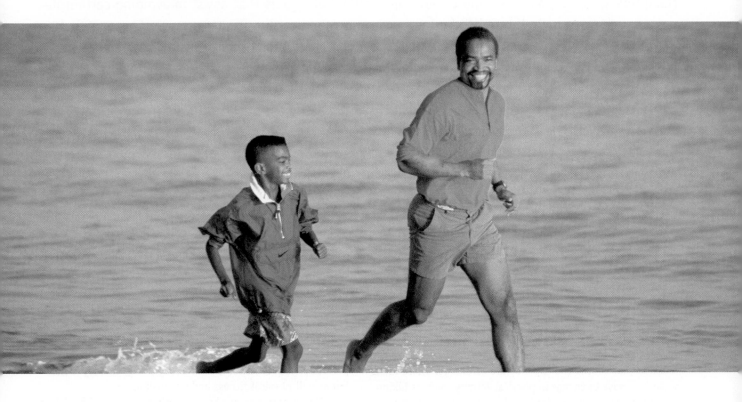

After studying this chapter, you should be able to

1. Describe the health benefits of physical activity.

2. Discuss the importance of healthy active living as it relates to the population health approach.

3. Discuss the concept of healthy active living versus physical activity, physical fitness, and exercise.

4. Define the terms *coronary heart disease* and *myocardial infarction*.

5. Compare the goals of health-related physical fitness prescriptions and sport-performance conditioning programs.

6. Describe the five components of health-related physical fitness.

7. Outline the seven components of wellness.

8. Outline the components of SuPeR SMART goal setting.

"Just do it." "Use it or lose it." "No pain, no gain." Chances are these slogans and clichés are very familiar to you—but what do they really mean to you and your health? Most of us realize the importance of being healthy but don't understand what is required at a personal level. For example, have you taken the time to evaluate your current health and fitness levels? What does it mean to you to be physically active? What will it take for you to maintain or enhance your current healthy behaviours?

This book contains the latest scientific information on how to evaluate your current level of physical fitness (Chapters 2 through 6, 11); to establish healthy eating habits and weight management (Chapters 7 and 8); to develop and maintain a physically active lifestyle as you age (Chapters 1, 12, 13, and 16); and to develop healthy behaviours that assist in avoiding certain illnesses such as sexually transmitted infections, cancer, and cardiovascular disease (Chapters 9, 10, 14, 15, and 16). A major theme of this text is the combined promotion of healthy eating and physical activity to improve overall well-being. Careful consideration of the material will provide answers to hundreds of nutrition, activity, and exercise-related questions.

In this first chapter, the benefits of healthy active living are outlined in detail, covering topics such as physical activity, physical fitness, wellness, and goal setting. Understanding the pervasive role that physical activity and physical fitness play in the maintenance of good health is a strong motivator for developing and sustaining a lifetime of healthy active living.

Health Benefits of Physical Activity

Why engage in physical activity? Almost all of us ask this question at some time in our lives. The answer is simple: Physical activity is good for you. In general, **physical activity** is considered any bodily movement produced by the body's muscles that causes the expenditure of energy. There are a variety of ways to engage in physical activity, such as hiking, biking, dancing, or gardening. Regular physical activity improves overall **physical fitness**—the body's ability to function at optimal efficiency with improved health and longevity. Health Canada's Physical Activity Unit (2005) defines regular physical activity as low-intensity activities such as snowshoeing, golfing, or walking, and suggests that adults acquire up to an hour a day of one or more of these lower-intensity activi-

ties. As fitness improves, Health Canada suggests stepping up to moderate-intensity activity for 30 to 60 minutes most days of the week, or 20 to 30 minutes of vigorous exercise four days a week. The Physical Activity Unit defines **exercise** as a specific physical activity, often called *training,* that uses the body's muscles, heart, and lungs. This type of activity could include group fitness classes, running, or playing basketball or soccer. A **healthy active lifestyle** is one that values and incorporates physical activity into everyday living, thereby increasing overall physical fitness and well-being.

The importance of physical activity and good health is emphasized in the Integrated Pan-Canadian Healthy Living Strategy developed by the federal, provincial, and territorial ministers of health. This initiative resulted in a report entitled the *Population Health Approach* (1999); the report states that two-thirds of Canadians between the ages of 25 and 55 are inactive. More than half the population is not engaging in the minimum requirement of 30 minutes of physical activity per day. The *Population Health Approach* (1999) focuses on the underlying reasons why Canadians are inactive, and then suggests strategies to overcome these conditions at several levels (see A Closer Look box: "A Population Health Approach"). It goes on to point out that each year three-quarters of deaths result from four groups of diseases: cardiovascular, cancer, diabetes, and respiratory. Two risk factors that lead to these diseases are physical inactivity and unhealthy eating. Health Canada (2005b) estimates that the economic burden caused by physical inactivity has reached $5.3 billion. Most Canadians can make improve-

physical activity Any bodily movement produced by the skeletal muscles that expends energy.

physical fitness The ability of the body to function at optimal efficiency with an improved physiological state that can lead to improved health and longevity.

exercise A specific physical activity (often called *training*) that causes the exertion of the muscles, heart, and lungs through various movements.

healthy active lifestyle A lifestyle that values and incorporates physical activity into everyday living.

ments to their health by engaging in 30 to 60 minutes of regular physical activity most days of the week (Bruce & Katzmarzyk, 2002; Katzmarzyk, 2002; Katzmarzyk & Craig, 2002; Katzmarzyk, Hebebrand, & Bouchard, 2002). A summary of these benefits is illustrated in Figure 1.1; a brief discussion of the major health benefits of physical activity follows.

Physical Activity Reduces the Risk of Heart Disease

Cardiovascular diseases (i.e., ailments of the heart and blood vessels) are a major cause of death in Canada. In fact, 22 percent of all male deaths and 19 percent of all female deaths are due to cardiovascular disease (Heart and Stroke Foundation, 2005; Morris, 1994). It is well established that regular physical activity can significantly reduce your risk of developing cardiovascular disease (Barrow, 1992; Bouchard, Shephard, Stephens, Sutton, & McPherson, 1990; Fagard, 1999; Health Canada, 2005b; Lee & Paffenbarger, 2000; Margen et al., 1992; Morris, 1994; Paffenbarger, Hyde, Wing, & Hsieh, 1986; Paffenbarger et al., 1994; Pollock & Wilmore, 1990; Powers & Demirel, 1998; Powers, Locke, & Demirel, 2001; Williams, 1997; Williams, 2001; Wood, 1994; Yamashita et al., 1999). Further, there is strong evidence that regular physical activity reduces the risk of death during a **myocardial infarction** (i.e., heart attack) (Lee & Paffenbarger, 2000; Lennon et al., 2004). The protective effect of physical activity training during a heart attack is illustrated in Figure 1.2. Notice that physical activity can reduce the magnitude of cardiac injury during a heart attack by 66 percent (Powers, Locke, & Demirel, 2001; Yamashita et al., 1999). Many specialists in preventive medicine argue that these facts alone are reason enough to engage in regular physical activity (Barrow, 1992; Paffenbarger et al.,

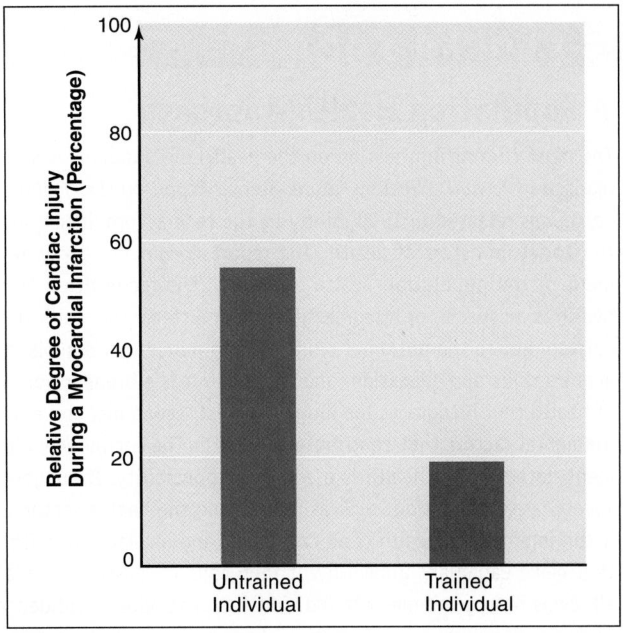

FIGURE 1.2 Regular endurance activities protect the heart against injury during a heart attack. This figure illustrates that during a myocardial infarction (i.e., heart attack) trained individuals suffer less cardiac (i.e., heart) injury than untrained individuals. Data are from research by Yamashita et al. (1999).

1994; Powell & Blair, 1994). Chapter 14 provides a detailed discussion of physical activity and cardiovascular disease.

Physical Activity Reduces the Risk of Diabetes

Diabetes is a disease characterized by high blood sugar (glucose) levels. Untreated diabetes can result in numerous health problems, including blindness and kidney dysfunction. Regular physical activity can reduce the risk of type 2 diabetes by improving the regulation of blood glucose (Helmrich, Ragland, & Paffenbarger, 1994; Pan et al., 1997; Rodnick, Holloszy, Mondon, & James, 1990). More is said about diabetes in Chapter 12.

Physical Activity Increases Bone Mass

The primary functions of the skeleton are to provide a mechanical lever system of interconnected bones to permit movement and to protect internal organs. Given these roles, it is important to maintain strong and healthy bones. The

myocardial infarction (MI) (also called a heart attack) Damage to the heart due to a reduction in blood flow, resulting in the death of heart muscle cells.

diabetes A metabolic disorder characterized by high blood glucose levels.

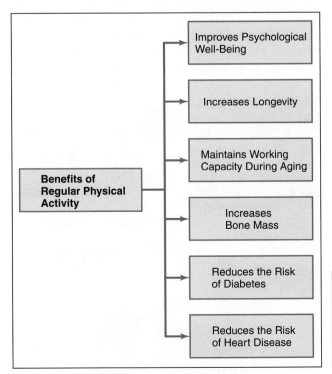

FIGURE 1.1 Benefits of regular physical activity.

A Population Health Approach

The most current information on the health of Canadians is summarized in *Toward a Healthy Future: Second Report on the Health of Canadians* released in 1999 jointly by the federal, provincial, and territorial ministers of health. The report documents a key element of the population health approach: the recognition that health is a capacity or resource rather than a state. This definition corresponds to the notion of being able to pursue one's goals, to acquire skills and education, and to grow—it is a broader notion of health that recognizes the range of social, economic, and environmental factors that contribute to health. The second key element noted is that health is a shared responsibility. It suggests several areas for action, such as revitalizing the health sector so it can improve the health of all Canadians, and reducing inequities that make Canadians unhealthy. It then calls for participation at all levels from government to individual so that public confidence in decision making and information sharing is increased, ensuring that those Canadians most affected by a health issue can contribute early in the planning process. Developing a population health approach requires building health alliances with sectors not traditionally thought of as health-oriented, such as finance, housing, education, recreation, and other social services. This innovative and interconnected framework is a strategy to achieve the greatest positive impact on population health.

The Federal Level: Collaborates on an international level to share information and develop the infrastructure to institutionalize the population health approach.

The Provincial Level: Collaborates across ministries to develop healthy public policies, health goals, and accountability frameworks that reflect the population health approach.

The Private-Sector Level: Provides a safe and healthy working environment and opportunities for continuous learning, and takes responsibility for protecting the environment.

The Local Level: Communities involve citizens in planning and providing high-quality services, and share information and resources that maximize health impacts.

The Individual Level: Individuals contribute by taking responsibility for their own health and well-being, making informed health decisions, and participating in community activities that have an impact on health.

Source: Federal, Provincial and Territorial Advisory Committee on Population Health. *Toward a Healthy Future: Second Report on the Health of Canadians.* "Health Canada Backgrounder: Health Services and Population Health—1999." Minister of Public Works and Government Services Canada.

loss of bone mass and strength (called **osteoporosis**) increases the risk of bone fractures. Although osteoporosis can occur in men and women of all ages, it is more common in the elderly, particularly among women.

Is there a link between physical activity and maintenance of good bone health? Yes! A key factor in regulating bone mass and strength is mechanical force applied by muscular activity. Indeed, numerous studies have demonstrated that regular physical activity increases bone mass and strength in young adults (Rankin, 1993; Taaffe, Robinson, Snow, & Marcus, 1997; Wheeler et al., 1995). Further, research on osteoporosis suggests that regular physical activity can prevent bone loss in the elderly and is also useful in the treatment of individuals with osteoporosis (Rankin, 1993; Taaffe et al., 1997; Wheeler et al., 1995).

Physical Activity Maintains Physical Working Capacity During Aging

Human aging is characterized by a gradual loss of physical working capacity. As we grow older there is a progressive decline in our ability to perform strenuous activities (e.g.,

running, cycling, or swimming). Although this process may begin as early as one's 20s, the most dramatic changes occur after approximately 60 years of age (Bouchard et al., 1990; Fleg & Lakatta, 1988; Hagberg, 1987). It is well established that regular physical activity can slow the rate of decline in physical working capacity while aging (Hagberg, 1987; Hammeren et al., 1992; Powers, Lawler, Criswell, Fu-Kong Lieu,

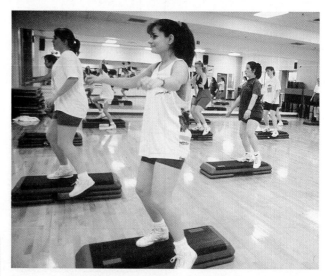

Regular physical activity and exercise can prevent the loss of bone mass.

osteoporosis The loss of bone mass and strength, which increases the risk of bone fractures.

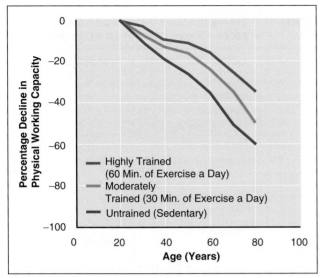

FIGURE 1.3 The relationship among age, physical activity, and decline in physical working capacity.

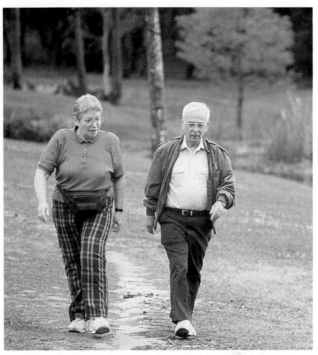

Regular physical activity has been shown to improve longevity.

& Martin, 1992). This fact is illustrated in Figure 1.3. Notice the differences in physical working capacity among highly trained, moderately trained, and inactive individuals during the aging process. The key point is that although a natural decline of ability occurs with age, regular physical activity can reduce the rate of this decline, resulting in an increased ability to enjoy a lifetime of physical recreation, health, and independence. Indeed, perhaps the most important benefit of regular physical activity may be the improved quality of life.

Physical Activity Increases Longevity

Although it is a controversial topic, growing evidence suggests that regular physical activity (combined with a healthy lifestyle) increases longevity (Bouchard et al., 1990; Franklin, 2001; Holloszy, 1993; Lee & Paffenbarger, 2000; Lee, Paffenbarger & Hennekens, 1997; Paffenbarger et al., 1986; Paffenbarger et al., 1994). For example, a classic study of Harvard alumni over the past 30 years reported that men with a sedentary (i.e., physically inactive) lifestyle have a 31-percent greater risk of death from all causes than men who engage in regular physical activity (Paffenbarger et al., 1986). This translates into a longer lifespan for those who are physically active. What factors are responsible for the increased longevity due to regular physical activity? The primary factor is that individuals who are regularly active have a lower risk of heart attack and cancer (Paffenbarger et al., 1986; Paffenbarger et al., 1994) (Chapters 9 and 14).

Physical Activity Improves Psychological Well-Being

Strong evidence indicates that regular physical activity improves psychological well-being in people of all ages.

Specifically, the mental health benefits of regular activity include a reduction in anxiety, depression, and reactivity to stress (Bouchard et al., 1990). These mental benefits lead to an improved sense of well-being in the physically active individual. We will further discuss the role of physical activity as a method for reducing psychological stress in Chapter 9.

How Much Physical Activity Is Required?

Physical activity doesn't have to be very hard to improve your health. Engaging in at least 10 minutes of physical activity several times throughout the day (for up to 60 minutes) will make a difference. After three months of regular physical activity you will notice a change.

Table 1.1 outlines the Public Health Agency of Canada's Physical Activity Unit's guidelines for most adults. The guidelines change slightly for children and special populations, which will be discussed in later chapters.

Physical Activity Training for Health-Related Physical Fitness

In general, physical fitness conditioning programs can be divided into two broad categories defined by their goals: sport-specific training (training that is meant to improve sport performance) and health-related physical fitness (the ability to

Very Light Effort	Light Effort 60 min.	Moderate Effort 30 to 60 min.	Vigorous Effort 20 to 30 min.	Maximum Effort 20 to 30 min.
Strolling Dusting	Light walking Volleyball Easy gardening Stretching	Brisk walking Biking Raking leaves Swimming Dancing Water aerobics	Aerobics Jogging Hockey Basketball Fast swimming Fast dancing	Sprinting Racing
How does it feel? How warm am I? What is my breathing like?				
No change from rest state	Starting to feel warm	Warmer	Quite warm	Very hot/perspiring heavily
Normal breathing	Slight increase in breathing rate	Greater increase in breathing rate	More out of breath	Completely out of breath
Range needed to stay healthy				

TABLE 1.1 Physical Activity and Effort Guidelines

Source: *Physical Activity Unit: Effort for Exercise*, Public Health Agency of Canada, 2005. Reproduced with the permission of the Minister of Public Works and Government Services Canada 2005.

function at optimal efficiency with physiological improvements that can lead to improved health and longevity). This textbook focuses on health-related physical fitness.

The overall goal of a total health-related physical fitness prescription is to optimize quality of life (Bouchard et al., 1990; Margen et al., 1992; Pollock & Wilmore, 1990). The specific goal of this type of fitness prescription is to reduce the risk of disease and to improve total physical fitness so that daily tasks can be completed with less effort and fatigue.

Although some conditioning programs aimed at improving sport performance may reduce the risk of disease, this is not their primary purpose. Instead, the single goal of a sport-conditioning program is to improve physical performance in a specific sport. However, even the "weekend" athlete who engages in total health-related physical fitness activities could also improve his or her physical performance in many sports. Specifically, health-related fitness improves sport performance by increasing cardiorespiratory endurance, muscular strength and endurance, and flexibility, and by reducing the risk of injury.

Components of Health-Related Physical Fitness

Exercise scientists (i.e., experts in exercise and physical fitness) do not always agree on all of the basic components of physical fitness. However, most do agree that the *five*

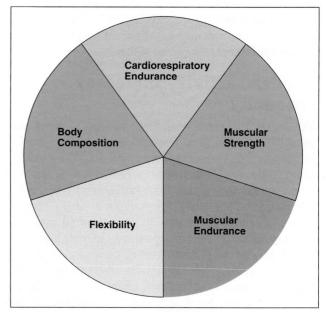

FIGURE 1.4 Components of health-related physical fitness.

major components of total health-related physical fitness (Figure 1.4) are:

1. cardiorespiratory endurance
2. muscular strength
3. muscular endurance
4. flexibility
5. body composition

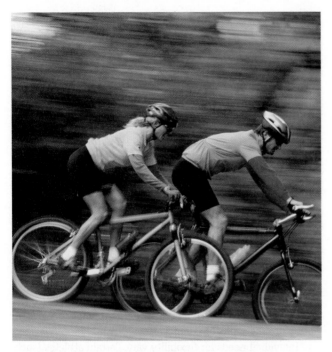

Individuals who have achieved a high level of cardiorespiratory endurance are capable of performing 30 to 60 minutes of vigorous activity without undue fatigue.

In addition to the health-related components of physical fitness, there are the skill-related components, which are sometimes called the *sport-related* or *skill-related components of fitness*. They are:

1. agility
2. balance
3. coordination
4. reaction time
5. speed
6. power
7. mental capability

These sport-related or skill-related components have at times been considered less important to overall health; however, these components of fitness are involved in all physical activity and are necessary for daily functioning. For example, physical agility and speed make it possible to quickly change direction or move out of the way when faced with an oncoming car. Mental capability or focus allows us to enjoy the relaxing and psychological benefits of walking through the park. Power gives us the ability to move quickly. Though these skills are certainly related to sport-specific training, it is obvious they have their place in a healthy active lifestyle as well.

Cardiorespiratory Endurance

Cardiorespiratory endurance (sometimes called *aerobic fitness* or *cardiorespiratory fitness*) is considered a key component of health-related physical fitness. It is a measure of the heart's ability to pump oxygen-rich blood to the working muscles during activity. It is also a measure of the muscles' ability to take up and use the delivered oxygen to produce the energy needed to continue physical activity. In practical terms, cardiorespiratory endurance is the ability to perform endurance-type activities (distance running, cycling, swimming, etc.). The individual who has achieved a high measure of cardiorespiratory endurance is generally capable of performing 30 to 60 minutes of vigorous activity without undue fatigue. Chapter 4 discusses the details of training designed to improve cardiorespiratory endurance.

Muscular Strength

Muscular strength is the maximal ability of a muscle to generate force (Powers & Howley, 2001; Robergs & Roberts, 2000; Williams, 1996). It is evaluated by how much force a muscle (or muscle group) can generate during a single maximal contraction. Practically, this means how much weight an individual can lift or move during one maximal effort.

Muscular strength is important in almost all sports. Athletes who participate in football, basketball, and hockey require a high level of muscular strength. Yet, even nonathletes require some degree of muscular strength to function in everyday life. For example, routine tasks around the home such as lifting bags of groceries and moving furniture require muscular strength. Resistance training (also called *weight* or *strength training*) results in an increase in the size and strength of muscles. The principles of developing muscular strength are presented in Chapter 5.

Muscular Endurance

Muscular endurance is defined as the ability of a muscle or muscle group to generate force over and over again or to sustain muscular contractions. Although muscular strength and muscular endurance are related, they are not the same. These two terms can be best distinguished by examples. An excellent example of muscular strength is a person lifting a heavy barbell during one maximal muscular effort. In contrast, muscular endurance is illustrated by a weight lifter performing multiple lifts or repetitions of a lighter weight.

Most successfully played sports require muscular endurance. For instance, tennis players, who must repeatedly swing their racquets during a match, require a high level of muscular endurance. Many everyday activities (e.g., waxing your car) also require some level of muscular endurance. Techniques of developing muscular endurance are also discussed in Chapter 5.

muscular strength The maximum amount of force that can be produced during one contraction.

muscular endurance The ability of a muscle or muscle group to generate force over and over again or to sustain muscular contractions.

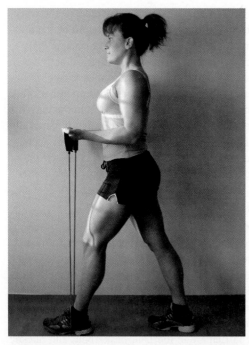

Resistance training can result in an increase in muscular strength.

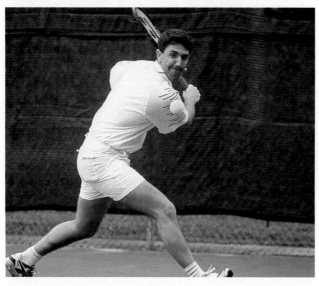

Tennis players require a high level of muscular endurance to play long matches.

Flexibility

Flexibility is the ability to move joints freely through their full range of motion. Flexible individuals can bend and twist at their joints with ease. Without routine stretching, muscles and

flexibility The ability to move joints freely through their full range of motion.

body composition The relative amount of fat and lean body tissue (muscle, organs, bone) found in the body.

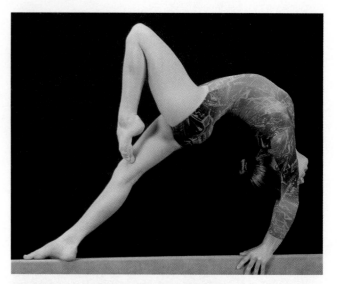

Gymnasts require great flexibility to be successful.

tendons shorten and become tight; this can limit the range of motion around joints and impair movement.

Individual needs for flexibility vary. Certain athletes (such as gymnasts and divers) require great flexibility in order to accomplish complex movements. The average individual requires less flexibility than an elite athlete; however, everyone needs some flexibility in order to perform activities of daily living. Research suggests that flexibility is useful in preventing some types of muscle–tendon injuries and may be useful in reducing low back pain (Cady, Bischoff, O'Connell, Thomas, & Allan, 1979; Cady, Thomas, & Karasky, 1985). Techniques for improving flexibility are discussed in Chapter 6.

Body Composition

The term **body composition** refers to the relative amount of fat and lean body tissue (muscle, organs, bone) found in your body. The rationale for including body composition as a component of health-related physical fitness is that having a high percentage of body fat (a condition known as *obesity*) is associated with an increased risk of coronary heart disease. Obesity also increases the risk of type 2 diabetes and contributes to joint stress during movement. In general, being "over-fat" elevates the risk of medical problems.

Lack of physical activity is shown to play a major role in gaining body fat. Conversely, regular physical activity is an important factor in promoting and maintaining lean muscle tissue. Assessment of body composition is discussed in Chapter 2, and the relationship between physical activity and weight maintenance is discussed in Chapter 8.

Wellness: A Healthy Lifestyle

Good health was once defined as the absence of disease. In the 1970s and 1980s many exercise scientists and health educators became dissatisfied with this limited definition of good health. These futuristic thinkers believed that health not only was the absence of disease but also included physical, emotional, and spiritual well-being. This concept of good health is called **wellness** (Margen et al., 1992) and is specifically defined as a state of optimal health that includes physical, emotional, intellectual, spiritual, social, environmental, and occupational health (Figure 1.5). In a broad sense, the term wellness means "healthy living."

Healthy living refers to health behaviours aimed at reducing one's risk of disease and accidents, achieving optimal physical health, and maximizing emotional, intellectual, spiritual, and social health (Heart and Stroke Foundation, 2005; Margen et al., 1992; Paffenbarger et al., 1994). It can be achieved by practising a healthy lifestyle, which includes regular physical activity, healthy eating, eliminating unhealthy behaviours, and cultivating emotional and spiritual soundness.

Physical Health

Physical health incorporates various physical characteristics and activities. Physical characteristics can include body size, shape, and susceptibility to illness or disease. Achieving wellness means developing and maintaining a body composition that is healthy for your age and sex. Making sure that you are engaging in healthy eating and visiting your health care provider on a regular basis are also a part of the interrelated dimensions of wellness. Physical activity can also positively affect your health by reducing your risk of certain diseases such as heart disease and type 2 diabetes. As well, it can improve your physical fitness and enhance overall mental health and longevity.

Emotional Health

Emotions play an important role in how you feel about yourself and others. *Emotional health* (also called *mental health*) includes your social skills and interpersonal relationships. Also included are your levels of self-esteem and your sense of self-efficacy (i.e., the belief in your ability to cope successfully with the routine stress of daily living).

The cornerstone of emotional health is *emotional stability*, which describes how well you deal with the day-to-day stresses of personal interactions and the physical environment. Although it is normal to experience some range of emotional highs and lows, the objective of achieving emotional wellness is to maintain emotional stability somewhere between an extreme high and an extreme low.

Intellectual Health

Intellectual health can be maintained by keeping your mind active through life-long learning. Although there are many ways to maintain an active mind, attending lectures, engaging in thoughtful discussions with friends or teachers, and reading are obvious ways to promote intellectual health. Maintaining good intellectual health can improve your quality of life by increasing your ability to define and solve problems. Further, continuous learning and thinking can provide you with a sense of fulfillment.

Spiritual Health

Spiritual health is often called the glue that holds an individual together. The term *spiritual* means different things to different people, but regardless of whether you define spiritual health as religious beliefs or the establishment of personal values, it is an important aspect of wellness and is closely linked to emotional health (Williams, 1996).

Optimal spiritual health is often described as the development of spiritual makeup to its fullest potential. This includes the ability to find a sense of purpose in life and to experience love, joy, pain, peace, and sorrow, and to care for and respect all living things (Williams, 1996). Anyone who has experienced a beautiful sunset or smelled the first scents of spring can appreciate the pleasure of maintaining optimal spiritual health (Williams, 1996).

Social Health

Social health is defined as the development and maintenance of meaningful interpersonal relationships. It involves the ability to get along with others and appreciate their individuality. Socially healthy people are able to show concern for their community and exhibit fairness and justice toward others. They also develop genuine friendships; foster close family ties; and engage in community activities. Having a sense of belonging to a large social unit and benefiting from the resultant feeling of emotional security is evidence of true social health.

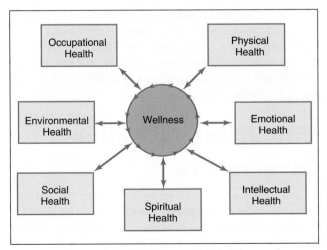

FIGURE 1.5 The wellness components and their interactions.

wellness A state of healthy living that includes physical, emotional, intellectual, spiritual, social, environmental, and occupational health.

Good Nutrition Is Essential to Achieving Physical Fitness and Wellness

A major theme of this book is that healthy eating is essential for developing and maintaining physical fitness and a state of wellness. Good nutrition means that an individual's dietary intake provides all of the components of food (called *nutrients*) needed to promote growth and repair body tissues. Additionally, a healthy dietary plan supplies the energy required to meet the body's daily needs.

Consuming too little of any nutrient can impair physical health and fitness and potentially result in disease (Powers & Howley, 2001). Therefore, eating well should be a goal for every-

one. In many of the chapters that follow, we provide nutritional information in the form of informational boxes such as this one. In addition, Chapter 7 is devoted entirely to nutrition.

Although consuming inadequate nutrients increases your risk of disease, consuming too much food (overeating) can be problematic as well. Overeating on a regular basis can lead to fat gain, resulting in obesity. As mentioned earlier, obesity increases your risk of coronary heart disease, some types of cancer, and type 2 diabetes. Chapter 8 discusses the relationship among nutrition, physical activity, and healthy weight management.

Environmental Health

Environmental wellness is the awareness of the precarious state of the earth. It deals with the preservation of natural resources as well as the protection of plant and animal wildlife. In the last few generations we have developed dependencies on automobiles and general industrialization that have created worldwide pollution.

Outdoor enthusiasts in large metropolitan cities can discuss at length the impact that gas-powered vehicles have had on their outdoor fun. On any given summer afternoon, many people consult their local radio stations or Environment Canada for the latest in smog alerts before venturing out for a run or a walk with their dogs.

The government recognizes the impact of the environment on health. In its draft *Report on Plans and Priorities: 2004–2005*, Environment Canada highlights clean air, toxic substances, and pollutants as critical issues that directly impact the health of Canadians. The agenda has made these issues Environment Canada's number-one priority as it seeks to promote the reduction of health risks and achieve physical improvements in things like air and water quality. These actions can reduce the incidence of health-related illnesses such as asthma and bronchial infections caused by air pollutants and *E.coli* outbreaks from contaminated drinking water.

The 10-year Action Plan on Clean Air has made substantial progress on a vehicles and fuels agenda, and Canada-wide standards on key air pollutants have also been created. However, the prevention of pollution and contamination is not just a government responsibility.

Environmental wellness includes being socially responsible and engaging in activities that protect the environment and wildlife: recycling, limiting the use of pesticides, carpooling, and conserving electricity and gas. The most comprehensive health and wellness plan cannot produce improvement if we do not have the highest-quality air, water,

and food. We must all take part in improving the quality of our environment—our physical health depends on it!

Occupational Health

Occupational health involves deriving personal satisfaction and confidence from your vocation and maintaining a satisfying balance between work and leisure. Since a majority of your time will likely be spent in the workplace, it is important that your career provide you with internal and external rewards that you personally value. For example, do you want a job that allows interaction with others? Do you prefer opportunities for advancement or leadership? How will your job affect your family now and in the future? Occupational health also involves a work environment that minimizes stress and exposure to health risks as well as accommodates personal weaknesses and strengths. Ergonomically correct workstations will assist in decreasing overuse injuries like carpal tunnel syndrome. Shift work that provides adequate rotation throughout the schedule and appropriate lighting during night work can minimize the harsh effects on the body and reduce potential injury. Proper labelling of chemicals can warn of potential danger to you or your unborn child. Comprehensive on-the-job training will instruct on back safety and health in order to keep you injury free. If you are overworked, underappreciated, and dissatisfied, and are continuously at risk or chronically injured, you will find that your entire well-being suffers.

Interaction of Wellness Components

No one component of wellness works in isolation; a strong interaction must occur among all seven of them. For example, poor physical health (such as chronic disease) can lead to poor emotional health (such as depression). Similarly, a lack of spiritual health—an inability to feel valuable—can contribute to poor emotional health and affect our relationships with family and friends. Simple steps to improving overall well-being can be as easy as being physically active with friends or encouraging family activities. This interaction will benefit not only your physical health, but also your emotional and social well-being. Being active in community works programs and volunteerism benefits the environment, helps others, and gives you a greater sense of belonging. Finding the activities to spice up your life and bring personal value and fulfillment creates strong spiritual wellness. These mind–body interactions are illustrated in Figure 1.5. Total wellness can be achieved only by a balance of physical, emotional, intellectual, spiritual, social, environmental, and occupational health.

Wellness Goals for the Nation

Healthy people are one of a nation's greatest resources. Poor health drains national resources by reducing worker productivity and increasing the amount of government money spent on health. Because of this, the Canadian government has established wellness goals for the nation. The government's Integrated Pan-Canadian Healthy Living Strategy seeks to improve the overall health of Canadians through all the stages of life and to reduce health disparities (Health Canada, 2005b). One of the objectives to improve the health of all age groups is to encourage active living. The concept of active living is based on the premise that the benefits of physical activity go beyond the prevention of disease. Active living values physical activity as an essential part of all the aspects and stages of life, and is characterized by the integration of all forms of physical activity in daily routines and leisure. For more details on the goals and objectives of the Integrated

Pan-Canadian Healthy Living Strategy, see the Health Canada website at **www.phac-aspc.gc.ca/hl-vs-strat**.

Living a Healthy Active Lifestyle

How does one practise a healthy active lifestyle? A good place to begin is with a personal assessment of your health-risk status. Laboratory 1.1 on page 16 is a lifestyle assessment inventory designed to increase your awareness of factors that affect your health. As you work on Laboratory 1.1, keep in mind that you have control over each of these factors, but that awareness alone does not result in change. A decision to alter your lifestyle to achieve total wellness is necessary—and is one that only you can make. Make a commitment today to improve the quality of your life by practising a healthy active lifestyle.

Physical activity, good nutrition, healthy weight management, stress management, and healthy behaviours are key components of a lifestyle that leads to wellness. Each of these issues is discussed in detail in Chapters 3 through 16.

Goal Setting and Motivation

Achieving a healthy active lifestyle or gaining a certain level of physical fitness requires time and effort. Unfortunately, many people who begin training programs stop before much progress has been achieved. Regular physical activity and physical fitness cannot be achieved in a matter of a few days. In general, 3 to 6 weeks of regular activity is required for any noticeable improvements in body composition, muscle strength and endurance, or cardiorespiratory endurance. Improvement will come if you are patient, diligent, and set realistic goals.

FITNESS AND WELLNESS FOR ALL

Wellness Issues Across the Population

The steps required to achieve wellness are the same across all populations. However, some individuals may experience difficulties in achieving wellness due to factors related to ethnicity, sex, age, and socioeconomic status. For example, in Canada type 2 diabetes was once virtually unknown among the Aboriginal population. Now the prevalence rate is at least three times the national average, with high rates occurring in all age groups (Health Canada, 2005a). The data available for some First Nations groups indicate a high rate of complications such as heart disease, hypertension, stroke, and lower limb amputations. Risk factors such as obesity

and physical inactivity are increasing while Aboriginal peoples experience the lowest access to physician and health professional services.

Type 2 diabetes is a critical health issue in the Aboriginal population for a variety of reasons other than prevalence rates. Other concerns include early onset, greater severity at diagnosis, high rates of complications, and lack of accessible services. Although wellness goals are similar across all populations, individual differences among people can present special challenges in achieving wellness.

The key to maintaining a lifetime of healthy active living is personal motivation. Motivation in this case can be viewed as the *energy required to maintain your desire* to engage in regular physical activity (Robergs and Roberts, 2000). The motivation to change from a sedentary lifestyle to a healthy active lifestyle requires behaviour modification and establishing goals. Without question, goal setting is the cornerstone to any kind of success. Establishing realistic goals provides a target for your efforts. Setting SuPeR SMART goals can help develop an achievable and realistic plan for personal success. The components for SuPeR SMART goals are outlined below.

Self-controllable. Whatever you choose as a goal has to be within your control. Weight loss is often a goal for individuals, but it is not necessarily self-controllable. Weight loss is an outcome of behaviours that can be modified or controlled. A more appropriate goal would be to increase the amount of fruit consumed in one day, or to limit the amount of sweets or processed foods eaten in a week. It could also include achieving a certain number of hours of physical activity per week.

Public. Making your goal visible on a daily basis will be a constant reminder of what you are trying to achieve. For example, keeping a calendar on the refrigerator and marking off the number of days when you engaged in vigorous activity can assist in your keeping track of your achievements.

Rewards. Rewarding yourself for accomplishments is important and can keep you motivated to stay on track. Remember, the reward should not be contrary to what you are trying to achieve, so treating yourself to a doughnut when your goal is to eat healthfully may not be the best idea. Instead, reward yourself with a healthy lunch with friends, a small shopping trip, or even a few extra minutes of sleep. Rewards should also not be so few and far between that they seem unattainable. Small pleasures at consistent intervals are an excellent motivator.

Specific. The desired outcome must be clear and precise. The desire to increase physical activity is not specific enough, and many people struggle with where to begin. Define what is meant by physical activity for you: is it moving from completely sedentary to active, or from moderately active to highly active? Each one will have a different prescription. Start by following the guidelines given by Canada's Physical Activity Guide. An example of goal setting using the guidelines for a sedentary person might be to accumulate the minimum of 30 to 60 minutes of moderate activity every day. To attain this, start out by engaging in 30 minutes of low-intensity activity a day. This can be achieved in 10-minute increments and with a variety of activities (see Table 1.1). After achieving and maintaining this goal for a specific

amount of time (i.e., 7 days), it will then be necessary to set a new goal that is consistent with achieving the desired 30 to 60 minutes of moderate-intensity activity each day.

Measurable. It is best if the outcome can be expressed in numbers; so, for the sedentary person, the goal of acquiring 20 to 30 minutes of physical activity every day has been set, with the ultimate goal being 30 to 60 minutes of moderate activity every day. Other quantifiable goals can be the number of fruit or vegetable servings consumed in one day, the amount of time spent on a project, or how often to engage in community activities.

Adjustable. Your goals and timelines need to be adjustable. Life can be unpredictable, and if you start to fall behind because of one stressor or another it is important to recognize that it's okay to be temporarily set back, as long as the setback isn't permanent. For example, you may have set the personal goal to quit smoking, you've outlined specific and measurable goals, and you are making progress. Then you encounter a personal stressor—a job change, or the loss of a family member—and you find yourself smoking to relieve the tension. This kind of setback is not uncommon. What is necessary is to identify why it happened, accept that this was a momentary disappointment, revamp your goals to meet your immediate needs, and start again.

Realistic. Whatever your desired goal is, it is important to make sure that achieving it is reasonable. Evaluating your circumstances—that is, your financial, environmental, physical, and emotional situations—is a part of successful goal setting. You may set a goal to climb Mount Everest in the next year—it's an admirable goal, but if you do not have the financial means to get there or the family or social networks supporting your efforts, it may not be realistic for your current situation. It does not mean that you cannot set a similar goal, such as planning and saving for a family vacation that may include hiking or climbing.

Time-based. Again, quantifiable numbers are important: without a specific date or deadline for achievement you simply have a wish, not a goal. Setting a realistic timeline requires accountability for your choices and actions. You do not want the timeline to be so unrealistic that if the goal is not achieved by the deadline you experience a sense of failure, thereby reducing your motivation to keep trying. Similarly, if the timeline is too far off in the future you can easily lose sight of what you are trying to achieve.

Whether you are trying to become more socially active, eat more healthfully, or become more physically active in order to improve physical fitness, your goals should be centred around the SuPeR SMART components and aimed at improving your overall well-being. More guidance in physical activity and physical fitness goal setting is provided in Chapters 3, 4, and 16.

Physical Fitness and Wellness: A Final Word

In this chapter, we discuss the benefits of regular physical activity and the importance of a healthy lifestyle to achieving wellness. The remainder of this book presents information that will help you set goals to increase your physical fitness, enrich your nutritional intake, and improve your health and wellness. Simply reading this book, however, will not accomplish these goals. Achieving physical fitness and wellness requires a personal commitment to regular activity and wise lifestyle choices. Indeed, there is no "magic pill" that you can take to make you healthy or improve your physical fitness. Start today and become physically active—your body will love you for it!

Summary

1. Physical activity offers many health benefits. Regular activity reduces the risk of coronary heart disease, some types of cancer, and type 2 diabetes, as well as increases bone mass and maintains physical working capacity during normal aging.

2. The five major components of "total" health–related physical fitness are

   a. cardiorespiratory endurance

   b. muscular strength

   c. muscular endurance

   d. flexibility

   e. body composition

3. The skill-related components of physical activity are

   agility

   balance

   coordination

   reaction time

   speed

   power

   mental capability

4. The term *wellness* means "healthy living." This state is achieved by practising a positive healthy lifestyle that includes regular physical activity, healthy eating, eliminating unhealthy behaviours (avoiding high-risk activities such as reckless driving, smoking, and illegal drug use), and maintaining good physical, emotional, intellectual, spiritual, social, environmental, and occupational health.

5. Total wellness can be achieved only by a balance of physical, emotional, intellectual, spiritual, social, environmental, and occupational health. The components of wellness do not work in isolation.

6. Setting goals is a key component in the maintenance of a lifetime of physical activity and achieving overall health and wellness.

7. SuPeR SMART goals comprise the following components:

   Self-controllable

   Public

   Rewards

   Specific

   Measurable

   Adjustable

   Realistic

   Time-based

Study Questions

1. Define the term *body composition*.
2. How much physical activity is required for healthy living?
3. Discuss the wellness concept.
4. Define *osteoporosis*.
5. List and discuss four major health benefits of regular physical activity.
6. Discuss fitness training for sport performance versus training for health-related fitness.
7. List and define the five components of health-related fitness.
8. List the seven skill-related components and how they are used every day.
9. Outline the SuPeR SMART strategies for setting exercise goals.
10. What causes a myocardial infarction?
11. List and define the seven components of wellness.

Suggested Reading

Armbruster, B., & Gladwin, L. (2001). More than fitness for older adults. *ACSM's Health and Fitness Journal, 5,* 6–12.

Fortier, M. D., Katzmarzyk, P. T., & Bouchard, C. (2002). Physical activity and seven-year changes in adiposity in Canada. *Canadian Journal of Applied Physiology, 27,* 449–462.

Hunt, M., Katzmarzyk, P. T., Pérusse, L., Rice, T., Rao, D. C., & Bouchard, C. (2002). Familial resemblance for seven-year changes in body mass and adiposity. *Obesity Research, 10,* 507–517.

Janssen, I., Katzmarzyk, P. T., & Ross, R. (2002). Body mass index, waist circumference and health risk: Evidence in support of current NIH guidelines. *Archives of Internal Medicine, 162,* 2074–2079.

Katzmarzyk, P. T., Craig, C. L., & Bouchard, C. (2002). Adiposity, adipose tissue distribution and mortality. *International Journal of Obesity and Related Metabolic Disorders, 26,* 1054–1059.

Tremblay, M. S., Katzmarzyk, P. T., & Willms, J. D. (2002). Temporal trends in overweight and obesity in Canada, 1981–1996. *International Journal of Obesity and Related Metabolic Disorders, 26,* 538–543.

Weblinks

Heart and Stroke Foundation of Canada

www.heartandstroke.ca

Contains the latest information about ways to reduce your risk of heart diseases. Includes information about physical activity and nutrition.

The Canadian Society for Exercise Physiology

www.csep.ca

Contains information about physical activity, health, and fitness.

Coalition for Active Living

www.activeliving.ca

Contains the latest information on a variety of health-related topics including nutrition, physical activity, and stress. Links to nutrition, fitness, and wellness topics.

Health Canada, Healthy Living

www.hc-sc.gc.ca

Contains information about the Canadian government's initiative to improve health and wellness for the Canadian people.

Canadian Council for Active Living at Work

www.cchalw-ccsvat.ca

Provides resources, tools, and expertise to active-living and health professionals in Canadian workplaces.

References

Barrow, M. (1992). *Heart talk: Understanding cardiovascular diseases.* Gainesville, FL: Cor-Ed Publishing.

Bouchard, C., Shephard, R., Stephens, T., Sutton, J., & McPherson, B. (Eds.). (1990). *Exercise, fitness, and health: A consensus of current knowledge.* Champaign, IL: Human Kinetics.

Bruce, M. & Katzmarzyk, P. T. (2002). Canadian population trends in leisure-time physical activity levels, 1981–1998. *Canadian Journal of Applied Physiology, 27,* 627–636.

Cady, L., Bischoff, D., O'Connell, E., Thomas, P., & Allan, J. (1979). Strength and fitness and subsequent back injuries in fire-fighters. *Journal of Occupational Medicine, 4,* 269–272.

Cady, L., Thomas, P., & Karasky, R. (1985). Programs for increasing health and physical fitness of fire-fighters. *Journal of Occupational Medicine, 2,* 111–114.

Fagard, R. (1999). Physical activity in the prevention and treatment of hypertension in the obese. *Medicine and Science in Sports and Exercise, 31,* S624–S630.

Fleg, J., & Lakatta, E. (1988). Role of muscle loss in the age-associated reduction in VO_2max. *Journal of Applied Physiology, 65,* 1147–1151.

Franklin, B. (2001). Improved fitness × Increased longevity. *ACSM's Health and Fitness Journal, 5,* 32–33.

Hagberg, J. (1987). Effect of training in the decline of VO_2max with aging. *Federation Proceedings, 46,* 1830–1833.

Hammeren, J., Powers, S., Lawler, J., Criswell, D., Martin, D., Lowenthal, D., & Pollock, M. (1992). Exercise training-induced alterations in skeletal muscle oxidative and antioxidant enzyme activity in senescent rats. *International Journal of Sports Medicine, 13,* 412–416.

Health Canada. (2005a). Aboriginal Diabetes Initiative: Diabetes among Aboriginal (First Nation, Inuit, Métis) People in Canada: The evidence. Retrieved February 2005 from www.hc-sc.qc.ca/fnihb-dqspni/cp.

Health Canada. (2005b). Healthy living. Retrieved February 2005 from www.hc-sc.gc.ca/english/lifestyles/healthyliving.

Helmrich, S., Ragland, D., & Paffenbarger, R. (1994). Prevention of non–insulin-dependent diabetes mellitus with physical activity. *Medicine and Science in Sports and Exercise, 26,* 824–830.

Holloszy, J. (1993). Exercise increases average longevity of female rats despite increased food intake and no growth retardation. *Journal of Gerontology, 48,* B97–B100.

Katzmarzyk, P. T. (2002). The Canadian obesity epidemic, 1985–1998. *Canadian Medical Association Journal, 166,* 1039–1040.

Katzmarzyk, P. T., & Craig, C. L. (2002). Musculoskeletal fitness and risk of mortality. *Medicine and Science in Sports and Exercise, 34,* 740–744.

Katzmarzyk, P. T., Hebebrand, J., & Bouchard, C. (2002). Spousal resemblance in the Canadian population: Implications for the obesity epidemic. *International Journal of Obesity and Related Metabolic Disorders, 26,* 241–246.

Lee, I., & Paffenbarger, R. (2000). Associations of light, moderate, and vigorous intensity physical activity with longevity: The Harvard Alumni Health Study. *American Journal of Epidemiology, 151,* 293–299.

Lee, I., Paffenbarger, R., & Hennekens, C. (1997). Physical activity, physical fitness, and longevity. *Aging–Milano, 9,* 2–11.

Lennon, S., Quindry, J., Hamilton, K., French, J., Staib, J., Mehta, J., & Powers, S. K. (2004). Loss of cardio protection after cessation of exercise. *Journal of Applied Physiology, 96,* 1299–1305.

Margen, S., et al. (Eds.). (1992). *The wellness encyclopedia.* Boston: Houghton Mifflin.

Morris, J. (1994). Exercise in the prevention of coronary heart disease: Today's best buy in public health. *Medicine and Science in Sports and Exercise, 26,* 807–814.

Paffenbarger, R., Hyde, R., Wing, A., & Hsieh, C. (1986). Physical activity, all cause mortality, longevity of college alumni. *New England Journal of Medicine, 314,* 605–613.

Paffenbarger, R., Kampert, J., I-Min Lee, Hyde, R., Leung, R., & Wing, A. (1994). Changes in physical activity and other lifeway patterns influencing longevity. *Medicine and Science in Sports and Exercise, 26,* 857–865.

Pan, X. R., et al. (1997). Effects of diet and exercise in preventing NIDDM in people with impaired glucose tolerance. *Diabetes Care, 20,* 537–544.

Pollock, M., & Wilmore, J. (1990). *Exercise in health and disease.* Philadelphia: W. B. Saunders.

Powell, K., & Blair, S. (1994). The public health burdens of sedentary living habits: Theoretical but realistic estimates. *Medicine and Science in Sports and Exercise, 26,* 851–856.

Powers, S., Demirel, H. A., et al. (1998). Exercise training improves myocardial tolerance to in vivo ischemia-reperfusion in the rat. *American Journal of Physiology, 275,* R1468–R1477.

Powers, S., & Howley, E. (2001). *Exercise physiology: Theory and application to fitness and performance* (4th ed.). St. Louis: McGraw-Hill.

Powers, S., Lawler, J., Criswell, D., Fu-Kong Lieu, & Martin, D. (1992). Aging and respiratory muscle metabolic plasticity: Effects of endurance training. *Journal of Applied Physiology, 72,* 1068–1073.

Powers, S., Locke, M., & Demirel, H. (2001). Exercise, heat shock proteins, and myocardial protection from I-R injury. *Medicine and Science in Sports and Exercise, 33,* 386–392.

Rankin, J. (1993). Diet, exercise, and osteoporosis. *Certified News (American College of Sports Medicine), 3,* 1–4.

Robergs, R., & Roberts, S. (2000). *Fundamental principles of exercise physiology: For fitness, performance, and health.* St. Louis: McGraw-Hill.

Rodnick, K., Holloszy, J., Mondon, C., & James, D. (1990). Effects of exercise training on insulin-regulatable glucose-transporter protein levels in rat skeletal muscle. *Diabetes, 39,* 1425–1429.

Taaffe, D., Robinson, T., Snow, C., & Marcus, R. (1997). High impact exercise promotes bone gain in well-trained female athletes. *Journal of Bone and Mineral Research, 12,* 255–260.

Wheeler, D., Graves, J., Miller, G., Vander Griend, R., Wronski, T., Powers, S. K., & Park, H. (1995). Effects of running on the torsional strength, morphometry, and bone mass of the rat skeleton. *Medicine and Science in Sports and Exercise, 27,* 520–529.

Williams, M. (1996). *Lifetime fitness and wellness.* Dubuque, IA: Wm. C. Brown.

Williams, P. (2001). Physical fitness and activity as separate heart disease risk factors: A meta-analysis. *Medicine and Science in Sports and Exercise, 33,* 754–761.

Williams, P. T. (1997). Relationship between distance run per week to coronary heart disease risk factors in 8283 male runners: The National Runners Health Study. *Archives of Internal Medicine, 157,* 191–198.

Wood, P. (1994). Physical activity, diet, and health: Independent and interactive effects. *Medicine and Science in Sports and Exercise, 26,* 838–843.

Yamashita, N., Hoshida, S., Otsu, K., Asahi, M., Kuzuya, T., & Hori, M. (1999). Exercise provides direct biphasic cardioprotection via manganese superoxide dismutase activation. *Journal of Experimental Medicine, 189,* 1699–1706.

Lifestyle Assessment Inventory

Name_____ Age _____ Sex _____ Date _____

The purpose of this lifestyle assessment inventory is to increase your awareness of areas in your life that increase your risk of disease, injury, and possibly premature death. A key point to remember is that you have control over each lifestyle area discussed.

Awareness is the first step in making change. After identifying the areas that require modification, you will be able to use the behaviour-modification techniques presented in Chapter 9 to bring about positive lifestyle changes.

DIRECTIONS

Put a check by each statement that applies to you. You may select more than one choice per category.

A. PHYSICAL FITNESS

_____ I engage in physical activity for a minimum of 20 to 30 minutes (at least 3 days per week).

_____ I play sports routinely (2 to 3 times per week).

_____ I walk for 15 to 30 minutes (3 to 7 days per week).

B. BODY FAT

_____ There is no place on my body where I can pinch more than 2.5 cm of fat.

_____ I am satisfied with the way my body appears.

C. STRESS LEVEL

_____ I find it easy to relax.

_____ I rarely feel tense or anxious.

_____ I am able to cope with daily stresses without undue emotional stress.

D. CAR SAFETY

_____ I have not had an auto accident in the past 4 years.

_____ I always use a seat belt when I drive.

_____ I rarely drive above the speed limit.

E. SLEEP

_____ I always get 7 to 9 hours of sleep.

_____ I do not have trouble going to sleep.

_____ I generally do not wake up during the night.

F. RELATIONSHIPS

_____ I have a happy and satisfying relationship with my partner.

_____ I have many close friends.

_____ I get a great deal of love and support from my family.

G. NUTRITION

_____ I generally eat 3 balanced meals and 2 healthy snacks per day.

_____ I rarely eat to the point of feeling uncomfortable.

_____ I rarely eat large quantities of fatty foods and sweets.

H. ALCOHOL USE

_____ I consume fewer than two drinks per day.

_____ I never get intoxicated.

_____ I never drink and drive.

I. TOBACCO USE

_____ I never smoke (cigarettes, pipe, cigars, etc.).

_____ I am not exposed to second-hand smoke on a regular basis.

_____ I do not use smokeless tobacco.

J. DRUG USE

_____ I never use illicit drugs.

_____ I never abuse legal drugs such as diet or sleeping pills.

K. SEXUAL PRACTICES

_____ I always practise safe sex (e.g., always using condoms or being involved in a monogamous relationship).

SCORING

1. **Individual areas:** If there are any unchecked areas in categories A through K, you can improve those aspects of your lifestyle.

2. **Overall lifestyle:** Add up your total number of checks. Scoring can be interpreted as follows:

   23–29 Very healthy lifestyle

   17–22 Average healthy lifestyle

   ≤16   Unhealthy lifestyle (needs improvement)

CHAPTER 2

Fitness Evaluation: Self-Testing

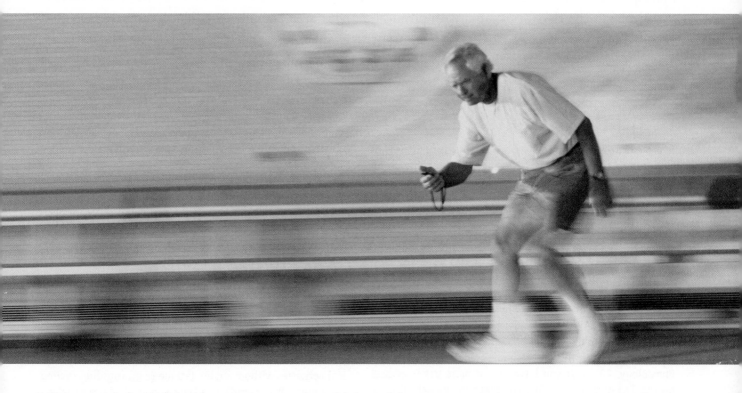

After studying this chapter, you should be able to

1. Explain the rationale for using field tests to assess cardiorespiratory endurance.

2. Explain the principle behind field testing of cardiorespiratory endurance using the modified Canadian Aerobic Fitness Test (mCAFT), Leger's 20-metre shuttle run, the 1.5-mile run test, the 1-mile walk test, the cycle ergometer test, and the step test.

3. Outline the design of the one-repetition maximum (1 RM) test for measurement of muscular strength.

4. Summarize the push-up and curl-up tests used to measure muscular endurance.

5. Define the term *flexibility* and describe two field tests used to assess it.

6. Explain the importance of body composition assessment in health-related physical fitness testing.

7. Describe how body composition is assessed using hydrostatic weighing, air displacement plethysmography (ADP), dual-energy X-ray absorptiometry (DXA), bioelectrical impedance analysis (BIA), skinfold measurements, waist girth, and body mass index (BMI).

An objective evaluation of your current physical fitness status is important prior to beginning an exercise program (American College of Sports Medicine, 1998, 2000; Barrow, 1992; Canadian Society for Exercise Physiology, 2003; Corbin, Welk, Lindsey, & Corbin, 2003; Getchell, 1998;

McGlynn, 1998; Pollock & Wilmore, 1990). This evaluation provides valuable information concerning your strengths and weaknesses and enables you to set reasonable fitness goals. Further, testing your initial physical fitness level also provides a benchmark against which you can compare future evaluations. Periodic retesting (every 3 to 6 months) provides motivating feedback as your training program progresses.

This chapter presents several physical fitness tests you can use for personal assessment. These tests are designed to evaluate each of the major components of health-related physical fitness: cardiorespiratory endurance, muscular strength, muscular endurance, flexibility, and body composition.

Although the risks associated with physical activity are generally less than the risks associated with living a sedentary lifestyle, it is important to evaluate your health status before engaging in any physical fitness test or before you become much more physically active.

Evaluating Health Status

Is a medical exam required before testing your fitness or beginning a fitness program? The answer is probably no for most healthy postsecondary-age individuals (American College of Sports Medicine, 1998, 2000). Although regular medical exams are encouraged for everyone, most people under 69 years of age generally do not require special medical clearance before beginning a low- to moderate-intensity physical activity program. However, if you have any concerns about your health, an examination by a physician is prudent prior to starting a physical activity program. Laboratory 2.1 contains the Physical Activity Readiness Questionnaire (PAR-Q), a useful screening questionnaire for people aged 15 to 69 who are becoming more active or beginning an exercise program (Canadian Society for Exercise Physiology, 2003). If you have one or more yes responses on the PAR-Q you can still participate in the activities to estimate your body composition, but you should not engage in any of the other tests to measure your physical fitness until you've contacted your physician and have been given approval to do so.

Should individuals over 69 years old have a medical exam at the beginning of an exercise program? The most conservative answer is yes. This is particularly true for obese and/or sedentary individuals.

Measuring Cardiorespiratory Endurance

As noted in Chapter 1, cardiorespiratory endurance is the ability of the heart and lungs to supply the working muscles with the nutrients needed to perform vigorous-intensity physical activities without undue fatigue (e.g., running, cycling, swimming). It is considered a key component of health-related

---

A CLOSER LOOK

Maximum Oxygen Uptake (VO$_2$max)

VO$_2$max, the maximal capacity to transport and utilize oxygen during exercise, is considered the most valid measurement of cardiorespiratory fitness (Powers & Howley, 2004; Robergs & Keteyian, 2002). In cardiorespiratory endurance testing, VO$_2$max is expressed as a function of body weight (called *relative VO$_2$max*). This means that "absolute" VO$_2$max (expressed in millilitres per minute; commonly written as ml·min^{-1}) is divided by the subject's body weight in kilograms. Therefore, relative VO$_2$max is expressed in millilitres (mL) of oxygen consumed per minute per kilogram of body weight (ml·kg^{-1}·min). Expressing VO$_2$max relative to body weight is necessary since body size influences cardiorespiratory performance. Specifically, a larger body (height or weight) requires more absolute aerobic power to do the same work as a smaller body. For example, two 20-year-old males derived the same value for absolute VO$_2$max, at 3212 ml·kg^{-1}·min^{-1}. One male weighed 55 kg, while the other weighed 75 kg. The male who weighed 55 kg has a relative VO$_2$max value of 58.4 ml·kg^{-1}·min^{-1}, while the male who weighed 75 kg has a relative VO$_2$max value of 42.8 ml·kg^{-1}·min^{-1}.

The higher the relative VO$_2$max, the greater the cardiorespiratory fitness. For example, a 20-year-old female student with a relative VO$_2$max of 53 ml·kg^{-1}·min^{-1} would be classified in the "superior" cardiorespiratory fitness category. In contrast, a 20-year-old woman with a VO$_2$max of 29 ml·kg^{-1}·min^{-1} would be classified in the "very poor" fitness category (Golding, Myers, & Sinning, 1989) (refer to Table 2.13 in Laboratory 2.6).

The Exercise ECG

The *electrocardiogram* (ECG, or sometimes EKG) is a common medical test that measures the electrical activity of the heart and can be used to diagnose several types of heart disease (Pollock & Wilmore, 1990; Pollock, Wilmore, & Fox, 1978). Although a resting ECG is useful for determining the heart's function, ECG monitoring during exercise is particularly useful in diagnosing hidden heart problems, because heart abnormalities often appear during periods of emotional or exercise stress (Pollock & Wilmore, 1990). An exercise ECG, commonly called an **exercise stress test**, is generally performed on a treadmill while a physician monitors the subject's heart rate, blood pressure, and ECG. The test begins with a brief warm-up period followed by a progressive increase in exercise intensity until the subject cannot continue or the physician stops the test for medical reasons. In general, the duration of the test varies as a function of the subject's fitness level. For example, poorly conditioned people may exercise for only 10 to 12 minutes, whereas well-conditioned subjects may work for up to 25 or 30 minutes. Therefore, the exercise stress test provides data not only about your cardiovascular health, but also about your cardiorespiratory endurance.

---

physical fitness. The most accurate means of measuring cardiorespiratory endurance is the laboratory assessment of *maximal oxygen consumption* (also called VO_2max or *aerobic power*) (Powers & Howley, 2004; Robergs & Keteyian, 2002). In simple terms, VO_2max is a measure of the endurance capacity of the cardiorespiratory system and exercising skeletal muscles. Direct measurement of VO_2max requires expensive laboratory equipment and is very time consuming; as such, it is impractical for general use. Alternatively, researchers have developed numerous methods for estimating VO_2max using simple field tests (Cooper, 1977, 1982; Fox, 1973).

Generally, these field tests are easy to administer and require less sophisticated and less expensive equipment. Results from these indirect measurements of cardiorespiratory endurance are somewhat less valid ($\pm 10-15$ percent) than direct measurements of VO_2max, but accuracy of the tests can be improved by avoiding strenuous activity and caffeine (or anything else that influences your heart rate) for 24 hours prior to the test and refraining from smoking or eating for 3 hours prior to the test. In most field tests, cardiorespiratory endurance is estimated from exercising or recovery heart rates or the time taken to complete the test, with age, sex, and body weight controlled. A lower heart rate in a submaximal exercise test indicates greater cardiorespiratory endurance. A lower recovery heart rate also indicates greater cardiorespiratory efficiency. Further, the less time it takes you to complete a field test, the greater your VO_2max.

Modified Canadian Aerobic Fitness Test (mCAFT)

A standard assessment of cardiorespiratory endurance promoted by the Canadian Society of Exercise Physiology (CSEP) is the modified Canadian Aerobic Fitness Test (mCAFT) (Canadian Society of Exercise Physiology, 1993). The validity of the mCAFT in predicting VO_2max has been established for males and females between ages 15 and 69 (Weller, Thomas,

exercise stress test A diagnostic test designed to determine if a subject's cardiovascular system responds normally to exercise.

Gledhill, Paterson, & Quinney, 1995). The physiological principle underlying the mCAFT is that more-fit individuals complete each stage of this test with a lower heart rate than less conditioned individuals. In this test, you complete one or more 3-minute sessions of stepping on double 20.3-cm steps at a predetermined pace based on your age and sex (see Figure 2.1). Using the protocol outlined above, heart rate is measured 5 to 10 seconds after each 3 minutes of stepping (see Figure 2.2). Depending upon your heart rate, you will proceed to the next stage or terminate the test. The final exercising heart rate is used along with your age and sex to determine an aerobic fitness score, which is then compared to the established *health benefit zone*. (See Laboratory 2.2 for more complete details on administering and interpreting the mCAFT.) The mCAFT is designed so that each person begins stepping at an intensity of 65 to 70 percent of the average VO_2max of a person 10 years older and then proceeds to an exercise intensity of 65 to 70 percent of the average VO_2max of a person their own age. If the second stage is completed without reaching the ceiling heart rate of 85 percent of the individual's predicted maximum heart rate, the individual proceeds to an exercise intensity equivalent to 65 to 70 percent of the average VO_2max of a person 10 years younger.

Leger's 20-Metre Shuttle Run

Another assessment of cardiorespiratory endurance promoted by the CSEP is Leger's 20-metre shuttle run (Canadian Society of Exercise Physiology, 1993). The validity of this test has been established with males and females 19 to 47 years of age (Leger & Gadboury, 1989). Since the Leger test involves a maximal protocol, it is not recommended for sedentary individuals or for individuals with musculoskeletal problems. The physiological principle underlying the Leger test, given

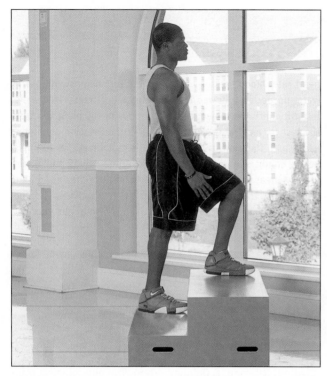

FIGURE 2.1 Subject performing the modified Canadian Aerobic Fitness Test (mCAFT).

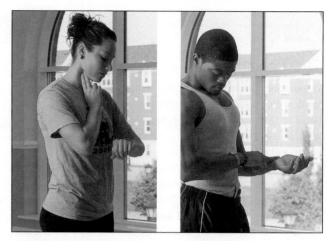

FIGURE 2.2 Subjects counting heart rate using the radial or carotid artery. Palpation of the radial artery (wrist) or carotid artery (neck) is a simple means of determining heart rate. The procedure is performed as follows. Locate your radial or carotid artery using your index finger. After finding your radial or carotid pulse, count the number of heart beats that occur during a 15-second period. Heart rate for 1 minute is calculated by multiplying the number of heart beats counted in 15 seconds by 4. For example, a 15-second heart rate count of 30 beats would indicate that the heart rate was 120 beats/min (i.e., $30 \times 4 = 120$). Alternatively, a 10-second count can be made. Heart rate for 1 minute is then calculated by multiplying the number of heart beats counted by 6. When palpating the carotid artery, apply limited pressure on the neck since too much force will result in a reflexic lowering of heart rate and therefore bias heart rate measurement.

that it involves a maximal protocol, is that more physically fit individuals are capable of reaching higher stages (speeds) of the test. In this test, you are required to run back and forth on a 20-metre course, touching a line at either end according to a predetermined cadence. The initial cadence is set at 8.5 km/hr and increases by 0.5 km/hr each minute. You have completed the test when you can no longer maintain the required pace. The running speed of the last stage you completed is used to predict your VO$_2$max. See Laboratory 2.3 for more complete details on administering and interpreting Leger's 20-metre shuttle run.

The 1.5-Mile Run Test

One of the simplest and most accurate means of evaluating cardiorespiratory endurance is the **1.5-mile run test**. This submaximal test, popularized by Dr. Kenneth Cooper, works on the physiological principle that people with a high level of cardiorespiratory fitness can run 1.5 miles (2.4 km) in less time than less-fit individuals (Cooper, 1977, 1982). (Note that the 1.5-mile run and 1-mile walk are not stated in metric, even in Canada.)

1.5-mile run test A field test designed to evaluate cardiorespiratory endurance. The objective of the test is to run/walk a 1.5-mile distance in the shortest possible time.

The 1.5-mile run test is an excellent assessment of cardiorespiratory endurance for physically active postsecondary-age individuals. Due to its intensity, however, the 1.5-mile run test is not well suited for sedentary people over 30 years of age, severely deconditioned people, individuals with joint problems, and individuals who are obese.

The objective of the test is to complete a 1.5-mile distance (preferably on a track) in the shortest possible time. The test is best conducted in moderate weather conditions (avoiding very hot or very cold days). For a reasonably physically fit individual, the 1.5-mile distance can be covered by running or jogging. For less-fit individuals, the test becomes a run/walk test. A good strategy is to try to keep a steady pace for the entire distance. In this regard, it may be beneficial to perform a practice test several days prior to testing to determine the optimal pace that can be maintained. Accurate timing of the test is essential, and use of a stopwatch is best. Laboratory 2.4 provides instructions for performing the test and recording and interpreting your score.

The 1-Mile Walk Test

Another field test to determine cardiorespiratory endurance is the **1-mile walk test**, which is particularly useful for sedentary individuals (Rippe, 1986; Rippe, Ward, Porcari, & Freedson, 1988; Ward & Rippe, 1988). It is a weight-bearing

Dehydration Can Negatively Impact a Cardiorespiratory Endurance Test

Approximately 60 to 70 percent of the body is water. Heavy sweating or the failure to drink enough fluids during the day can lower body water levels and result in dehydration. Water is involved in every vital process of the body, so dehydration can impair physical performance. For example, dehydration results in reduced blood volume and elevated heart rate during submaximal exercise. This dehydration-induced high heart rate during submaximal exercise will result in an underestimation of VO_2max during submaximal fitness tests (e.g., a

cycle ergometer or step test) (Powers & Howley, 2004). Further, dehydration can negatively impact endurance performance during field tests of VO_2max (e.g., a 1.5-mile run) (Powers & Howley, 2004; Roitman, 2001). Therefore, because dehydration can impair exercise performance, cardiorespiratory endurance tests should be performed only when the test subjects are adequately hydrated.

See Chapter 7 for more details on the maintenance of normal body water levels.

---

test, however, so individuals with joint problems should not participate.

The 1-mile walk test works on the same principle as the 1.5-mile run test. That is, individuals with high levels of cardiorespiratory fitness will complete a 1-mile walk (1.6 km) in a shorter time than those who are less conditioned. This test also is best conducted in moderate weather conditions, preferably on a track. Subjects should try to maintain a steady pace over the distance. Again, accurate timing is essential. Laboratory 2.5 provides instructions for performing the test and interpreting and recording your score.

The Cycle Ergometer Test

For those with access to a *cycle ergometer* (a stationary exercise bicycle that provides pedalling resistance via friction applied to the wheel), a **cycle ergometer test** is an excellent means of evaluating cardiorespiratory endurance (Figure 2.3). This test is recommended for individuals with joint problems, due to the non–weight bearing nature of cycling. Further, because this type of test can be performed indoors, it has advantages over outdoor fitness tests during very cold or hot weather.

Although numerous types of cycle ergometers exist, the most common type is *friction braked,* which incorporates a belt wrapped around the wheel. The belt is loosened or tightened to provide a change in resistance (reducing or elevating pedalling difficulty). The work performed on a cycle ergometer is commonly expressed in units called *kilopond metres per minute (KPM)* or in watts. It is not important to understand the details of these units, but you should recognize that KPMs and watts are measurement units that represent the amount of work performed. For example, a workload of 300 KPM (50 watts) on the cycle ergometer would be considered a submaximal (involving a light load) work rate for almost everyone, whereas a load of 3000 KPM (500 watts) would represent a high work rate for even highly conditioned individuals. Laboratory 2.6 provides instructions for performing the test and interpreting and recording your score.

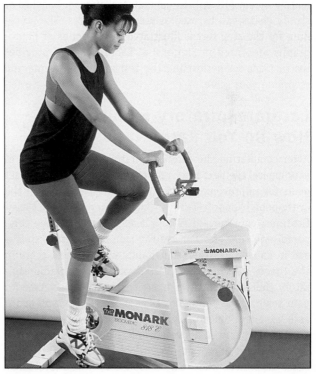

FIGURE 2.3 Friction-braked cycle ergometers can be used to evaluate cardiorespiratory endurance.

This submaximal cycle test works on the principle that individuals with high cardiorespiratory endurance levels have a lower exercise heart rate for a standard workload than less fit individuals (Fox, 1973; Pollock et al., 1978).

1-mile walk test A field test designed to evaluate cardiorespiratory endurance. The objective of the test is to complete a 1-mile walk in the shortest possible time.

cycle ergometer test A field test performed on a cycle ergometer designed to evaluate cardiorespiratory endurance.

The Step Test

Another test to determine cardiorespiratory endurance is the **step test**. This test is similar to the mCAFT in that it involves stepping to a cadence and is based on the principle that individuals with a higher level of cardiorespiratory fitness will have a lower heart rate during recovery from 3 minutes of bench stepping than less-conditioned individuals (Getchell, 1998; Powers & Howley, 2004). The difference is that only one step is used. The mCAFT also includes a protocol for one step (40.6 cm) for young, physically fit individuals. An advantage of this test is that it can be performed indoors and can be used by people at all fitness levels. Further, the step test does not require expensive equipment and can be performed in a short amount of time.

Step height for men and women should be approximately 46 cm (18 in.). In general, locker-room benches or sturdy chairs can be used as stepping devices. The procedure for the step test is illustrated in the series of photographs presented in Figure 2.4. Laboratory 2.7 provides instructions for performing the test and interpreting and recording your score.

Cardiorespiratory Endurance: How Do You Rate?

After completing the cardiorespiratory endurance test of your choice, the next step is to interpret your results and set goals for improvement. If your results placed you in the "very poor," "poor," "fair," or "needs improvement" classifications, your current fitness level is below average compared with that of other healthy men or women of similar age in Canada. On the other hand, a fitness test score in the "good" category means that your current cardiorespiratory endurance is between average and above average for your sex and age group. The fitness categories "very good" and "excellent" mean that your level of cardiorespiratory conditioning is well above average. The "excellent" (from health benefit zone) and "superior" rating is reserved for those individuals whose cardiorespiratory fitness level ranks in the top 15 percent of people in their age group. A key point here is that regardless of how low your current cardiorespiratory fitness level may be, you can improve it by adopting and adhering to a regular exercise program.

As mentioned above, testing your initial cardiorespiratory fitness level provides a benchmark against which you can compare future evaluations. Performing additional fitness tests as your fitness level improves is important because this type of positive feedback provides motivation to maintain regular physical activity habits (Barrow, 1992; Getchell, 1998; Howley & Franks, 2003; McGlynn, 1998).

step test A field test that involves bench stepping designed to evaluate cardiorespiratory endurance.

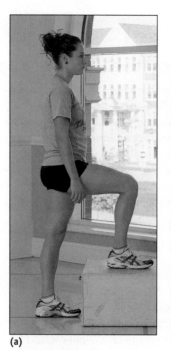
(a)

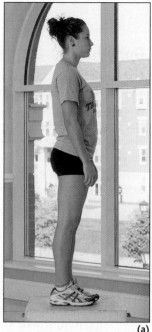
(a)

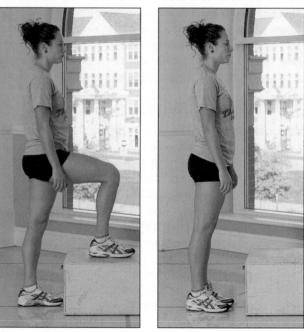
(c)

(d)

FIGURE 2.4 Step test to evaluate cardiorespiratory endurance. Subjects step up onto a 46-cm-high surface (18 in.) (a), (b), and then down (c), (d), once every 2 seconds.

Evaluation of Muscular Strength

As noted in Chapter 1, muscular strength is the maximum amount of force you can produce during one contraction (Roitman, 2001). Muscular strength is important for success not only in athletes, but also in the average person in performing routine tasks at work or home. Strength can be measured using the **one-repetition maximum (1 RM) test,** which measures the maximum amount of weight that can be lifted one time. It is also possible to estimate the 1 RM by performing multiple repetitions using a submaximal weight. Methods for directly measuring and estimating the 1 RM are discussed in Laboratory 2.8.

The 1 RM Test

Although the 1 RM test for muscular strength is widely accepted (Pollock & Wilmore, 1990), it is considered unsuitable for older individuals or deconditioned people. The major concern is risk of injury. The 1 RM test should therefore be attempted only after several weeks of strength training, which results in improvements in skill and strength and reduces the risk of injury during the test. An older or sedentary individual would require approximately 6 weeks of training prior to the 1 RM test, whereas a physically active postsecondary-age student could perform the 1 RM test after 1 to 2 weeks of training.

The 1 RM test is designed to test muscular strength in selected muscle groups and is performed in the following manner. Begin with a 5- to 10-minute warm-up using the muscles to be tested. For each muscle group, select an initial weight that you can lift without undue stress. Then gradually add weight until you reach the maximum weight that you can lift one time.

If you can lift the weight more than once, add more weight until you reach a level of resistance at which you can perform only one repetition. Remember that a true 1 RM is the maximum amount of weight that you can lift one time.

Figures 2.5 through 2.8 illustrate four common lifts used to measure strength. Three of these (bench press, biceps curl, and shoulder press) use upper-body muscle groups; the fourth lift (leg press) measures leg strength. Your muscle strength score is the percentage of body weight lifted in each exercise. To compute your strength score in each lift, divide your 1 RM weight in kilograms by your body weight

one-repetition maximum (1 RM) test   Measurement of the maximum amount of weight that can be lifted one time.

in kilograms and multiply by 100. For example, suppose a 75-kg man has a bench press 1 RM of 90 kg.

This man's muscle strength score for the bench press is computed as

$$\frac{\text{RM weight}}{\text{body weight}} \times 100 = \text{muscle strength score}$$

Therefore,

$$\text{muscle strength score } \frac{90 \text{ kg}}{75 \text{ kg}} \times 100 = 120$$

In Laboratory 2.8, you can record and interpret your strength scores.

Estimating 1 RM Using a 10 RM Test

Determining 1 RM is relatively easy for an experienced weight lifter, but measurement of 1 RM for an inexperienced lifter

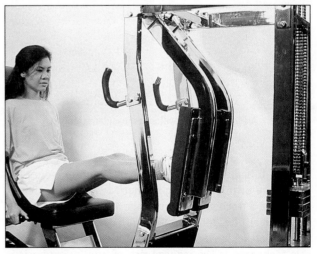

FIGURE 2.5 A leg press to evaluate muscular strength.

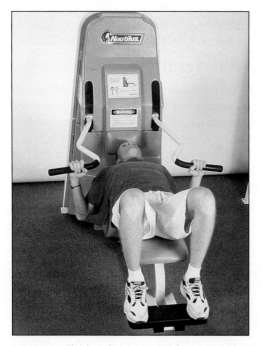

FIGURE 2.6 The bench press to evaluate muscular strength.

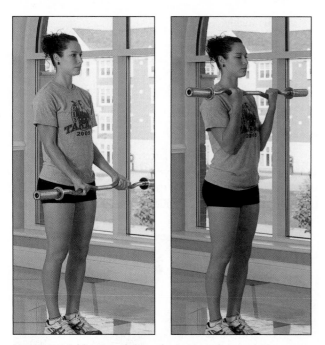

FIGURE 2.7 A biceps curl to evaluate muscular strength.

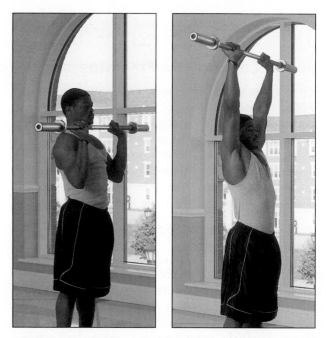

FIGURE 2.8 The shoulder or "military" press to evaluate muscular strength.

is often difficult and there is a risk of injury. To reduce the possibility of injury during strength testing, researchers developed a method to estimate the 1 RM using a series of submaximal lifts. Although the use of submaximal lifts to estimate 1 RM is slightly less accurate, the advantage of this technique is the reduced risk of injury. Emphasis is placed on using correct body alignment; form is never sacrificed for additional weight.

Estimating 1 RM in any particular lift (e.g., bench press) is achieved using the following procedure (Roitman, 2001). Testing begins with the individual performing 10 repetitions using a light weight. Depending on the ease with which these repetitions are completed, the instructor then adds more weight and the individual performs another 10 repetitions. This process continues until a weight is reached that can be lifted only 10 times (called the 10 RM). In general, an experienced instructor can aid the individual by supervising the process so that the 10 RM weight can be discovered in fewer than five trials (Roitman, 2001). A rest period of approximately 5 minutes should separate each trial to permit adequate time for recovery.

After determining the 10 RM, the 1 RM can be estimated using Table 2.16 (see Laboratory 2.8). For example, if an individual's 10 RM for a particular lift is 45 kg, then the estimate for the 1 RM would be 61.2 kg. This was determined by locating the number closest to 45 kg in the 10 repetitions column (i.e., 45.0 kg) in Table 2.16 and then locating the 1 RM weight in the left-hand column for this row.

Note that the 1 RM can also be estimated using fewer than 10 repetitions (i.e., 7–9 repetitions). For example, a beginning weight lifter can sometimes develop muscle fatigue and fail to complete 10 repetitions during a testing period. In this case, if the individual completes as many as 7 to 9 repetitions with a given weight, the 1 RM still can be estimated using Table 2.16. For instance, if an individual completes 7 repetitions with 50 kg, the estimate for 1 RM is 61.4 kg. As in the previous example, the estimated 1 RM was determined by locating the number closest to 50 kg in the 7 repetitions column (i.e., 49.6 kg) in Table 2.16, and then locating the 1 RM weight in the left-hand column for this row.

After determining the estimated 1 RM, the individual's muscle strength score is determined using the formula discussed in the previous section. That is,

$$\text{muscle strength score} = \frac{1 \text{ RM weight}}{\text{body weight}} \times 100$$

In Laboratory 2.8, you can record and interpret your muscle strength scores.

Muscular Strength: How Do You Rate?

When you have completed your muscular strength test, the next step is to interpret your results (see Laboratory 2.8) and set goals for improvement. Similar to the fitness categories used for cardiorespiratory endurance, the fitness categories for muscular strength range from very poor (lowest) to superior (highest). If your current strength level is classified as average or below, don't be discouraged; you can improve! A key point in maintaining your motivation to exercise regularly is the establishment of goals. Record short-term and long-term goals for improvement. After 6 to 12 weeks of training, perform a retest to evaluate your progress. Reaching a short-term goal provides added incentive to continue your exercise program.

Measurement of Muscular Endurance

Muscular endurance is the ability of a muscle or muscle group to generate force over and over again. Although an individual might have sufficient strength to lift a heavy box from the ground to the back of a truck, he or she might not have sufficient muscular endurance to perform this task multiple times. Because many everyday tasks require submaximal but repeated muscular contractions, muscular endurance is an important facet of health-related physical fitness.

Two simple tests advocated by CSEP to assess muscular endurance are push-ups and curl-ups. Push-ups are a measure of muscular endurance of the upper body, including muscles from the shoulder, arm, and chest; curl-ups evaluate abdominal muscle endurance.

In the curl-up, the trunk is not raised more than 30 to 40 degrees above the mat (attained when the shoulders are lifted approximately 15 to 25 cm above the mat; see Figure 2.9) (Sparling, 1997; Faulkner, Sprigings, McQuarrie, & Bell, 1989) so that only abdominal muscles are recruited; less stress is therefore placed on the lower back than by the conventional sit-up. For this reason, the curl-up test is used instead of sit-ups to evaluate abdominal muscle endurance. Furthermore, sit-ups involve the abdominal muscles *and* hip flexors.

Instructions to perform push-ups and curl-ups correctly as well as normative tables according to age groups and sex are presented in Laboratory 2.9. If you are currently experiencing back pain, you should not perform push-ups or curl-ups.

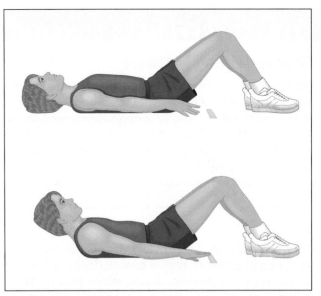

FIGURE 2.9 The position and movement pattern for the performance of a curl-up.

Muscular Endurance: How Do You Rate?

The fitness categories for muscular endurance range from "needs improvement" (lowest) to "excellent" (highest). If your muscular endurance test score placed you in the "needs improvement" or "fair" classification, your present muscular endurance level is below average compared with other men or women of your age group. On the other hand, a fitness test score in the "good" category means that your current muscular endurance is average. You may still want to improve this classification. The fitness category "very good" means that your muscular endurance level is likely above average. Finally, the fitness category labelled "excellent" is at the top of the rankings. At the "very good" and "excellent" zones, you most likely want to keep doing the physical activities and training you are currently doing to maintain your muscular endurance.

If you scored poorly on either the push-up or the curl-up test, do not be discouraged. Establish your goals and begin doing push-ups and curl-ups on a regular basis (see Chapter 5 for the exercise prescription for muscular endurance). Your ability to perform curl-ups and push-ups will increase within the first 3 to 4 weeks of training and will continue to improve for weeks to come.

Assessment of Flexibility

Flexibility, the ability to move joints freely through their full range of motion, can decrease as one gets older due to tightening of muscles and/or tendons. Loss of flexibility can occur due to muscle disuse and lack of muscular training. The key to maintaining flexibility is a program of regular stretching (Chapter 6).

Individual needs for flexibility are variable. Some athletes, such as gymnasts, require great flexibility in order to perform complex movements in competition (Barrow, 1992; Corbin et al., 2003; Howley & Franks, 2003; Robergs & Keteyian, 2002). In general, nonathletes require less flexibility than athletes. Some flexibility, however, is required for everyone in order to perform common activities of daily living or recreational pursuits.

Flexibility is joint-specific. That is, a person might be flexible in one joint but lack flexibility in another. Although no single test is representative of total body flexibility, measurements of trunk and shoulder flexibility are most commonly evaluated.

Trunk Flexibility

The **sit and reach test** measures the ability to flex the trunk, which means stretching the lower back muscles and the muscles in the back of the thigh (hamstrings). Figure 2.10 illustrates the sit and reach test using a sit and reach box. Instructions to perform the sit and reach test correctly as well as normative data for comparison are included in Laboratory 2.10.

sit and reach test A field test that measures the flexibility of the muscles in the lower back and in the back of the thigh.

Shoulder Flexibility

As the name implies, the shoulder flexibility test evaluates the shoulder's range of motion (flexibility). Figure 2.11 illustrates this test. It is performed on both shoulders.

Flexibility: How Do You Rate?

It is not uncommon for active and inactive individuals to be classified as average or below average for trunk and shoulder flexibility. In fact, only individuals who regularly perform stretching exercises are likely to possess flexibility levels that exceed the average. Regardless of your current flexibility classification, your flexibility goal should be to reach a classification of above average (i.e., good, very good, or excellent).

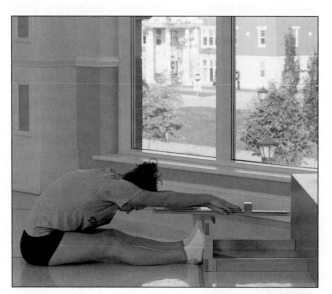

FIGURE 2.10 The sit and reach test to evaluate trunk flexibility.

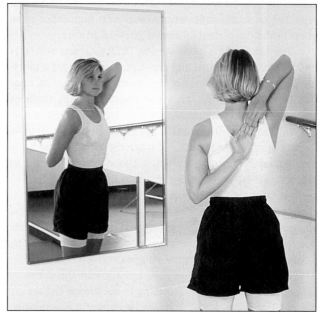

FIGURE 2.11 The shoulder flexibility test.

Assessment of Body Composition

Assessments of body composition generally attempt to quantify body weight into its basic components. In assessments of the health-related components of physical fitness, estimates of body fat are considered most important. Recall that a high percentage of body fat is associated with an increased risk of heart disease, several types of cancer, type 2 diabetes, and other diseases. Several methods of assessing body composition have been developed, with significant progress made in the development and refinement of most techniques (Malina, Bouchard, & Bar-Or, 2004).

A technique once considered the gold standard for laboratory assessment of body fat in humans is **hydrostatic weighing.** This technique involves weighing the individual both on land and in water (Lohman et al., 1997; Pollock & Wilmore, 1990; Powers & Howley, 2004). The two body weights are then entered into a simple formula to calculate percentage body fat.

Based on the same premise as underwater weighing, a new technique called **air displacement plethysmography (ADP)** has become popular in recent years to measure body composition. Figure 2.12 shows a Bod Pod®, which measures total body volume from which an estimate of body fat can be made. The major assumption of hydrostatic weighing and ADP is that the density of fat and fat-free mass (all components of the body except fat) is constant. Thus, with estimates of total body volume (either in water or air) and recognizing that density = mass / volume, an estimate of fat can be determined (see Malina et al. [2004] for more details).

Dual-energy X-ray absorptiometry (DXA) measures bone mineral content as well as lean and fat tissue. This technique does not rely on the same assumption as underwater weighing and ADP. Some consider DXA the new gold standard for laboratory assessment of body composition.

Hydrostatic weighing, ADP, and DXA are time-consuming and require expensive equipment. Thus, these procedures are rarely employed to assess body composition in post-secondary physical fitness courses.

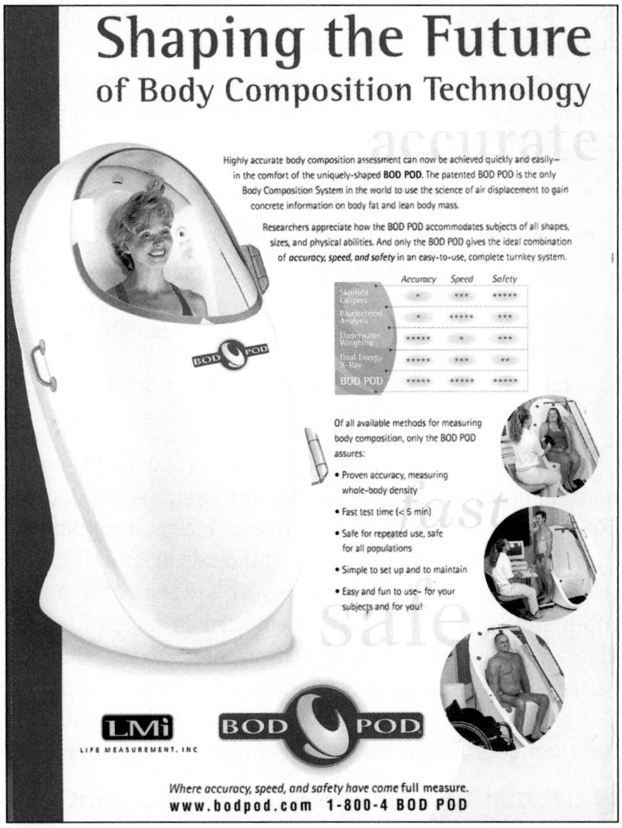

Estimation of Body Composition: Field Techniques

Several quick and inexpensive field techniques exist to evaluate body composition (DiGirolamo, 1986; Howley & Franks, 2003; Van Itallie, 1988).

Bioelectrical impedance analysis
Bioelectrical impedance analysis (BIA) is a convenient, rapid, non-invasive technique used to provide an estimate of body composition (Malina et al., 2004). The rationale for this technique is based on the fact that lean tissue has a greater electrolyte and water content than fat tissue. As such, a weak electrical current is passed through the body to measure impedance to the flow, resulting in an estimate of body fat. When using this test, it is important for the body to be

FIGURE 2.12 Determining body composition using the Bod Pod®.

normally hydrated since fluctuations would result in less accurate estimates of lean body mass. Body fat can then be determined from this two-compartment model that assumes body weight equals lean body mass plus fat mass.

Skinfold measurements
An inexpensive method to assess body composition that involves measuring subcutaneous (beneath the skin) fat is **skinfold measurements.**

Subcutaneous fat is measured using an instrument called a skinfold caliper. Since approximately 50 percent of body fat lies just beneath the skin (Pollock & Wilmore, 1990; Powers & Howley, 2004; Williams, 1996), measurement of representative samples provides a means of estimating overall body fatness. Skinfold measurements to determine body fat are

hydrostatic weighing A method of determining body composition that involves weighing an individual on land and in water.

air displacemnt plethysmography (ADP) A method of determining body composition in which body volume is measured in an enclosed chamber.

dual-energy X-ray absorptiometry (DXA) A method used to estimate fat, lean, and bone mineral content.

bioelectrical impedance analysis (BIA) A convenient, rapid, non-invasive technique used to provide an estimate of body composition.

skinfold measurements A field test in which measurement of representative samples of subcutaneous fat provides a means of estimating overall body fatness.

reliable but generally have a ±3 to 4 percent margin of error (Pollock & Wilmore, 1990; Powers & Howley, 2004).

The accuracy of determining body fat from skinfold measurements can be improved by (Canadian Society for Exercise Physiology, 2003):

- identifying each skinfold site accurately
- aligning each skinfold accurately
- forming the skinfold firmly prior to applying the calipers
- maintaining a firm hold on the skinfold while the measurement is taken
- releasing the caliper jaws completely prior to reading the skinfold measurement.

Body fatness can be estimated from 5 standard skinfold measurements (Canadian Society for Exercise Physiology, 2003).These sites include the triceps, biceps, subscapular, iliac crest, and medial calf. For standardization, all measurements are made on the right side of the body. Alternatively, skinfold measurements can be summed to provide an overall indication of body fatness. Then, when reassessed, pre- and post-measurements can be compared. Complete details of how to take these measurements and interpret your health risk are presented in Laboratory 2.11.

Waist girth
Recent evidence suggests that **waist girth** can be used to determine the risk of disease associated with high body fat (Van Itallie, 1988). The rationale for this technique is that a high percentage of fat in the abdominal region is associated with an increased risk of disease (such as heart disease or hypertension, and hyperlipidemia) (Reeder et al., 1986). A waist circumference of greater than 100 cm in males and 88 cm in females is used to define health risk (Crespo & Smit, 2003). Details of waist girth assessment and health risk tables are presented in Laboratory 2.11.

Body mass index
Research indicates that **body mass index (BMI)**, despite its many limitations, is a useful technique for placing people into health-risk categories of normal or too much body fat (DiGirolamo, 1986; Van Itallie, 1988). BMI is simply the ratio of the body weight in kilograms divided by height in metres squared:

$$BMI = \frac{weight\ (kg)}{height\ (m)^2}$$

For example, if an individual weighs 64.5 kg and is 1.72 m tall, their BMI would be computed as follows:

$$\frac{64.5\ kg}{(1.72\ m)^2} = \frac{64.5}{2.96} = 21.8$$

waist girth The measurement taken at the smallest point of the waist, usually at the level of the umbillicus (navel).

body mass index (BMI) The ratio of body weight (kg) divided by height squared (m²).

Table 2.1 shows weight classifications for males and females according to BMI. Figure 2.13 illustrates the distribution of BMI in Canada.

Although it is simple to calculate BMI, the result has limited meaning. First, it is not a measure of body composition but rather a ratio of height to weight. As such, this method can over- or underestimate body fatness. For example, an individual with a low percentage of body fat but a high level of muscularity would typically have a relatively high BMI, which would incorrectly suggest health risk. Conversely, an individual with a high level of body fat and low level of muscularity may have a "normal" BMI even though the level of body fat puts this individual at health risk. Therefore, this technique should be used only when other more sensitive techniques are not available. Alternatively, BMI can be used in conjunction with other field techniques.

Height/weight tables The Metropolitan Life Insurance Company has published a series of height/weight tables designed to determine whether a person is overweight. In these tables, overweight is defined as having a body weight greater than what is considered normal for a specific height. Although the idea that a simple table could be used to deter-

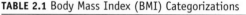

	BMI (kg/m²)
Underweight	<18.5
Normal weight	18.5–24.9
Overweight	25–29.9
Obese	≧ 30.0

TABLE 2.1 Body Mass Index (BMI) Categorizations

Source: Adapted from Statistics Canada: Community Health Surveys.

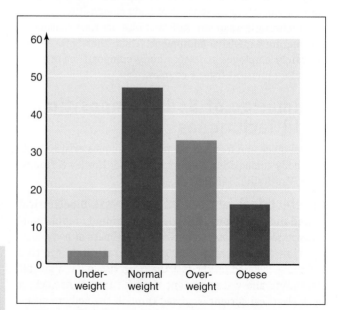

FIGURE 2.13 BMI distribution among Canadian adults, ages 20 to 64 years, based on the 2001 Canadian Community Health Survey.

mine an individual's ideal body weight is attractive, several problems affect this procedure. The major problem with this approach is that the tables do not indicate how much of the body weight is fat. For example, an individual can exceed the ideal body weight on such a chart by being heavily muscled *or* by being over-fat. Therefore, this approach to a determination of an "ideal" body weight is not recommended.

Body Composition: How Do You Rate?

The determination of your health benefit zone differs from the determination of other components of health-related physical fitness. As noted in Laboratory 2.11, the *health benefit zone* is based on a points system of various combinations of healthy and unhealthy estimates of BMI, sum of 5 skinfolds, waist girth, and sum of 2 skinfolds. None of these measures gives you a percentage body fat. However, if desired, you can use skinfold measurements along with standard regression equations to determine a percentage body fat. It is as effective, however, to monitor changes in your sum of skinfolds over time as it is to use percentage body fat to determine changes in your level of fat. Obviously, an increase in your sum of skinfolds is equal to an increase in body fat. Your goal should be to reach and maintain an optimal level of body fat, a level at which you are at the least health risk.

Table 2.2 presents body composition categories for men and women. Research suggests that a range of 10 to 20 percent body fat is an optimal health and fitness goal for men; the optimal range for women is 15 to 25 percent. These ranges in body fat provide little risk of disease associated with body fatness and permit individual differences in body shape, physical activity patterns, and nutritional intake.

Percentage Body Fat	Body Composition Fitness Category
Men	
<10%	Low body fat
10–20%	Optimal range of body fat
21–25%	Moderately high body fat
26–31%	High body fat
>31%	Very high body fat
Women	
<15%	Low body fat
15–25%	Optimal range of body fat
26–30%	Moderately high body fat
31–35%	High body fat
>35%	Very high body fat

TABLE 2.2 Body Composition Fitness Categories for Men and Women
Data from Lohman (29).

Body fat levels above the optimal range are associated with an increased risk of disease and are therefore undesirable.

What is less obvious is that a body fat lower than the recommended optimal range is also undesirable. Indeed, body fat below the optimal range may also increase the risk of health problems. This is because extremely low body fat is often associated with poor nutrition and a loss of muscle mass. This is clearly undesirable. The relationships among nutritional intake, physical activity, and body composition are discussed in detail in Chapter 8.

Summary

1. Prior to beginning a physical fitness program (or performing a fitness evaluation), you should complete the PAR-Q. If you respond yes to one or more of the questions, you should consult your physician prior to engaging in physical activity.
2. An objective evaluation of your current physical fitness status is important before beginning an exercise training program. Further, periodic retesting can provide feedback about your training progress.
3. Cardiorespiratory endurance is the ability of the heart and lungs to pump oxygen-rich blood to working muscles; this translates into the ability to perform endurance-type physical activities. Field tests to evaluate cardiorespiratory endurance include the Modified Canadian Aerobic Fitness Test (mCAFT), Leger's 20-metre shuttle run, the 1.5-mile run test, the 1-mile walk test, the cycle ergometer test, and the step test.
4. Muscular strength is the maximum amount of force you can produce during one contraction. The most popular method of evaluating muscular strength is the one-repetition maximum (1 RM) test. The 10 RM test can also be used to estimate 1 RM.
5. Muscular endurance is the ability of a muscle group to generate force over and over again or to sustain muscle contractions. Two commonly used methods of evaluating muscular endurance are the push-up test and the curl-up test.
6. Flexibility is defined as the ability to move joints freely through their full range of motion. Although flexibility is joint-specific, two popular means of evaluating flexibility are the trunk flexibility (sit and reach) test and the shoulder flexibility test.
7. Body composition is an important component of health-related physical fitness because a high percentage of body fat is associated with an increased risk of disease. In the field, body fat can be estimated indirectly using skinfold measurements, waist girth, or body mass index (BMI). Health risk can be estimated from a combination of these measures.

Study Questions

1. Why should the PAR-Q be completed prior to physical fitness testing?

2. What are the principles that underlie field tests used to measure cardiorespiratory endurance?

3. Describe the following field tests used to evaluate cardiorespiratory endurance: mCAFT, Leger's test, the 1.5-mile run test, the 1-mile walk test, the cycle ergometer test, and the step test.

4. Discuss the one-repetition maximum (1 RM) test for measuring muscular strength. What safety concerns are associated with this test? What is an alternative method for measuring strength?

5. Explain how the push-up and curl-up tests are used to evaluate muscular endurance.

6. Discuss the concept that flexibility is joint-specific.

7. Identify two field tests used to examine flexibility.

8. How can skinfold measurements be taken to increase the validity of the measurements?

9. How can measurement of the waist girth and body mass index (BMI) be used to assess body composition?

10. How are skinfold measurements, waist girth, and BMI used to estimate health risk?

Suggested Reading

American College of Sports Medicine. (2000). *Guidelines for exercise testing* (6th ed.). Philadelphia: Lea and Febiger.

Canadian Society for Exercise Physiology. (1987). *Canadian standardized test of fitness interpretation and counselling manual*. Ottawa: Author.

Canadian Society for Exercise Physiology. (1993). *Professional fitness and lifestyle consultant (PFLC) resource manual*. Ottawa: Author.

Canadian Society for Exercise Physiology. (2003). *The Canadian physical activity, fitness & lifestyle approach (CPAFLA): CSEP-health & fitness program's health-related appraisal and counselling strategy* (3rd ed.). Ottawa: Author.

Roitman, J. (Ed.) (2001). *ACSM's resource manual for guidelines for exercise testing and prescription*. Philadelphia: Lippincott, Williams & Wilkins.

Weblinks

Canadian Society for Exercise Physiology

www.csep.ca

A Canadian resource that promotes the generation, synthesis, transfer, and application of knowledge and research related to exercise physiology (encompassing physical activity, fitness, health, and human performance).

American College of Sports Medicine

www.acsm.org

A U.S. resource that promotes the generation, synthesis, transfer, and application of knowledge and research related to exercise physiology (encompassing physical activity, fitness, health, and human performance).

Health Canada

www.hc-sc.gc.ca/english/lifestyles/physical_activity.html

Contains information regarding the promotion of physical activity for the Canadian population.

Cooper Institute

www.cooperinst.org

Contains information regarding physical fitness and physical activity testing.

References

American College of Sports Medicine. (1998). *Resource manual for exercise testing and prescription*. Philadelphia: Lea and Febiger.

American College of Sports Medicine. (2000). *Guidelines for exercise testing* (6th ed.). Philadelphia: Lea and Febiger.

Barrow, M. (1992). *Heart talk: Understanding cardiovascular diseases*. Gainesville, FL: Cor-Ed Publishing.

Canadian Society for Exercise Physiology. (1993). *Professional fitness and lifestyle consultant (PFLC) resource manual*. Ottawa: Author.

Canadian Society for Exercise Physiology. (2003). *The Canadian physical activity, fitness & lifestyle approach (CPAFLA): CSEP health & fitness program's health-related appraisal and counselling strategy* (3rd ed.). Ottawa: Author.

Cooper, K. (1977). *The aerobics way*. New York: Bantam Books.

Cooper, K. (1982). *The aerobics program for total well-being*. New York: M. Evans.

Corbin, C., Welk, G., Lindsey, R., & Corbin, W. (2003). *Concepts of physical fitness*. St. Louis, MO: McGraw-Hill.

Crespo, C. J., & Smit, E. (2003). Prevalence of overweight and obesity in the United States. In R. E. Andersen (Ed.), *Obesity: Etiology, assessment, treatment and prevention*. Champaign, IL: Human Kinetics.

DiGirolamo, M. (1986, March). Body composition—roundtable. *Physician and Sports Medicine*, 144–162.

Faulkner, R., Sprigings, E. J., McQuarrie, A., & Bell, R. D. (1989). A partial curl-up protocol for adults based on two procedures. *Canadian Journal of Sports Sciences*, 14, 135–141.

Fox, E. (1973). A simple technique for predicting maximal aerobic power. *Journal of Applied Physiology, 35*, 914–916.

Getchell, B. (1998). *Physical fitness: A way of life* (5th ed.). Needham Heights, MA: Allyn and Bacon.

Golding, L., Myers, C., & Sinning, W. (1989). *Y's way to physical fitness: The complete guide to fitness testing and instruction* (3rd ed.). Champaign, IL: Human Kinetics.

Howley, E., & Franks, B. D. (2003). *Health fitness instructor's handbook* (4th ed.). Champaign, IL: Human Kinetics.

Lamb, D., & Williams, M. (1991). *Ergogenics: Enhancement of performance in exercise and sport.* Vol. 4. Dubuque, IA: Brown and Benchmark.

Leger, L., & Gadboury, C. (1989). Validity of the 20 m shuttle run test with 1 min stages to predict VO$_2$max in adults. *Canadian Journal of Sport Sciences, 14(1),* 21–26.

Lohman, T. (1987). The use of skinfold to estimate body fatness in children and youth. *Journal of Alliance for Health, Physical Education, Recreation, and Dance, 58,* 98–102.

Lohman, T., et al. (1997). Body fat measurement goes high-tech: Not all are created equal. *ACSM's Health and Fitness Journal, 1(1),* 30–35.

Malina, R. M., Bouchard, C., & Bar-Or, O. (2004). *Growth, maturation, and physical activity.* Champaign, IL: Human Kinetics.

McGlynn, G. (1998). *Dynamics of fitness: A practical approach* (5th ed.). Dubuque, IA: Wm. C. Brown.

Pollock, M., & Wilmore, J. (1990). *Exercise in health and disease* (3rd ed.). Philadelphia: W. B. Saunders.

Pollock, M., Wilmore, J., & Fox, S. (1978). *Health and fitness through physical activity.* New York: John Wiley and Sons.

Powers, S., & Howley, E. (2004). *Exercise physiology: Theory and application to fitness and performance* (5th ed.). St. Louis: McGraw-Hill.

Reeder, B. A., Senthilselvan, A., Després, J-P., Angel, A., Liu, L., Wang, H., & Rabkin, S. W. (1997). The association of cardiovascular disease risk factors with abdominal obesity in Canada. *Canadian Medical Association Journal, 157(1 suppl),* S39–S45.

Rippe, J. (1986). Walking for fitness: A roundtable. *Physician and Sports Medicine, 14,* 144–159.

Rippe, J., Ward, A., Porcari, J., & Freedson, P. (1988). Walking for fitness and health. *Journal of the American Medical Association, 259,* 2720–2724.

Robergs, R., & Keteyian, S. (2002). *Fundamental principles of exercise physiology: For fitness, performance, and health.* St. Louis: McGraw-Hill.

Roitman, J. (Ed.) (2001). *ACSM's resource manual for guidelines for exercise testing and prescription.* Philadelphia: Lippincott, Williams & Wilkins.

Sparling, P. (1997). Field testing for abdominal muscular fitness; speed versus cadence sit-ups. *ACSM's Health and Fitness Journal, 1(4),* 30–33.

Van Itallie, T. (1988). Topography of body fat: Relationship to risk of cardiovascular and other diseases. In T. Lohman et al. (Eds.) *Anthropometric standardization reference manual.* Champaign, IL: Human Kinetics.

Ward, A., & Rippe, J. (1988). *Walking for health and fitness.* Philadelphia: J. B. Lippincott.

Weller, I. M., Thomas, S. G., Gledhill, N., Paterson, D., & Quinney, A. (1995). A study to validate the Modified Canadian Aerobic Fitness Test. *Canadian Journal of Applied Physiology, 20(2),* 211–221.

Williams, M. (1996). *Lifetime fitness and wellness.* Dubuque, IA: Wm. C. Brown.

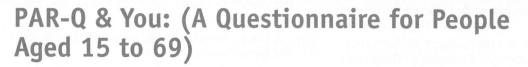

LABORATORY 2.1

PAR-Q & You: (A Questionnaire for People Aged 15 to 69)

Name _____ Age _____ Sex _____ Date _____

Regular physical activity is fun and healthy, and increasingly more people are starting to become more active every day. Being more active is very safe for most people. However, some people should check with their doctor before they start becoming much more physically active.

If you are planning to become much more physically active than you are now, start by answering the 7 questions in the box below. If you are between the ages of 15 and 69, the PAR-Q will tell you if you should check with your doctor before you start. If you are over 69 years of age, and you are not used to being very active, check with your doctor.

Common sense is your best guide when you answer these questions. Please read the questions carefully and answer each one honestly: check YES or NO.

YES	NO	
____	____	1. Has your doctor ever said that you have a heart condition *and* that you should only do physical activity recommended by a doctor?
____	____	2. Do you feel pain in your chest when you do physical activity?
____	____	3. In the past month, have you had chest pain when you were not doing physical activity?
____	____	4. Do you lose your balance because of dizziness or do you ever lose consciousness?
____	____	5. Do you have a bone or joint problem (for example, back, knee, or hip) that could be made worse by a change in your physical activity?
____	____	6. Is your doctor currently prescribing drugs (for example, water pills) for your blood pressure or heart condition?
____	____	7. Do you know of *any other reason* why you should not do physical activity?

If you answered YES to one or more questions:

Talk with your doctor by phone or in person BEFORE you start becoming much more physically active or BEFORE you have a fitness appraisal. Tell your doctor about the PAR-Q and which questions you answered YES.

- You may be able to do any activity you want—as long as you start slowly and build up gradually. Or you may need to restrict your activities to those which are safe for you. Talk with your doctor about the kinds of activities you wish to participate in and follow his/her advice.
- Find out which community programs are safe and helpful for you.

If you answered NO to all questions:

If you answered NO honestly to *all* PAR-Q questions, you can be reasonably sure that you can

- start becoming much more physically active—begin slowly and build up gradually. This is the safest and easiest way to go.
- take part in a fitness appraisal—this is an excellent way to determine your basic fitness so that you can plan the best way for you to live actively. It is also highly recommended that you have your blood pressure evaluated. If your reading is over 144/94, talk with your doctor before you start becoming much more physically active.

DELAY BECOMING MUCH MORE ACTIVE:

- if you are not feeling well because of a temporary illness such as a cold or a fever—wait until you feel better; or
- if you are or may become pregnant—talk to your doctor before you start becoming more active.

Please Note: If your health changes so that you answer YES to any of the above questions, tell your fitness or health professional. Ask whether you should change your physical activity plan.

Informed use of the PAR-Q: The Canadian Society for Exercise Physiology, Health Canada, and their agents assume no liability for persons who undertake physical activity, and if in doubt after completing this questionnaire consult your doctor prior to physical activity.

FITNESS AND HEALTH PROFESSIONALS MAY BE INTERESTED IN THE INFORMATION BELOW:

The following companion forms are available for doctors' use by contacting the Canadian Society for Exercise Physiology (address below):

The **Physical Activity Readiness Medical Examination (PARmed-S)**—to be used by doctors with people who answer yes to one or more questions on the PAR-Q.

The **Physical Activity Readiness Medical Examination for Pregnancy (PARmed-X for Pregnancy)**—to be used by doctors with pregnant patients who wish to become more active.

REFERENCES

Arraix, G. A., Wigle, D .T., & Mao, Y. (1992). Risk Assessment of Physical Activity and Physical Fitness in the Canada Health Survey Follow-Up Study. **I. Clin. Epidemiol,** 45(4), 419–428.

Mottola, M., & Wolfe, L. A. (1994). Active Living and Pregnancy, In A. Quinney, L. Gavin, T. Wall (Eds.) *Toward Active Living: Proceedings of the International Conference on Physical Activity, Fitness and Health.* Champaign, IL: Human Kinetics.

PAR-Q Validation Report, British Columbia Ministry of Health, 1978.

Thomas, S., Reading, J., & Shephard, R. J. (1992). Revision of the Physical Activity Readiness Questionnaire (PAR-Q). **Can I. Spt. Sci,** 17(4), 338–345.

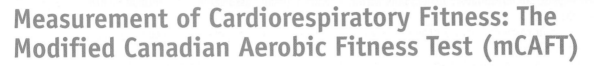

LABORATORY 2.2

Measurement of Cardiorespiratory Fitness: The Modified Canadian Aerobic Fitness Test (mCAFT)

Name_____ Age _____ Sex _____ Date _____

DIRECTIONS

The objective of this test is to complete as many stages of the mCAFT as possible without reaching your ceiling heart rate (85 percent of predicted heart rate maximum). You should participate in this test only after completing Laboratory 2.1 (i.e., obtaining medical clearance).

Prior to beginning the test, you should practise the required stepping sequence first without the music, then with the music. The stepping sequence is as follows (described with right foot starting):

- Step up with your right foot onto the first step.
- Step up with your left foot onto the second step.
- Step up with your right foot onto the second step so that your feet are now together.
- Step down with your left foot onto the first step.
- Step down with your right foot to the ground.
- Step down with your left foot to the ground so that your feet are once again together.
- Repeat.

It helps to follow the required stepping sequence if you think of "step, step, up; step, step, down" or "up, 2, 3, down 2, 3." You may start with either your left or right foot. No more than two practice sessions of each are recommended. Ensure that your feet are placed completely at the top step (i.e., that your calves are not hanging over the back of the step or toes over the front) and that your legs fully extend and back is straight during each phase of the stepping sequence. The prescribed cadence must be maintained.

As noted earlier in this chapter, the mCAFT is designed so that each person begins stepping at an intensity of 65 to 70 percent of the average VO_2max of a person 10 years older. See Table 2.3 to determine the stage where you should begin. Table 2.4 shows the cadence for each of the stages of the mCAFT. Instructions and time signals to start and stop stepping as well as for the measurement of heart rate for 10 seconds are vocalized on the CD/cassette tape that your instructor is using for this laboratory. Remember when measuring your heart rate to start counting immediately after the command "count" and continue counting until the first sound of the command "stop." The first count is 1. Depending upon your heart rate you will proceed to the next stage or terminate the test. See Table 2.5 for ceiling post-exercise heart rates.

Once the test is completed, you will use your final exercising heart rate along with your age, sex, and body weight to determine an aerobic fitness score. The score is calculated using the following equation:

$$\text{Aerobic Fitness Score} = 10\,(17.2 + [1.29 \times O_2\text{cost*}] - [0.9 \times \text{weight (kg)}] - [0.18 \times \text{age (yrs)}])$$

---

* O_2 cost for each stepping cadence is listed for males and females in Table 2.6.

Your aerobic fitness score can then be compared to the established health benefit zone presented in Table 2.7. Your health benefit zone score can be interpreted as follows:

Excellent—your cardiorespiratory fitness falls within a range generally associated with optimal health benefits.

Very good—your cardiorespiratory fitness falls within a range generally associated with considerable health benefits.

Good—your cardiorespiratory fitness falls within a range generally associated with many health benefits.

Fair—your cardiorespiratory fitness falls within a range generally associated with some health benefits. Progressing from here to the "good" zone and beyond requires accumulating 30 minutes or more of physical activity over most days of the week. This is a very important step to improving your cardiorespiratory fitness and health benefits.

Needs improvement—your cardiorespiratory fitness falls within a range generally associated with health risks. Try to accumulate 30 minutes or more of physical activity on most days of the week.

Fill in your data in the appropriate places below:

Weight _____ kg

Age _____ yrs

Last stepping stage completed _____

Final heart rate _____ beats·min^{-1}

O$_2$cost for last stepping stage completed _____ ml·kg^{-1}·min^{-1}

Aerobic fitness score = 10 (17.2 + [1.29 × _____ (O$_2$cost)] − [0.9 × _____

(weight)] − [0.18 × _____ age (yrs)])

Aerobic fitness score = _____

Health benefit zone = _____

Age	Starting Stage	
	Males	Females
60–69	1	1
50–59	2	1
40–49	3	2
30–39	3	3
20–29	4	3
15–19	4	3

TABLE 2.3 The mCAFT Starting Stage by Age and Sex

Source: *The Canadian Physical Activity, Fitness & Lifestyle Approach: CSE-Health & Fitness Program's Health-Related Appraisal and Counselling Strategy*, 3rd edition, copyright 2003. Reprinted with permission of the Canadian Society for Exercise Physiology.

Stage	Cadence (footplants/min)	
	Males	Females
1	66	66
2	84	84
3	102	102
4	114	114
5	132	120
6	144	132
7	118*	144
8	132*	118*

*One-step pattern to a step 40.6 cm in height. All other stages: two-step pattern on two 20.3-cm steps.

TABLE 2.4: The mCAFT Stages of the Modified Protocol

Source: *The Canadian Physical Activity, Fitness & Lifestyle Approach: CSE-Health & Fitness Program's Health-Related Appraisal and Counselling Strategy*, 3rd edition, copyright 2003. Reprinted with permission of the Canadian Society for Exercise Physiology.

Heart Rate*								
Age	10-Sec. Count	Monitor Reading	Age	10-Sec. Count	Monitor Reading	Age	10-Sec. Count	Monitor Reading
15	29	174	34	26	158	53	23	142
16	28	173	35	26	157	54	23	141
17	28	173	36	26	156	55	23	140
18	28	172	37	26	156	56	23	139
19	28	171	38	26	155	57	23	139
20	28	170	39	25	154	58	23	138
21	28	169	40	25	153	59	23	137
22	28	168	41	25	152	60	22	136
23	28	167	42	25	151	61	22	135
24	28	167	43	25	150	62	22	134
25	27	166	44	25	150	63	22	133
26	27	165	45	25	149	64	22	133
27	27	164	46	24	148	65	22	132
28	27	163	47	24	147	66	22	131
29	27	162	48	24	146	67	21	130
30	27	162	49	24	145	68	21	129
31	27	161	50	24	145	69	21	128
32	26	160	51	24	144			
33	26	159	52	24	143			

*85 percent of predicted maximum (220−age). Determined for each age and to balance accuracy and safety, rounding of 10-second counts was determined as follows: ≤ .8 round down; > .8 round up.

TABLE 2.5 The mCAFT Ceiling Post-Exercise Heart Rates

Source: *The Canadian Physical Activity, Fitness & Lifestyle Approach: CSE-Health & Fitness Program's Health-Related Appraisal and Counselling Strategy*, 3rd edition, copyright 2003. Reprinted with permission of the Canadian Society for Exercise Physiology.

	Females		Males	
Stage	Stepping Cadence	O_2 Cost	Stepping Cadence	O_2 Cost
1	66	15.9	66	15.9
2	84	18.0	84	18.0
3	102	22.0	102	22.0
4	114	24.5	114	24.5
5	120	26.3	132	29.5
6	132	29.5	144	33.6
7	144	33.6	118*	36.2
8	118*	36.2	132*	40.1

*Single step (all others double step). O_2 cost is measured in ml·kg^{-1}·min^{-1}.

TABLE 2.6 The mCAFT O_2 Cost in ml·kg^{-1}·min^{-1} and Stepping Cadence in footplants·min^{-1} for the Different Stages

Source: *The Canadian Physical Activity, Fitness & Lifestyle Approach: CSE-Health & Fitness Program's Health-Related Appraisal and Counselling Strategy*, 3rd edition, copyright 2003. Reprinted with permission of the Canadian Society for Exercise Physiology.

Age 15–19

Zone	Gender	M	F
Excellent		574+	490+
Very good		524–573	437–489
Good		488–523	395–436
Fair		436–487	368–394
Needs improvement		<436	<368

Age 20–29

Zone	Gender	M	F
Excellent		556+	472+
Very good		506–555	420–471
Good		472–505	378–419
Fair		416–471	350–377
Needs mprovement		<416	<350

Age 30–39

Zone	Gender	M	F
Excellent		488+	454+
Very good		454–487	401–453
Good		401–453	360–400
Fair		337–400	330–359
Needs improvement		<337	<330

Age 40–49

Zone	Gender	M	F
Excellent		470+	400+
Very good		427–469	351–399
Good		355–426	319–350
Fair		319–354	271–318
Needs improvement		<319	<271

Age 50–59

Zone	Gender	M	F
Excellent		418+	366+
Very good		365–417	340–365
Good		301–364	310–339
Fair		260–300	246–309
Needs improvement		<260	<246

Age 60–69

Zone	Gender	M	F
Excellent		384+	358+
Very good		328–383	328–357
Good		287–327	296–327
Fair		235–286	235–295
Needs improvement		<235	<235

TABLE 2.7 The mCAFT Determination of Health Benefit Zone from Aerobic Fitness Score

Source: *The Canadian Physical Activity, Fitness & Lifestyle Approach: CSE-Health & Fitness Program's Health-Related Appraisal and Counselling Strategy,* 3rd edition, copyright 2003. Reprinted with permission of the Canadian Society for Exercise Physiology.

Measurement of Cardiorespiratory Fitness: Leger's 20-Metre Shuttle Run

Name_____ Age _____ Sex _____ Date _____

DIRECTIONS

The objective of this test is to complete as many stages of the shuttle run as possible. Since this is a test of maximal performance, you should participate only after completing Lab 2.1 (i.e., obtaining a medical clearance). It is important to warm up with a 5-minute light jog followed by 5 minutes of dynamic stretching of the major muscle groups, particularly the leg muscles.

In this test you are required to run back and forth keeping in time with a recorded cadence on a 20 metre path, touching the line at either end. As noted previously, the starting speed of the test is 8.5 km/hr and increases 0.5 km/hr each minute. You will stop the test when you can no longer keep up with the required pace. The running speed of the stage you last completed is called your *maximal aerobic speed (MAS)* and is used to predict your VO_2max using the equation listed below:

$$VO_2max = -24.4 + (6.0 \times MAS)$$

Once you've determined your VO_2max, interpret your score using the data presented in Table 2.8. Fill in your data in the appropriate places below:

Age _____ yrs

Number of stages completed _____

Maximal aerobic speed (MAS)* _____ km/hr

VO_2max = –24.4 + (6.0 × _____ MAS)

VO_2max = _____ mL/kg/min

VO_2max rating = _____

_____

* Remember that the initial speed of the test was 8.5 km/hr and increased 0.5 km/hr each minute.

Interpreting your test results is simple. Table 2.9 contains norms for cardiorespiratory endurance using the 1.5-mile run test. Find your sex, age group, and finish time in the table and then locate your fitness category on the left side of the table. Consider the following example: Johnny Jones is 21 years old and completes the 1.5-mile run in 13 minutes and 25 seconds (13:25). Using Table 2.9, locate Johnny's age group and time column. Note that a finish time of 13:25 for the 1.5-mile run would place Johnny in the "average" fitness category.

			Women		
Age	Low	Fair	Average	Good	High
20–29	≤28	29–34	35–40	41–46	≥47
30–39	≤27	28–34	35–38	39–45	≥46
40–49	≤25	26–31	32–37	38–43	≥44
50–65	≤21	22–28	29–34	35–40	≥41
			Men		
20–29	≤37	38–41	42–50	51–55	≥56
30–39	≤33	34–37	38–42	43–50	≥51
40–49	≤29	30–35	36–40	41–46	≥47
50–59	≤25	26–30	31–38	39–42	≥43
60–69	≤21	22–25	26–33	34–37	≥38

TABLE 2.8 Normative VO_2max mL/kg/min Data for Women and Men

Source: CSEP, Professional Fitness & Lifestyle Consultant Resource Manual.

Fitness Category	Age (years)					
	13–19	20–29	30–39	40–49	50–59	60+
Men						
Very poor	>15:30	>16:00	>16:30	>17:30	>19:00	>20:00
Poor	12:11–15:30	14:01–16:00	14:46–16:30	15:36–17:30	17:01–19:00	19:01–20:00
Average	10:49–12:10	12:01–14:00	12:31–14:45	13:01–15:35	14:31–17:00	16:16–19:00
Good	9:41–10:48	10:46–12:00	11:01–12:30	11:31–13:00	12:31–14:30	14:00–16:15
Excellent	8:37–9:40	9:45–10:45	10:00–11:00	10:30–11:30	11:00–12:30	11:15–13:59
Superior	<8:37	<9:45	<10:00	<10:30	<11:00	<11:15
Women						
Very poor	>18:30	>19:00	>19:30	>20:00	>20:30	>21:00
Poor	16:55–18:30	18:31–19:00	19:01–19:30	19:31–20:00	20:01–20:30	20:31–21:31
Average	14:31–16:54	15:55–18:30	16:31–19:00	17:31–19:30	19:01–20:00	19:31–20:30
Good	12:30–14:30	13:31–15:54	14:31–16:30	15:56–17:30	16:31–19:00	17:31–19:30
Excellent	11:50–12:29	12:30–13:30	13:00–14:30	13:45–15:55	14:30–16:30	16:30–18:00
Superior	<11:50	<12:30	<13:00	<13:45	<14:30	<16:30

Times are given in minutes and seconds. (> = greater than; < = less than)

From Cooper, K. *The aerobics program for total well-being.* Bantam Books, New York, 1982. Copyright © 1982 by Kenneth H. Cooper. Used by permission of Bantam Books, a division of Bantam Doubleday Dell Publishing Group, Inc.

TABLE 2.9 Fitness Categories for Cooper's 1.5-Mile Run Test to Determine Cardiorespiratory Endurance

LABORATORY 2.4

Measurement of Cardiorespiratory Fitness: The 1.5-Mile Run Test

Name_____ Age _____ Sex _____ Date _____

DIRECTIONS

The objective of the test is to complete the 1.5-mile distance as quickly as possible. The run can be completed on an oval track or any properly measured course. Remember, you should attempt this test only if you have completed Laboratory 2.1.

Prior to the test, perform a 5- to 10-minute warm-up. It is best to try to find a speed (intensity) that you can maintain for the duration of the test. If you become extremely fatigued during the test, slow your pace—do not overstress yourself! If you feel faint or nauseated, or experience any unusual pains in your upper body, stop and notify your instructor.

On completion of the test, cool down and record your time and fitness category, using the information in Table 2.9.

Ambient conditions:

*Temperature: _____   *Relative Humidity: _____

Finish Time: _____   Fitness Category: _____

---

* The purpose of recording the temperature and relative humidity is to provide a record of the amount of heat stress during the test. High heat and relative humidity could have a negative impact on your test score.

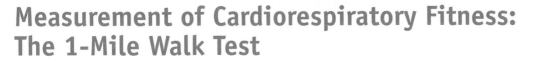

LABORATORY 2.5

Measurement of Cardiorespiratory Fitness: The 1-Mile Walk Test

Name_____ Age _____ Sex _____ Date _____

DIRECTIONS

The objective of the test is to walk the 1-mile distance as quickly as possible. The walk can be completed on an oval track or any properly measured course. Remember, you should attempt this test only if you have completed Laboratory 2.1.

Prior to the test, perform a 5- to 10-minute warm-up. As noted earlier in this chapter, you are advised to maintain a speed that you can walk for the duration of the test. If you become extremely fatigued during the test, slow your pace—do not overstress yourself! If you feel faint or nauseated, or experience any unusual pains in your upper body, stop and notify your instructor.

On completion of the test, cool down and record your time and fitness category. Table 2.10 contains norms for scoring cardiorespiratory fitness using the 1-mile walk test. Find your age group and finish time in the table and then locate your fitness category on the left side of it.

Ambient conditions:

*Temperature: _____   *Relative Humidity: _____

Finish Time: _____   Fitness Category: _____

---

* The purpose of recording the temperature and relative humidity is to provide a record of the amount of heat stress during the test. High heat and relative humidity could have a negative impact on your test score.

Fitness Category	Age (years)			
	13–19	20–29	30–39	40+
Men				
Very poor	>17:30	>18:00	>19:00	>21:30
Poor	16:01–17:30	16:31–18:00	17:31–19:00	18:31–21:30
Average	14:01–16:00	14:31–16:30	15:31–17:30	16:01–18:30
Good	12:30–14:00	13:00–14:30	13:30–15:30	14:00–16:00
Excellent	<12:30	<13:00	<13:30	<14:00
Women				
Very poor	>18:01	>18:31	>19:31	>20:01
Poor	16:31–18:00	17:01–18:30	18:01–19:30	19:31–20:00
Average	14:31–16:30	15:01–17:00	16:01–18:00	18:01–19:30
Good	13:31–14:30	13:31–15:00	14:01–16:00	14:31–18:00
Excellent	<13:30	<13:30	<14:00	<14:30

Because the 1-mile walk test is designed primarily for older or less conditioned individuals, the fitness categories listed here do not include a "superior" category.

Modified from *Rockport Fitness Walking Test*. Copyright © 1993. The Rockport Company, Inc. All rights reserved. Reprinted by permission of The Rockport Company, Inc.

TABLE 2.10 Fitness Classification for 1-Mile Walk Test

Cycle Ergometer Test to Determine Cardiorespiratory Fitness

Name_____ Age _____ Sex _____ Date _____

DIRECTIONS

The cycle ergometer test is conducted as follows:

- Warm up for 3 minutes while pedalling the cycle at 60 revolutions per minute (RPM) with no load against the pedals.
- After completion of the warm-up, begin the fitness test. Set the load on the cycle ergometer using Table 2.11 and perform 5 minutes of cycling.
- During the last minute of exercise, measure your heart rate for 15 seconds (see Figure 2.2). Accurate measurement of your heart is critical for the test to be a valid assessment of cardiorespiratory endurance.

Remember you should complete this test only if you have satisfied the requirements in Laboratory 2.1 (i.e., you have obtained medical clearance).

Cool down for 3 to 5 minutes using unloaded pedalling. Record your heart rate (15-second count) below and compute your relative VO_2max using Table 2.12. After calculating your relative VO_2max, locate your fitness category in Table 2.13.

Test 1 Date: _____

Heart rate (15-second count) during minute 5 of test: _____

Fitness category: _____

Gender	Age (years)	Pedal Speed (RPM)	Load (watts)
Male	Up to 29	60	150 (900 KPM)
	30 and up	60	50 (300 KPM)
Female	Up to 29 (or poorly conditioned)	60	100 (600 KPM)
	30 and up (or poorly conditioned)	60	50 (300 KPM)

TABLE 2.11 Work Rates for Submaximal Cycle Ergometer Test

Locate your 15-second heart rate in the left-hand column, below; then find your estimated VO_2max in the appropriate column on the right. For example, the second column from the left contains absolute VO_2max (expressed in mL/min) for male subjects using the 900-KPM work rate. The third column from the left contains the absolute VO_2max (expressed in mL/min) for women using the 600-KPM work rate, and so on. After determining your absolute VO_2max, calculate your relative VO_2max (mL/kg/min) by dividing your VO_2max expressed in mL/min by your body weight in kilograms. For example, if your body weight is 70 kilograms and your absolute VO_2max is 2631 mL/min, your relative VO_2max is approximately 38 mL/kg/min (i.e., 2631 divided by 70 = 37.6). After computing your relative VO_2max, use Table 2.13 to identify your fitness category.

	Estimated Absolute VO_2max (mL/min)		
15-Sec. Heart Rate	Men: 900–KPM Work Rate (mL/min)	Women: 600–KPM Work Rate (mL/min)	Men or Women: 300–KPM Work Rate (mL/min)
28	3560	2541	1525
29	3442	2459	1475

TABLE 2.12 Cycle Ergometer Fitness Index for Men and Women

continued

| 15-Sec. Heart Rate | Estimated Absolute VO$_2$max (mL/min) | | |
	Men: 900–KPM Work Rate (mL/min)	Women: 600–KPM Work Rate (mL/min)	Men or Women: 300–KPM Work Rate (mL/min)
30	3333	2376	1425
31	3216	2293	1375
32	3099	2210	1325
33	2982	2127	1275
34	2865	2044	1225
35	2748	1961	1175
36	2631	1878	1125
37	2514	1795	1075
38	2397	1712	1025
39	2280	1629	—
40	2163	1546	—
41	2046	1463	—
42	1929	1380	—
43	1812	1297	—
44	1695	1214	—
45	1578	1131	—

TABLE 2.12 *continued*

| Age Group (years) | Fitness Categories Based on VO$_2$max (mL/kg/min) | | | | | |
	Very Poor	Poor	Average	Good	Excellent	Superior
Men						
13–19	<35	36–39	40–46	47–53	54–59	>60
20–29	<33	34–38	39–45	46–52	53–58	>59
30–39	<32	33–37	38–43	44–49	50–53	>54
40–49	<30	31–36	37–41	42–48	49–52	>53
50–59	<28	29–32	33–38	39–45	46–49	>50
60+	<24	25–29	30–34	35–39	40–44	>45
Women						
13–19	<28	29–34	35–40	41–44	45–52	>52
20–29	<30	31–33	34–38	39–42	43–51	>51
30–39	<28	29–31	32–36	37–42	43–45	>45
40–49	<25	26–28	29–34	35–39	40–42	>42
50–59	<23	24–25	26–30	31–34	35–38	>38
60+	<22	23–24	25–29	30–34	35–36	>36

Modified from Golding, L., C. Myers, and W. Sinning. Y's way to physical fitness: The complete guide to fitness testing and instruction. 3rd ed. Human Kinetics, Champaign, IL, 1989.

TABLE 2.13 Cardiorespiratory Fitness Norms for Men and Women Based on Estimated VO$_2$max Values Determined by the Cycle Ergometer Test

LABORATORY 2.7

Measurement of Cardiorespiratory Fitness: Step Test

Name_____ Age _____ Sex _____ Date _____

DIRECTIONS

Prior to engaging in this test, complete Laboratory 2.1. Record your heart rates below and use Table 2.14 to determine your fitness category.

Recovery heart rate post exercise (beats)

1–1.5 min: _____

2–2.5 min: _____

3–3.5 min: _____

Total: _____ (recovery index)

Fitness category: _____

The test is conducted as follows:

- Select a partner to assist you with the step test. Your partner is responsible for timing the test and helping you to maintain the proper stepping cadence. The exercise cadence is 30 complete steps (up and down) per minute during a 3-minute exercise period, which can be maintained by a metronome or voice cues from your partner ("up, up, down, down"). Thus, you need to make one complete step cycle every 2 seconds (i.e., set the metronome at 60 tones/minute and step up and down with each sound). Note that it is important that you straighten your knees during the "up" phase of the test (see Figure 2.4 on page 24).
- After completing the test, sit quietly on a chair or on the step bench. Find your pulse and count your heart rate for 30-second periods during the following recovery times:
  - 1 to 1.5 minutes post exercise
  - 2 to 2.5 minutes post exercise
  - 3 to 3.5 minutes post exercise
- Your partner should assist you in timing the recovery period and recording your recovery heart rates. Note that the accuracy of this test depends on the faithful execution of 30 steps per minute during the test and the valid measurement of heart rate during the appropriate recovery times.

To determine your fitness category, add the three 30-second heart rates obtained during recovery; this is called the *recovery index*. Table 2.14 contains norms for step test results in a postsecondary-age population (18–25 years). For example, a male student with a recovery index of 165 beats would be classified as having average cardiorespiratory endurance.

3-Minute Step Test Recovery Index					
Fitness Category	**Women**	**Men**	**Fitness Category**	**Women**	**Men**
Superior	95–120	95–117	Average	154–174	148–165
Excellent	121–135	118–132	Poor	175–204	166–192
Good	136–153	133–147	Very poor	205–233	193–217

Fitness categories are for postsecondary-age men and women (ages 18–25 years) at the University of Florida who performed the test on a 45-cm bench.

TABLE 2.14 Norms for Cardiorespiratory Fitness Using the Sum of Three Recovery Heart Rates Obtained Following the Step Test

LABORATORY 2.8

Measurement of Muscular Strength: The 1 RM Test and Estimating 1 RM Using a 10 RM Test

Name_____ Age _____ Sex _____ Date _____

DIRECTIONS

Prior to engaging in these strength tests, complete Laboratory 2.1. Directions for determining 1 RM using a 10 RM test are provided earlier in the chapter on page 26, and using Table 2.16 on the next page. After performance of your 1 RM test, compute your muscular strength scores as follows:

$$\frac{1 \text{ RM weight}}{\text{body weight}} \times 100 = \text{muscular strength score}$$

Record your muscular strength scores below and use Table 2.15 to determine your fitness category. Table 2.15 contains strength score norms for postsecondary-age men and women in each of these lifts. Using Table 2.15, a muscle strength score of 120 on the bench press places a postsecondary-age man in the "good" category.

Body weight: _____ **kg**

1 RM Test

Exercise	1 RM (kg)	Muscular Strength	Fitness Category
Bench press	_____	_____	_____
Biceps curl	_____	_____	_____
Shoulder press	_____	_____	_____
Leg press	_____	_____	_____

	Fitness Category					
Exercise	Very Poor	Poor	Average	Good	Excellent	Superior
Men						
Bench press	<23	23–44	45–50	51–59	60–68	>68
Biceps curl	<14	14–18	19–25	26–27	28–36	>36
Shoulder press	<18	18–23	24–30	31–36	37–50	>50
Leg press	<73	73–90	91–95	96–104	105–109	>109
Women						
Bench press	<18	18–31	32–34	35–36	37–50	>50
Biceps curl	<7	7–15	16–18	19–25	26–27	>27
Shoulder press	<9	9–21	22–25	26–27	28–36	>36
Leg press	<45	45–59	60–65	66–79	80–86	>86

Norms are from Williams (1996).

TABLE 2.15 Norms for Muscle Strength Scores Using a 1 RM Test

Estimated 1 RM (kg)	Weight (kg) Lifted During 7 Reps	Weight (kg) Lifted During 8 Reps	Weight (kg) Lifted During 9 Reps	Weight (kg) Lifted During 10 Reps	Estimated 1 RM (kg)	Weight (kg) Lifted During 7 Reps	Weight (kg) Lifted During 8 Reps	Weight (kg) Lifted During 9 Reps	Weight (kg) Lifted During 10 Reps
2.3	1.9	1.8	1.7	1.7	106.6	86.4	83.7	81.0	78.3
4.5	3.7	3.6	3.4	3.4	108.9	88.2	85.5	82.7	80.0
6.8	5.5	5.4	5.2	5.0	111.1	90.0	87.2	84.5	81.7
9.1	7.3	7.1	6.9	6.7	113.4	91.9	89.0	86.2	83.4
11.3	9.2	8.9	8.6	8.3	115.7	93.7	90.8	87.9	85.0
13.6	11.0	10.7	10.3	10.0	117.9	95.5	92.6	89.6	86.7
15.9	12.9	12.5	12.1	11.7	120.2	97.4	94.4	91.4	88.4
18.1	14.7	14.2	13.8	13.3	122.5	99.2	96.2	93.1	90.0
20.4	16.6	16.0	15.5	15.0	124.7	101.1	97.9	94.8	91.7
22.7	18.4	17.8	17.2	16.7	127.0	102.9	99.7	96.5	93.3
24.9	20.2	19.6	19.0	18.3	129.3	104.7	101.5	98.2	95.0
27.2	22.0	21.4	20.7	20.0	131.5	106.5	103.3	100.0	96.7
29.5	23.9	23.1	22.4	21.7	133.8	108.4	105.1	101.7	98.3
31.8	25.7	24.9	24.1	23.4	136.1	110.2	106.8	103.4	100.0
34.0	27.6	26.7	25.9	25.0	138.3	112.1	108.6	105.1	101.7
36.3	29.4	28.5	27.6	26.7	140.6	113.9	110.4	106.9	103.4
38.6	31.3	30.3	29.3	28.3	142.9	115.8	112.2	108.6	105.0
40.8	33.1	32.1	31.0	30.0	145.2	117.6	113.9	110.3	106.7
43.1	34.9	33.8	32.7	31.7	147.4	119.4	115.7	112.0	108.4
45.4	36.7	35.6	34.5	33.3	149.7	121.2	117.5	113.8	110.0
47.6	38.6	37.4	36.2	35.0	152.0	123.1	119.3	115.5	111.7
49.9	40.4	39.2	37.9	36.7	154.2	124.9	121.1	117.2	113.4
52.2	42.3	41.0	39.6	38.3	156.5	126.8	122.8	118.9	115.0
54.4	44.1	42.7	41.4	40.0	158.8	128.6	124.6	120.7	116.7
56.7	45.9	44.5	43.1	41.7	161.0	130.5	126.4	122.4	118.3
59.0	47.8	46.3	44.8	43.4	163.3	132.3	128.2	124.1	120.0
61.2	49.6	48.1	46.5	45.0	165.6	134.1	130.0	125.8	121.7
63.5	51.4	49.8	48.3	46.7	167.8	135.9	131.8	127.6	123.4
65.8	53.3	51.6	50.0	48.4	170.1	137.8	133.5	129.3	125.0
68.0	55.1	53.4	51.7	50.0	172.4	139.6	135.3	131.0	126.7
70.3	57.0	55.2	53.4	51.7	174.6	141.5	137.0	132.7	128.4
72.6	58.8	57.0	55.2	53.3	176.9	143.3	138.9	134.4	130.0
74.8	60.6	58.7	56.9	55.0	179.2	145.1	140.7	136.2	131.7
77.1	62.5	60.6	58.6	56.7	181.4	147.0	142.4	137.9	133.4
79.4	64.3	62.3	60.3	58.3	183.7	148.8	144.2	139.6	135.0
81.7	66.1	64.1	62.1	60.0	186.0	150.6	146.0	141.6	136.7
83.9	68.0	65.9	63.8	61.7	188.2	152.5	147.8	143.1	138.3
86.2	69.8	67.7	65.5	63.4	190.5	154.3	149.5	144.8	140.0
88.5	71.7	69.4	67.2	65.0	192.8	156.2	151.3	146.5	141.7
90.7	73.5	71.2	68.9	66.7	195.0	158.0	153.1	148.2	143.4
93.0	75.3	73.0	70.7	68.4	197.3	159.8	154.9	150.0	145.0
95.3	77.2	74.8	72.4	70.0	199.6	161.7	156.7	151.7	146.7
97.5	79.0	76.6	74.1	71.7	201.9	163.5	158.4	153.4	148.4
99.8	80.8	82.9	75.8	73.3	204.1	165.3	160.3	155.1	150.0
102.0	82.7	80.1	77.6	75.0	206.4	167.2	162.0	156.9	151.7
104.3	84.5	81.9	79.3	76.7					

TABLE 2.16 Estimating the 1 RM from the 10 RM

LABORATORY 2.9

Measurement of Muscular Endurance: The Push-Up and Curl-Up Tests

Name_____ Age _____ Sex _____ Date _____

DIRECTIONS

Prior to completing these tests, you should have completed Laboratory 2.1.

THE PUSH-UP TEST

Males: Start by positioning yourself on the ground (Figure 2.14a). Your hands should be below your shoulders pointing forward and your legs extended in a straight line. Push your body up by straightening your elbows and using your toes as a pivot. Lower your body until your chin touches the mat. Neither your stomach nor thighs should contact the ground. It is important to keep your back straight and to lower your entire body to the ground as a unit. Repeat.

Females: Start by positioning yourself on the ground as in Figure 2.14c. Your hands should be below your shoulders pointing forward and your legs extended in a straight line. Push yourself up by straightening your elbows and using your knees as a pivot point. Your lower legs remain in contact with the floor. Keep your upper body in a straight line. Lower your body until your chin touches the mat. Your stomach should not contact the mat. Repeat.

The push-up test is performed as follows:

- Select a partner to count your push-ups and assist with monitoring your form. Warm up with a few push-ups. Give yourself a 2- to 3-minute recovery period after the warm-up and prepare to start the test.
- On the command "go," start performing push-ups. Your partner counts your push-ups aloud and observes your body alignment. Remember, only those push-ups performed correctly will be counted toward your total; therefore, use the proper form and make every push-up count. Push-ups are performed consecutively and without a time limit. The test is terminated when you are unable to maintain proper form over 2 consecutive repetitions. The test may also be terminated when you are visibly straining. Remember to exhale on effort; that is, during the upward phase of the push-up.

After completion of the push-up test, use Table 2.17 to determine your health benefit zone, and then record your data in the appropriate space provided.

THE CURL-UP TEST

The protocol for the curl-up test is as follows:

- Select a partner to count your curl-ups; lie on your back with knees bent 90 degrees. Keep your heels in contact with the mat.
- Extend your arms so that your fingertips touch a strip of tape perpendicular to the body (Figure 2.15). A second strip of tape is located toward the feet and parallel to the first (10 centimetres apart). The curl-up is accomplished by raising your trunk (i.e., curling upward) until your fingertips touch the second strip of tape and then returning to the starting position.
- The curl-up test is not timed and is performed at a slow and controlled cadence of 25 curl-ups per minute. This cadence is guided by the aid of a metronome set at 50 beats per minute (curl up on one beat and down on the second).

- On the command "go," start performing curl-ups in cadence with the metronome. Perform as many curl-ups as you can to a maximum of 25 in 1 minute. The test is terminated in less than 1 minute if you experience undue discomfort, you are unable to maintain the required cadence, or if you are unable to perform the proper curl-up technique. See Table 2.17 to determine your health benefit zone, and then record your score in the appropriate space below.

After completion of the push-up and curl-up tests, record your scores and fitness classifications (Table 2.17).

Number of push-ups: _____ Fitness category: _____

Number of curl-ups: _____ Fitness category: _____

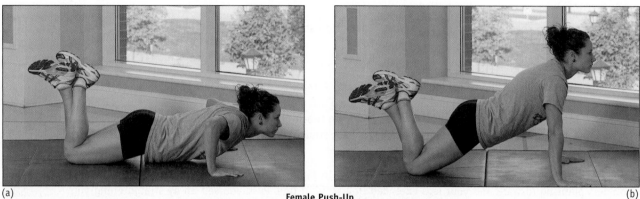

(a)   Female Push-Up   (b)

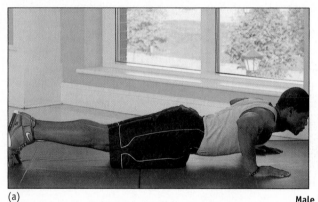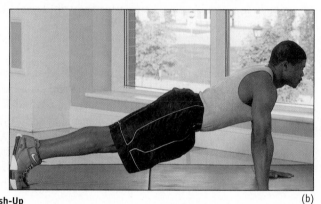

(a)   Male Push-Up   (b)

FIGURE 2.14 Push-ups.

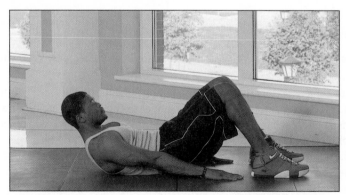

Partial Curl-Up

FIGURE 2.15 Partial curl-up.

Age (years) 15–19

Zone	Gender	Push-Ups (#) M	F	Trunk Fwd Flexion (cm) M	F	Partial Curl-Up (#) M	F
ZONE	Excellent	≥ 39	≥ 33	≥ 39	43	25	25
	Very good	29–38	25–32	34–38	38–42	23–24	23–24
	Good	23–28	18–24	29–33	34–37	21–22	21–22
	Fair	18–22	12–17	24–28	29–33	16–20	16–20
	Needs improvement	≤17	≤11	≤23	≤28	≤15	≤15

Age (yrs) 20–29

Zone	Gender	Push-Ups (#) M	F	Trunk Fwd Flexion (cm) M	F	Partial Curl-Up (#) M	F
ZONE	Excellent	≥36	≥30	≥40	≥41	25	25
	Very good	26–35	21–29	34–39	37–40	23–24	23–24
	Good	22–27	15–20	30–33	33–36	21–22	19–22
	Fair	17–21	10–14	25–29	28–32	13–20	13–18
	Needs improvement	≤16	≤9	≤24	≤27	≤12	≤12

Age (yrs) 30–39

Zone	Gender	Push-Ups (#) M	F	Trunk Fwd Flexion (cm) M	F	Partial Curl-Up (#) M	F
ZONE	Excellent	≥30	≥27	≥38	≥41	25	25
	Very good	22–29	20–26	33–37	36–40	23–24	22–24
	Good	17–21	13–19	28–32	32–35	21–22	16–21
	Fair	12–16	8–12	23–27	27–31	13–20	11–15
	Needs improvement	≤11	≤7	≤22	≤26	≤12	≤10

Age (yrs) 40–49

Zone	Gender	Push-Ups (#) M	F	Trunk Fwd Flexion (cm) M	F	Partial Curl-Up (#) M	F
ZONE	Excellent	≥22	≥24	≥35	≥38	25	25
	Very good	17–21	15–23	29–34	34–37	22–24	21–24
	Good	13–16	11–14	24–28	30–33	16–21	13–20
	Fair	10–12	5–10	18–23	25–29	11–15	6–12
	Needs improvement	≤9	≤4	≤17	≤24	≤10	≤5

Age (yrs) 50–59

Zone	Gender	Push-Ups (#) M	F	Trunk Fwd Flexion (cm) M	F	Partial Curl-Up (#) M	F
ZONE	Excellent	≥21	≥21	≥35	≥39	25	25
	Very good	13–20	11–20	28–34	33–38	20–24	16–24
	Good	10–12	7–10	24–27	30–32	14–19	9–15
	Fair	7–9	2–6	16–23	25–29	9–13	4–8
	Needs improvement	≤6	≤1	≤15	≤24	≤8	≤3

Age (yrs) 60–69

Zone	Gender	Push-Ups (#) M	F	Trunk Fwd Flexion (cm) M	F	Partial Curl-Up (#) M	F
ZONE	Excellent	≥18	≥17	≥33	≥35	25	≥18
	Very good	11–17	12–16	25–32	31–34	16–24	11–17
	Good	8–10	5–11	20–24	27–30	10–15	6–10
	Fair	5–7	1–4	15–19	23–26	4–9	2–5
	Needs improvement	≤4	≤1	≤14	≤23	≤3	≤1

TABLE 2.17 Healthy Musculoskeletal Fitness: Norms and Health Benefit Zones by Age Groups and Gender

Source: *The Canadian Physical Activity, Fitness & Lifestyle Approach: CSE-Health & Fitness Program's Health-Related Appraisal and Counselling Strategy*, 3rd edition, copyright 2003. Reprinted with permission of the Canadian Society for Exercise Physiology.

LABORATORY 2.10

Assessment of Flexibility: Trunk Flexion (Sit and Reach Test) and the Shoulder Flexibility Test

DIRECTIONS

Remember to complete Laboratory 2.1 prior to engaging in these tests.

TRUNK FLEXION (SIT AND REACH TEST)

A brief warm-up followed by a few minutes of stretching is recommended prior to performance of the test. Start by sitting upright with your feet, shoes removed, flat against the box. Keeping your feet flat on the box and your legs straight, extend your hands, palms down, as far forward as possible without jerking and hold this position for 2 seconds. Lowering the head assists in reaching the maximum potential distance. Knees should not bend, nor should they be held in place. Avoid bouncing and jerking movements; the sit and reach test should involve a slow, controlled reach. Repeat this procedure 2 times. Your score on the sit and reach test is the distance, measured to the nearest centimetre, between the edge of the sit and reach box closest to you and the tips of your fingers during the best of your three stretching efforts.

After completing the test, record your scores in the appropriate space below.

SHOULDER FLEXIBILITY TEST

A brief warm-up period followed by a few minutes of stretching is recommended prior to performance of the shoulder flexibility test. While standing, raise your right arm and reach down your back as far as possible. At the same time, extend your left arm behind your back and reach upward toward your right hand. The objective is to try to overlap your fingers as much as possible. Your rating on this test is simply based on whether or not your fingers can touch and overlap.

If your fingers are not able to touch during this test, your rating is "below average." If your fingers are just able to touch, your rating is "average." Finally, if your fingers are able to overlap, your rating is "above average."

After completing the test with the right hand up, repeat the test in the opposite direction (left hand up). It is common to be more flexible on one side than on the other.

Again, to prevent injury, avoid rapid or jerky movements during the test. After completion of the test, record your results in the appropriate space.

After completion of the sit and reach test and the shoulder flexibility test, record your scores and fitness classifications (Table 2.17 in Laboratory 2.9).

Test 1 Date: _____

Sit and reach score (cm): _____
Fitness category: _____
Shoulder flexibility (cm): _____
Fitness category: _____

LABORATORY 2.11

Assessment of Health Risk Based on Anthropometric Measurements

Name_____ Age _____ Sex _____ Date _____

SKINFOLD MEASUREMENTS

The skinfold calipers are held in your right hand while the left hand (thumb and forefinger) holds the skinfold. The calipers should always be applied perpendicular to the skinfold. The calipers are applied 1 cm below the fold, firmly grasped between your thumb and forefinger. Complete all 5 skinfold measurements before repeating them. If the difference between the two measurements is greater than 0.4 mm, a third measurement should be taken. If two measurements are taken, the average is used as the final value. If three measurements are taken, the median value is used as the final value.

To make each measurement, hold the skinfold between your thumb and index finger. Slowly release the tension on the skinfold calipers while you continue to hold approximately 1 cm above the calipers. Continue to hold the skinfold with your fingers and fully release the tension on the calipers; then, simply read the number (the skinfold thickness in millimetres) from the gauge. Release the calipers and then your grasp of the skinfold and allow the tissue to relax.

TRICEPS SKINFOLD

To determine the location of the triceps skinfold, the upper arm is measured from the tip of the *acromion process* (shoulder) to the tip of the *olecranon process* (elbow) with the arm bent at a right angle (see Figure 2.16). Once the midpoint of the right arm is located, a skinfold can be raised along the midline of the back arm with arm extended alongside the body (see Figure 2.17).

BICEPS SKINFOLD

With the right arm extended, palm facing forward, a fold of skin is raised at the midpoint (as determined above) of the midarm so that it runs vertically along the midline of the front of the arm (see Figure 2.18).

SUBSCAPULAR SKINFOLD

With shoulders relaxed and arms extended alongside the body, the subscapular skinfold is raised 1 cm below the inferior angle of the right scapula (see Figure 2.19). This skinfold runs downward and outward at a 45-degree angle to the spine.

ILIAC CREST SKINFOLD

In a standing position with the right arm raised so that the right hand touches the right shoulder, the iliac crest skinfold is raised 3 cm above the right ilium at the midline (mid-axillary line) of the body so that the skinfold runs forward and slightly downward (see Figure 2.20).

MEDIAL CALF SKINFOLD

With the right foot placed on an elevated surface such that the knee is at a 90° angle, the point of greatest calf is determined (see Figure 2.21). At this point, the medial calf skinfold is raised so that it runs vertically along the midline (see Figure 2.22).

WAIST GIRTH

The waist girth measurement should be made while standing, using a nonelastic tape. It is important that bulky clothing not be worn during the measurement, because it could bias the measurement. During measurement, the tape should be placed snugly around the waist but not press into the skin. Record your measurements to the nearest 0.5 cm.

Place the tape at the level of the umbilicus or at the level of noticeable waist narrowing (navel; Figure 2.23). Take your measurement at the end of a normal expiration. Record your data in the appropriate space.

After completing the skinfold measurements, total the 5 values and use Tables 2.18, 2.19, and 2.20 to determine your health risk. Record your rating in the appropriate place.

Working in pairs and using the directions above, measure and record one another's skinfolds and waist girth. Record your values in the appropriate spaces below.

Height (m): _____
Weight (kg): _____
Body mass index (kg/m^2): _____
Waist circumference (cm): _____
Skinfolds: _____

Skinfold	Test 1	Test 2	Test 3	Final
Triceps (mm)	_____	_____	_____	_____
Bicep (mm)	_____	_____	_____	_____
Subscapular (mm)	_____	_____	_____	_____
Iliac crest (mm)	_____	_____	_____	_____
Medial calf (mm)	_____	_____	_____	_____
Sum of 5 skinfolds (mm):	_____			
Sum of 2 skinfolds* (mm):	_____			
Health benefit zone:	_____			

---

* Sum of subscapular and iliac crest.

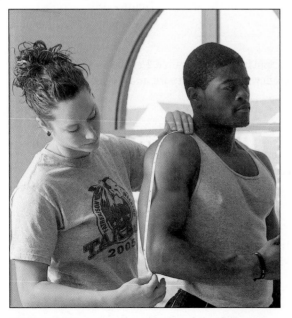

FIGURE 2.16 Measuring the midpoint of the right arm.

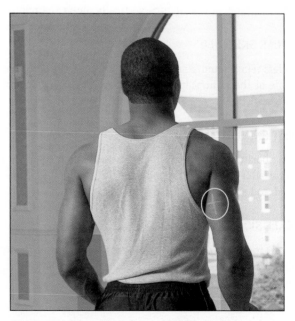

FIGURE 2.17 Where the triceps skinfold should be taken.

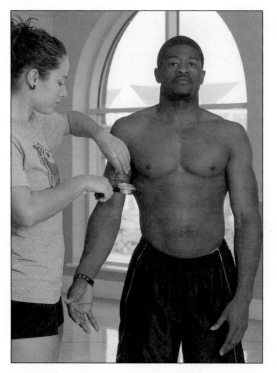

FIGURE 2.18 Where the biceps skinfold should be taken.

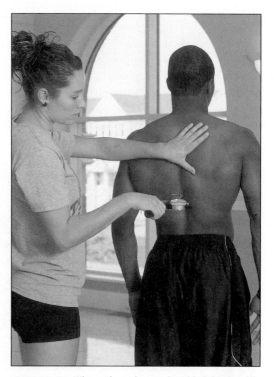

FIGURE 2.19 Where the subscapular skinfold should be taken.

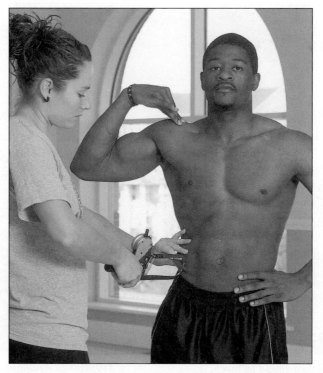

FIGURE 2.20 Where the iliac crest skinfold should be taken.

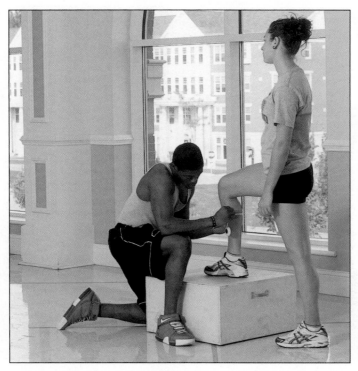

FIGURE 2.21 Measuring the midpoint of the medial calf.

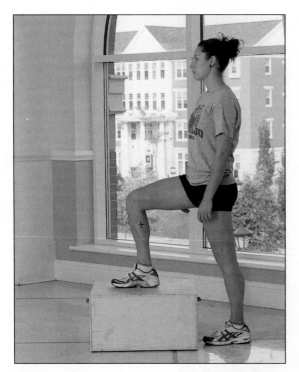

FIGURE 2.22 Where the medial skinfold should be taken.

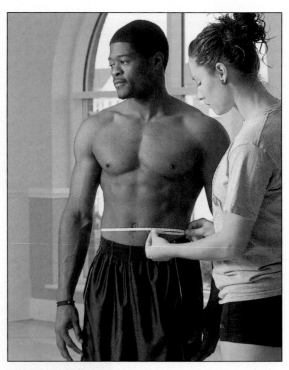

FIGURE 2.23 Measuring waist girth.

Age (yrs) 15–19

**Measures	BMI		SO5S		WG		SO2S	
Sex	M	F	M	F	M	F	M	F
	18	17	25	36	67	61	11	13
	19	18	27	40	68	63	12	14
	19	19	28	43	64	64	13	16
	20	19	29	46	70	65	13	17
	20	19	31	49	72	65	14	18
	20	20	32	51	72	66	15	19
	21	20	33	54	73	67	15	20
	21	20	35	56	74	67	16	21
	21	21	36	58	75	68	17	22
	22	21	38	61	76	68	17	23
	22	22	40	63	77	69	18	24
	22	22	42	66	78	70	19	26
	22	22	44	69	79	70	21	27
	23	23	47	72	80	71	22	29
	23	23	51	77	81	72	24	31
	24	24	54	83	82	72	27	33
	25	25	61	89	84	74	28	37
	26	26	69	97	88	77	32	42
	28	28	82	116	95	81	42	49

Age (yrs) 20–29

**Measures	BMI		SO5S		WG		SO2S	
Sex	M	F	M	F	M	F	M	F
	19	18	26	37	71	61	13	13
	20	18	29	40	73	63	14	14
	21	19	30	43	75	64	16	16
	21	19	32	46	76	65	17	17
	22	20	34	49	77	65	18	18
	22	20	36	51	78	66	19	19
	22	20	38	53	79	66	20	20
	23	21	40	56	81	67	21	21
	23	21	43	58	81	68	23	22
	23	21	46	60	82	69	25	23
	24	22	49	63	83	70	27	24
	24	22	52	65	84	71	28	26
	25	22	55	69	85	72	30	27
	25	23	58	72	86	73	32	29
	26	23	62	76	87	75	35	31
	27	24	68	81	89	77	38	33
	27	25	74	86	91	78	41	36
	28	26	82	95	93	81	46	42
	30	28	94	111	97	86	54	48

TABLE 2.18 Health Benefit Zones by Age and Sex: Body Weight, Adiposity, and Fat Distribution*

Source: *The Canadian Physical Activity, Fitness & Lifestyle Approach: CSE-Health & Fitness Program's Health-Related Appraisal and Counselling Strategy*, 3rd edition, copyright 2003. Reprinted with permission of the Canadian Society for Exercise Physiology.

Age (yrs) 30–39

**Measures	BMI		S05S		WG		S02S	
Sex	M	F	M	F	M	F	M	F
	20	19	28	40	75	63	14	14
	21	19	32	45	77	64	17	15
	22	20	35	48	79	65	19	17
	22	20	38	52	80	66	20	18
	23	21	41	55	81	68	22	20
	23	21	44	58	82	69	24	21
	24	22	46	61	83	70	26	23
	24	22	49	63	83	71	27	24
	24	22	52	66	85	72	29	25
	25	23	55	69	86	73	31	27
	25	23	58	72	87	74	33	28
	26	23	60	76	88	75	35	30
	26	24	63	79	89	76	37	32
	27	24	67	83	90	77	39	34
	28	25	71	88	92	79	42	36
	28	26	76	93	94	81	45	39
	29	27	82	99	96	83	48	43
	30	29	89	109	99	86	53	48
	32	31	101	128	106	91	59	59

Age (yrs) 40–49

**Measures	BMI		S05S		WG		S02S	
Sex	M	F	M	F	M	F	M	F
	21	19	28	42	78	65	15	14
	22	20	37	48	80	67	20	16
	23	20	40	51	82	68	22	18
	23	21	44	56	84	69	24	20
	24	21	46	59	85	70	26	21
	24	22	48	62	86	72	27	23
	25	22	51	66	87	73	29	25
	25	23	53	69	88	74	31	26
	25	23	56	73	89	75	32	28
	26	24	58	77	91	76	34	29
	26	24	60	81	92	77	35	32
	27	25	63	86	93	78	36	34
	27	25	66	90	94	80	38	37
	28	26	69	94	96	81	40	40
	28	27	72	98	98	83	42	43
	29	28	75	105	100	85	44	46
	30	29	79	113	102	88	47	50
	31	31	86	125	105	92	50	56
	32	34	97	150	114	99	56	65

TABLE 2.18 *Continued*

Age (yrs) 50–59

**Measures		BMI		S05S		WG		S02S	
Sex		M	F	M	F	M	F	M	F
		21	20	31	48	83	67	17	16
		22	21	36	54	85	69	20	19
		23	22	40	60	87	71	22	22
		24	22	44	65	88	73	24	24
		24	23	46	69	89	75	26	26
		24	23	48	73	90	76	27	28
		25	23	51	75	91	78	29	29
		25	24	53	78	92	79	30	30
		25	24	55	81	93	80	32	31
		26	25	58	84	94	81	33	33
		26	25	60	87	95	83	35	35
		27	26	62	90	95	84	36	37
		27	26	65	93	96	85	38	39
		28	27	68	97	98	86	40	41
		28	28	71	101	99	88	43	44
		29	29	74	106	101	90	45	46
		30	30	77	112	103	92	47	49
		31	31	81	121	105	95	49	53
		32	34	88	138	109	103	54	60

Age (yrs) 60–69

**Measures		BMI		S05S		WG		S02S	
Sex		M	F	M	F	M	F	M	F
		21	20	33	45	82	66	17	16
		22	21	38	54	84	69	21	18
		23	22	41	61	87	73	23	22
		24	22	45	65	88	75	25	24
		25	23	48	67	91	77	27	25
		25	23	50	70	92	78	28	28
		25	24	52	72	92	79	29	29
		26	24	54	76	93	80	31	31
		26	25	56	80	94	81	32	33
		27	25	58	82	95	82	33	34
		27	26	59	85	96	83	34	36
		27	26	61	87	97	84	35	38
		28	27	63	93	99	85	37	40
		28	28	65	98	101	86	38	42
		28	28	69	100	103	88	40	44
		29	29	72	103	104	90	42	46
		30	30	76	112	105	93	45	49
		31	32	81	123	107	98	48	54
		33	34	91	139	112	103	55	60

* Based on data from the Canada Fitness Survey, 1981

** BMI: Body mass index = Body weight (kg) ÷ Height^2(m)

  S05S: Sum of (five) skinfolds (mm) = Triceps + biceps + subscapular + iliac crest + medial calf

WG: Waist girth (cm)

S02S: Sum of (two) trunk skinfolds (mm) = subscapular + iliac crest

    Estimated health benefit zones according to trends in morbidity and mortality data

TABLE 2.18 *Continued*

Scoring of Body Composition Assessments

BMI healthy and SO5S healthy	8 points	WG healthy and SO2S healthy	8 points
BMI unhealthy and SO5 healthy	8 points	WG healthy and SO2S unhealthy	4 points
BMI healthy and SO5S unhealthy	3 points	WG unhealthy and SO2S healthy	2 points
BMI unhealthy and SO5S unhealthy	0 points	WG unhealthy and SO2S unhealthy	0 points

Corresponding Health Benefit Zones for Healthy Body Composition

16 points	Excellent
12 points	Very good
7–11 points	Good
4–5 points	Fair
0–3 points	Needs improvement

TABLE 2.19 Determination of Health Benefit Zones

Source: *The Canadian Physical Activity, Fitness & Lifestyle Approach: CSE-Health & Fitness Program's Health-Related Appraisal and Counselling Strategy*, 3rd edition, copyright 2003. Reprinted with permission of the Canadian Society for Exercise Physiology.

Health Benefit Zone

Excellent	⇑	Your body composition falls within a range that is generally associated with optimal health benefits.
Very good	⇑	Your body composition falls within a range that is generally associated with considerable health benefits.
Good	⇑	Your body composition falls within a range that is generally associated with many health benefits.
Fair	⇑	Your body composition falls within a range that is generally associated with some health benefits but also some health risks. *Progressing from here into the GOOD zone is a very significant step to increasing the health benefits associated with your body composition.*
Needs improvement	⇑	Your body composition falls within a range that is generally associated with considerable health risks. *Try to achieve and maintain a healthy body composition by enjoying regular physical activity and healthy eating.*

TABLE 2.20 Benefits of Healthy Body Composition

Source: *The Canadian Physical Activity, Fitness & Lifestyle Approach: CSE-Health & Fitness Program's Health-Related Appraisal and Counselling Strategy*, 3rd edition, copyright 2003. Reprinted with permission of the Canadian Society for Exercise Physiology.

CHAPTER 3

General Principles of Exercise for Health and Fitness

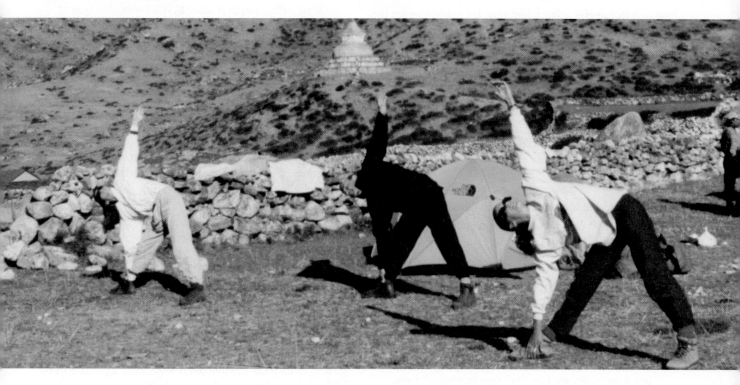

After studying this chapter, you should be able to

1. Outline the FITT principle.

2. Describe the principles of physical fitness and training: overload, progression, specificity, recuperation, and reversibility.

3. Describe the three main principles involved in a workout.

4. Outline the physiological objectives of a warm-up and a cool-down.

5. Explain why individualizing the workout is important in the exercise prescription principles.

6. Discuss how much physical activity and exercise is required to reach the *threshold for health benefits*.

As discussed in Chapter 1, exercise—a specific physical activity often called *training*—is part of a healthy lifestyle related to increased longevity and improved quality of life. The principles of an exercise prescription for health and fitness will be discussed in this chapter, including progression, specificity, and recuperation. Establishing realistic and achievable goals to improve physical fitness in conjunction with the FITT principle (frequency, intensity, time, and type) will also be outlined, and the chapter will address the questions of how much training is needed, how often to train, and how hard to train. The basic principles contained in this chapter can be applied to men and women of all ages and fitness levels. The individual components of health-related fitness are covered in Chapters 4, 5, and 6, which detail the development of cardiorespiratory endurance, muscular strength and endurance, and flexibility.

Principles of Training to Improve Physical Fitness

Research in exercise science has provided guidelines for the development of a safe and efficient program to improve personal fitness (Corbin & Lindsey, 1997; Fleck & Kraemer, 1997; Getchell, 1997; Hagan, 2000; Hockey, 1996; Pollock & Wilmore, 1990; Powers & Howley, 2001; Williams, 1996). Although the specifics of a physical activity or training program should be tailored to the individual based on age, sex, ability, and preference, the general **exercise prescription guidelines** or the FITT principles are the same for everyone:

Frequency—How often to exercise. This is guided by one's goals, personal needs, and ability. The best way to get started is to consult Health Canada's Physical Activity Unit (see **www.phac-aspc.gc.ca/pau-uap/ fitness/about.html**). The Physical Activity Unit publishes various guides where the number of sessions and amount of time dedicated to each session are outlined based on type of activity and age.

Intensity—How hard to exercise. Exercising harder or more intensely than one is capable of can affect the enjoyment of that activity, or, worse, lead to injury. A beginner would want to start easy to moderate and progress toward longer, more vigorous activity. This is where goal setting can be most beneficial. See Chapter 1 and the discussion of SuPeR SMART goals.

Time—How long to exercise. There is an important relationship between exercise intensity and exercise time. The more vigorous the activity, the less time is needed to obtain the health-related benefits. The Physical Activity Unit suggests only 20 to 30 minutes of vigorous activity. A beginner may want to start with 10 to

15 minutes of low to moderate activity, and after achieving 30 to 60 minutes of moderate activity every day pursue more intense or longer periods of exercise.

Type—What physical activity to choose. The type of physical activity should be based on the concept of enjoyment and success. It should meet the needs of one's current situation and physical capability, and fit realistically with future goals. People are more likely to keep participating in an activity when they experience a level of enjoyment and success.

The following section describes the principles of overload, progression, specificity, recuperation, and reversibility. Combining these principles and the FITT principles will assist in developing an exercise prescription that will enhance one's fitness and health.

Overload Principle

The **overload principle** is a key component of all conditioning programs (American College of Sports Medicine, 1991; Corbin & Lindsey, 1997; Fleck & Kraemer, 1997; Getchell, 1997; Hagan, 2000; Hockey, 1996; Pollock & Wilmore, 1990; Powers & Howley, 2001; Williams, 1996). In order to improve physical fitness, the body or specific muscles must be stressed beyond what they are used to. For example, for a skeletal muscle to increase in strength it must work against a heavier load than what it has been working against. In this case, we achieve an overload by increasing the intensity of the exercise (i.e., by using heavier weights). Note, however, that overload can also be achieved by increasing the duration of the exercise. For instance, to increase muscular endurance, a muscle must be worked over a longer duration than what it has been doing (by performing a higher number of repetitions). Another practical example of the overload principle applied to health-related physical fitness is the improvement of flexibility. To increase the range of motion at a joint, we must either stretch the muscle to a longer length or hold the stretch for a longer time.

Although improvement in physical fitness requires application of overload, this does not mean that training sessions must be exhausting. The often heard quote "No pain, no gain" is not accurate. It suggests that if your training sessions don't leave you in agony you won't see any results. The reality is that improvement in physical fitness can be achieved without punishing training sessions (Pollack & Wilmore, 1990).

exercise prescription guidelines Guidelines that incorporate regular exercise in accordance with the FITT principles that can be tailored to individual needs. It incorporates fitness goals, type of exercise, warm-up, workout (primary conditioning), and cool-down.

overload principle Stressing the body or a specific muscle beyond what it is used to, in order to improve physical strength.

Progression Principle

The **progression principle** states that overload should be increased gradually and in phases that occur between training blocks. A typical training program is a 3- to 4-week block. The first 2 to 3 weeks are called the *working weeks*. In the last week, known as *active recovery*, the working load is a bit lighter, and incorporates rest into the training program. The next block would increase the working load above the level of the previous working week block; the active recovery week is then repeated, and so the cycle moves on. This type of progression allows the muscles, heart, and lungs to be stimulated and adapt, improve, and then re-stimulate for more progress. It is important that the overload not be increased too slowly or too rapidly if optimum fitness improvement is to result. Progression that is too slow will result in limited improvement in physical fitness. Increasing the exercise overload too rapidly may result in chronic fatigue and injury. Muscle or joint injuries that occur because of too much activity or exercise are called *overuse injuries*. Activity-induced injuries can come either from short bouts of high-intensity activity or long bouts of low-intensity activity. (See Chapter 13 for information on the care and prevention of injuries.)

What is a safe rate of progression during a training program? A definitive answer to this question is not possible, because individuals vary in their tolerance for training overload. However, a common-sense guideline for improving physical fitness and avoiding overuse injuries is the **10-percent rule**, incorporated into a block of progression. In short, this rule states that the training intensity or duration of exercise should not be increased more than 10 percent per week. For example, a runner running 20 minutes per day could increase his or her daily exercise to 22 minutes per day (10 percent of 20 = 2) the following week. This progression should be followed for 2 to 3 weeks, and then the runner should spend 1 week running the original 20 minutes per day. The next 2- to 3-week block would potentially have the participant running 24 minutes per day.

The traditional 10-percent training rule can be detrimental if followed in a straight linear fashion, which can lead to overtraining and injury. However, the training blocks can easily incorporate the 10-percent rule and accommodate active recovery and progression.

The **variety principle** calls for alternating low-, medium, and high-intensity workouts. This type of program challenges the body and assists in making progress. Variations of low- to high-intensity exercises can be incorporated into blocks of training. The first 2 to 3 weeks can alternate high- to moderate-intensity activities, and the active recovery week would incorporate moderate- to low-intensity activities. Note that those moving from sedentary to active would want to limit high-intensity activities to no more than 2 weeks in the beginning training blocks. Once progress is made, the intensity of the physical activity can increase.

When an individual reaches his or her desired level of physical fitness (i.e., the goal as defined by one of the fit-

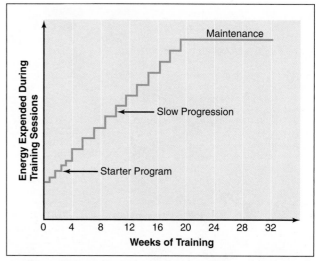

FIGURE 3.1 The progression and maintenance of exercise training during the first several months after beginning an exercise program. (From Pollock, M. L., Wilmore, J. H., and Fox, S. M., III. *Health and Fitness Through Physical Activity*. New York: Prentice-Hall, 1978. Copyright © 1978. Reprinted by permission of Allyn and Bacon.)

ness tests described in Chapter 2), it is no longer necessary to increase the training intensity or duration. Indeed, once a desired level of fitness has been achieved, physical fitness can be maintained by regular exercise at a constant level (Figure 3.1). Exercising to sustain a certain level of physical fitness is called a *maintenance program*.

Specificity Principle

Another key principle of training is the **specificity principle**, which states that the exercise training effect is specific to those muscles involved in the activity (Roberts & Alspaugh, 1972). You would not expect your arms to become trained following a 10-week jogging program!

Specificity of training also applies to the types of adaptations that occur in the muscle. Though increases in strength are related to endurance, the reverse is not true. So, engaging in regular resistance training will improve muscle strength and endurance. However, regular cardiorespiratory training will not necessarily improve your ability to lift heavy weights. Therefore, resistance training is specific to improving muscular strength (Abernethy, Jurimae, Logan, Taylor, & Thayer, 1994).

progression principle Placing gradual and increasing stress on the body, producing positive changes.

10-percent rule   Intensity or time of activity should not be increased more than 10 percent per week.

variety principle Training blocks that alternate between low, medium, and high intensity to challenge the body and facilitate improvements.

specificity principle The effect of training is specific to those muscles involved in the activity.

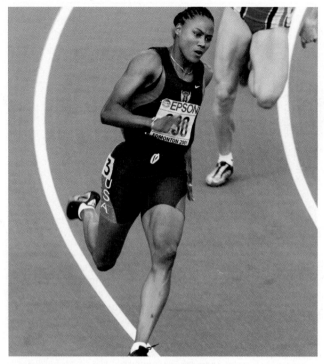

Running illustrates the principle of specificity because it promotes improvements in muscular endurance in the legs.

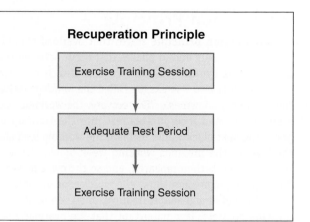

FIGURE 3.2 Recuperation principle. This principle of training requires that adequate rest periods separate training sessions.

Consider the following simple illustration of exercise specificity. Suppose you want to improve your ability to run a distance of 5 kilometres. In this case, specific training should include running 5 or more kilometres several times a week. This type of training would improve muscular endurance in your legs but would not result in large improvements in leg strength (Roberts & Alspaugh, 1972).

Recuperation Principle

Because the principle of overload requires exercise stress to improve physical fitness, it follows that exercise training places a stress on the body. During the recovery period between training sessions the body adapts to the stress by increasing endurance or becoming stronger. Therefore, a period of rest is essential for achieving maximal benefit from training. This needed rest period between training sessions is called the **recuperation principle** (Figure 3.2).

How much rest is required between heavy exercise training sessions? One or two days is adequate for most individuals (Powers & Howley, 2004). Failure to get enough rest

recuperation principle The body requires recovery periods between exercise training sessions in order to adapt to the stress of exercise. Therefore, a period of rest is essential for achieving maximal benefit from exercise.

overtraining Results from exercising too hard, too fast, or too frequently with an inadequate amount of rest between sessions.

reversibility principle Fitness gains made through training will be lost when training is stopped for long periods of time or permanently.

between sessions may result in **overtraining**. Overtraining may lead to chronic fatigue and injuries, chronic injury, or illness. (See A Closer Look: "Too Much Exercise Increases Your Risk of Colds"; the J-curve demonstrates how high-intensity and long-duration exercise can increase the risk of illness.) Overuse can also lead to injuries such as *plantar fasciitis,* where the heel and/or the ball of the foot becomes tender or painful. This is common with repetitive weight-bearing exercises such as running or aerobics (see also Chapter 13).

Shin splints is another common problem in repetitive weight-bearing exercises. *Shin splints* is a broad term for any pain that occurs below the knee and above the ankle and can range from stress fractures to severe inflammation in the muscular compartments of the lower leg.

Runner's knee is a common overuse injury that describes a series of problems involving the muscles, tendons, and ligaments around the knee resulting in pain when downward pressure is applied.

Overtraining can also come in the form of a "workout hangover." Common symptoms are sore and stiff muscles or a feeling of general fatigue the morning after a training session. The cure is to increase the duration of rest between workouts, reduce the intensity of workouts, or both. Although too much high-intensity activity is the primary cause of the overtraining syndrome, failure to consume a well-balanced diet can contribute to the feeling (see Nutritional Links to Health and Fitness: "Diet and the Workout Hangover").

Reversibility Principle

Although rest periods between training sessions are essential for maximal benefit from exercise, long intervals between workouts (that is, several days or weeks) can result in a reduction in fitness levels (Coyle et al., 1984). Maintenance of physical fitness requires regular exercise sessions. In other words, physical fitness cannot be stored. The loss of fitness due to inactivity is an example of the **reversibility principle**. The old adage "What you don't use, you lose" is true when applied to physical fitness.

Too Much Exercise Increases Your Risk of Colds

Recent research indicates that intense exercise training (i.e., over-training) reduces the body's immunity to disease (Nieman, 1997b). In contrast, light to moderate exercise training boosts the immune system and reduces the risk of infections (Nieman, 1997b). The relationship between exercise training and the risk of developing an upper respiratory tract infection (e.g., a cold) is shown in the figure in this box. The J-shaped curve in the figure indicates that moderate exercise training reduces the risk of infection, whereas high-intensity and long-duration exercise training increase the risk of infection.

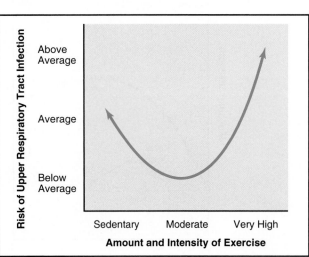

This J-shaped curve illustrates the relationship between physical activity and colds. Note that moderate physical activity reduces your risk of infection, whereas long-duration or high-intensity exercise increases your risk of disease. (Redrawn from Nieman, D. [1997]. Moderate exercise boosts the immune system: Too much exercise can have the opposite effect. *ACSM's Health and Fitness Journal, 1 [5]*: 14–18.)

How quickly is fitness lost when training is stopped? The answer depends on which component of physical fitness you are referring to. For example, after cessation of resistance training, the loss of muscular strength is relatively slow (Abernethy et al., 1994; Costill & Richardson, 1993). In contrast, after you stop performing endurance exercise, the loss of muscular endurance is relatively rapid (Coyle et. al., 1984). Figure 3.3 on the next page illustrates this point. Note that 8 weeks after stopping resistance training, only 10 percent of muscular strength is lost (Costill & Richardson, 1993). In contrast, 8 weeks after cessation of endurance training, 30 to 40 percent of muscular endurance is lost (Coyle et al., 1984).

Exercise Prescription Principles

It is important to remember that the FITT principle described at the beginning of this chapter provides the framework for every person's training program. It is equally important to remember that individualizing the training program is also necessary (Corbin & Lindsey, 1997; Fleck & Kraemer, 1997; Getchell, 1997; Hagan & Hutton, 2000; Hockey, 1996; Powers & Howley, 2001; Pollack & Wilmore, 1990; Williams, 1996). In other words, healthy exercise prescription guidelines will incorporate regular physical activity or exercise in accordance with the FITT principles, which should be tailored to individual needs such as sex, age, ability, and preference. As discussed later in this chapter, it will also include fitness goals, the type of exercise, a warm-up, a workout (primary conditioning period), and a cool-down.

Table 3.1 lists the frequency guidelines given by Health Canada's Physical Activity Unit. (Refer to Table 1.1 on page 6 for specific examples.) As the individual increases the intensity of activity, he or she is able to limit the amount of time spent doing that activity. The guidelines also adapt to fit the circumstances of children, youth, older adults, and pregnant women. For example, the Physical Activity Unit prescribes that children and youth increase their vigorous-intensity activity by 30 minutes and moderate-intensity physical activity by 60 minutes while reducing physical inactivity by 90 minutes a day. The guidelines for pregnant women can be found on the Physical Activity Unit's website; a more detailed discussion of this and other special populations' needs is provided in Chapters 12 and 16.

As noted above, all exercise prescriptions should include fitness goals, the type of exercise, a warm-up, a workout (primary conditioning period), and a cool-down (Figure 3.4). The following sections provide a general introduction to each of these components.

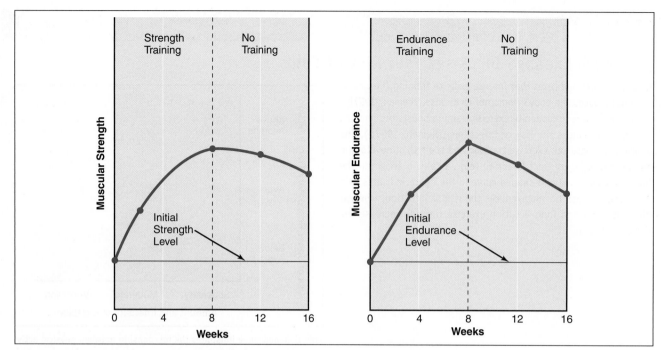

FIGURE 3.3 Retention of muscular strength and endurance after training is stopped.

Fitness Goals

As mentioned in Chapter 1, establishing short- and long-term fitness goals is an important part of the exercise prescription. The components of SuPeR SMART goal setting (see page 12 help to attain fitness goals, to improve self-esteem, and to provide the incentive needed to make a lifetime commitment to regular physical activity and exercise.

A logical and common type of fitness goal is a performance goal. You can establish performance goals in each component of health-related physical fitness. Table 3.2 illustrates a hypothetical example of how Susie Jones might establish short- and long-term performance goals using fitness testing (Chapter 2) to determine when she has

reached her objective. The column labelled "current status" contains Susie's fitness ratings based on tests performed prior to starting her exercise program. After consultation with her instructor, Susie established short-term goals that she hopes to achieve within the first 8 weeks of training. Note that the short-term goals are not fixed in stone and can be modified if the need arises. Susie's long-term goals are the fitness levels that she hopes to reach within her first 18 months of training. Similar to short-term goals, long-term goals can be modified to meet changing needs or circumstances.

In addition to performance goals, consider establishing physical activity adherence goals. That is, set a goal to be

Adults	Frequency
Endurance	4 to 7 days a week of continuous physical activities of moderate to vigorous intensity for heart and lungs.
Flexibility	4 to 7 days a week of gentle stretching activities to loosen and relax muscles and keep joints mobile.
Strength	2 to 4 days a week of resistance activities to strengthen muscles and improve posture, muscle tone, and bone density.
Older Adults	
Endurance	4 to 7 days a week to accumulate 30 to 60 minutes of moderately intense physical activity. This can be achieved through 10-minute sessions in a variety of activities.
Flexibility	Every day. It is important to keep muscles and joints agile to avoid falls and injury.
Strength and Balance Activities	2 to 4 days a week to keep muscles strong and improve balance and posture.

TABLE 3.1 Healthy Active Living—Frequency of Physical Activity

Source: *Physical Activity Unit: Effort for Exercise*, Public Health Agency of Canada, 2005. Reproduced with the permission of the Minister of Public Works and Government Services Canada, 2005.

Diet and the Workout Hangover

Can a poor diet contribute to fatigue and overtraining? Yes! Failure to consume the recommended amount of water, carbohydrates, fats, proteins, vitamins, and minerals can lead to chronic fatigue (Lamb & Williams, 1991). Of particular importance to people engaged in regular training are dietary carbohydrates. Because heavy training uses carbohydrates as a primary fuel source (Powers & Howley, 2001), diets low in carbohydrates can result in a depletion of muscle carbohydrate stores and lead to a feeling of chronic fatigue. To maintain muscle carbohydrate stores, these nutrients should make up 55 to 60 percent of the total energy consumed (Lamb & Williams, 1991; Powers & Howley, 2001). See Chapter 7 for a complete discussion of nutrition for physical fitness.

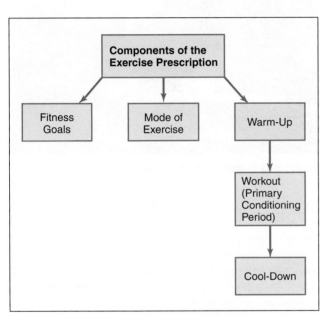

FIGURE 3.4 Components of the exercise prescription.

Fitness Category	Cardiorespiratory Endurance
Current status	Walking once a week
Short-term goal	Walking three times a week for 20 minutes
Long-term goal	Walking seven times a week for 45 minutes

TABLE 3.2 Illustration of Short- and Long-Term Performance Goals

physically active a specific number of days per week. Physical activity adherence goals are important because fitness will improve only if you are active on a regular basis!

In writing your personal fitness goals, consider the following guidelines:

Set Realistic Goals—The most important rule in setting goals is that you must be realistic. After a thorough self-evaluation, set fitness goals that you can reach. Because failure to reach goals is discouraging, establishing realistic short-term goals is critical to the success of your fitness program. Goals can be as simple as how many days a week you will be active, and for how long. Keeping a detailed record can provide positive feedback and monitor success.

Establish Short-Term Goals First—Reaching short-term fitness goals is a great motivation to continue exercising. Therefore, establishing realistic, timed short-term goals is critical. The SuPeR SMART goals listed in Chapter 1 are *quantifiable,* which means that they are precise and their achievement can be measured. Table 3.3 gives good examples of timed and measurable short- and long-term goals. After reaching a short-term goal it is important to establish a new one. Unless you keep overloading on a continual basis your body will adapt and you will quickly plateau—progress will slow or even stop.

Set Realistic Long-Term Goals—Many factors need to be considered in establishing long-term goals: finances, family and social support, personal health, ability, limitations, and many more. Our fitness goals need to be flexible in order to handle the daily events that can impede our efforts. They also need to be within our control; that is, based on our behaviour and not on an outcome that we may have no control over. When creating our long-term fitness goals we need to recognize our physical limitations and set realistic goals based on our individual needs—not on the performance or achievement of other people.

Establish Lifetime Maintenance Goals—In addition to short- and long-term goals, consider establishing a fitness maintenance goal to last a lifetime. A maintenance goal is established when your fitness goals have been met and your focus becomes remaining physically active and fit. This topic is covered in detail in Chapter 16.

List Goals in Writing—A key to meeting goals is to write them down and put them in a place where you can see them every day. Goals can be forgotten if they are not verifiable. Further, remember that all goals should be periodically re-evaluated and modified if necessary. Just because goals are in writing does not mean that they cannot be changed. A simple way to keep track is by putting check marks on a calendar for the days when physical activity has been completed. This will help keep motivation high and will be a quick check to see if fitness goals are being met.

Recognize Obstacles to Achieving Goals—If you do not make your fitness goals a serious priority, you will keep putting them off until they no longer exist. Once you begin your fitness program, be prepared to make mistakes (such as skipping workouts and losing motivation) and to backslide a bit (and have your fitness level decline temporarily). This is normal. However, once you realize that you have stopped making progress toward your goals, you must get back on track as soon as you can.

The importance of fitness goals cannot be overemphasized. Goals provide structure and motivation for a personal fitness program. Keys to maintaining a lifelong fitness program are discussed again in Chapter 16.

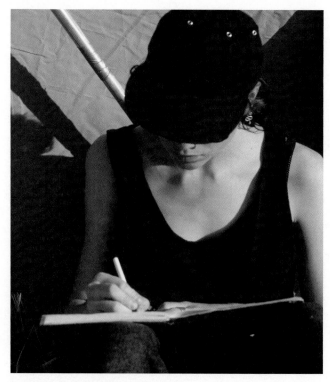

Keeping track of physical activity will ensure sufficient motivation.

Type of Exercise

Every fitness prescription includes at least one **type of exercise**—that is, a specific exercise to be performed. For example, to improve cardiorespiratory fitness you could select from several endurance exercises such as running, swimming, cycling, or aerobics. Key factors to consider when selecting a type of exercise are enjoyment, availability of the activity, and risk of injury.

Type of exercise can be classified as either high-impact or low-impact based on the amount of stress placed on joints during the activity. Activities that place a large amount of pressure on joints are called *high-impact activities* (e.g., sprinting), whereas *low-impact activities* are less stressful (e.g., strolling). Because of the strong correlation between high-impact types of exercise and injuries, many fitness

type of exercise   The specific type of exercise to be performed.

Fitness Category	Current Status	Short-Term Goal	Long-Term Goal
Cardiorespiratory fitness	Poor	Average	Excellent
Muscular strength	Poor	Average	Excellent
Muscular endurance	Very poor	Average	Good
Flexibility	Poor	Average	Good
Body composition	High fat	Moderately high	Optimal

TABLE 3.3 Timed and Measurable Short- and Long-Term Goals

The fitness categories are the five components of health-related physical fitness. The current status, short-term goals, and long-term goals are the fitness norms presented in Chapter 2.

experts recommend low-impact activities for beginners or for those individuals susceptible to injury (such as participants who are older, obese, or pregnant). High-impact activities include running, basketball, and high-impact aerobic dance. Low-impact activities include walking, cycling, swimming, and low-impact aerobic dance.

Warm-Up

A **warm-up** is a brief (5- to 15-minute) period of activity that precedes a workout. It generally involves light calisthenics or a low-intensity form of the actual type of exercise and often includes dynamic range-of-motion stretching as well (Chapter 6). The purpose of a warm-up is to elevate muscle temperature and increase blood flow to those muscles that will be engaged in the workout (DeVries & Housh, 1994; Powers & Howley, 2001). Another purpose of the warm-up is to psychologically prepare to be active. A warm-up can also reduce the strain on the heart imposed by rapidly engaging in heavy exercise, and may reduce the risk of muscle and tendon injuries. However, this is not the time to focus on increasing flexibility—that comes later. You simply want to warm up.

Workout (Primary Conditioning Period)

Regardless of the type of exercise (described earlier), the major components of the exercise prescription that make up the workout (also called the *primary conditioning period)* are frequency, intensity, and time (duration) of exercise (Figure 3.5). The **frequency of exercise** is the number of times per week that you intend to be active. In general, the recommended frequency of exercise to improve most components of health-related physical fitness is 3 to 7 times per week for 30 to 60 minutes (Barrow, 1992; Bouchard, Shepard, Stephens, Sutton, & McPherson, 1990; Morris, 1994; Pollock & Wilmore, 1990; Public Health Agency of Canada, 2005).

The **intensity of exercise** is the amount of physiological stress or overload placed on the body. The method for determining the intensity of activity varies with the type of exercise performed. For example, because heart rate increases linearly with energy expenditure (effort) during exercise, measurement of heart rate has become a standard means of determining exercise intensity during training to improve cardiorespiratory endurance. Although heart rate can also be used to gauge exercise intensity during strength training, the number of repetitions that can be performed before muscular fatigue occurs is more useful. For instance, a load that can be lifted only 3 to 8 times before fatigue is an example of high-intensity resistance training. In contrast, a load that can be lifted more than 10

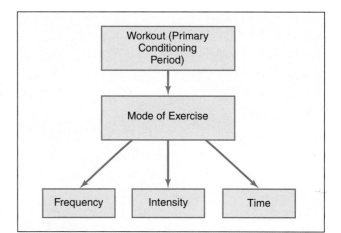

FIGURE 3.5 The components of the workout: the frequency, intensity, and time (duration) of exercise.

to 15 times without resulting in muscular fatigue is an illustration of low-intensity resistance training.

Finally, flexibility is improved by stretching muscles beyond their normal length. Intensity of stretching is monitored by the degree of tension or discomfort felt during the stretch. Low-intensity stretching results in minor tension (or limited discomfort) on the muscles and tendons. In contrast, high-intensity stretching places great tension or moderate discomfort on the muscle groups being stretched. For best results, it is recommended that flexibility training be done every day. However, 3 times a week will bring added health benefits (Hagan & Hutton, 2000; Public Health Agency of Canada, 2005).

A key aspect of the primary conditioning period is the **time (duration) of physical activity**—that is, the amount of time invested in performing the primary workout. Note that the time of activity does not include the warm-up or cool-down. In general, research has shown that 20 to 30 minutes per session (performed at least 3 times per week) is the minimum time required to significantly improve physical fitness (Hagan & Hutton, 2000; Public Health Agency of Canada, 2005).

warm-up A brief period of activity that precedes a workout so that muscle temperature and blood flow increase.

frequency of exercise The number of times per week that one intends to be active.

intensity of exercise The amount of physiological stress or overload placed on the body during exercise.

time (duration) of physical activity The amount of time invested in performing the primary workout.

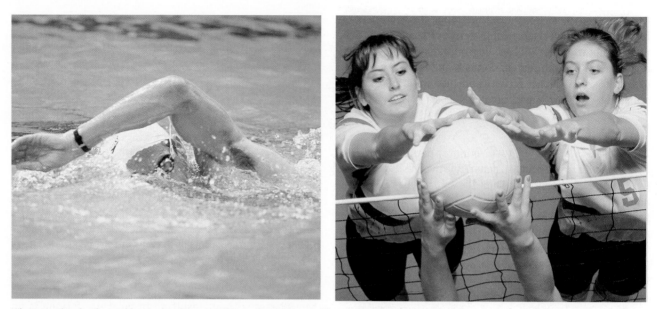

Whereas swimming is considered a low-impact activity, volleyball is considered a high-impact activity.

Cool-Down

The **cool-down** (sometimes called a *warm-down*) is a 5- to 15-minute period of low-intensity exercise that immediately follows the primary conditioning period. For instance, a period of slow jogging might be used as a cool-down following a running workout. A cool-down period accomplishes several goals (Figure 3.6). In addition to its goal of lowering body temperature after high-intensity activities, one primary purpose of a cool-down is to allow blood to be returned from the muscles back toward the heart (Fleck & Kraemer, 1997; Hagan & Hutton, 2000; Pollock & Wilmore, 1990; Powers & Howley, 2001). During exercise, large amounts of

cool-down A 5- to 15-minute period of low-intensity activity that immediately follows the primary conditioning period.

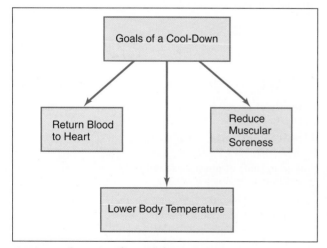

FIGURE 3.6 Purposes of a cool-down.

blood are pumped to the working muscles. On cessation of exercise, blood tends to remain in large blood vessels located around the exercised muscles (a process called *pooling*). Failure to redistribute pooled blood after exercise could result in lightheadedness or even fainting. Prevention of blood pooling is best accomplished by low-intensity exercise using those muscles utilized during the workout. The cool-down is the best time to focus on lengthening muscles and improving flexibility. Flexibility exercises should be held for longer periods, 30 to 60 seconds, and repeated 2 to 3 times. All the major muscles used during primary conditioning should be focused on while stretching.

Finally, some fitness experts argue that post-exercise muscle soreness may be reduced as a result of a cool-down (Robergs & Roberts, 2000). Although a cool-down period may not eliminate muscular soreness entirely, it seems possible that the severity of exercise-induced muscle soreness may be reduced in people who perform a thorough cool-down (Robergs & Roberts, 2000).

Individualizing the Workout

A key point to remember about fitness prescription principles is that each should be tailored to the needs and objectives of the individual. Although the same general principles of exercise training (FITT) apply to everyone, no two people are the same. Therefore, the fitness prescription principles should consider such factors as the individual's general health, age, fitness status, musculoskeletal condition, and body composition. Other considerations include enjoyment, accessibility, resources, and time commitment or practicality. For example, you wouldn't incorporate swimming 3 times a week if you did not have regular access to a pool. However, if you enjoy walking, making a fitness prescription that incorporates walking 3 times a week ensures accessibility and offers plenty of resource options. More will be said about individualizing workouts in later chapters.

How Much Physical Activity Is Enough?

Students often ask how much physical activity is enough to provide health benefits. Although even low levels of physical activity can provide some health benefits, growing evidence indicates that moderate- to high-intensity levels are required to provide major health benefits (Blair et al., 1992; Bouchard et al., 1990; Lee & Paffenbarger, 2000; Morris, 1994; Paffenbarger et al., 1994; Williams, 2001). The theoretical relationship between physical activity and health benefits is illustrated in Figure 3.7. Note that the minimum level of physical activity or exercise required to achieve some of the health benefits is called the **threshold for health benefits**. Most experts believe that 20 to 60 minutes of continuous moderate- to high-intensity exercise performed 3 to 5 days per week will surpass the threshold for health benefits and will reduce many of the risk factors associated with premature death (Blair et al., 1992; Lee & Paffenbarger, 2000; Pollock et al., 1998). Importantly, any one of many exercise modalities (e.g., running, swimming, cycling) can be used to achieve the exercise thresholds for health benefits. Obviously, the guidelines presented in this chapter are aimed at improving the health and fitness of the general population. An elite athlete would tailor his or her fitness prescription to meet the demands of the sport. Similarly, the general population can tailor the fitness prescription and suggestions from Figures 3.1 and 3.2 to meet their individual goals and needs.

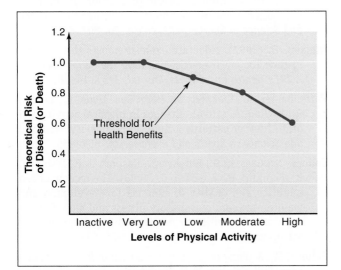

FIGURE 3.7 The relationship between physical activity and improved health benefits. Note that as the level of regular physical activity is increased, the theoretical risk of disease (or death) is decreased. (From Blair et al., 1992; Lee & Paffenbarger, 2000; and Williams, 2001.)

threshold for health benefits   The minimum level of physical activity required to achieve the health benefits of exercise.

Summary

1. The FITT prescription refers to the frequency, intensity, time, and type of exercise needed to improve fitness.
2. The overload principle states that in order to improve physical fitness, the body or muscle group used during exercise must be stressed beyond what is accustomed.
3. The principle of progression states that overload should be increased gradually during the course of a physical fitness program.
4. The principle of specificity states that gains occur to the part of the body that is specifically overloaded.
5. The need for a rest period between training sessions is called the recuperation principle.
6. Physical fitness can be lost due to inactivity; this is often called the reversibility principle.
7. The components of the fitness prescription guidelines include fitness goals, the type of exercise or activity, the warm-up, the workout (primary conditioning period), and the cool-down.
8. All physical activity training programs should be tailored to meet the objectives of the individual. Therefore, the fitness guidelines should consider the individual's age, health, fitness status, musculoskeletal condition, and body composition.
9. The minimum level of physical activity required to achieve the health benefits is called the threshold for health benefits.

Study Questions

1. Define *overtraining* and *recuperation principle*.
2. What are the general purposes of a cool-down and a warm-up?
3. Describe the components of the fitness prescription guidelines.
4. How does the progression principle apply to the fitness prescription?
5. Define the FITT principle.
6. Discuss the overload principle.
7. Define the term *threshold for health benefits*.
8. What happens to physical fitness if you stop training?
9. Explain why the fitness prescription guidelines should be individualized.

Suggested Reading

Howley, E. T. (2000). You asked for it: Is rigorous exercise better than moderate activity in achieving health-related goals? *ACSM's Health and Fitness Journal, 4(2),* 6.

Maughan, R. (Ed.) (1999). *Basic and applied sciences for sports medicine.* Oxford, England: Butterworth-Heinemann.

Powers, S., & Howley, E. (2001). *Exercise physiology: Theory and application to fitness and performance* (4th ed.). St. Louis: McGraw-Hill.

Roitman, J. (2001). *ACSM's resource manual for exercise testing and prescription.* Philadelphia: Lippincott, Williams & Wilkins.

Weblinks

Heart and Stroke Foundation of Canada

www.heartandstroke.ca

Contains the latest information about ways to reduce your risk of heart disease. Site includes information about physical activity and nutrition.

Canada's Physical Activity Guide

www.phac-aspc.gc.ca/pau-uap/paguide

Contains information about exercise, health, and fitness for children, adults, pregnant women, and older adults.

Canadian Institute for Health Information

www.cihi.ca

Contains the latest information on a variety of health-related topics, including nutrition, exercise, and stress.

Statistics Canada—Health

www.statcan.ca/english/ads/82-003-XPE

Compilation of statistics relating to the health of the Canadian population.

References

Abernethy, P., Jurimae, J., Logan, P., Taylor, A., & Thayer, R. (1994). Acute and chronic response of skeletal muscle to resistance exercise. *Sports Medicine, 17,* 22–28.

American College of Sports Medicine. (1991). *Guidelines for exercise testing and prescription.* Philadelphia: Lea and Febiger.

Barrow, M. (1992). *Heart talk: Understanding cardiovascular diseases.* Gainesville, FL: Cor-Ed Publishing.

Blair, S., Kohl, H. W., Gordon, N., & Paffenbarger, R. (1992). How much physical activity is good for health? *Annual Review of Public Health, 13,* 99–126.

Bouchard, C., Shephard, R., Stephens, T., Sutton, J., & McPherson, B. (Eds.) (1990). *Exercise, fitness, and health: A consensus of current knowledge.* Champaign, IL: Human Kinetics.

Corbin, C., & Lindsey, R. (1997). *Concepts of physical fitness and wellness.* Dubuque, IA: Brown and Benchmark.

Costill, D., & Richardson, A. (1993). *Handbook of sports medicine: Swimming.* London: Blackwell Publishing.

Coyle, E., Martin, W., Sinacore, D., Joyner, M., Hagberg, J., & Holloszy, J. (1984). Time course of loss of adaptations after stopping prolonged intense endurance training. *Journal of Applied Physiology, 57,* 1857–1864.

DeVries, H., & Housh, T. (1994). *Exercise physiology* (5th ed.). Dubuque, IA: Brown and Benchmark.

Fleck, S., & Kraemer, W. (1997). *Designing resistance training programs.* Champaign, IL: Human Kinetics.

Getchell, B. (1997). *Physical fitness: A way of life.* Needham Heights, MA: Allyn and Bacon.

Hagan, M., & Hutton, J. (2000). *The Canadian Association of Fitness Professionals: Fitness instructor specialist manual.* CAN-FIT-PRO.

Hockey, R. (1996). *Physical fitness: The pathway to healthful living.* St. Louis: Times Mirror/Mosby.

Howley, E. T. (2000). You asked for it: Is rigorous exercise better than moderate activity in achieving health-related goals? *ACSM's Health and Fitness Journal, 4(2),* 6.

Lamb, D., & Williams, M. (1991). *Ergogenics: Enhancement of performance in exercise and sport.* Vol. 4. Madison, WI: Brown and Benchmark.

Lee, I., & Paffenbarger, R. (2000). Associations of light, moderate, and vigorous intensity physical activity with longevity. *American Journal of Epidemiology, 151,* 293–299.

McGlynn, G. (1996). *Dynamics of fitness: A practical approach.* Dubuque, IA: Wm. C. Brown.

Morris, J. (1994). Exercise in the prevention of coronary heart disease: Today's best buy in public health. *Medicine and Science in Sports and Exercise, 26,* 807–814.

Nieman, D. (1997). Moderate exercise boosts the immune system: Too much exercise can have the opposite effect. *ACSM's Health and Fitness Journal, 1(5),* 14–18.

Paffenbarger, R., Kampert, J., I-Min Lee, Hyde, R., Leung, R., & Wing, A. (1994). Changes in physical activity and other lifeway patterns influencing longevity. *Medicine and Science in Sports and Exercise, 26,* 857–865.

Pollock, M., Gaesser, G., Butcher, J., Despres, J. P., Dishman, R., Franklin, B., & Garber, C. (1998). The recommended quantity and quality of exercise for developing and maintaining cardiorespiratory fitness and muscular fitness, and flexibility in healthy adults. *Medicine and Science in Sports and Exercise, 30,* 975–991.

Pollock, M., & Wilmore, J. (1990). *Exercise in health and disease.* Philadelphia: W. B. Saunders.

Powers, S., & Howley, E. (2001). *Exercise physiology: Theory and application to fitness and performance* (4th ed.). St. Louis: McGraw-Hill.

Public Health Agency of Canada. (2005). Physical Activity Unit. www.phac-aspc.gc.ca/pau-uap/paguide/. Retrieved February 2005.

Robergs, R., & Roberts, S. (2000). *Fundamental principles of exercise physiology: For fitness, performance, and health.* St. Louis: McGraw-Hill.

Roberts, J., & Alspaugh, J. (1972). Specificity of training effects resulting from programs of treadmill running and bicycle ergometer riding. *Medicine and Science in Sports, 4,* 6–10.

Williams, M. (1996). *Lifetime fitness and wellness.* Dubuque, IA: Wm. C. Brown.

Williams, P. (2001). Physical fitness and activity as separate heart disease risk factors: A meta-analysis. *Medicine and Science in Sports and Exercise, 33,* 754–761.

CHAPTER 4

Exercise Prescription Principles: Cardio-respiratory Endurance

4

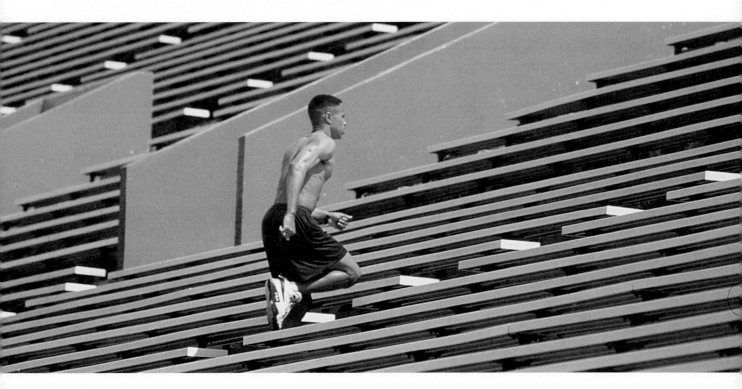

After studying this chapter, you should be able to

1. Explain the benefits of improving cardiorespiratory endurance.

2. Contrast the anaerobic and aerobic energy systems involved in the production of adenosine triphosphate for muscular contraction.

3. Discuss the role of the circulatory and respiratory systems during exercise.

4. Define VO_2max.

5. Identify the major changes that occur in skeletal muscles, the circulatory system, and the respiratory system in response to training.

6. List several types of training used to improve cardiorespiratory endurance.

7. Outline the three components of an exercise training session.

8. Outline the FITT principles designed to improve cardiorespiratory endurance.

9. Design an exercise program for yourself to improve cardiorespiratory endurance, beginning at the starter phase and finishing with the maintenance phase.

Canadians' current interest in cardiorespiratory training began in 1971, when the participACTION program was inaugurated thanks largely to the efforts of long-time volunteer Dr. Russ Kisby (Diekmeyer, 2004). Federal funding for participACTION was established in 1972, when Canadians were informed through a social marketing campaign that a typical 60-year-old Swede was more physically fit and healthier than the average 35-year-old Canadian. Similar television and print ads followed, with impressive results. Data from participACTION reported an increase in "regularly active" Canadians, from 5 percent in 1971 to 35 percent in 1995 (Diekmeyer, 2004). Canadians were advised to simply "get moving," to "just do it," and to "walk a block a day." Unfortunately, the funding for participACTION dwindled over the years and the non-profit organization ultimately closed its doors in 2002. The legacy lives on, however—in people's memories and in the methods used to prescribe exercise for improving physical fitness.

In a similar way, the publication of Dr. Kenneth Cooper's best-selling fitness book *Aerobics* fuelled interest in improving physical fitness (Cooper, 1968). After the book's appearance, the term **aerobics** became commonly used to describe all forms of exercise designed to improve cardiorespiratory endurance (such as jogging, walking, cycling, and swimming). Because aerobic exercise has proven effective in promoting weight loss (Ross & Janssen, 2001; Wong et al., 2004) and reducing the risk of cardiovascular disease (Kohl, 2001), many exercise scientists consider cardiorespiratory endurance the most important component of health-related physical fitness.

In the first three chapters of this book we discussed the health benefits of physical activity and physical fitness; self-testing to evaluate physical fitness; and the general principles of training. In the next three chapters we describe how to design a comprehensive, scientifically based exercise program to promote health-related physical fitness. This chapter describes techniques for promoting cardiorespiratory endurance. Before we discuss the exercise prescription for cardiorespiratory endurance, however, it is important to review the benefits of cardiorespiratory endurance and some basic concepts concerning how your body works during aerobic exercise.

Benefits of Cardiorespiratory Endurance

The benefits of cardiorespiratory endurance are many. A key advantage is that people with high levels of cardiorespiratory endurance have a lower risk of heart disease and increased longevity. Other health benefits include a reduced risk of type 2 diabetes, lower blood pressure, and increased bone density in weight-bearing bones (Kesaniemi et al., 2001).

aerobics   A common term that describes all forms of exercise designed to improve cardiorespiratory fitness (e.g., jogging, walking, cycling, and swimming).

Another positive factor associated with developing cardiorespiratory endurance is that as fitness improves, energy for work and play increases. This translates into the ability to perform more work with less fatigue. Indeed, people with high levels of cardiorespiratory endurance often state that one of the reasons why they exercise is that they feel better as a result.

Development of cardiorespiratory endurance through regular exercise also improves self-esteem (Dunn, Trivedi, & O'Neal, 2001). Self-esteem increases for several reasons. First, starting and maintaining a regular physical activity program provides a strong sense of accomplishment. Second, regular physical activity improves muscle tone and assists in weight maintenance. Combined, these factors result in an improved appearance and self-esteem. Finally, people with high levels of cardiorespiratory endurance sleep better than less fit individuals (Gambelunghe, Rossi,

Mariucce, Tantucci, & Ambrosini, 2001). Specifically, fit individuals tend to sleep longer and without interruptions (i.e., they enjoy more restful sleep). This activity-related improved sleep results in a better night's rest and a more complete feeling of being mentally restored.

Physiological Basis for Developing Cardio-respiratory Endurance

Energy to Perform Exercise

The prolonged type of exercise necessary to develop cardiorespiratory endurance requires an enormous amount of energy supplied to the working muscles. Where do muscles get the energy to contract during exercise? The answer is from the chemical energy released by the breakdown of food (such as carbohydrates, proteins, and fat). However, food energy cannot be used directly for energy by the muscles. Instead, the energy released from the breakdown of food is used to manufacture another biochemical compound, called **adenosine triphosphate (ATP)**, a high-energy compound synthesized and stored in small quantities in muscle and other cells. The breakdown of ATP results in the release of energy that can be used to fuel muscular contraction. ATP is the only compound in the body that can provide this immediate source of energy. Therefore, for muscles to contract during exercise, a supply of ATP must be available.

Two "systems" in muscle cells can produce ATP. One system does not require oxygen and is called the **anaerobic** (without oxygen) system. The second system requires oxygen and is called the **aerobic** (with oxygen) system.

Anaerobic ATP Production   Most of the anaerobic ATP production in muscle occurs in a metabolic process called **glycolysis**, which breaks down carbohydrates (sugars) in cells. The end result of glycolysis is the anaerobic production of ATP and often the formation of **lactic acid**. Because lactic acid is often a byproduct of glycolysis, this pathway for ATP production is called the lactic acid system. The lactic acid system can use only carbohydrates as an energy source. Carbohydrates are supplied to muscles from *glucose* (blood sugar) and *glycogen* (muscle stores of glucose). Conceptually, it is convenient to think of the lactic acid system as the energy pathway that produces ATP at the beginning of exercise and during short-term (10–90 seconds), high-intensity exercise. For instance, most of the ATP required to sprint 400 metres (which may require 60–80 seconds) would be derived from the lactic acid system. During this type of intense exercise, muscles produce large amounts of lactic acid because the lactic acid system is operating at high speed. The accumulation of lactic acid in muscles results in fatigue and explains the decline in running speed of a 400-metre runner toward the finish line.

Aerobic ATP Production   Exercise lasting longer than 60 seconds requires ATP production by the aerobic system. Therefore, activities of daily living and many types of exercise depend on aerobic ATP production.

Whereas the anaerobic lactic acid system uses only carbohydrates as a food source, aerobic metabolism can use all three foodstuffs (fats, carbohydrates, and protein) to produce ATP. In a healthy individual consuming a balanced dietary intake, protein plays a limited role as an energy source during exercise; therefore, carbohydrates and fats are the primary sources. In general, at the beginning of exercise carbohydrate is the principal foodstuff broken down during aerobic ATP production. During prolonged exercise (i.e., longer than 20 minutes in duration), there is a gradual shift from carbohydrate to fat as an energy source. Figure 4.1 clearly demonstrates that the longer an individual exercises, the more fat he or she will use as an energy source. For example, at 60 minutes of aerobic exercise more than 50 percent of the energy is derived from fat. Regardless of the combination of energy sources used, the total calories burned remains at the same rate for each minute of additional exercise.

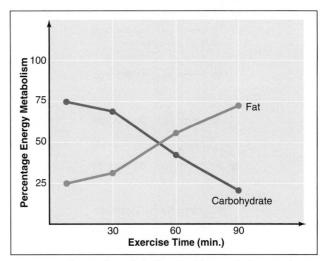

FIGURE 4.1 Changes in carbohydrate and fat use during 90 minutes of aerobic exercise.

adenosine triphosphate (ATP)   A high-energy compound synthesized and stored in small quantities in muscle and other cells. The breakdown of ATP results in a release of energy that can be used to fuel muscular contraction.

anaerobic   Means "without oxygen"; in cells pertains to energy-producing biochemical pathways that do not require oxygen to produce energy.

aerobic   Means "with oxygen"; in cells pertains to energy-producing biochemical pathways that use oxygen to produce energy.

glycolysis   Metabolic process in which carbohydrates are broken down to ATP.

lactic acid   A byproduct of glucose metabolism, produced primarily during intense exercise.

The Energy Continuum   Although it is common to speak of aerobic versus anaerobic exercise, in reality the energy to perform many types of physical activities comes from both sources. Figure 4.2(a) illustrates the anaerobic–aerobic energy continuum as a function of the exercise duration. Anaerobic energy production dominates during short-term activities, whereas aerobic energy production is greatest during long-term activities. For example, maximal exercise of 10 seconds in duration uses anaerobic energy sources almost exclusively. On the other end of the energy spectrum, notice that aerobic energy production dominates during 30 minutes of continuous exercise. Running a maximal-effort 800-metre race (2–3 minutes) is an example of an activity that obtains the required energy almost equally from aerobic and anaerobic energy sources.

Figure 4.2(b) applies the anaerobic–aerobic energy continuum to various physical activities. Weight lifting, gymnastics, and football are activities that use anaerobic energy production almost exclusively. Boxing and skating (1500 metres) require an equal contribution of anaerobic and aerobic energy production. Finally, cross-country skiing and jogging are activities in which aerobic energy production dominates.

Exercise and the Cardiorespiratory System

The term **cardiorespiratory system** refers to the cooperative work of the circulatory and respiratory systems. Together, these systems are responsible for the delivery of oxygen and nutrients as well as for the removal of waste products (e.g.,

cardiorespiratory system   Refers to the cooperative work of the circulatory (heart, blood, vascular system) and respiratory (lungs) systems.

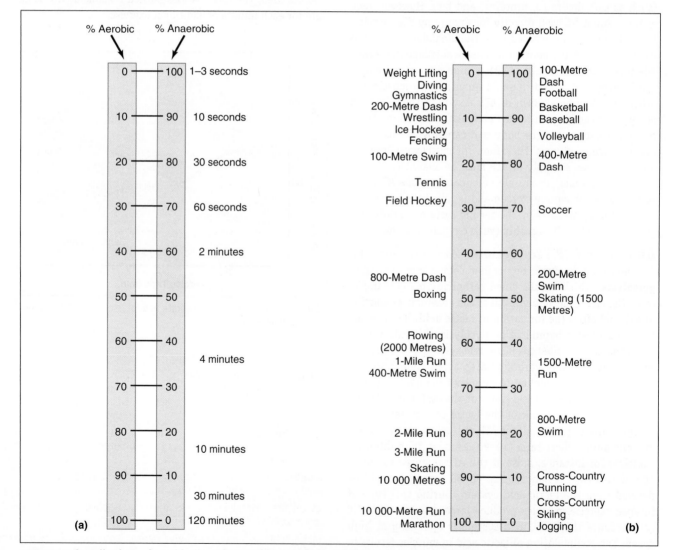

FIGURE 4.2 Contributions of aerobically and anaerobically produced ATP to energy metabolism during exercise. (a) Contributions as a function of exercise duration. (b) Contributions for various physical activities.

carbon dioxide) from tissues. Physical activity poses a major challenge to the cardiorespiratory system by increasing the muscles' demand for oxygen and nutrients. The cardiorespiratory system must meet this demand to allow the individual to continue participating. In the following sections we present a brief overview of cardiorespiratory function during physical activity.

The Circulatory System

The circulatory system is a closed loop comprising the heart and blood vessels. The pump in this system is the heart, which generates pressure to move blood through the system with each contraction (heartbeat). Figure 4.3 illustrates that the heart can be considered two pumps in one. The right side pumps oxygen-depleted (deoxygenated) blood through the lungs (a pathway called the **pulmonary circuit**), while the left side pumps oxygen-rich (oxygenated) blood to tissues throughout the body (a pathway called the **systemic circuit**).

In the systemic circuit, blood carrying oxygen leaves the heart in **arteries**, which branch to form microscopic vessels called *arterioles;* arterioles eventually branch into beds of smaller vessels called *capillaries*. **Capillaries** are thin-walled vessels that permit the exchange of gases (oxygen and carbon dioxide) and nutrients between the blood and tissues. After this exchange, blood passes from the capillaries into microscopic vessels called *venules*. As venules move back toward the heart, they increase in size and form **veins**, which carry oxygen-depleted blood back to the heart.

Venous blood (blood carried by veins) from all parts of the body returns to the right side of the heart and is pumped through the lungs. In the lungs, oxygen is loaded into the blood and carbon dioxide is removed. The oxygen-rich blood is returned to the left side of the heart and pumped to all body tissues by the systemic circuit.

The amount of blood the heart pumps per minute is called **cardiac output**. Cardiac output can be calculated by multiplying **heart rate** (number of heartbeats per minute) and **stroke volume** (how much blood is pumped per heartbeat, generally expressed in millilitres). During exercise, cardiac output can be increased by increasing heart rate or stroke volume or both. Stroke volume does not increase beyond low-intensity physical activity rates. Therefore, the increase in cardiac output needed for moderate-intensity and greater physical activity is achieved by increases in heart rate alone. (Changes in cardiac output in response to exercise are discussed later in this chapter.)

Maximal cardiac output declines in men and women after approximately 20 years of age, primarily due to a decrease in maximal heart rate. The decrease in maximal heart rate (HR_{max}) with age can be estimated by the formula

$$HR_{max} = 220 - age \text{ (in years)}$$

According to this formula, a 20-year-old individual would have a maximal HR of 200 beats per minute (220 – 20 = 200), whereas a 60-year-old would have a maximal HR of 160 beats per minute (220 – 60 = 160).

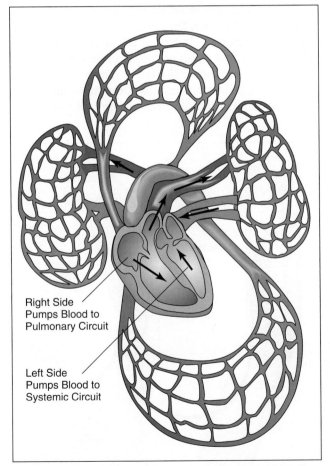

Right Side
Pumps Blood to
Pulmonary Circuit

Left Side
Pumps Blood to
Systemic Circuit

FIGURE 4.3 The concept of the heart as "two pumps in one."

Source: From Wilmore, J. H., & Costill, D. L. (1994). *Physiology of sport and exercise.* (p. 173). Champaign, IL: Human Kinetics. Copyright © 1994 by Jack H. Wilmore and David L. Costill. Reprinted with permission.

pulmonary circuit The blood vascular system that circulates deoxygenated blood from the right side of the heart, through the lungs, and back to the left side of the heart.

systemic circuit The blood vascular system that circulates oxygenated blood from the left side of the heart, throughout the body, and back to the right side of the heart.

arteries The blood vessels that transport blood away from the heart.

capillaries Thin-walled vessels that permit the exchange of oxygen and carbon dioxide and nutrients between the blood and tissues.

veins Blood vessels that transport blood toward the heart.

cardiac output The amount of blood the heart pumps per minute.

heart rate Number of heartbeats per minute.

stroke volume The amount of blood pumped per heartbeat.

What Nutrients Are Most Important for Endurance Performance?

Whether you're an athlete or a fitness enthusiast, nutrition is fundamental to your performance. A balanced eating plan that accounts for the type and level of activity is essential for cardiorespiratory endurance. Your eating plan should not vary considerably from a normal diet—that is, it should include plenty of fluids and low-fat, high-carbohydrate foods for energy. Tailor the caloric content of your eating plan to reflect the amount of energy you expend during workouts. Carbohydrates should constitute at least 60 percent of the calories you consume, because they are the most critical supply of energy. Since muscles replenish stored carbohydrates most efficiently within the first 2 hours following physical activity, you should consume 200 to 400 calories as soon as possible after physical activity. Some good things to eat as a source of complex carbohydrates include the following:

2 pieces of fruit
250 mL nonfat yogurt + 250 mL fruit topping
28 g cereal + 125 mL skim milk
1 low-fat muffin + 125 mL skim milk
375 mL fruit juice
250 mL grapes + 1/2 bagel
250 mL vegetable soup + 1 slice bread

The intake of fluids is critical during exercise. Fluids are necessary to maintain blood volume and to replenish water lost through sweating. Because thirst is not a good regulator of fluid balance over the short term, fluids should be consumed before, during, and after your workout. Consume about 200 mL of water 30 minutes before the workout, 100 to 200 mL every 15 minutes during the workout, and 500 mL for every pound lost during the workout.

Blood Pressure

Blood is moved through the circulatory system by pressure generated by the pumping heart. The pressure that blood exerts against the walls of arteries is called *blood pressure*. Measurement of arterial blood pressure is generally attained by a *sphygmomanometer* (Figure 4.4). During contraction of the heart (called *systole*), arterial blood pressure reaches its highest value. Blood pressure during systole is called **systolic blood pressure**; the normal resting systolic blood pressure for a young male adult is approximately 120 mm Hg. Women may register 10 to 20 mm Hg lower. During the relaxation phase of the heart (called *diastole*), blood pressure declines and reaches its lowest value. Blood pressure during diastole is called **diastolic blood pressure**; normal diastolic blood pressure for a young male adult is approximately 80 mm Hg. Again, women may register 10 to 20 mm Hg lower. The reason why women's blood pressure is typically lower than men's relates to the general difference in height. More specifically, males are usually taller than females, and blood pressure is higher in taller individuals (Malina, Bouchard, & Bar-Or, 2004). It is important to measure both systolic and diastolic blood pressure because it is the combination of these two pressures that determines your mean (average) arterial pressure.

The walls of arteries are elastic, and expand during the contraction of the heart. The increase in blood pressure during systole causes a pulsation in the arteries that can be felt by placing your finger on the skin near a major artery, such as the carotid or radial arteries. (Since there is pulsation that can be felt in your thumb, the thumb should not be used when determining your heart rate.) One pulse

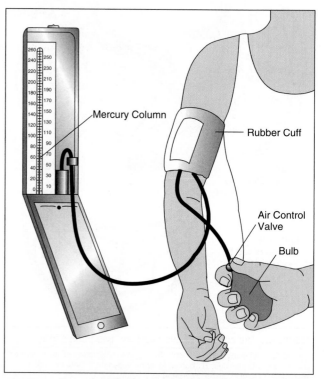

FIGURE 4.4 Measuring blood pressure using a sphygmomanometer.

---

systolic blood pressure   The pressure of the blood in the arteries at the level of the heart during the contraction phase of the heart (systole).

diastolic blood pressure   The pressure of the blood in the arteries at the level of the heart during the resting phase of the heart (diastole).

represents one heartbeat. This technique can be used to count your heart rate during or after physical activity (discussed in Chapter 2).

Approximately 13 percent of all Canadians aged 12 and older have high blood pressure, or **hypertension** (Statistics Canada, 2000/01). Systolic blood pressure of 140 mm Hg and diastolic blood pressure of 90 mm Hg are "threshold" blood pressure values; all higher values indicate hypertension. The threshold values for hypertension are currently under debate. In fact, some suggest that a blood pressure greater than 120/80 may indicate hypertension. The percentage of the population with hypertension increases with the age group examined, as shown in Figure 4.5 (Statistics Canada, 2000/01). Further, the percentage of females with high blood pressure is less than males in the 25-to-34 and 35-to-44 age groups. In the 45-to-54, 55-to-64, 65-to-74, and 75-years-and-over age groups a greater percentage of females have hypertension.

Hypertension is a serious health problem because it increases the risk of heart attack and stroke (Heart & Stroke Foundation, 2005). As noted in Chapter 1, regular physical activity reduces blood pressure in many individuals. Therefore, physicians often prescribe light exercise in addition to a healthy nutritional intake (see Chapter 7) for people with hypertension in an effort to lower their blood pressure.

The Respiratory System

The primary purpose of the respiratory system (also called the *pulmonary system*) is to provide a means of supplying oxygen to and removing carbon dioxide from the blood. This is achieved by bringing oxygen-rich air into the lungs, which we do by breathing. Oxygen then moves from the lungs into the blood, and carbon dioxide moves from the blood into the lungs and is then exhaled.

Maximal Cardiorespiratory Function: VO_2max

The body's maximum ability to transport and use oxygen during exercise (called **VO_2max**, or *maximal aerobic power*) was introduced in Chapter 2. VO_2max is considered by many exercise physiologists to be the most valid measurement of cardiorespiratory endurance. Indeed, graded exercise tests designed to measure VO_2max are often conducted by fitness experts to determine an individual's cardiorespiratory endurance. As noted in Chapter 2, these tests require expensive equipment to measure oxygen consumption and are usually conducted on a treadmill or stationary exercise cycle. The graded exercise tests are also called *incremental exercise tests*.

Figure 4.6 illustrates the change in oxygen consumption (called *oxygen uptake*) at every intensity (work rate) during a typical incremental exercise test. Note that oxygen uptake increases in a straight line with respect to exercise intensity until VO_2max is reached. Thus, VO_2max represents a "physiological ceiling" for the ability of the cardiorespiratory system to transport oxygen and for the muscles to use it.

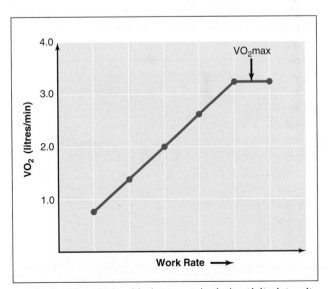

FIGURE 4.6 The relationship between physical activity intensity (work rate) and VO_2.

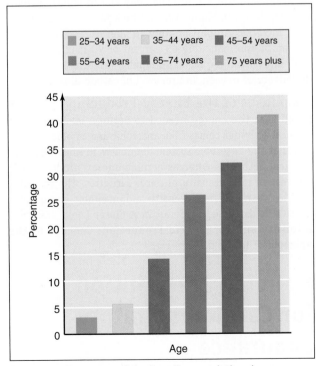

FIGURE 4.5 Percentage of the Canadian population, by age group, with high blood pressure.

Source: Adapted from Statistics Canada CANSIM database, Table 105-0010.

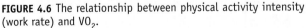

hypertension (high blood pressure)   Usually considered to be a blood pressure of greater than 140 for systolic or 90 for diastolic.

VO_2max   Maximum aerobic power is an indication of the fitness of the cardiorespiratory system. Specifically, it refers to the highest oxygen consumption achieved during an exercise test.

Physiological Responses to Exercise

Circulatory Responses   Physical activity increases the body's need for oxygen. To meet this need, blood flow (and therefore oxygen delivery) to working muscles must increase in proportion to the demand. Increased oxygen transport to skeletal muscle is accomplished by increasing cardiac output and redistributing the blood flow toward the working muscles. The change in cardiac output, heart rate, and blood pressure in response to physical activity of various intensities is illustrated in Figure 4.7. Note that the heart rate and cardiac output increase in a straight line as the intensity of the physical activity intensity increases.

Since heart rate increases as a function of physical activity intensity, it is useful for monitoring the intensity of exercise or the amount of physiological stress. For instance, a person riding a bicycle or running can stop exercising and quickly check his or her heart rate (the pulse) to measure how hard he or she is working. Because it is easy to check heart rate during physical activity, this has become the standard means of determining physical activity intensity. Also, note in Figure 4.7 that heart rate and cardiac output reach a plateau when VO_2max is achieved. Again, VO_2max represents the physiological ceiling of the body's ability for delivery and utilization of oxygen in working muscles.

It is important to also consider the changes in blood pressure in response to physical activity of varying intensity. The key point in Figure 4.7 is that systolic blood pressure increases as the physical activity intensity rises; in contrast, the diastolic blood pressure remains relatively unchanged from the resting

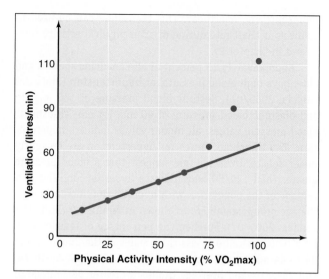

FIGURE 4.8 The ventilatory response to physical activity. Each point on the graph represents the amount of ventilation required at a specific physical activity intensity. Points lying on the straight line indicate rates below the anaerobic threshold.

state. The rise in systolic blood pressure with greater physical activity intensity provides the increased driving pressure to push blood toward the working muscles.

Respiratory Responses   The responsibility of the respiratory system during physical activity is to maintain constant arterial oxygen and carbon dioxide levels. Therefore, because physical activity increases oxygen consumption and carbon dioxide production, the breathing rate must increase to bring more oxygen into the body and to remove carbon dioxide. Notice in Figure 4.8 that breathing (called *ventilation*) increases proportionately to physical activity intensity up to approximately 65 percent of VO_2max. At higher work rates breathing increases rapidly, resulting in increases in delivery of oxygen and removal of carbon dioxide.

Responses of the Energy-Producing Systems
Recall that the energy needed to perform many types of physical activities comes from anaerobic and aerobic sources, and that the anaerobic system dominates in high-intensity physical activities whereas aerobic energy production is greatest in low-intensity physical activities. The relationship between exercise intensity and anaerobic energy production is discussed in detail in A Closer Look: "Exercise Intensity and Lactic Acid Production: Concept of the Anaerobic Threshold."

Exercise Prescription for Cardiorespiratory Endurance

After assessing your health status and evaluating your current cardiorespiratory endurance (Chapter 2), you are ready to develop an exercise prescription to improve your car-

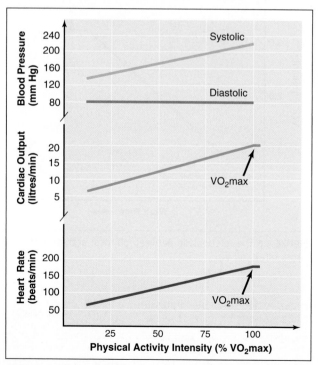

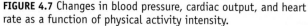

FIGURE 4.7 Changes in blood pressure, cardiac output, and heart rate as a function of physical activity intensity.

dioresperatory fitness. As discussed, the exercise training session comprises three primary elements: warm-up, workout (primary conditioning period), and cool-down.

Warm-Up

Every workout should begin with a warm-up. For an activity such as jogging, the warm-up might consist of the following:

1. 1 to 3 minutes of light calisthenics or large body movements
2. 1 to 3 minutes of walking at a pace that elevates heart rate by 20 to 30 beats/minute above rest
3. 2 to 4 minutes of light stretching (optional; see Chapter 6 for details)
4. 2 to 5 minutes of jogging at a slow pace to gradually elevate the heart rate toward the desired target heart rate (discussed later in the section on intensity).

If the workout is to consist of exercise modes other than jogging, the same general warm-up routine could be followed by substituting other exercise modes, as in steps 2 and 4. For instance, if cycling is the primary mode of exercise, low-intensity cycling exercise would take the place of walking and jogging in steps 2 and 4.

Workout: Primary Conditioning Period

The components of an exercise prescription to improve cardiovascular endurance follow the FITT principles—frequency, intensity, time (duration), and type of exercise.

Frequency Although cardiorespiratory endurance gains can be achieved with as few as two exercise sessions per week, the general recommendation for exercise frequency is 3 to 5 sessions per week to achieve near-optimal gains in cardiorespiratory fitness with minimal risk of injury (ACSM, 2001). If you remain injury-free while training, 5 days per week is advocated; otherwise, an individual should stick to the lower recommendation of 3 days per week. It is unlikely that greater health or fitness benefits will be obtained from exercising more than 5 days per week.

anaerobic threshold The level of intensity above which the aerobic system cannot supply enough energy and the body fatigues quickly. Specifically, the work intensity during graded, incremental exercise at which there is a rapid accumulation of blood lactic acid.

A CLOSER LOOK

Exercise Intensity and Lactic Acid Production: Concept of the Anaerobic Threshold

High-intensity exercise results in an increased production of lactic acid. The relationship between exercise intensity and blood levels of lactic acid is illustrated in the figure in this box. Note that blood levels of lactic acid during exercise remain low until an exercise intensity of 50 to 60 percent of VO_2max is achieved. However, exercise above 50 to 60 percent of VO_2max results in a rapid accumulation of blood lactic acid. The exercise intensity that results in an increased rate of muscle lactic acid accumulation is called the **anaerobic threshold** (Svendahl & MacIntosh, 2003).

During exercise above the anaerobic threshold, muscles begin to produce large amounts of lactic acid, resulting in muscular fatigue. This explains why exercise below the anaerobic threshold can be tolerated for a long period, whereas exercise above the anaerobic threshold results in rapid fatigue. Those of us who have experimented with finding the maximum speed that we can maintain while running or cycling have had experience with the anaerobic threshold. We learn that there are some speeds we can tolerate for the full duration of the exercise session. Attempts to "pick up the pace" result in muscle fatigue that forces us to slow our pace. This is because the maximal speed we can maintain represents an exercise intensity close to but below the anaerobic threshold. Accordingly, prolonged exercise sessions (i.e., 20–60 minutes in duration) aimed at improving cardiorespiratory endurance are generally performed at exercise intensities below the anaerobic threshold.

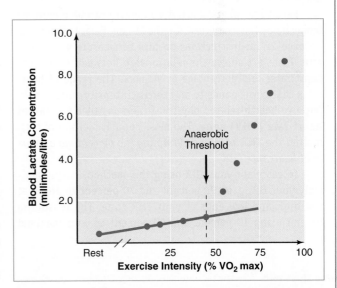

The relationship between blood lactic acid concentration and exercise intensity. Points lying on the straight line indicate physical activity work rates below the anaerobic threshold.

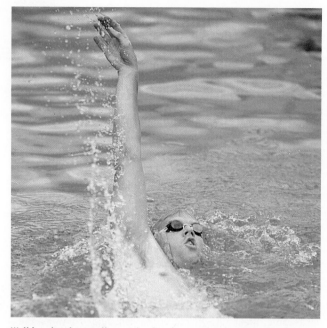

THR (beats/minute*)	% VO$_2$max	% HR$_{max}$
186	90	93
180	85	90
173	80	87
166	75	83
160	70	80
153	65	76
146	60	73
140	55	70
134	49	67

Heart rate based on an HR$_{max}$ of 200 beats/minute.

TABLE 4.1 The Relationship of Target Heart Rate (THR) to Percentage VO$_2$max and Percentage HR$_{max}$ for a 20-Year-Old Individual

Source: Adapted from Fox, E., Bowers, R., & Foss, M. (1989). The physiological basis for exercise and sport. Dubuque, IA: Brown and Benchmark.

Walking, jogging, cycling, and swimming are popular modes of physical activity that can be used to improve cardiorespiratory endurance.

Intensity Cardiorespiratory endurance begins to improve when the training intensity is approximately 50 percent of VO$_2$max. This work rate is called the **training threshold**. Cardiorespiratory fitness can also be improved by exercising at VO$_2$max; however, this intensity of exercise is not realistic since most people could exercise for only 1 to 2 minutes at this rate. To ensure a sufficient length of time, the recommended range of exercise intensity for improving health-related cardiorespiratory endurance is between 50 and 85 percent VO$_2$max.

Recall that physical activity intensity can be monitored indirectly by the measurement of heart rate. Refer to Figure 2.2 on page 22 for instructions on how to measure your heart rate. Table 4.1 shows the relationship between exercising heart rates and percentage of VO$_2$max. The range of heart rates that corresponds to an exercise intensity sufficient to improve health-related physical fitness is called the **target heart rate (THR) zone**. The most popular method of estimating the THR zone is *determining the percentage of maximal heart rate (HR$_{max}$)*.

To calculate your THR using this method, simply multiply your HR$_{max}$ by 90 percent and 70 percent to arrive at the high and low ends of your THR zone. The reasoning behind using 70 percent and 90 percent of your maximal

heart rate to compute your target rate is based on the relationship between percentage HR$_{max}$ and percentage VO$_2$max (Table 4.1). Note that 70 percent of HR$_{max}$ represents the heart rate associated with an exercise intensity that is close to 50 percent VO$_2$max (the lower end of the training-sensitive zone), and that 90 percent of the HR$_{max}$ represents 85 percent VO$_2$max (the upper end of the recommended training-sensitive zone).

For example, the maximal HR of a 20-year-old student can be estimated by the formula

$$HR_{max} = 220 - 20 = 200 \text{ beats/min}$$

The THR is then computed as

$$200 \text{ beats/min} \times 0.70 = 140 \text{ beats/min}$$
$$200 \text{ beats/min} \times 0.90 = 180 \text{ beats/min}$$
$$THR = 140 \text{ to } 180 \text{ beats/min}$$

In this example, the THR to be maintained during a workout to improve cardiorespiratory endurance is between 140 and 180 beats/minute; this range of exercise intensities is sometimes called the *training-sensitive zone*.

It is important to remember that your THR will change as you get older due to the decrease in maximal heart rate. This point is illustrated in Figure 4.9. For instance, while the THR for a 20-year-old is between 140 and 180 beats per minute, the THR for a 60-year-old is 108 to 139 beats per minute.

Another way to estimate the exercise intensity is to use the Borg Rating of Perceived Exertion Scale (Borg, 1998). *Perceived exertion* refers to how hard you think you are exercising. The collected efforts of breathing, sweating, and muscle exertion determine how hard the heart is working to circulate blood. Thus, it is reasonable to assume that a subjective rating of these efforts correlates to heart rate.

training threshold A training intensity above 50 percent of VO$_2$max where there is an improvement in cardiorespiratory fitness.

target heart rate (THR) zone The range of heart rates that corresponds to an exercise intensity of approximately 50 to 85 percent VO$_2$max and results in improvements in aerobic capacity.

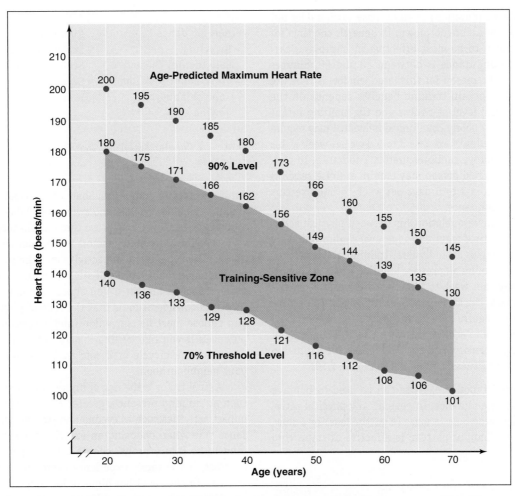

FIGURE 4.9 Target heart rate zones for individuals of ages 20 through 70. The zones cover 70 to 90 percent of maximum heart rate, which is indicated above the zones for selected ages.

Source: Used with permission from Nieman, D. C. (1995). *Fitness and sports medicine: A health-related approach*. Palo Alto, CA: Bull Publishing Co.

Instructions for Using the Rating of Perceived Exertion (RPE) Scale During exercise, rate your perception of your efforts (exertion) using the scale listed below. Consider all sensations and feelings of physical stress, effort, and fatigue. Do not focus on only one factor such as leg pain or shortness of breath.

Look at the rating scale when you are exercising. Find the best descriptor of your effort on the right and choose the associated number on the left. Your RPE multiplied by 10 is a rough estimate of your heart rate during exercise. For example, if your RPE is 13, your heart rate could be estimated by multiplying 13 by 10 to get 130 beats per minute. This is a very rough estimate of the intensity of the physical activity you are engaged in. You can use this information to work harder (or less hard) until you reach your target heart rate zone.

When using the RPE scale, be honest about your feelings of exertion without thinking about the actual workload. It is important to rate your own feeling of effort and not compare yourself to someone else.

6 No exertion at all
7 Extremely light
8
9 Very light*
10
11 Light
12
13 Somewhat hard**
14
15 Hard (heavy)
16
17 Very hard***
18
19 Extremely hard****
20 Maximal exertion

* 9 corresponds to "very light" exercise; for a healthy person, it is like walking slowly at his or her own pace for some minutes.

** 13 "somewhat hard" exercise, but it feels okay to continue.

*** 17 "very hard" is very strenuous; a healthy person can still go on, but he or she has to really push. It feels very heavy and the person is very tired.

**** 19 "extremely hard"; this is the most strenuous exercise most people have ever experienced.

Source: Borg-RPE-scale® from G. Borg (1998), Borg's perceived exertion and pain scales. Champaign, IL: Human Kinetics. © Gunnar Borg, 1970, 1985, 1994, 1998. Used with permission of Dr. G. Borg. For correct usage of the scale, the exact design and instructions given in Borg's folders must be followed.

Time The *time* (duration) of an exercise session does not include the warm-up or cool-down. In general, the time for exercising shown to be most effective in improving cardiorespiratory endurance is between 20 and 60 minutes (ACSM, 2001). The reason for this large window is that the time required to obtain training benefits depends on the individual's initial level of fitness and the training intensity. For example, a poorly conditioned individual may require only 20 to 30 minutes of exercise 3 to 5 days per week at his or her THR to improve cardiorespiratory endurance. In contrast, a highly trained person may require exercise sessions of 40 to 60 minutes 3 to 5 days per week to improve cardiorespiratory endurance.

There is an inverse relationship between physical activity intensity and time required to improve cardiorespiratory fitness. For example, an individual training at 50 percent of VO_2max may require an exercise duration of 40 to 60 minutes 3 to 5 days per week to improve cardiorespiratory fitness. In contrast, the same person exercising at 70 percent of VO_2max may require only 20 to 30 minutes of exercise 3 to 5 days per week to achieve the same effect. A summary of the frequency, intensity, and time guidelines for improving cardiorespiratory fitness is provided in Figure 4.10.

Type Several types of exercise can be used to improve cardiorespiratory endurance. In general, any physical activity that uses a large muscle mass (e.g., the legs) in a slow, rhythmical, continuous pattern is effective at improving

cross training The use of a variety of physical activities for improving cardiorespiratory endurance.

Aerobic dance	Running
Bicycling	Skating (ice or roller)
Calisthenics (heavy)	Stair climber
Cross-country skiing	Swimming
Rope skipping	Walking
Rowing	

TABLE 4.2 Popular Activities That Promote Cardiorespiratory Endurance

cardiorespiratory endurance. Some of the most common are walking, jogging, cycling, and swimming. Table 4.2 lists several activities shown to improve cardiorespiratory endurance.

There are several key factors to consider when choosing an exercise type. First, the activity must be something you enjoy doing! Your chances of sticking with an exercise program are much greater if you choose an activity you like. A second consideration is that the type of physical activity you choose must be convenient and accessible. For example, even if you like cycling it may not be possible if you do not own a bicycle or if safe trails are not available in your neighbourhood.

A final factor is the risk of injury. High-impact activities such as running present a greater risk of injury than low-impact activities such as cycling and swimming. A common-sense rule when choosing an exercise type is that if you tend to be injury prone, choose a low-impact activity. In contrast, if you rarely experience exercise-related injuries, feel free to choose either high- or low-impact activities.

Historically, most exercise prescriptions for improving cardiorespiratory endurance have used only one type of activity. There is now a trend toward using **cross training** (i.e., a variety of physical activities) for improving the cardiorespiratory system. Many fitness experts think that participating in only one type of physical activity may be perceived as boring and leads to dropout. Cross training may also reduce the frequency of injury by avoiding overuse of the same muscle groups. (Cross training is discussed later in this chapter.)

Safety: Improving Cardiorespiratory Endurance without Injury
What is the optimal combination of exercise frequency, intensity, and time to promote cardiorespiratory endurance while minimizing risk of injury? The FITT principles are illustrated in Figure 4.11; these are modified slightly to minimize risk of injury. The optimal frequency of training sessions to minimize risk of injury while still improving cardiorespiratory fitness is 3 to 4 days per week. The optimal exercise intensity to improve cardiorespiratory fitness without increasing the risk of injury is between 60 and 80 percent of VO_2max (73–87 percent HR_{max}). Further, the optimal time is 20 to 30 minutes per training session. These factors are highly related and should be considered along with the type of training being done. The risk of injury is minimized when a variety of physical activities are performed (see "Cross Training" later in this chapter).

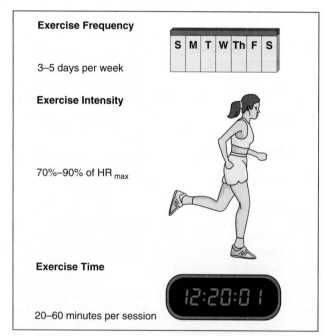

Exercise Frequency

S M T W Th F S

3–5 days per week

Exercise Intensity

70%–90% of HR_{max}

Exercise Time

12:20:01

20–60 minutes per session

FIGURE 4.10 The suggested frequency, intensity, and time of physical activity necessary for improving cardiovascular endurance.

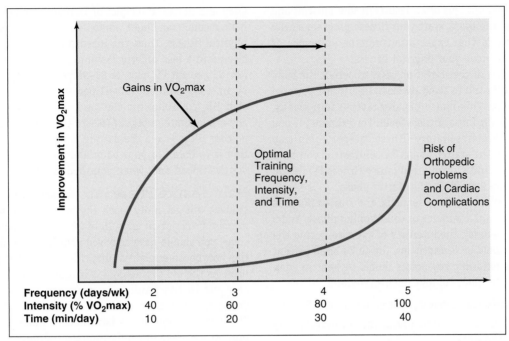

FIGURE 4.11 The effects of increasing frequency, intensity, and time on the improvements in VO_2max versus the increased risk of injury.

Cool-Down

Every training session should conclude with a cool-down (5–15 minutes of light physical activity and stretching). One purpose of the cool-down is to promote blood return to the heart, thereby preventing blood from pooling in the arms and legs, which could result in dizziness or fainting. Another purpose of the cool-down is to return the muscles to their normal length. A cool-down may also decrease muscle soreness and cardiac irregularities that sometimes occur after a vigorous workout. Although cardiac irregularities are rare in healthy individuals, it is prudent to cool down and reduce this risk.

A general cool-down consisting of at least 5 minutes of light physical activity (such as walking and calisthenics) should be followed by 5 to 30 minutes of stretching exercises. In general, stretching exercises should focus on the muscles used in training. The type and time of the stretching session depends on your flexibility goals (Chapter 6).

Starting and Maintaining a Cardiorespiratory Endurance Program

Two key elements in any physical fitness program are the individual's specific short- and long-term goals. Without these, motivation to continue training is hard to maintain. Many fitness experts agree that the lack of goals is a major contributor to the high dropout rates seen in many organized fitness programs (Mullineaux, Barnes, & Barnes, 2001). It pays to establish short- and long-term fitness goals *before* you start your training program.

If your training plans include several weight-bearing activities such as running, walking, aerobic dance, and so on, it is important to exercise in good shoes. Good running, walking, or aerobics shoes are expensive (costs range from $50–$150). Investing in quality, well-designed shoes is important for comfort and injury prevention. Look for a well-cushioned shoe with the following features: soft, comfortable upper material; adequate toe room (as indicated by comfort); well-padded heel and firm ankle collar; firm arch support; and a heel lift (a wedge that raises the heel about 1.5 cm higher than the sole). Many athletic shoe stores have well-trained sales personnel to assist you in the selection process.

Developing an Individualized Exercise Prescription

Regardless of your initial fitness level or your choice of physical activity, the exercise prescription for improving cardiovascular endurance usually has three stages: the starter phase, the slow progression phase, and the maintenance phase.

Starter Phase The quickest way to extinguish enthusiasm for an exercise program is to try to accomplish too much too soon. Many people begin an exercise program with great excitement and anticipation of improved physical fitness and weight loss. Unfortunately, this early excitement can lead to exercising too hard for too long during the very first training session. This often results in sore muscles and undue fatigue. Therefore, start your fitness program slowly and be realistic in your expectations for the outcomes. It takes time to improve your physical fitness.

The objective of the starter phase is to permit the body to adapt gradually and to avoid soreness, injury, and personal discouragement. This phase usually lasts 2 to 6 weeks, depending on your initial fitness level. For example, if you are in a poor cardiorespiratory fitness category, you may need 6 weeks in the starter phase. In contrast, if you have a relatively high initial cardiorespiratory fitness level, you may require only 2 weeks in the starter phase.

Similar to other workout sessions, the starter program includes a warm-up, a workout or conditioning phase, and a cool-down. In general, the intensity of exercise during the starter phase should be relatively low (up to 70 or 80 percent of HR_{max}). The following key points should be kept in mind during the starter phase of an exercise program:

1. Start at an exercise intensity that is comfortable for you.
2. Increase your training time (duration) or intensity only when comfortable.
3. Be aware of new aches or pains. Pain is a symptom of injury and indicates that rest is required to allow the body to repair itself. (See Chapter 13 for a discussion of injury prevention and treatment.)

Slow Progression Phase
The slow progression phase may last 12 to 20 weeks, with exercise progression more rapid than during the starter phase. The intensity can be gradually elevated, and the frequency and time of exercise increased, depending on fitness goals and the presence of injuries. In general, this stage should involve an exercise frequency of 3 to 4 times per week and an exercise time of 20 to 30 minutes per session. Exercise intensity should range between 70 and 90 percent HR_{max} (50–85 percent VO_2max), depending on your personal fitness goals.

A common question students frequently ask is what component of the FITT principles to focus on first when increasing the workload of a training program. First, increase the frequency of your workouts from 3 to 4 days per week; then from 4 to 5 days per week. Remember, there is little benefit and greater risk when training more than 5 days per week. Next, increase the length of your workout sessions from 20 to 22 minutes, then 22 to 24 minutes, and so forth until you reach 40 minutes. Finally, increase the intensity of your workouts from 50 percent VO_2max (67 percent HR_{max}) to 55 percent VO_2max (70 percent HR_{max}), then to 60 percent VO_2max (73 percent HR_{max}), and so forth until you reach 85 percent VO_2max (90 percent HR_{max}). Remember that training at a higher intensity than 85 percent VO_2max is difficult and associated with an increased risk of injury. Also keep in mind that it is recommended you increase the intensity or time of your workout in only 10-percent increments. As noted in

Chapter 3 in the "Principles of Training" section, alternating hard, medium, and light workouts is recommended to increase physical fitness. Thus, the intensity of the workout may be altered in a less orderly fashion so that a "hard" workout (74–85 percent VO_2max, or 83–90 percent HR_{max}) is followed by an "easy" workout (50–61 percent VO_2max, or 67–74 percent HR_{max}). Following the hard and easy workout is usually a "moderate" workout (62–73 percent VO_2max, or 75–82 percent HR_{max}), and the pattern is repeated. A final suggestion is to listen to your body and progress with increasing your workload only when your body is ready.

Maintenance Phase
The average postsecondary-age student will generally reach the maintenance phase of the exercise prescription after 16 to 28 weeks of training. At this stage, you should have achieved your fitness goal. The objective now becomes maintaining this new level of physical fitness. As the old saying goes, "Fitness is not something you can put in the bank." To maintain cardiorespiratory endurance, you must continue to train on a regular basis. The key question now is how much training is required to prevent a decline in cardiorespiratory fitness.

The primary factor in maintaining cardiorespiratory fitness is the intensity of exercise (Laursen & Jenkins, 2002). If the exercise intensity and length of exercise session each remain the same as during the final weeks of the slow progression phase, frequency can be reduced to as few as 2 days per week without a significant loss in VO_2max. Alternatively, if frequency and intensity remain the same as during the final weeks of the slow progression phase, time can be reduced to as few as 20 to 25 minutes per session. In contrast, when frequency and time are held constant, a one-third decrease in intensity results in a significant decline in VO_2max. To summarize, if exercise intensity is maintained, the exercise frequency and time necessary to maintain a given level of cardiorespiratory fitness can be substantially reduced without a loss in cardiorespiratory endurance.

Sample Exercise Prescriptions
As mentioned above, the exercise prescription must be tailored to the individual. The key factor to consider when designing a personal training program is your current level of physical fitness. Programs designed for people with good or excellent cardiorespiratory endurance start at a higher level and progress more rapidly compared with programs designed for people in poor physical condition. Tables 4.3 through 4.5 illustrate three sample cardiorespiratory training programs designed for postsecondary-aged people beginning a fitness program. Table 4.3 contains an exercise prescription that might be appropriate for people with very poor or poor cardiorespiratory endurance. Table 4.4 illustrates a sample program designed for people with good or average cardiorespiratory endurance, while Table 4.5 contains a program aimed at people with a cardiorespiratory fitness rating of excellent or

Week No.	Phase	Duration (min/day)	Intensity (% of HR_{max})	Frequency (days/wk)
1	Starter	10	60	3
2	Starter	10	60	3
3	Starter	12	60	3
4	Starter	12	70	3
5	Starter	15	70	3
6	Starter	15	70	3
7	Slow progression	20	70	3
8	Slow progression	20	70	3
9	Slow progression	25	70	3
10	Slow progression	25	70	3
11	Slow progression	30	70	3
12	Slow progression	30	70	3
13	Slow progression	35	70	3
14	Slow progression	35	70	3
15	Slow progression	40	70	3
16	Slow progression	40	70	3
17	Slow progression	40	75	3
18	Slow progression	40	75	3
19	Slow progression	40	75	3
20	Slow progression	40	75	3–4
21	Slow progression	40	75	3–4
22	Slow progression	40	75	3–4
23	Maintenance	30	75	3–4
24	Maintenance	30	75	3–4
25	Maintenance	30	75	3–4
26	Maintenance	30	75	3–4

TABLE 4.3 Sample Cardiorespiratory Endurance Training Program Designed for People in the Very Poor or Poor Fitness Category

General guidelines:
1. Begin each session with a warm-up.
2. Don't progress to the next level until you feel comfortable with your current level of exercise.
3. Monitor your heart rate during each training session.
4. End each session with a cool-down.
5. Be aware of aches and pains. If you are injury prone, choose a low-impact activity and limit your exercise duration to 20 to 30 minutes per session.

greater. Note that these programs are merely sample programs, and can be modified to meet your individual fitness levels and goals. If you feel that none of these training programs meet your training needs, use Laboratory 4.1 to develop your personal exercise prescription. After designing your cardiorespiratory training program, use Laboratory 4.2 to keep a record of your physical activity habits.

Training Techniques

Endurance training is a generic term that refers to any type of exercise aimed at improving cardiorespiratory endurance. Over the years, numerous endurance training techniques

have evolved including cross training; long, slow distance training; interval training; and fartlek training.

Cross Training

As previously mentioned, cross training is a popular form of training that uses several different types of physical activities. It may mean running one day, swimming another day, and cycling another day. One advantage of cross training is that it reduces the boredom of performing the same kind of activity day after day. Further, it may reduce the risk of injuries by avoiding overuse of the same body parts. A disadvantage of cross training is the lack of training specificity for the musculoskeletal system. However, the cardiorespiratory system

Week No.	Phase	Duration (min/day)	Intensity (% of HR_{max})	Frequency (days/wk)
1	Starter	10	70	3
2	Starter	15	70	3
3	Starter	15	70	3
4	Starter	20	70	3
5	Slow progression	25	70	3
6	Slow progression	25	75	3
7	Slow progression	25	75	3
8	Slow progression	30	75	3
9	Slow progression	30	75	3
10	Slow progression	35	75	3
11	Slow progression	35	75	3
12	Slow progression	40	75	3
13	Slow progression	40	75	3
14	Slow progression	40	75	3
15	Slow progression	40	80	3
16	Slow progression	40	80	3–4
17	Slow progression	40	80	3–4
18	Slow progression	40	80	3–4
19	Maintenance	30	80	3–4
20	Maintenance	30	80	3–4
21	Maintenance	30	80	3–4
22	Maintenance	30	80	3–4

TABLE 4.4 Sample Cardiorespiratory Endurance Training Program Designed for People in the Average or Good Fitness Category

General guidelines:
1. Begin each session with a warm-up.
2. Don't progress to the next level until you feel comfortable with your current level of exercise.
3. Monitor your heart rate during each training session.
4. End each session with a cool-down.
5. Be aware of aches and pains. If you are injury prone, choose a low-impact activity and limit your exercise duration to 20 to 30 minutes per session.

long, slow distance training Continuous exercise that requires a steady, submaximal exercise intensity, generally around 70 percent HR_{max}.

interval training Repeated sessions or intervals of relatively intense exercise.

(heart, blood, lungs) will improve in efficiency. For example, jogging does not improve swimming endurance as much as swimming because the arm muscles are not trained during jogging. Similarly, swimming does not improve jogging endurance as effectively as jogging. In general, to improve musculoskeletal endurance in a particular activity, training should consist of exercises similar to that activity.

Long, Slow Distance Training

Long, slow distance training, or *continuous training*, requires a steady, submaximal exercise intensity (i.e., generally around 70 percent HR_{max}). It is one of the most popular cardiorespiratory training techniques and can be applied to any type of exercise. During the progression phase of the exercise program, an individual may find this type of training enjoyable because the exercise intensity does not increase. If injuries are not a problem, there is no reason why the duration of the training cannot be extended to 40 to 60 minutes per session. An advantage of continuous training is that risk of injury is lower than in more intensive training.

Interval Training

Interval training refers to repeated sessions or intervals of relatively intense exercise. The duration of the intervals can be varied, but a 1- to 5-minute duration is common. Each interval is followed by a rest period, which should be equal to, or slightly longer than, the interval duration. For example, if you are running 400-metre intervals on a track, and it takes approximately 90 seconds to complete each run, your rest period between each run should be at least 90 seconds.

Week No.	Phase	Duration (min/day)	Intensity (% of HR_{max})	Frequency (days/wk)
1	Starter	15	75	3
2	Starter	20	75	3
3	Slow progression	25	75	3
4	Slow progression	30	75	3
5	Slow progression	35	75	3
6	Slow progression	40	75	3
7	Slow progression	40	75	3–4
8	Slow progression	40	75	3–4
9	Slow progression	40	80	3–4
10	Slow progression	40	80	3–4
11	Slow progression	40	80	3–4
12	Slow progression	40	80–85	3–4
13	Slow progression	40	80–85	3–4
14	Slow progression	40	80–85	3–4
15	Maintenance	30	80–85	3–4
16	Maintenance	30	80–85	3–4
17	Maintenance	30	80–85	3–4
18	Maintenance	30	80–85	3–4

TABLE 4.5 Sample Cardiorespiratory Endurance Training Program Designed for People in the Excellent Fitness Category

General guidelines:
1. Begin each session with a warm-up.
2. Don't progress to the next level until you feel comfortable with your current level of exercise.
3. Monitor your heart rate during each training session.
4. End each session with a cool-down.
5. Be aware of aches and pains. If you are injury prone, choose a low-impact activity and limit your exercise duration to 20 to 30 minutes per session.

Interval training is a common training technique among athletes who have already established a strong base of cardiorespiratory endurance training and wish to attain much higher fitness levels in order to be more competitive in a particular sport. With correct spacing of exercise and rest periods, more work can be accomplished with interval training than with long, slow distance training. A major advantage of interval training is the variety of workouts it allows, which may reduce the tedium associated with some other forms of training. A risk of this type of training is injury associated with high-intensity training.

Fartlek Training

Fartlek is a Swedish word meaning "speed play," and refers to a popular form of training for long-distance runners. **Fartlek training** is similar to interval training, but it is not as rigid in its work-to-rest interval ratios. It consists of inserting sprints into long, slow running done on trails, roads, golf courses, and the like. An advantage of fartlek training is that these workouts provide variety and reduce the possibility of boredom associated with long continuous types of training. Again, the risk of this type of training is the possibility of injury with the high-intensity phases.

Aerobic Exercise Training: How the Body Adapts

How does the body adapt to aerobic exercise training? Cardiorespiratory endurance training induces changes in the cardiovascular and respiratory systems, the skeletal muscles and the energy-producing systems, VO_2max, flexibility, and body composition.

Cardiovascular System

Several adaptations occur in the cardiovascular system as a result of endurance training (Powers & Howley, 2004). First, although training does not alter maximal heart rate, a decrease in submaximal exercising heart rate occurs. This reduction in heart rate occurs because stroke volume at submaximal loads is greater. In other words, the heart is able to

fartlek training *Fartlek* is a Swedish word meaning "speed play," and refers to an interval-type training in which sprints are inserted into long, slow runs.

Frequently Asked Questions About Aerobic Workouts

What is a simple way to judge my workout intensity?

A very simple way to gauge intensity is the talk test. You should be able to talk without gasping for air while exercising. If you cannot, you should slow down. In contrast, if your intensity allows you to laugh and sing, then you need to work harder.

Is it better to exercise for several short sessions, or for one longer period?

Either approach can be beneficial. Regardless, you need to warm up for 5 to 15 minutes and cool down for 5 to 15 minutes no matter the session length. So if you exercise for one 60-minute period, 30 to 50 minutes of that time should be for aerobic training, with the remainder for warm-up and cool-down. If you exercise for shorter periods, make sure to get at least 15 to 20 minutes of aerobic training.

Should I train my muscles in addition to doing aerobic activity?

Yes. Resistance training is an important part of any physical fitness program because strength will help protect you from injuries. Moreover, when you are strong it is easier to maintain proper form.

Can steam, the sauna, or a hot tub be helpful after a workout?

After a workout, blood vessels in the skin are open because blood is sent to the skin to aid in cooling the body. Additional heat will open the blood vessels even more, which diverts blood from critical areas such as the brain, the heart, and muscles. Therefore, adding heat to the body immediately after physical activity is not a wise thing to do. However, if you have thoroughly cooled down and your heart rate has returned to near its normal resting rate, you may use steam, the sauna, or a hot tub to help relax. However, if you feel any weakness or dizziness, get out immediately.

What is step aerobics?

Step aerobics is a form of aerobic activity performed on a step or platform approximately 10 to 25 cm in height. It was developed to provide aerobic training without high impact. It is done in a small area, so in a given space more people can do it than aerobic dance.

How good are exercise gadgets?

Trends and fads come and go in the fitness industry. Some gadgets are useful and help you to reach your fitness goals, and others are worthless. Before buying a new gadget, follow the guidelines in this text to determine if the equipment is useful. In general, the best piece of cardiovascular training equipment is the one that you will actually use. If you are simply concerned with which modality burns the most calories, the best piece is the one that you use for the *longest amount of time*.

Is the meal before a workout important, and what should it be?

Most of the energy expended during a workout will come from the food you ate the previous day. Energy from that food was stored in your muscles and liver. Since some energy also comes from food consumed the day of your workout, the pre-workout meal is important as well. Keep in mind that the food you consume prior to a workout should be (1) easily digestible to keep from upsetting your stomach and preventing your workout and (2) high in complex carbohydrates to replace the energy expended in the workout.

Does it matter what I eat after I work out?

Yes, the types of food you eat or drink have an effect on the replenishment of your glycogen stores, as noted in the Nutritional Links to Health and Fitness on page 86. Ideally, within the first 15 minutes after your workout you should eat or drink foods high in carbohydrates (see the Nutritional Links box for examples) so that your body's muscle glycogen stores can be replenished.

Are fluids important during and after my workout?

It is important to consume fluids throughout the day to ensure your body is adequately hydrated. Current recommendations are to consume at least 2 L per day (Manitoba Milk Producers, Nutritional Education Department, 2005). Keep in mind that fluids are obtained from the foods and drinks you consume. Physical activity, particularly in hot or humid environments, increases the body's need for fluids. As such, it is recommended to drink 100 to 250 mL for every 15 to 20 minutes of physical activity, more if you're sweating heavily or exercising in a hot or humid environment (Manitoba Milk Producers, 2005). A good method of ensuring that your body is adequately hydrated is to monitor the amount and colour of your urine: plenty of pale urine during the day is a sign of adequate fluid intake. (See also Nutritional Links to Health and Fitness on page 86.)

What is the best time of day to exercise?

The same principle that applies to choosing exercise equipment applies here: The best time of day to exercise is the time you are most likely to maintain your workout routine. The best time to work out is when you want to exercise, so pick a time of day that works best for you.

Should I train if I'm sick?

Generally, if the sickness is above the neck (sinus, headache, sore throat, etc.), light-intensity exercise for 20 to 30 minutes should be okay. Take it easy, and if you feel any weakness or dizziness stop immediately. Remember to respect others by wiping off any equipment you use when you are finished and by washing your hands frequently.

---

pump more blood with each heartbeat. Further, endurance exercise results in an increase in maximal stroke volume (SV) with a corresponding increase in maximal cardiac output (because maximal cardiac output = maximal HR × maximal SV). Resting heart rate also lowers in response to cardiorespiratory endurance training. Again, this change occurs because of an improved stroke volume. An increased maximal cardiac output results in an increased oxygen delivery capacity to the working muscles and improved exercise tolerance.

Respiratory System

Endurance exercise may improve lung function by increasing the volume of the lungs and improving the efficiency of oxygen and carbon dioxide exchange. However, there is no scientific evidence to support this belief. Although endurance training does not alter the structure or function of the respiratory system, it does increase respiratory muscle endurance (Powers, Criswell, Lieu, Dodd, & Silverman, 1992; Powers, Grinton, Lawler, Criswell, & Dodd, 1992). That is, the diaphragm and other key muscles of respiration can work harder and longer without fatigue. This improvement in respiratory muscle endurance may reduce the sensation of breathlessness during physical activity and eliminate the pain in the side (often called a *stitch*) sometimes associated with exercise.

Skeletal Muscles and Energy-Producing Systems

Endurance training increases the muscles' capacity for aerobic energy production. The practical result of an improvement in muscle aerobic capacity is an improved ability to use fat as an energy source and an increase in muscular endurance (Powers & Howley, 2004). Note that these changes occur only in the muscles used during the training activity. For example, endurance training using a stationary exercise cycle results in an improvement in muscular endurance in leg muscles, with little effect on arm muscles. Finally, although endurance training improves muscle tone, it does not result in large increases in muscle size or muscular strength.

VO$_2$max

Recall that VO$_2$max is considered the best single measure of cardiorespiratory fitness. Therefore, improvement in VO$_2$max is an important physiological adaptation that occurs in response to endurance training. In general, 12 to 15 weeks of endurance exercise results in a 10- to 30-percent improvement in VO$_2$max (Powers & Howley, 2004). This improvement is due to a combination of improved aerobic capacity in skeletal muscles and increased maximal cardiac output. The net result is increased oxygen delivery and use by skeletal muscles during physical activity. Therefore, an increase in VO$_2$max translates to improved muscular endurance and less fatigue during routine daily activities.

How much VO$_2$max increases after endurance training is dependent on several factors: (1) fitness status at the beginning of the training program, (2) intensity of the training program, and (3) nutritional status during the training program. In general, people who start exercise programs with high VO$_2$max values improve less than those with low initial values. For example, a person entering an endurance training program with a high VO$_2$max may achieve as little as a 5-percent improvement over a 12-week period, whereas an individual with a low VO$_2$max may improve as much as 30 percent (Figure 4.12). The explanation is that a physiological ceiling or limit for improvement in VO$_2$max exists. Thus, the people who

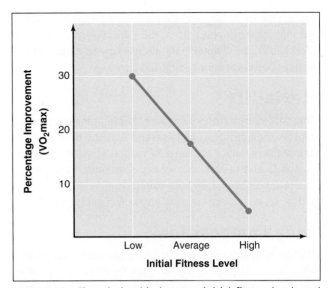

FIGURE 4.12 The relationship between initial fitness levels and improvements in VO$_2$max after a 12-week training period.

enter fitness programs with relatively high VO$_2$max values are probably closer to their limits than the people who enter programs with low VO$_2$max values.

The magnitude of the exercise-induced increase in VO$_2$max is directly related to the intensity of the training program (Laursen & Jenkins, 2002). High-intensity training programs result in greater VO$_2$max gains than low-intensity and short-duration programs (Figure 4.13). A plateau exists in the relationship between training intensity and improvement in VO$_2$max at higher training intensity. Once a high intensity of training is reached, increasing the intensity does not result in further improvement in fitness. Furthermore, training at extremely high intensities may increase the risk of injury and illness.

Finally, failure to maintain proper nutritional habits during an endurance training program will impair

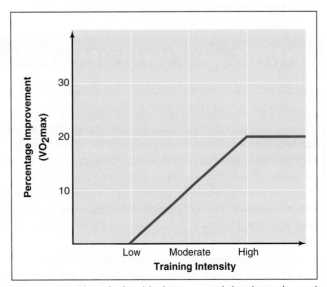

FIGURE 4.13 The relationship between training intensity and improvements in VO$_2$max following a 12-week training period.

improvements in VO$_2$max. Proper nutrition means an eating plan that provides all of the necessary nutrients for good health. In Chapter 7 we discuss how to construct the eating plan needed for health and fitness.

Flexibility

Most cardiorespiratory endurance training programs do not improve flexibility. In fact, several months of endurance training may reduce the range of motion at some joints due to muscle and tendon shortening. Therefore, to prevent a loss of flexibility, stretching exercises should always be a part of an endurance training program (Chapter 6).

Body Composition

Cardiorespiratory endurance training generally results in a reduction in the percentage of body fat (Powers & Howley, 2004). However, a loss of body fat in response to endurance training is not guaranteed. Whether or not an individual loses body fat is a result of many factors, including nutritional intake and the amount of physical activity performed. More is said about this topic in Chapter 8.

Motivation to Maintain Cardiorespiratory Fitness

Every year, millions of people make the decision to start an exercise routine. Unfortunately, more than half of those who begin a cardiorespiratory fitness program quit within the first 6 months (Mullineaux et al., 2001). Although there are many reasons for this high dropout rate, lack of time is commonly cited as a major one. Although finding time for physical activity in a busy schedule is difficult, it is not impossible. The key is to schedule a regular time for physical activity and to stick with it. A small investment in time to be physically active can reap large improvements in fitness and health. Think about the time required to improve cardiorespiratory fitness in the following way. There are 168 hours in every week. All you need is three 30-minute workouts per week to improve cardiorespiratory fitness. Including the associated warm-ups, cool-downs, and showers, this is about 3 hours per week, which is less than 2 percent of the total week. This leaves you with 165 hours per week to accomplish all of the other things you need to do. The bottom line is that with time management, anyone can find time to be physically active.

In order for you to keep your commitment to develop cardiorespiratory fitness, exercise must be fun. Therefore, choose a training technique that you enjoy. Further, your chosen exercise should be convenient. Failure to meet either of these criteria increases your risk of becoming an exercise dropout.

One of the things that makes exercise enjoyable is the interaction with friends. Therefore, exercising with a partner is an excellent idea because it makes physical activity more fun and helps maintain your sense of commitment to a regular exercise routine. In choosing an exercise partner, choose someone that you enjoy interacting with and someone who is a good exercise role model.

Another technique that may help you to maintain commitment to your training program is keeping a record of your training. This assists you in keeping track of your training progress and serves as a motivating factor when you notice improvements in your fitness level.

Finally, it is normal and expected to experience some discomfort and soreness with your first several exercise sessions. Don't let this discourage you. In a short time the soreness will fade and the discomfort associated with physical activity will begin to disappear. As your fitness level improves, you will start to feel and look better. Although reaching and maintaining a reasonable level of cardiorespiratory endurance requires time and effort, the rewards will be well worth your efforts.

FITNESS AND WELLNESS FOR ALL

Wellness Issues Across the Population

Don't Let a Disability Stop You!

Although any type of temporary or permanent disability can certainly be a disincentive to be physically active, you can take comfort in knowing that even with most disabilities you can obtain all of the benefits of cardiorespiratory endurance training. Swimming and other water activities are popular ways to take away the burden of supporting your body weight and safely exercise capable muscle groups. Physical activity in water is beneficial for several reasons:

- Exercising in water eliminates the dangers of falling.
- Flexibility exercises are much easier to do in water.

- Water provides resistance that allows capable muscle groups to work at an intensity that provides progressive overload to the cardiorespiratory system.
- A variety of water aids, including hand paddles, pull-buoys, flotation belts, and kick boards, can be used to help maintain buoyancy and balance as well as help you work in the water.

You must take responsibility for knowing about the medical complications associated with your disability and for knowing how you can prevent or control those complications. Finally, remember that the potential for drowning always exists; never swim or work out in the water while alone.

Summary

1. Benefits of cardiorespiratory endurance include a lower risk of disease, feeling better, increased capacity to perform everyday tasks, and improved self-esteem.
2. Adenosine triphosphate, which is required for muscle contraction, can be produced in muscles by two systems: anaerobic (without oxygen) and aerobic (with oxygen).
3. Anaerobic ATP production occurs mostly through a metabolic process called glycolysis. Glycolysis results in the breakdown of carbohydrates to ATP and the formation of lactic acid. The anaerobic system is the primary energy producer for physical activities lasting 10 to 90 seconds.
4. Aerobic ATP production takes over where the anaerobic system stops and is used for longer-lasting physical activities. In this system, carbohydrates and fats are most often used to produce ATP.
5. The term *cardiorespiratory system* refers to the cooperative work of the circulatory and respiratory systems. The primary function of the circulatory system is to transport blood carrying oxygen and nutrients to body tissues. The principal function of the respiratory system is to load oxygen into and remove carbon dioxide from the blood.
6. The maximum capacity to transport and utilize oxygen during exercise is called VO_2max; many exercise physiologists consider VO_2max the most valid measurement of cardiorespiratory endurance.
7. Cardiac output, systolic blood pressure, and heart rate increase as a function of exercise intensity. Breathing (ventilation) also increases in proportion to exercise intensity.
8. A key factor in prescribing exercise to improve cardiorespiratory endurance is knowledge of the individual's initial level of physical fitness and health status.
9. Three primary elements make up the exercise training session: warm-up, workout, and cool-down.
10. The components of the workout include the frequency, intensity, time, and type of exercise.
11. The recommended frequency of exercise sessions to improve cardiorespiratory endurance is 3 to 5 times per week.
12. The intensity of the exercise is one in which the target heart rate is the range of exercise heart rates that lies between 70 and 90 percent of maximal heart rate.
13. The time of each exercise session is 20 to 60 minutes. This time is for the workout (conditioning period) only and does not include time for warm-up or cool-down.
14. In general, the type of exercise to be used to increase cardiorespiratory endurance is one that uses a large muscle mass in a slow, rhythmical, continuous pattern.
15. Establishing short- and long-term fitness goals is essential before beginning a training program to increase your commitment and likelihood of sticking with the program.
16. Regardless of your initial fitness level, an exercise prescription for improving cardiorespiratory endurance has three phases: the starter phase, the slow progression phase, and the maintenance phase.
17. Common training techniques to improve cardiorespiratory endurance include cross training; long, slow distance training; interval training; and fartlek training.
18. Aerobic exercise training results in an improvement in cardiorespiratory fitness (VO_2max) and muscular endurance and can result in a reduction in percentage body fat.
19. Maintaining a regular exercise routine requires time management and the choice of physical activities you enjoy.

Study Questions

1. Describe the two energy pathways used to produce muscle ATP during physical activity.
2. Which energy pathway (aerobic or anaerobic) is predominantly responsible for production of ATP during the following activities: 100-metre dash, 800-metre run, 10 000-metre run, tennis, football, and weight lifting?
3. What is meant by the term *cardiorespiratory system*? List the major functions of the circulatory and respiratory systems.
4. Why is the heart considered "two pumps in one"?
5. Define the following terms:
   adenosine triphosphate (ATP)
   cross training
   hypertension
   target heart rate
6. Graph the changes in heart rate, blood pressure, cardiac output, and ventilation as a function of exercise intensity.
7. Define VO_2max.
8. Define the *anaerobic threshold*. What is the practical significance of the anaerobic threshold for exercise?
9. What physiological changes occur as a result of cardiorespiratory endurance training?
10. Will cardiorespiratory endurance training alone result in improvement in all components of health-related physical fitness? Why or why not?
11. What information is necessary to develop an individualized exercise prescription?
12. Describe the guidelines that must be met to improve aerobic capacity.

13. What effect does type of training have on increasing aerobic capacity?

14. What range in frequency of exercise is needed to improve aerobic capacity?

15. Define the *training threshold* and give the range of intensities considered necessary to elicit an increase in VO_2max.

16. What training techniques are generally used in exercise programs for improving cardiorespiratory endurance?

Suggested Reading

American College of Sports Medicine. (1998). American College of Sports Medicine position stand: The recommended quantity and quality of exercise for developing and maintaining cardiorespiratory and muscular fitness and flexibility in healthy adults. *Medicine and Science in Sports and Exercise, 30*, 975–991.

Neiman, D. C. (1995). *Fitness and sports medicine: A health-related approach* (3rd ed.). Palo Alto, CA: Bull Publishing.

Pollock, M. L., & Wilmore, J. H. (1998). *Exercise in health and disease* (3rd ed.). Philadelphia: W. B. Saunders.

Powers, S., & Howley, E. (2004). *Exercise physiology: Theory and application to fitness and performance* (5th ed.). Dubuque, IA: McGraw-Hill.

Warburton, D. E., Gledhill, N., & Quinney, A. (2001a). Musculoskeletal fitness and health. *Canadian Journal of Applied Physiology, 26(2)*, 217–237.

Warburton, D. E., Glendhill, N., & Quinney A. (2001b). The effects of changes in musculoskeletal fitness on health. *Canadian Journal of Applied Physiology, 26(2)*, 161–216.

Weblinks

Canadian Society for Exercise Physiology
www.csep.ca
A Canadian resource that promotes the generation, synthesis, transfer, and application of knowledge and research related to exercise physiology (encompassing physical activity, fitness, health, and human performance).

American College of Sports Medicine
www.acsm.org
A U.S. resource that promotes the generation, synthesis, transfer, and application of knowledge and research related to exercise physiology (encompassing physical activity, fitness, health, and human performance).

Health Canada
www.hc-sc.gc.ca
Contains the latest information regarding the health of Canadians.

Health Canada (Heart/Cardiovascular)
www.hc-sc.gc.ca/english/diseases/heart.html
Contains the latest information on the cardiorespiratory health of Canadians.

Heart and Stroke Foundation of Canada
www.heartandstroke.ca
Contains information on the risk factors for heart disease and ways to modify one's lifestyle to reduce risk.

Heart Information Organization
www.heartinfo.org
Provides timely and trustworthy patient guides about heart attack, blood pressure, cholesterol, stroke, nutritional intake, and more.

References

ACSM. (2001). *ACSM's resource manual for guidelines for exercise testing and prescription* (4th ed.). Philadelphia: Lippincot, Williams & Wilkins.

Borg, G. (1998). *Borg's perceived exertion and pain scales.* Champaign, IL: Human Kinetics.

Cooper, K. H. (1968). *Aerobics.* New York: Bantam Books.

Diekmeyer, P. (2004). Health Canada should reinstate ParticipAction funding: Advertising convinced a generation of Canadians to get fit. Diekmeyer Report, Retrieved September 2005 from www.peterdiekmeyer.com/010130.html.

Dunn, A. L., Trivedi, M. H., & O'Neal, H. A. (2001). Physical activity dose-response effects on outcomes of depression and anxiety. *Medicine and Science in Sports and Exercise, 33(6)*, S587–S597.

Gambelunghe, C., Rossi, R., Mariucci, G., Tantucci, M., & Ambrosini, M. V. (2001). Effects of light physical exercise on sleep regulation in rats. *Medicine and Science in Sports and Exercise, 33(1)*, 57–60.

Heart and Stroke Foundation of Canada. (2005). *Risk factors: Coronary heart disease risk factor.* Retrieved from ww1.heartandstroke.ca/Page.asp?PageID=110&ArticleID=589&Src=heart.

Kesaniemi, Y. A., Danforth, E., Jensen, M. D., Kopelman, P. G., Lefebvre, P., & Reeder, B. A. (2001). Dose-response issues concerning physical activity and health: An evidence-based symposium. *Medicine and Science in Sports and Exercise, 33(6)*, S351–S358.

Kohl, H. W. (2001). Physical activity and cardiovascular disease: Evidence for a dose response. *Medicine and Science in Sports and Exercise, 33(6)*, S472–S483.

Laursen, P. B., & Jenkins, D. G. (2002). The scientific basis for high-intensity interval training: Optimising training programmes and maximising performance in highly trained endurance athletes. *Sports Medicine 32(1)*, 53–73.

Malina, R. M., Bouchard, C., & Bar-Or, O. (2004). *Growth, maturation, and physical activity.* Champaign, IL: Human Kinetics.

Manitoba Milk Producers, Nutrition Education Department. (2005). *Sport nutrition: Tips on food intake and fluid replacement to help athletes gain the "winning edge" in competition!* Dairy Farmers of Canada.

Mullineaux, D. R., Barnes, C. A., & Barnes, E. F. (2001). Factors affecting the likelihood to engage in adequate physical activity to promote health. *Journal of Sports Sciences, 19(4),* 279–288.

Powers, S., Criswell, D., Lieu, F.-K., Dodd, S., & Silverman, H. (1992). Exercise-induced cellular alterations in the diaphragm. *American Journal of Physiology, 263,* R1093–R1098.

Powers, S., Grinton, S., Lawler, J., Criswell, D., & Dodd, S. (1992). High intensity exercise training–induced metabolic alterations in respiratory muscles. *Respiration Physiology, 89,* 169–177.

Powers, S., & Howley, E. (2004). *Exercise physiology: Theory and application to fitness and performance* (5th ed.). Dubuque, IA: McGraw-Hill.

Ross, R., & Janssen, I. (2001). Physical activity, total and regional obesity: Dose-response considerations. *Medicine and Science in Sports and Exercise, 33(6),* S345–S641.

Statistics Canada. (2000/01). *High blood pressure, by age group and sex, household population aged 12 and over, Canada 2000/01.* Retrieved from www.statcan.ca/englishfreepub/82-221-XIE/00502/tables/html/1265.htm.

Svendahl, K., & MacIntosh, B. R. (2003). Anaerobic threshold: The concept and methods of measurement. *Canadian Journal of Applied Physiology 28(2),* 299–323.

Wong, S. L., Katzmarzyk, P. T., Nichaman, M. Z., Church, T. S., Blair, S. T., & Ross, R. (2004). Cardiorespiratory fitness is associated with lower abdominal fat independent of body mass index. *Medicine and Science in Sports and Exercise, 36(2),* 286–291.

LABORATORY 4.1

Developing Your Personal Exercise Prescription

Name_____ Age _____ Sex _____ Date _____

Using Tables 4.3 through 4.5 as models, develop your personal exercise prescription based on your current physical fitness level and goals. Record the appropriate information in the spaces provided below. Monitor your fitness levels periodically and adjust your prescription accordingly.

Week No.	Phase	Time (min/day)	Intensity (% of HR_{max})	Frequency (days/wk)	Exercise Type	Comments
1						
2						
3						
4						
5						
6						
7						
8						
9						
10						
11						
12						
13						
14						
15						
16						

LABORATORY 4.2

Cardiorespiratory Training Log

(Note: Make additional copies as needed.)

Name_____ Age _____ Sex _____ Date _____

In the spaces below keep a record of your training program. Exercise heart rate can be recorded as the range of heart rates measured at various times during the training session. Use the comments section to record any useful information concerning your exercise session, such as weather conditions, time of day, how you felt, and so on.

Date	Activity	Warm-Up Time	Exercise Time	Cool-Down Time	Exercise Heart Rate	Comments

CHAPTER 5

Exercise Prescription Principles: Muscular Strength and Endurance

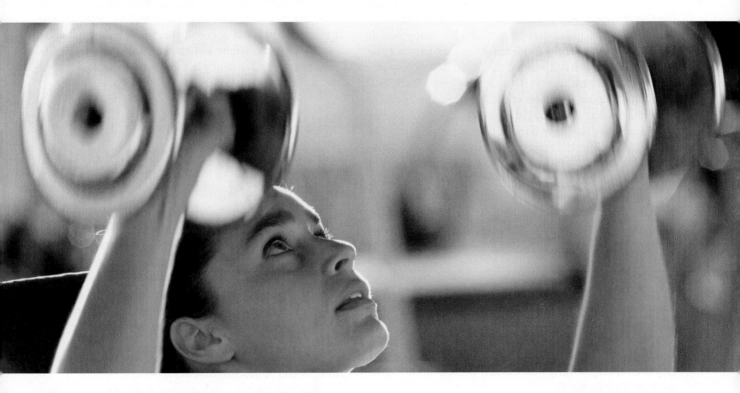

After studying this chapter, you should be able to

1. Explain the benefits of developing muscular strength and endurance.
2. Describe how muscles contract.
3. Distinguish the three muscle fibre types.
4. Describe physical activities that require a predominance of slow-twitch or fast-twitch muscle fibres.
5. Identify the major changes that occur in skeletal muscles in response to strength training.
6. List the factors that determine muscle strength and endurance.
7. Outline the principles used to design strength and endurance training programs.
8. Distinguish among the training programs for improving strength and endurance.
9. Design a program for improving strength and endurance.
10. Identify the safety precautions for strength and endurance training.

Lifting weights or performing other types of resistance exercises to build muscular strength and endurance is commonly referred to as *resistance training* or *strength training*. In addition to a brief overview of the benefits associated with developing muscular strength and endurance, this chapter discusses the principles and techniques employed in strength training programs.

Benefits of Muscular Strength and Endurance

Musculoskeletal fitness is related to health in males and females (Payne, Gledhill, Katzmarzyk, Jamnik, & Ferguson, 2000). In fact, regular strength training has many health benefits. For example, the incidence of low back pain, a common problem in men and women, can be reduced with appropriate strengthening exercises for the lower-back and abdominal muscles (Mannion et al., 2001). Further, muscle-strengthening exercises may reduce the occurrence of joint or muscle injuries that may happen during physical activity (Stone, 1990; Kibler, Chandler, & Stracener, 1992). As discussed in Chapter 1, strength training can postpone the age-related decreases in muscle strength experienced by sedentary older individuals (Tarpenning, Hamilton-Wessler, Wiswell, & Hawkins, 2004), as well as contribute to the prevention of the bone-wasting condition *osteoporosis* (Snow-Harter & Marcus, 1991). Favourable results of muscular strength training in the elderly may also be important in the prevention of falls (Chilibeck et al., 2002).

Another positive aspect of strength training is the improvement in personal appearance and self-esteem associated with increased muscular tone and strength (Dunn, Trivedi, & O'Neal, 2001). Increased muscular strength has many practical benefits in daily activities, such as an improved ability to carry heavy boxes, perform routine yard work, or do housework.

One of the most important benefits of strength training is that increasing muscle size results in an elevation in resting energy expenditure. *Resting energy expenditure,* called **resting metabolic rate,** is the total amount of energy the body requires to perform all necessary functions associated with maintaining life. For example, resting metabolic rate includes the energy required to drive the heart and respiratory muscles and to build and maintain body tissues. In other words, you can consider resting metabolic rate the "engine" of the body.

How does strength training influence resting metabolic rate? Strength training increases muscle mass, and since muscle tissue requires energy even at rest, then muscular enlargement increases resting energy expenditure. An increase of 0.5 kg of muscle elevates resting metabolism approximately 2 to 3 percent. This increase can be magnified with larger gains in muscle. For instance, a 2.5-kg increase in muscle mass would result in a 10- to 15-percent increase in resting metabolic rate. Changes in resting metabolic rate of this magnitude can play an important role in maintaining a desirable body weight and composition throughout life. Therefore, strength training is a key component of any physical fitness program.

Physiological Basis for Developing Strength and Endurance

The human body contains approximately 600 skeletal muscles. The primary function of skeletal muscles is to provide force for bodily movement. The body and its parts move when the appropriate muscles shorten and apply force to the bones. Skeletal muscles also assist in maintaining posture and regulating body temperature during cold exposure (for example, heat is produced through the mechanism of shivering). Because all physical activities require the use of skeletal muscles, some understanding of their structure and function is essential prior to discussing the principles of strength and endurance training programs.

Muscular strength and endurance are related, but they are not the same thing. *Muscular strength* is defined as the ability of a muscle to generate maximal force. In simple terms, muscular strength is the amount of weight that an individual can lift during one maximal effort. In contrast, *muscular endurance* is defined as the ability to generate force over and over again, or the ability to maintain a static position for a length of time. In general, increasing muscular strength will increase muscular endurance as well. However, training aimed at improving muscular endurance does not always improve muscular strength. Techniques to improve muscular strength and endurance are discussed later in this chapter.

Muscle Structure and Contraction

Muscle Structure Skeletal muscle is a collection of long thin cells called *fibres*. Each muscle fibre is composed of 100 to 1000 contractile units called *myofibrils* (Malina, Bouchard, & Bar-Or, 2004). Within each myofibril are

resting metabolic rate The amount of energy the body requires to perform all necessary functions associated with maintaining life.

elongated structures called *myofilaments*. These myofilaments interact and slide past one another during a muscle contraction.

Muscle fibres are surrounded by a dense layer of connective tissue called *fascia* that holds the individual fibres together and separates muscle from surrounding tissues (Figures 5.1 and 5.2).

Muscles are attached to bone by connective tissues known as *tendons*. Muscular contraction causes the tendons to pull on the bones, thereby causing movement. The major muscle groups are illustrated in Figure 5.3.

Muscle Contraction   Muscle contraction is regulated by signals coming from motor nerves. Motor nerves originate in the spinal cord and send nerve fibres to individual muscles throughout the body. A motor nerve and an individual muscle fibre meet and make contact at a *neuromuscular junction*. The relationship between a motor nerve and skeletal muscle fibres is illustrated in Figure 5.4. Note that each motor nerve branches and then connects with numerous individual muscle fibres. The motor nerve and all of the muscle fibres it controls is called a **motor unit.**

A muscle contraction begins when a message to contract (called a *nerve impulse*) reaches the neuromuscular junction (Figure 5.4). The arrival of the nerve impulse triggers the contraction process by permitting the interaction of contractile proteins in muscle.

Because the nerve impulse initiates the contractile process, it is logical that the removal of the nerve signal from the muscle would "turn off" the contractile process. Indeed, when a motor nerve ceases to send signals to a muscle, the contraction stops. Occasionally, an uncontrolled muscular contraction occurs, resulting in a muscle cramp.

Types of Muscle Contractions

Muscle contractions are classified into two major categories: dynamic and static. **Dynamic contractions** (also called *isotonic contractions*) are those that result in movement of a body part. Most physical activity, exercise, or sports skills utilize dynamic contractions. For example, lifting a dumbbell (Figure 5.5, top) involves movement of a body part and is classified as a dynamic contraction. A **static contraction** (also called *isometric contraction*) requires the development of muscular tension but results in no movement of body

motor unit   A motor nerve and the muscle fibres it controls.

dynamic contractions   Muscle contractions in which there is movement of a body part.

static contractions   Muscle contractions in which muscular tension is developed but no movement of body parts takes place.

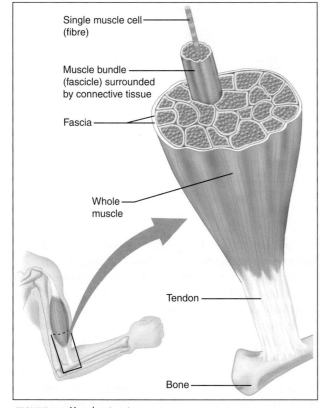

FIGURE 5.1 Muscle structure.

Source: Johnson, M. (2001). *Human biology*. San Francisco: Benjamin Cummings.

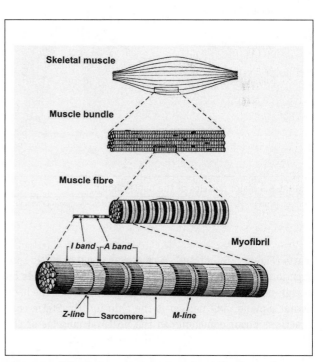

FIGURE 5.2 Schematic representation of a skeletal muscle, muscle fibre, myofibril, and sarcomere. The most important bands and lines on the myofibril are shown.

Source: From Malina, R. M., Bouchard C. , & Bar-Or, O. (2004). *Growth maturation and physical activity*. (2nd ed.), 139, Figure 7.1. Copyright 2004 by Robert M. Malina, Claude Bouchard and Oded Bar-Or. Reprinted with permission from Human Kinetics (Champaign, IL).

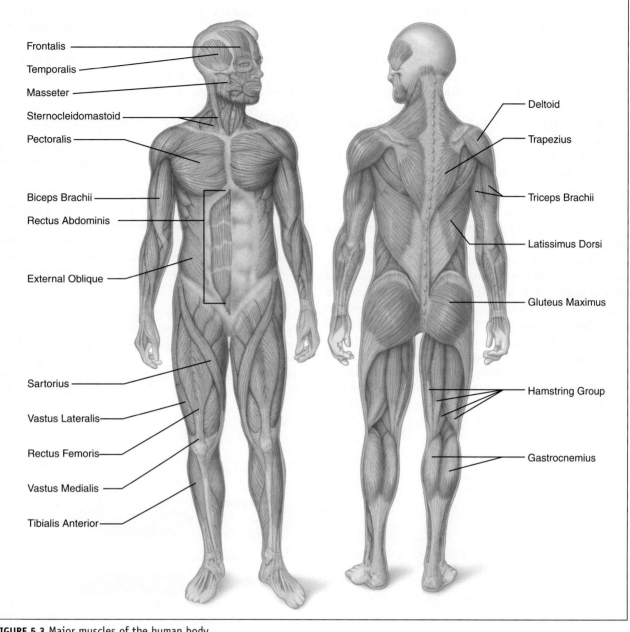

FIGURE 5.3 Major muscles of the human body.

Source: Johnson, M. (2001). *Human biology*. San Francisco: Benjamin Cummings.

parts (Figure 5.5, bottom). A classic example of static contraction is an individual hanging from his or her hands on a chin-up bar; the muscle is developing tension but the body is not moving, and neither is the chin-up bar. Static contractions occur commonly in the postural muscles of the body during sitting or standing; for instance, static contractions are responsible for holding the head upright.

Dynamic contractions can be further subdivided into concentric, eccentric, and isokinetic contractions. **Concentric contractions** are dynamic muscle contractions that result in the muscle shortening. The upward movement of the arm in Figure 5.6 is an example of a concentric contraction. In contrast, **eccentric contractions** are defined as contractions in which the muscle exerts force while it lengthens. For example, an eccentric contraction occurs when an individual resists the pull of a weight during the lowering phase of weight lifting (Figure 5.6). Here, the muscle is developing

concentric contractions   Dynamic contractions that result in muscle shortening.

eccentric contractions   Dynamic contractions that result the muscle lengthening.

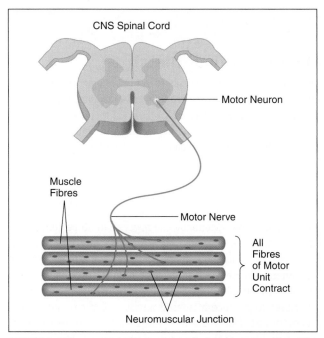

FIGURE 5.4 The concept of a motor unit. A motor nerve from the central nervous system is shown innervating several muscle fibres. With one impulse from the motor nerve, all fibres contract.

Source: Fox, E., Bowers, R., & Foss, M. (1997). *The physiological basis of physical education and athletics*. Madison, WI: Brown and Benchmark.

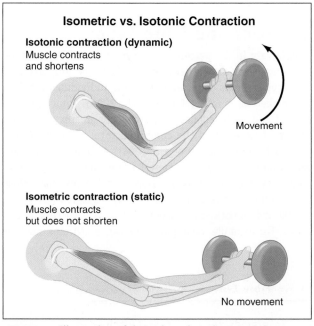

FIGURE 5.5 Illustration of dynamic and static contractions.

Source: Powers, S., & Howley, E. (2001). *Exercise physiology: Theory and application to fitness and performance*. Dubuque, IA: McGraw-Hill.

tension, but the force developed is not great enough to prevent the weight from being lowered.

Isokinetic contractions are concentric or eccentric contractions performed at a constant speed. That is, the speed of muscle shortening or lengthening is regulated at a fixed,

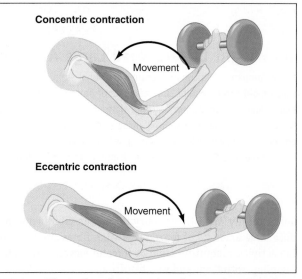

FIGURE 5.6 Illustration of concentric and eccentric contractions.

Source: Adapted from Powers, S., & Howley, E. (2001). *Exercise physiology: Theory and application to fitness and performance*. Dubuque, IA: McGraw-Hill.

controlled rate. This type of muscle contraction is generally accomplished by a resistance-training machine that controls the rate of muscle shortening or muscle lengthening.

Muscle Fibre Types

There are three types of skeletal muscle fibres: slow twitch, fast twitch, and intermediate. These fibre types differ in their speeds of contraction and in fatigue resistance (Pette, 2001). Because most human muscles contain a mixture of all three fibre types and the mixture is primarily genetically determined, it is important to understand each before discussing the strength-training process (Malina et al., 2004).

Slow-Twitch Fibres (Type I)
As the name implies, **slow-twitch fibres** contract slowly and produce a small amount of force. Further, these fibres are highly resistant to fatigue. Slow-twitch fibres, which are red in appearance, have the capacity to produce large quantities of ATP aerobically, making them suited to low-intensity prolonged physical activities like walking or slow jogging. Because of their resistance to fatigue, most postural muscles are composed primarily of slow-twitch fibres.

Fast-Twitch Fibres (Type IIA)
Fast-twitch fibres contract rapidly, generate great amounts of force, and fatigue quickly. These fibres are white and have a low aerobic capacity, but they are well equipped to produce ATP

isokinetic contractions Concentric or eccentric dynamic contractions performed at a constant speed.

slow-twitch fibres Muscle fibres that contract slowly and are highly resistant to fatigue.

fast-twitch fibres Muscle fibres that contract rapidly and fatigue quickly.

anaerobically. With their ability to shorten rapidly and produce large amounts of force, fast-twitch fibres are used during activities requiring rapid or forceful movement, such as jumping, sprinting, and weight lifting.

Intermediate Fibres (Type IIB)
Intermediate fibres, although more red in colour, possess a combination of the characteristics of fast- and slow-twitch fibres. They contract rapidly, produce great force, and are fatigue resistant due to a well-developed aerobic capacity. Intermediate fibres contract more quickly and produce more force than slow-twitch fibres, but contract more slowly and produce less force than fast-twitch fibres. They are more fatigue resistant than fast-twitch fibres but less fatigue resistant than slow-twitch fibres. Quite simply, they are an "intermediate" fibre. Table 5.1 summarizes the properties of all three fibre types.

Recruitment of Muscle Fibres During Physical Activities

Many types of physical activity use only a small fraction of the muscle fibres available in a muscle group. For example,

intermediate fibres Muscle fibres that possess a combination of the characteristics of fast- and slow-twitch fibres.

recruitment The process of involving more muscle fibres to increase muscular force.

walking at a slow speed may use fewer than 30 percent of the muscle fibres in the legs. More intense physical activity, however, requires more force. In order for a muscle group to generate more force, a greater number of muscle fibres must be called into play. The process of involving more muscle fibres to produce increased muscular force is called fibre **recruitment.** Figure 5.7 illustrates the order of recruitment of muscle fibres as the intensity of physical activity increases. Note that during low-intensity physical activity, only slow-twitch fibres are used. As the intensity increases, progressive recruitment of fibres occurs, from slow-twitch to intermediate fibres and finally to fast-twitch fibres. High-intensity activities like strength training recruit large numbers of fast-twitch fibres.

Genetics and Fibre Type

People vary in the percentage of type I, type IIA, and type IIB fibres their muscles contain. In fact, the proportion of fibre types varies considerably among individuals within a given skeletal muscle (Malina et al., 2004). Typically, adolescent and adult females have a slightly greater proportion of type I fibres than the combined total of type IIA and type II B fibres (Malina et al., 2004). Although adolescent males have slightly more type I fibres than the combination of type IIA and type IIB fibres, adult males have close to an equal ratio (Malina et al., 2004). Research has shown a relationship between muscle fibre type and success in athletics. For example, champion endurance athletes, such as

Property	Fibre Type		
	Slow-Twitch	**Intermediate**	**Fast-Twitch**
Contraction speed	Slow	Intermediate	Fast
Resistance to fatigue	High	Intermediate	Low
Predominant energy system	Aerobic	Combination aerobic and anaerobic	Anaerobic
Force generation	Low	Intermediate	High

TABLE 5.1 Properties of Human Skeletal Muscle Fibre Types

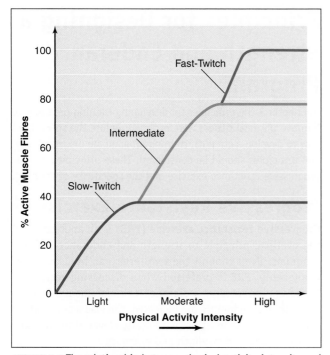

FIGURE 5.7 The relationship between physical activity intensity and recruitment of muscle-fibre type.

Source: Adapted from Powers, S., & Howley, E. (2001). *Exercise physiology: Theory and application to fitness and performance*. Dubuque, IA: McGraw-Hill.

marathon runners, have a predominance of slow-twitch fibres. This is logical, because endurance sports require muscles with high fatigue resistance. In contrast, elite sprinters, such as 100-metre runners, possess a predominance of fast-twitch fibres. Because of the interrelationship among genetics, fibre type, and athletic success, some researchers have jokingly suggested that if you want to be a champion athlete, you must pick your parents wisely!

Factors That Determine Muscular Strength

Two primary physiological factors determine the amount of force a muscle can generate: the size of the muscle and the number of fibres recruited during the contraction.

Muscle Size
The primary determinant of how much force a muscle can generate is its size. The larger the muscle, the greater the force it can produce. Although there is no difference in the chemical makeup of muscle in men and

anabolic steroids Synthetic hormones (usually testosterone) that cause the body to produce muscle and prevent muscle breakdown.
androgenic steroids Weaker anabolic steroids.

A CLOSER LOOK

Anabolic Steroid Use

The use of *anabolic–androgenic steroids* continues to be a concern. **Anabolic steroids** are synthetic hormones (usually testosterone) that cause the body to produce muscle and prevent muscle breakdown. **Androgenic steroids** refer to a weaker anabolic steroid. Contrary to popular opinion, not only athletes use anabolic steroids. In fact, a study of more than 16 000 Canadian students in Grades 6 through 12 (ages 11 to 18) reported that 2.8 percent of the respondents had used anabolic–androgenic steroids in the past year (Melia, Pipe, & Greenberg, 1996). Many students used steroids to alter body build as opposed to improving athletic performance. Of the 29.4 percent who reported they injected their steroids, 29.2 percent shared needles—this statistic is of particular concern given the increased risk of contracting HIV created by exposure to shared needles.

The fierce competition in bodybuilding and sports in which strength and power are necessary for success has driven men and women to risk serious health consequences in order to gain an edge over their competitors. The use of steroids has been associated with many health risks. Peterson (2002) listed the following 10 negative side effects:

1. **Heightened risk of injury**—steroid use elevates the risk of tendon and ligament injury, because muscle tissue strengthens more quickly than connective tissue.

2. **Unbecoming conduct**—steroid use causes increased aggressive behaviour.

3. **Increased risk for heart disease**—steroid use increases "bad" cholesterol (LDL-C) and decreases "good" cholesterol (HDL-C).

4. **Beleaguered complexion**—steroid use may cause severe acne from enlarged oil glands that secrete more frequently.

5. **Blood clots**—steroid use promotes increased blood stickiness; therefore, there is an increased risk of heart attack and stroke.

6. **Arrested development**—steroid use may cause premature closure of the growth plates in children and adolescents.

7. **Liver toxicity**—steroid use causes an increased risk of cysts and tumours; since the liver is the main site to clear steroids from the body, an excessive intake can be toxic.

8. **Loss of hair**—steroid use may cause men prone to baldness to lose their hair faster.

9. **Reduced sex drive**—steroid use may reduce sex drive; testicles may atrophy, sperm production may decrease, and production of reproductive hormones may decrease.

10. **Masculinizing/feminizing effects**—in women, steroid use may cause an enhancement of male characteristics including deepening of voice, increase in facial hair, and development of a "manly" shape. Further, a woman's breasts may reduce in size and her menstrual cycle can be disrupted. In men, breast-like tissue may develop.

women, men are generally stronger than women because men have a greater muscle mass (i.e., larger muscles). The larger muscle mass in men is primarily due to hormonal differences between the sexes; men have higher levels of the male sex hormone testosterone. The fact that testosterone promotes an increase in muscle size has led some athletes to attempt to improve muscular strength with various androgenic drugs (for more information, see A Closer Look: "Anabolic Steroid Use").

Muscle Fibre Recruitment   As noted previously, the number of muscle fibres recruited influences the production of muscle force. The more muscle fibres stimulated, the greater the muscle force generated, because the force generated by individual fibres is additive (Figure 5.8).

Muscle fibre recruitment is regulated voluntarily through the nervous system. That is, we determine how many muscle fibres to recruit by making a decision about how much effort to put into a particular movement. For instance, when we choose to make a minimal effort in lifting an object, we recruit only a few motor units, and the muscle develops limited force. However, if we make a decision to exert our maximal effort in lifting a heavy object, many muscle fibres are recruited and great force is generated (Figure 5.8).

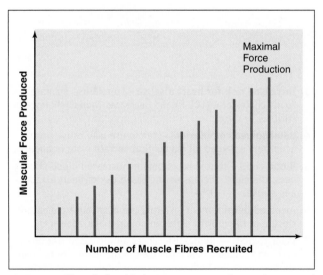

FIGURE 5.8 The relationship between motor unit recruitment and muscular force production.

progressive resistance exercise (PRE)   The application of the overload principle to strength and endurance training programs.

specificity of training   The development of muscular strength and endurance is specific to the muscle group exercised and the training intensity.

Principles for Designing a Strength and Endurance Program

In Chapter 3 the principles for developing training programs to improve physical fitness were outlined. Before the specifics of how to develop a strength training program are discussed, several principles should be considered. These principles include progressive resistance exercise and the specificity of training.

Progressive Resistance Exercise

Progressive resistance exercise (PRE) is an application of the overload principle to strength and endurance training programs. Even though the two terms can be used interchangeably, PRE is preferred when discussing resistance training. Progressive resistance exercise means that as strength and endurance are increased, the load against which the muscle works must be periodically elevated to continue to realize gains in strength and endurance.

Specificity of Training

The principle of **specificity of training** means that development of muscular strength and endurance is specific to the muscle group that is exercised and the training intensity. First, only the muscles trained will improve in strength and endurance. For example, if an individual wishes to improve the strength of the supporting musculature of the lower back, strengthening the arm muscles would not be effective for reaching that goal. The specific muscles involved with movement of the lower back should be trained instead. Second, the training intensity determines whether the muscular adaptation is primarily an increase in strength or endurance. High-intensity training (e.g., lifting heavy weights for 4 to 6 reps) results in an increase in muscular strength and size with some improvements in muscular endurance. Conversely, high-repetition, low-intensity training (e.g., lifting light weights 15 reps or more) promotes an increase in muscular endurance, with limited improvements in muscular size and strength (see Figure 5.9).

Designing a Training Program for Increasing Muscle Strength

There are numerous approaches to the design of resistance-training programs. Any program that adheres to the basic principles described earlier will result in an improvement in strength and endurance. However, the type of resistance-training program you develop for yourself depends on your

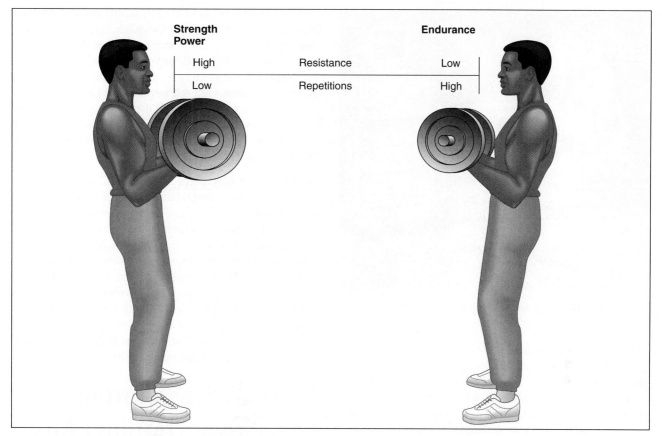

Strength Power		Endurance
High	Resistance	Low
Low	Repetitions	High

FIGURE 5.9 The strength–endurance continuum.

goals and the types of equipment available to you. Other considerations in the development of a resistance-training program include safety, strength versus endurance, and types of programs.

Safety Concerns

The need for safety while resistance training should be emphasized. Resistance training can be performed safely, if the following guidelines are adhered to:

1. When using free weights (like barbells), have spotters (helpers) assist you in the performance of exercises. They can help you if you are unable to complete a lift.
2. Ensure the collars on the ends of the bars of free weights are tightly secured to prevent the weights from falling off. Dropping weight plates can result in serious injuries.
3. Warm up prior to resistance training. Generally, 5 to 10 minutes of large body movements suffice.
4. Breathe regularly during resistance training. Avoid holding your breath. A recommended breathing pattern is to exhale while lifting the weight and inhale while lowering. Also, breathe through your nose and mouth. The static nature of resistance training can lead to breath holding (called a **valsalva manoeuvre**), which can reduce blood flow to the brain and cause dizziness and

fainting. In an individual at high risk for coronary disease, the manoeuvre could be extremely dangerous and should always be avoided.

5. Slow and controlled movements may reduce the risk of injury.
6. Use light weights in the beginning so body alignment and the proper manoeuvre can be achieved in each exercise. This is particularly true when lifting free weights.
7. Do not sacrifice body alignment and proper technique to lift heavier weights or to perform more push-ups, curl-ups, chin-ups, or other resistance training exercises.

Training to Improve Strength versus Endurance

Resistance-training programs specifically designed to improve strength and programs designed to improve muscular endurance differ mainly in the number of repetitions and sets (i.e., the number of lifts performed) and the amount of

valsalva manoeuvre Breath holding during an intense muscle contraction; can reduce blood flow to the brain and cause dizziness and fainting.

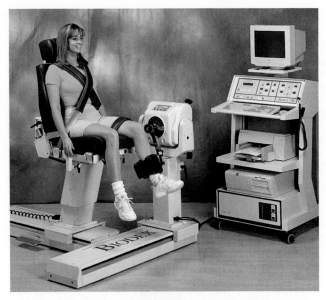

A commercially available isokinetic strength-training device.

resistance (Fleck & Kraemer, 1997). A resistance-training program using low repetitions and high resistance results in the greatest strength gains, whereas a program using high repetitions and low resistance results in the greatest improvement in muscular endurance. It is important to appreciate that low-repetition/high-resistance training increases not only strength, but also muscular endurance. In contrast, resistance training using high repetitions and low resistance improves endurance, but has little effect on strength.

Types of Resistance-Training Programs

Resistance-training programs can be divided into three general categories classified by the type of muscle contraction involved: dynamic (isotonic), static (isometric), and isokinetic.

Dynamic Programs
Dynamic programs, like dynamic contractions, involve contracting a muscle against a movable load (although usually a free weight or weights mounted by cables or chains to form a weight machine, it can also involve whole body exercises such as push-ups, curl-ups, and chin-ups). Dynamic programs are very popular and are the most common type of resistance-training program in use today.

Static Programs
A static strength-training program is based on the concept of contracting a muscle at a fixed angle against an immovable object, using static contraction.

Two important aspects of static training make it different from dynamic training. First, in static training the development of strength and endurance is specific to the joint angle at which the muscle group is trained (Kitai, 1989). Therefore, if static techniques are used, static contractions at several different joint angles are needed to gain strength and endurance throughout a full range of motion. In contrast, because dynamic contractions generally involve the full range of joint motion, strength is developed over the full movement pattern.

Isokinetic Programs
Recall that isokinetic contractions are dynamic contractions performed at a constant speed. Isokinetic training is a relatively new strength training method, so limited research exists to describe its strength benefits compared with those of static and dynamic programs. Isokinetic exercises require the use of machines that govern the speed of movement during muscle contraction. The first isokinetic machines available were very expensive and used primarily in clinical settings for injury rehabilitation. Recently, less expensive machines use a piston device (much like a shock absorber on a car) to limit the speed of movement throughout the range of the exercise.

Exercise Prescription for Resistance Training: An Overview

The general concepts of the frequency, intensity, time, and type of exercise required to improve physical fitness were discussed in Chapter 3. Although these same concepts apply to improving muscular strength and endurance via resistance training, the terminology used to monitor the intensity and time is unique. For example, the intensity of resistance training is measured not by heart rate but by the number of "repetition maximums." Similarly, the time of resistance training is monitored not by duration but by the number of repetitions and sets performed.

The intensity of exercise in dynamic and isokinetic strength-training programs is measured by the concept of the **repetition maximum (RM).** The RM is the maximal load that a muscle group can lift a specified number of times before tiring. For example, 6 RM is the maximal load that can be lifted 6 times.

The number of repetitions (reps) performed consecutively without resting is called a **set.** In the example of 6 RM, 1 set = 6 reps. Because the amount of rest required between sets varies among individuals depending on level of fitness, the time of strength training is measured by the number of sets performed, not by duration.

Although disagreement exists as to the optimum number of reps and sets required to improve strength and endurance, some general guidelines can be provided. Table 5.2 presents an overview of these guidelines.

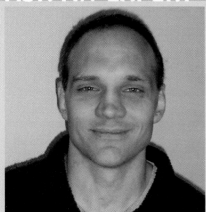

Philip Chilibeck, Ph.D.

Resistance Training

Dr. Chilibeck is an Associate Professor in the College of Kinesiology at the University of Saskatchewan. His main research interests are the adaptation of muscle and bone to exercise and nutritional interventions. Dr. Chilibeck's research has involved a variety of populations including healthy young adults, older adults, individuals with spinal cord injury, and individuals with conditions that affect bone mineral status. Here, Dr. Chilibeck responds to a few common questions about strength training.

Q: How many sets are optimal during strength training for improving strength?

A: The number of sets you choose depends on your level of training. For beginners, 1 to 2 sets per exercise are adequate for improving strength. Strength in untrained individuals increases rapidly at the beginning of a training program; therefore, only a small stimulus is required for strength development. One to two sets would also be optimal for safety and increasing compliance to programs for beginners. People with more advanced training backgrounds benefit the most from multiple-set routines (e.g., sets per exercise could vary from approximately 3 to 6). When one adapts to a training stimulus, an increased stimulus, or progressive overload, is necessary to continue to increase strength. For an advanced program, optimal strength development would occur with a relatively high number of sets, low repetitions per set, high loads or resistance, and a long rest interval between sets. Usually, advanced programs use a principle called "periodization," where training with heavy loads, low repetitions, and high sets is alternated with periods of training with lighter loads, higher repetitions, and fewer sets. This prevents overtraining and allows for optimal strength development.

Q: After starting a training program several months ago, my strength gains have plateaued. What can I do to further increase my strength?

A: In my opinion the best way to overcome a strength plateau is to introduce more variety in a training program. Do not use the same exercises for too long. Variety can be introduced by altering any of the following: starting positions for exercises (e.g., incline or decline bench press), number of sets or repetitions, load, speed of movement, rest periods between sets, and type of exercise for a specific muscle group. A general guide to follow is that something about your training program should be changed every 2 to 3 weeks. Free weights (barbells and dumbbells) are better to use than machines to achieve greater variety. One should also keep a training log or diary to record weight/resistance used, sets, and repetitions. Using a training diary allows you to better achieve goals, acts as a motivational tool, and allows you to better track your progress. If you find from your training log that you cannot increase your resistance or number of repetitions per set for a given exercise, then it is probably time to introduce a different exercise for that muscle group.

Q: Is creatine beneficial for increasing muscle mass and strength?

A: There is a mixture of results from studies of creatine, with some showing no beneficial effects; however, most studies indicate it is beneficial to use creatine for increasing strength and lean tissue mass. There is controversy on whether there is a true increase in muscle mass (protein) or whether the muscle retains more water when creatine is ingested. The increase in strength with creatine supplementation may either come from a direct increase in muscle mass (i.e., stimulation of protein synthesis or inhibition of protein degradation) or from a higher store of phosphocreatine, which is an immediate energy source within the muscle that could allow one to train with a greater volume (i.e., a higher number of repetitions, sets, or resistance). This would indirectly lead to an increased muscle mass as the muscle adapts to a higher volume of training. Creatine supplementation usually involves a "loading phase," where one loads the muscle by ingesting 15 to 20 grams of creatine per day for 5 to 7 days, and a "maintenance" phase, where one ingests 3 to 5 grams of creatine per day to maintain the high "loaded" level of creatine in the muscle. Recent studies indicate that a constant moderate dose of creatine (i.e., 5 to 7 grams per day) can also be effective. Ingesting creatine in combination with carbohydrate or protein-containing foods is more effective than taking creatine by itself. The ingestion of other food will increase the amount of insulin released in the body, and this stimulates the uptake of creatine into muscle. There may be "responders" and "non-responders" to creatine supplementation; that is, it may be beneficial for some people, but not for others. Studies indicate that people with a low meat intake (e.g., vegetarians) may respond better to creatine supplementation. The safety of creatine supplementation continues to be debated. Most studies indicate that creatine supplementation is relatively safe, but there will always be questions about long-term effects of high doses of creatine. The ethics of using creatine as a legal ergogenic aid will also continue to be debated.

Plyometric Training Is Not for Everyone

You may have heard the term *plyometrics* used in reference to training for athletes. Athletes use this technique to develop explosive power. Plyometric training is performed by quickly stretching a muscle prior to initiating a maximal contraction. Plyometric training is based on the principle that stretching a muscle prior to contraction enables a greater force to be generated by the muscle. A common example is the vertical jump. When you attempt to jump as high as possible, you almost always bend your knees quickly and "rebound" in order to maximize your jump height. You can certainly jump higher by using this "rebound" than by starting the jump with your knees already bent. This is effectively what plyometric training does.

The most common method of plyometric training is called "drop jumping"—dropping from a height and rebounding (see the illustration). This exercise requires the athlete to drop (not jump) to the ground from a platform or box, and then immediately jump. The drop prestretches the muscles, and the jump overloads the muscles with the ensuing concentric contraction. The exercise is more effective the shorter the time the feet are in contact with the ground. The amount of load placed on the muscles is determined in part by the height of the drop, which should be in the range of 30 to 75 cm. Drop jumping is a relatively high-impact form of

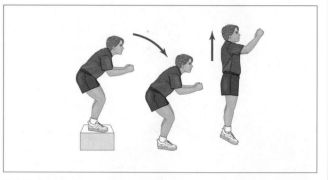

A drop jump.

training and should not be introduced until after an athlete has used lower-impact alternatives, such as two-footed jumping on the ground.

Because of the dynamic nature of plyometric training, there is great potential for injury to muscles and joints. For a basic fitness program, there is no need to include a high-risk type of training when a low-risk activity will accomplish the same goal. This training technique is best reserved for athletes looking for a competitive edge and for closely supervised rehabilitation programs.

		Novice	Intermediate	Advanced
Strength	Repetitions	8–12	6–12	1–12
	Sets	1–3	multi	multi
	Intensity	60–70% 1 RM	70–80% 1 RM	70–100% 1 RM
	Frequency	2–3 days/week	2–4 days/week	4–6 days/week
Endurance	Repetitions	10–15	10–15	10–25
	Sets	1–3	multi	multi
	Intensity	50–70% 1 RM	50–70% 1 RM	30–80% 1 RM
	Frequency	2–3 days/week	2–4 days/week	4–6 days/week

TABLE 5.2 Recommendations for Number of Repetitions and Sets for Strength and Endurance Training

Source: Adapted from Kraemer, W. J., & Ratamess, N. A. (2004). Fundamentals of resistance training: Progression and exercise prescription. *Medicine and Science in Sports and Exercise, 36(4),* 674–688.

To improve strength, the novice weight lifter should use 1 to 3 sets of 8 to 12 repetitions (Kraemer & Ratamess, 2004). The advanced weight lifter generally uses a higher intensity with multiple sets of 1 to 12 repetitions (Kraemer & Ratamess, 2004).

The concept of progressive resistance applied to a strength-training program involves increasing the amount of

weight to be lifted or resistance used a specific number of reps and sets. As your training progresses and you become stronger, the amount of weight lifted or resistance used must be increased. A good guideline is that once 12 reps can be performed, the load should be increased to a level at which 8 reps are again maximal. Figure 5.10 illustrates the relationship between strength improvement and various

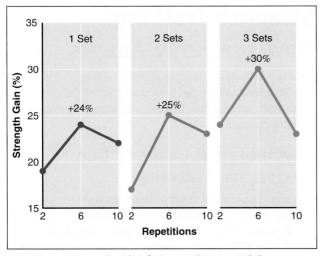

FIGURE 5.10 Strength gains from a resistance training program consisting of various sets and repetitions. All programs were performed 3 days per week for 12 weeks. Note that the greatest strength gains (130-percent improvement) were obtained using 3 sets of 6 reps per set.

Source: Adapted from Fox, E., Bowers, R., & Foss, M. (1998). *Fox's physiological basis of exercise and sports.* Boston: WCB-McGraw-Hill.

combinations of reps and sets. A key point in Figure 5.10 is that programs involving 3 sets result in the greatest strength gains. This is because the third set requires the greatest effort and thus is the greatest overload for the muscle. Although it may seem that adding a fourth set should elicit even greater gains, 4 or more sets results in overtraining and decreased benefits (Kraemer & Ratamess, 2004).

To improve muscular endurance, 1 to 3 sets of 10 to 15 reps (Table 5.2) for each exercise are recommended. Muscular endurance can be improved by either increasing the number of reps progressively while maintaining the same load, or increasing the amount of resistance while maintaining the same number of reps. The advantage of the latter is that muscular strength would also improve.

What role does training frequency play in the development of strength? Most research suggests that 2 to 3 days of training per week is optimal for strength gains (Powers & Howley, 2004). Once the desired level of strength has been achieved, one high-intensity training session per week is considered sufficient to maintain the new level of strength. The optimal frequency of training to improve muscular endurance is 2 to 6 days per week depending on individual goals and level of experience (see Table 5.2) (Leveritt, Abernethy, Barry, & Logan, 1999).

Starting and Maintaining a Resistance-Training Program

You should begin your resistance-training program with short- and long-term goals. Identifying goals is an important

means of maintaining interest and enthusiasm for strength training. A key point is to establish realistic short-term goals that can be reached in the first several weeks of training. Reaching these goals usually provides the motivation needed to continue training.

Developing an Individualized Exercise Prescription

An exercise prescription for strength training has three stages: the starter phase, the slow progression phase, and the maintenance phase.

Starter Phase The primary objective of the starter phase is to build strength gradually without developing undue muscular soreness or injury. This can be accomplished by starting your resistance-training program slowly—beginning with light resistance, a high number of repetitions, and only 2 sets per exercise. The recommended frequency of training during this phase is twice per week. The duration of this phase varies from 1 to 3 weeks, depending on your initial fitness level. A sedentary person might spend 3 weeks in the starter phase, whereas a relatively well-trained person may spend only 1 to 2 weeks.

Slow Progression Phase This phase may last 4 to 20 weeks depending on your initial strength and long-term goal. The transition from the starter phase to the slow progression phase involves three changes in the exercise prescription: increasing the frequency of training from 2 to 3 or 4 days per week; increasing the amount of resistance, decreasing the number of repetitions; and increasing the number of sets performed to 3 sets.

The objective of the slow progression phase is to gradually increase muscular strength until you reach your desired level. After reaching your strength goal, your long-term objective becomes maintenance.

Maintenance Phase After reaching your strength goals, the problem becomes how to maintain your strength. The bad news is that maintaining strength requires a lifelong resistance-training effort. Strength is lost if you do not continue to resistance train. The good news is that the effort required to maintain muscular strength is less than the initial effort needed to gain it. As little as one workout per week is all that is required to maintain strength. A sample exercise prescription incorporating all three training phases follows.

Sample Exercise Prescription for Resistance Training

Getting Started Similar to training to improve cardiorespiratory endurance, the exercise prescription for improving muscular strength must be tailored to the individual. Before starting a program, keep in mind the guidelines and precautions in Table 5.3.

TABLE 5.3 Guidelines and Precautions to Follow Prior to Beginning a Strength-Training Program

Details of the Prescription As mentioned earlier, the time of the starter and slow progression phases varies depending on initial level of fitness. When the strength goals of the program are reached, the maintenance phase begins. This period utilizes the same routine as used during the progression phase but may be done only once per week.

Sample Strength-Training Exercises The dynamic strength-training program contains 12 exercises designed to provide a whole-body workout. Although specific machines are used in the following examples, barbells or whole-body exercises may also be used. It is important to remember that safety, maintaining body alignment, and proper lifting technique are especially important when using barbells.

A resistance-training program is described and illustrated in Exercises 5.1 through 5.12. This selection of exercises is designed to provide a comprehensive strength-training program that focuses on the major muscle groups. Many more exercises exist; some use the same muscle groups as those covered here, but simply use a different kind of resistance (e.g., dumbbells or the body). Be aware of which muscle groups are involved in an exercise in order to avoid overtraining one muscle group (Figure 5.3). Note that it is not necessary to perform all 12 exercises in one workout session; you can perform half of the exercises on one day and the remaining exercises on an alternate day.

Use Laboratory 5.1 on page 131 to keep a record of your training progress. Remember: maintenance and review of your training progress will help motivate you to continue your strength-training program!

hypertrophy An increase in muscle fibre size.
hyperplasia An increase in the number of muscle fibres.

Strength Training: How the Body Adapts

What physiological changes occur as a result of strength training? How quickly can muscular strength be gained? Do men and women differ in their responses to resistance-training programs?

Physiological Changes Due to Resistance Training

Programs designed to improve muscular strength can do so only by increasing muscle size or by increasing the number of muscle fibres recruited. In fact, both these factors are altered by strength training (Fleck & Kraemer, 1997). Strength-training programs increase muscular strength first by altering fibre recruitment patterns due to changes in the nervous system, and then by increasing muscle size (Figure 5.11).

How do muscles increase in size? Muscle size is increased primarily through an increase in fibre size, called **hypertrophy** (Fleck & Kraemer, 1997). The formation of new muscle fibres, a process called **hyperplasia,** is not involved in postnatal muscle growth. It should be noted that the increase in muscle size due to strength training depends on nutritional intake, the muscle fibre type (fast-twitch fibres may hypertrophy more than slow-twitch fibres), blood levels of testosterone, and the type of training program.

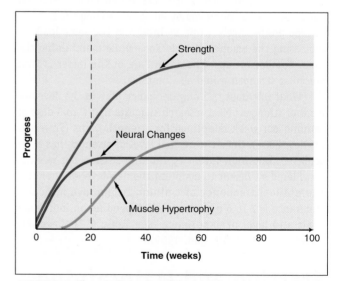

FIGURE 5.11 The relative roles of the nervous system and muscular adaptation in strength development. Strength training increases muscular strength first through changes in the nervous system and then by increasing muscle size.

Source: Wilmore, J. H., & Costill, D. L. (1994). *Physiology of sport and exercise.* Champaign, IL: Human Kinetics.

Dynamic Strength-Training Exercises

Exercise 5.1 Lower Back Extension

Purpose: To strengthen the muscles of the lower back and buttocks.

Movement: Position the thighs and upper back against the padded bars (a). Buckle the strap around the thighs. Slowly press backward against the padded bar until the back is fully extended (b). Slowly return to the original position.

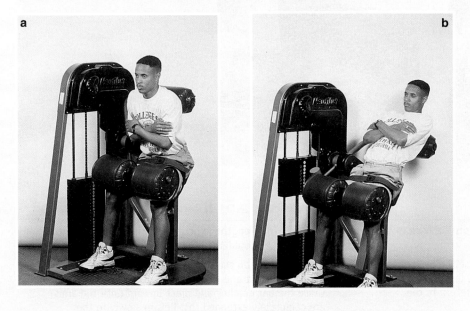

Exercise 5.2 Hip and Back

Purpose: To strengthen the muscles of the hip and lower back.

Movement: Lying on the left side, grasp the handles at both sides for stability. Place the back of the knees against the padded bars (a). Press the legs back until fully extended (b). Slowly return to the original position.

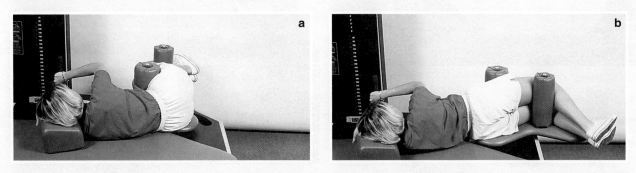

Exercise 5.3 Leg Extension

Purpose: To strengthen the muscles in the front of the upper leg.

Movement: Sitting in a nearly upright position, grasp the handles on the side of the machine (a). Extend the legs until they are completely straight (b) and then slowly return to the starting position.

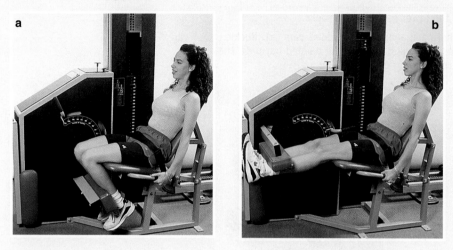

Exercise 5.4 Leg Curl

Purpose: To strengthen the muscles on the back of the upper leg and buttocks.

Movement: Lying on the left side, place the back of the feet over the padded bar (a). Curl the legs to at least a 90-degree angle (b) and then slowly return to the original position.

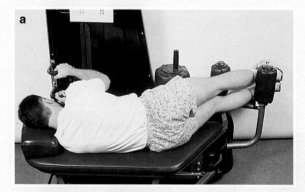

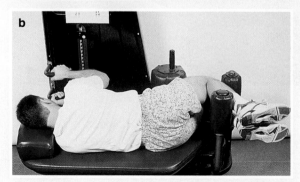

Exercise 5.5 Bench Press

Purpose: To strengthen the muscles in the chest, the front of the shoulders, and the back of the upper arm.

Movement: Lie on the bench with the bench press bar above the chest and the feet flat on the foot rest (a). Grasp the bar handles and press upward until the arms are completely extended (b). Return slowly to the original position. **Caution:** Do not arch the back while performing this exercise.

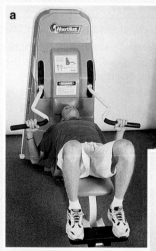

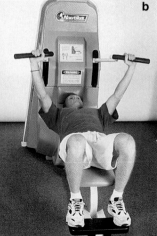

Exercise 5.6 Chest Press

Purpose: To strengthen the muscles of the chest and shoulder.

Movement: With the elbows bent at a 90-degree angle and the forearms against the pads (a), press the arms forward as far as possible, leading with the elbows (b). Slowly return to the original position.

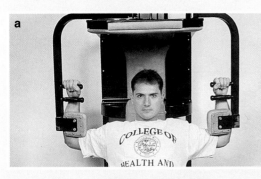

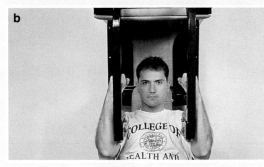

Exercise 5.7 Upper Back

Purpose: To strengthen the muscles of the upper back.

Movement: Sit in the machine with elbows bent and the backs of the arms resting against the padded bars (a). Press the arms back as far as possible, drawing the shoulder blades together (b). Slowly return to the original position.

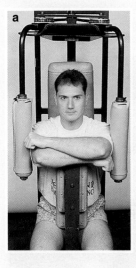
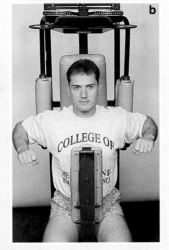

Exercise 5.8 Torso Twist

Purpose: To strengthen the muscles on the sides of the abdomen.

Movement: Sitting upright with the elbows behind the padded bars, twist the torso as far as possible to one side (a). Slowly return to the original position and repeat to the other side (b).

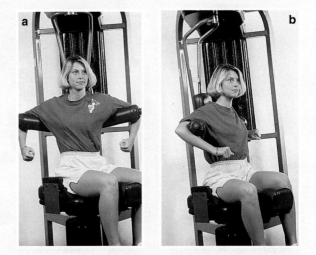

Exercise 5.9 Triceps Extension

Purpose: To strengthen the muscles on the back of the upper arm.

Movement: Sit upright with elbows bent (a). With the little-finger side of the hand against the pad, fully extend the arms (b) and then slowly return to the original position.

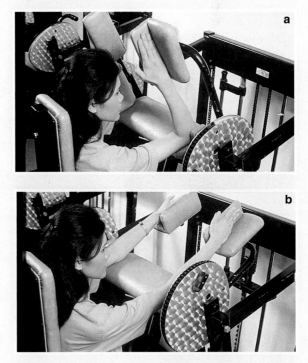

Exercise 5.10 Pullover

Purpose: To strengthen the muscles of the chest, shoulder, and side of the trunk.

Movement: Sit with elbows against the padded end of the movement arm and grasp the bar behind your head (a). Press forward and down with the arms, pulling the bar overhead and down to the abdomen (b). Slowly return to the original position.

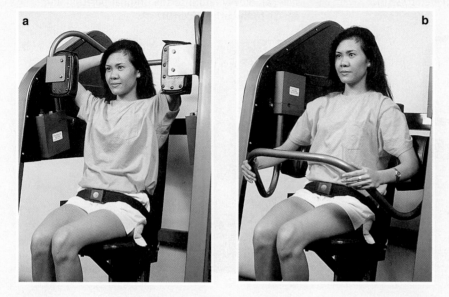

Exercise 5.11 Biceps Curl

Purpose: To strengthen the muscles in the front of the upper arm that cause flexion at the elbow.

Movement: Holding the grips with palms up and arms extended (a), curl up as far as possible (b) and slowly return to the starting position.

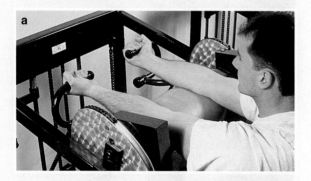

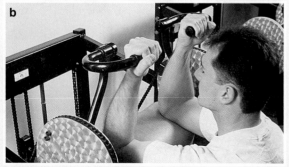

Exercise 5.12 Abdominal Curl

Purpose: To strengthen the abdominal muscles.

Movement: Place hands on the abdomen (a) and curl forward, bringing the chest toward the knees (b). Slowly return to the upright position.

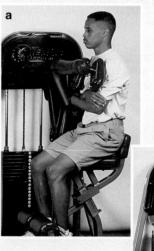

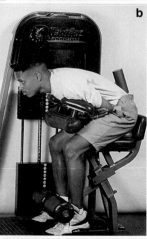

Whole-Body Strength-Training Exercises

Exercise 5.13 Push-Ups

Purpose: To strengthen the muscles of the upper body including muscles in the chest, shoulders, and arms.

Movement: With the body as straight as possible, lower your body by bending at the elbow until you are almost touching the floor. Exhale as you straighten your arms to return to the starting position.

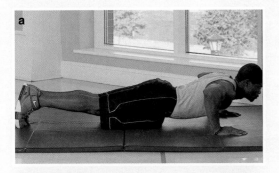

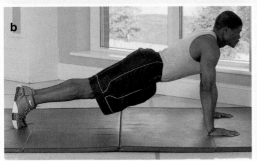

Exercise 5.15 Curl-Ups

Purpose: To strengthen the abdominal muscles.

Movement: Begin lying on your back with your arms folded over your chest or at your side, knees bent with feet flat on the floor. Curl up your trunk by raising your head and shoulders off the floor. Lower to the starting position.

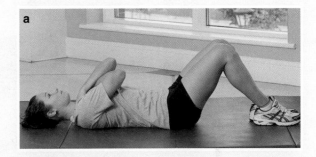

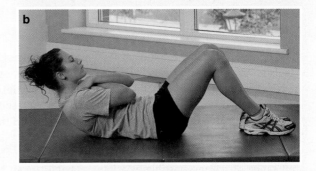

Exercise 5.14 Dips

Purpose: To strengthen the muscles of the arms and shoulders.

Movement: Using a bench or step, keep your hips close to the bench. Begin with your hands directly under your shoulders and arms straight. Lower your body as far as you can, then straighten to return to the starting position.

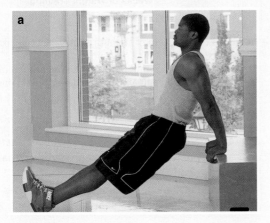

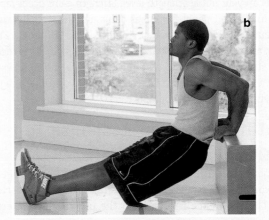

Exercise 5.16 Reverse Crunches

Purpose: To strengthen the abdominal muscles.

Movement: Begin lying on your back with your knees bent and over your hips. Contract your abdominal muscles so that your lower back is flattened and pressed to the floor. Then pull your hips up and toward your chest as far as you can go. Lower to the starting position.

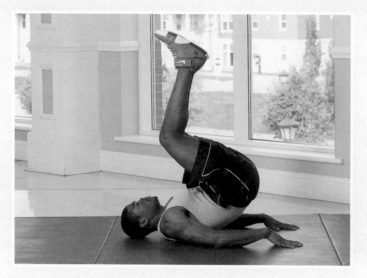

Although regular strength training does not result in improvements in cardiorespiratory fitness (Leveritt et al., 1999), it can provide positive changes in body composition and flexibility. For most men and women, rigorous resistance training results in an increase in muscle mass and a loss of body fat, with the end result of a decrease in percentage body fat.

If resistance-training exercises are performed over the full range of motion possible at a joint, flexibility can be improved (Kraemer & Ratamess, 2004). Many diligent weight lifters have excellent flexibility.

Rate of Strength Improvement with Resistance Training

How rapidly does strength improvement occur? The answer depends on your initial strength level. Strength gains occur rapidly in untrained people, whereas gains are more gradual in individuals with relatively higher strength levels (Figure 5.12). Indeed, an exciting point about resistance training for a novice is that strength gains occur very quickly (Enoka, 1997). These rapid strength gains often provide motivation to continue a regular resistance-training program.

Sex Differences in Response to Weight Training

In terms of absolute strength, men tend to be stronger than women because men generally have a greater muscle mass. The difference is greater in the upper body, where

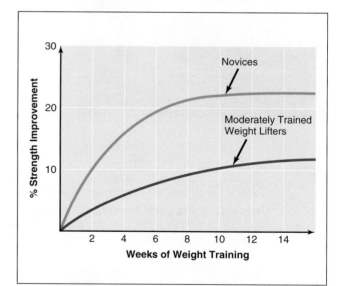

FIGURE 5.12 Time course of strength improvement in novice weight lifters versus moderately well-trained weight lifters. The rate of improvement and the total percentage strength improvement is greater in novices compared with moderately trained weight lifters.

men are approximately 50 percent stronger than women; men are approximately 30 percent stronger than women in the lower body.

Do men and women differ in their responses to resistance-training programs? In short, no (Shephard, 2000). On

Frequently Asked Questions About Resistance Training

How much rest is necessary between training sessions?
Getting the correct amount of rest is as important as doing the proper exercises! Resistance training depletes energy stores and damages muscle fibres. With the proper rest, water intake, and nutrition, the muscles grow stronger by replenishing and repairing themselves. You should also try to get 6 to 8 hours of sleep per night. If you do not get the proper rest, your muscles will not reach their potential. Depending on the muscle groups used and the intensity and volume of training, you may need 24 to 72 hours to recover and allow muscles to repair themselves.

What is the best kind of equipment for resistance training?
No particular kind of resistance-training equipment is "better" than any other. All exercise accessories have advantages and disadvantages. As discussed earlier in this chapter, equipment should be safe and provide the ability to overload the muscle groups you want to train. Remember, the best piece of equipment is the one that you use regularly.

Should I use free weights or machines?
This argument has been ongoing for years. Free weights indirectly work more muscles (those needed for stability and balance), and they allow a larger range of motion. Machines isolate muscles better and can be safer since you don't need a spotter. Most people who train use both, and many others use whatever type is available. Keep in mind that strength gains can be accomplished by doing exercises with neither, such as push-ups, pull-ups, one-legged squats, lunges, and so on. Each exercise or piece of equipment works the muscles at a slightly different angle. Experiment to find what works for you.

Should I train a muscle if it's sore?
No. If your legs are still sore from the last leg workout, take at least another day off before working the same muscle group again. But if you want to work an upper-body muscle group, that's okay.

Will doing aerobics retard muscle growth?
If you're training for maximum muscle mass, aerobics will slow muscle growth. However, if you are developing an all-purpose fitness program, aerobics and resistance training are necessary.

Should I use a lifting belt?
Most people don't need to use a lifting belt. Using a belt all the time actually weakens the abdominals and the lower back by making them work less. Weight belts are recommended for max squats or heavy lifting above the head.

I have reached a plateau in strength gains. What can I do?
First, you could be overtraining. Try taking a week off, and when you come back take it easy for a few weeks while re-evaluating your workout. Second, make sure your caloric intake is adequate and rich in nutrients. Don't overeat—doing so will not build muscle. Third, if you have been using the same routine/exercise for every workout, change your routine and use different muscle groups. Remember, the muscles will respond only if overloaded. Finally, you may be hitting your genetic limits. Taking a break, eating more, and changing your workout should help when you hit a strength plateau.

What exercises should I avoid?
Any exercise can cause an injury when done improperly. Again, safety is a primary concern, so go slow, don't bounce, and don't cheat. Maintain body alignment. Do not sacrifice body alignment to lift heavier weights. If you feel any pain during any exercise, STOP!

What is periodization?
Periodization, or cycling, is a training method in which you cycle your routine in an attempt to keep muscles growing and getting stronger. It is commonly performed by varying the intensity and volume of lifting (reps and sets). It is a valuable training method for athletes. For example, as an athlete's off-season training program progresses, the intensity of the workout is increased and repetitions are reduced. However, for most fitness programs periodization is unnecessary.

Will unexercised muscle turn into fat?
No! Muscle and fat are different types of tissue. In any given area of the body, muscle mass and fat stores can become smaller or larger. However, neither one is converted to the other. Fat is gained with excessive caloric intake and/or a reduction in caloric expenditure. Muscle mass can be increased only with resistance training.

I don't want to look like a bodybuilder. Should I still lift weights?
YES! For most people, adding muscle is very difficult. Hard work, eating well, and having the right genetics are needed to get the bodybuilder look. It also takes years to put on the kind of mass that you see in magazines. If you find yourself getting larger muscles than you'd like, you can stop training and they will shrink due to lack of work.

---

a percentage basis, women gain strength as rapidly as men during the first 12 weeks of a strength-training program (see Figure 5.13 on the next page). However, as a result of long-term resistance training, men generally exhibit a greater increase in muscle size than women. This occurs because men have 20 to 30 times more testosterone (a male sex hormone that builds muscles) than do women.

Motivation to Maintain Strength and Endurance

The problems associated with starting and maintaining a strength-training program are similar to those associated with cardiorespiratory training. You must find time to train regularly, so effective time management is critical.

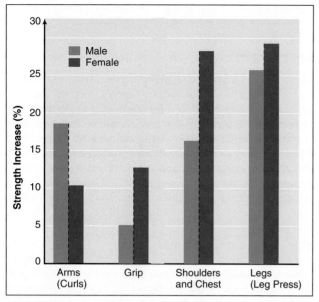

FIGURE 5.13 A comparison of strength gains for men and women. In relation to beginning strength levels, the increase in strength for women over the first 12 weeks of training is equal to or greater than that seen in men for most muscle groups.

Source: Adapted from Wilmore, J. (1975). Body composition and strength development. *Journal of Physical Education Research, 46(1),* 38–40.

Another key feature of any successful exercise program is that training must be fun. Making resistance training fun involves several elements. First, find an enjoyable place to work out. Locate a facility that contains the type of resistance equipment that you want to use and provides a pleasant and motivating environment. Second, develop an enjoyable strength-training routine. Designing a routine that is too hard may be good for improving strength but does not assist your desire to train. Therefore, design a program that is challenging, but fun. Further, resistance training is more enjoyable if you have a regular training partner. Select a friend who is highly motivated and has strength abilities similar to yours.

Although the benefits of resistance training are numerous, recent studies have shown that improved appearance, elevated self-esteem, and the overall feeling of well-being that result from regular resistance training are the most important factors in motivating people to continue to train regularly. Looking your best and feeling good about yourself are excellent reasons to maintain a regular strength-training program.

Summary

1. Maintaining/obtaining adequate muscular strength and endurance is important to reduce low back pain, reduce the incidence of exercise-related injuries, decrease the risk of osteoporosis, and aid in maintenance of functional capacity, which normally decreases with age.
2. *Muscular strength* refers to the ability of a muscle to generate maximal force. In simple terms, this refers to the amount of weight an individual can lift during one maximal effort. In contrast, *muscular endurance* is defined as the ability of a muscle to generate force over and over again or to maintain a static position for a length of time. In general, increasing muscular strength will increase muscular endurance as well. In contrast, improving muscular endurance does not result in significant improvements in muscular strength.
3. Skeletal muscle is composed of a collection of long thin cells (fibres). Fibres are composed of contractile units called myofibrils. Myofibrils are composed of myofilaments. Muscles are attached to bone by thick connective tissue (tendons). Therefore, muscle contraction results in the tendons pulling on bone, thereby causing movement.
4. Muscle contraction is regulated by signals coming from motor nerves. Motor nerves originate in the spinal cord and send nerve fibres to individual muscles throughout the body. The motor nerve and all of the muscle fibres it controls are called a *motor unit*.
5. Dynamic contractions result in movement of a body part. Static contractions involve the development of force but result in no movement of body parts. Concentric contractions are dynamic muscle contractions involving muscle shortening. In contrast, eccentric contractions are dynamic contractions in which the muscle lengthens. Isokinetic contractions are concentric or eccentric muscle contractions performed at a constant speed.
6. Human skeletal muscle can be classified into three major types: slow-twitch fibres (type I), fast-twitch fibres (type IIA), and intermediate fibres (type IIB) Slow-twitch fibres shorten slowly but are highly fatigue resistant. Fast-twitch fibres shorten and fatigue rapidly. Intermediate fibres possess a combination of the characteristics of slow- and fast-twitch fibres.
7. The process of involving more muscle fibres to produce increased muscular force is called *fibre recruitment*.
8. The percentages of slow-, intermediate-, and fast-twitch fibres vary among individuals. A relationship exists between muscle fibre type and success in athletics. For example, champion endurance athletes (e.g., marathon runners) have a high percentage of slow-twitch fibres, while champion sprint athletes have a high percentage of fast-twitch fibres.
9. Two primary physiological factors determine the amount of force that can be generated by a muscle: the size of the muscle and the neural influences (i.e., number of fibres recruited).
10. Muscle size is increased primarily because of an increase in fibre size (hypertrophy).
11. The overload principle states that a muscle will increase in strength or endurance only when a workload greater than normal has been applied.
12. Progressive resistance exercise (PRE) is the application of the overload principle to strength and endurance exercise programs.

13. A resistance-training program using low repetitions/high resistance results in strength gains, whereas a resistance-training program using high repetitions/low resistance results in muscular endurance gains.

14. Dynamic programs, like a dynamic contraction, involve the concept of contracting a muscle against a movable load (usually a free weight or weights mounted by cables or chains to form a weight machine). A static strength-training program is based on the concept of contracting a muscle at a fixed angle against an immovable object. Isokinetic exercises require the use of machines that govern the speed of movement during muscle contraction throughout the range of motion.

15. To begin a strength-training program, divide the program into three phases: starter phase—2 to 3 weeks with 2 workouts per week using 1 to 3 sets of 8 to 12 reps; slow progression phase—20 weeks with 2 to 4 workouts per week using 3 sets of 6 to 12 reps; and maintenance phase—continues for life with 1 workout per week using 3 sets of 6 to 12 reps.

Study Questions

1. Define the following terms:

   anabolic steroid
   hypertrophy
   motor unit
   progressive resistance exercise
   static contraction
   valsalva manoeuvre

2. List three reasons why training for muscular strength and endurance is important.

3. List and discuss the characteristics of slow-twitch (type I), fast-twitch (type IIA), and intermediate (type IIB) skeletal muscle fibres.

4. Discuss the pattern of muscle fibre recruitment with increasing intensities of contraction.

5. Discuss the relationship of muscle fibre type to success in various types of athletic events.

6. What factors determine muscle strength?

7. Why do people use steroids? What are some of the consequences of steroid use?

8. What physiological changes occur as a result of strength training?

9. Compare and contrast the overload principle and progressive resistance exercise.

10. Discuss specificity of training.

11. Compare and contrast the differences in training to increase strength versus training to increase endurance.

12. Define *repetition maximum*.

13. Distinguish between *concentric* and *eccentric* contractions.

14. Describe each of the following types of muscle contraction: isokinetic, static, and dynamic.

15. List at least five safety precautions for resistance training.

Suggested Reading

American College of Sports Medicine. (1998). The recommended quantity and quality of exercise for developing and maintaining cardiorespiratory and muscular fitness, and flexibility in healthy adults. *Medicine and Science in Sports and Exercise, 30,* 975–991.

Kraemer, W. J., & Ratamess, N. A. (2004). Fundamentals of resistance training: Progression and exercise prescription. *Medicine and Science in Sports and Exercise, 36(4),* 674–688.

Malina, R. M., Bouchard, C., & Bar-Or, O. (2004). Skeletal muscle tissue. In *Growth, Maturation, and Physical Activity*. Champaign, IL: Human Kinetics.

Payne, N., Gledhill, N., Katzmarzyk, P. T., Jamnik, V., & Ferguson, S. (2000). Health implications of musculoskeletal fitness. *Canadian Journal of Applied Physiology, 25(2),* 114–126.

Weblinks

Canadian Society for Exercise Physiology
www.csep.ca
A Canadian resource that promotes the generation, synthesis, transfer, and application of knowledge and research related to exercise physiology (encompassing physical activity, fitness, health, and human performance).

American College of Sports Medicine
www.acsm.org
A U.S. resource that promotes the generation, synthesis, transfer, and application of knowledge and research related to exercise physiology (encompassing physical activity, fitness, health, and human performance).

Lumen: Welcome to the Bone Box
www.meddean.luc.edu/lumen/MedEd/GrossAnatomy/learnem/bones/main_bone.htm
Contains information related to human anatomy, specifically in regard to the structure and maintenance of the skeleton.

Lumen: Master Muscle List
www.meddean.luc.edu/lumen/MedEd/GrossAnatomy/
dissector/mml
Contains information related to human anatomy, specifically in regard to the structure and maintenance of the musculature.

The New England Wellness Web
www.newellness.com/physfitn/strntrng.htm
Contains information on strength training for women.

Health World Strength Training
www.healthy.net/fitness/training/strength.asp
Contains information on strength training.

References

Chilibeck, P. D., Davison, K. S., Whiting, S. J., Suzuki, Y., Janzen, C. L., & Peloso, P. (2002). The effect of strength training combined with bisphosphonate (etidronate) therapy on bone mineral, lean tissue, and fat mass in postmenopausal women. *Canadian Journal of Physiology and Pharmacology, 80(10)*, 941–950.

Dunn, A. L., Trivedi, M. H., & O'Neal, H. A. (2001). Physical activity dose-response effects on outcomes of depression and anxiety. *Medicine and Science in Sports and Exercise 33(6)*, S587–S597.

Enoka, R. M. (1997). Neural adaptations with chronic physical activity. *Journal of Biomechanics 30(5)*, 447–455.

Fleck, S. J., & Kraemer, W. J. (1997). *Designing resistance training programs*. Champaign, IL: Human Kinetics.

Kibler, W. B., Chandler, T. J., & Stracener, E. S. (1992). Musculoskeletal adaptations and injuries due to overtraining. In *Exercise and Sports Sciences Reviews* (J. O. Holloszy, Ed.) (Vol. 20). Baltimore: Williams and Wilkins.

Kitai, T. A. (1989). Specificity of joint angle in isometric training. *European Journal of Applied Physiology, 58*, 744.

Kraemer, W. J., & Ratamess, N. A. (2004). Fundamentals of resistance training: Progression and exercise prescription. *Medicine and Science in Sports and Exercise, 36(4)*, 674–688.

Leveritt, M., Abernethy, P. J., Barry, B. K., & Logan, P. A. (1999). Concurrent strength and endurance training: A review. *Sports Medicine, 28(6)*, 413–427.

Malina, R. M., Bouchard, C., & Bar-Or, O. (2004). *Growth, maturation, and physical activity*. Champaign, IL: Human Kinetics.

Mannion, A. F., Junge, A., Taimela, S., Muntener, M., Lorenzo, K., & Dvorak, J. (2001). Active therapy for chronic low back pain, Part 3: Factors influencing self-rated disability and its change following therapy. *Spine, 26(8)*, 920–929.

Melia, P., Pipe, A., & Greenberg, L. (1996). The use of anabolic-androgenic steroids by Canadian students. *Clinical Journal of Sport Medicine: Official Journal of the Canadian Academy of Sports Medicine, 6(1)*, 9–14.

Payne, N., Gledhill, N., Katzmarzyk, P. T., Jamnik, V., & Ferguson, S. (2000). Health implications of musculoskeletal fitness. *Canadian Journal of Applied Physiology, 25(2)*, 114–126.

Peterson, J. A. (2002). 10 negative side effects of taking steroids. *ACSM's Health & Fitness Journal, 6(6)*, 44.

Pette, D. (2001). Perspectives: Plasticity of mammalian skeletal muscle. *Journal of Applied Physiology, 90(3)*, 1119–1124.

Powers, S., & Howley, E. (2004). *Exercise physiology: Theory and application to fitness and performance* (5th ed.). Dubuque, IA: McGraw-Hill.

Shephard, R. J. (2000). Exercise and training in women, Part 1: Influence of gender on exercise and training responses. *Canadian Journal of Applied Physiology, 25(1)*, 19–34.

Snow-Harter, C., & Marcus, R. (1991). Exercise, bone mineral density, and osteoporosis. In *Exercise and Sports Sciences Reviews* (J. O. Holloszy, Ed.) (Vol. 19). Baltimore: Williams and Wilkins.

Stone, M. H. (1990). Muscle conditioning and muscle injuries. *Medicine and Science in Sports and Exercise, 22*, 457–462.

Tarnopolsky, M. A., Atkinson, S. A., MacDougall, J. D., Chesley, A., Phillips, S., & Schwarcz, H. P. (1992). Evaluation of protein requirements for trained strength athletes. *Journal of Applied Physiology, 73(5)*, 1986–1995.

Tarpenning, K. M., Hamilton-Wessler, M., Wiswell, R. A., & Hawkins, S. A. (2004). Endurance training delays age of decline in muscle strength and muscle morphology. *Medicine and Science in Sports and Exercise, 36(1)*, 74–78.

LABORATORY 5.1

Strength-Training Log

Name_____ Age _____ Sex _____ Date _____

The purpose of this log is to provide a record of progress in building strength in the upper and lower body.

DIRECTIONS

Record the date, number of sets, reps, and the weight for each of the exercises listed in the left column.

St/RP/Wt = Sets/Reps/Weights
Example: 2/6/35 = 2 sets of 6 reps, each with 35 kg.

DATE							
Exercise	St/Rp/Wt	St/Rp/Wt	St/Rp/Wt	St/Rp/Wt	St/Rp/Wt	St/Rp/Wt	St/Rp/Wt
Lower back extension							
Hip and back							
Leg extension							
Leg curl							
Bench press							
Chest press							
Upper back							
Torso twist							
Triceps extension							
Pullover							
Biceps curl							
Abdominal curl							

CHAPTER 6

Exercise Prescription Principles: Flexibility

6

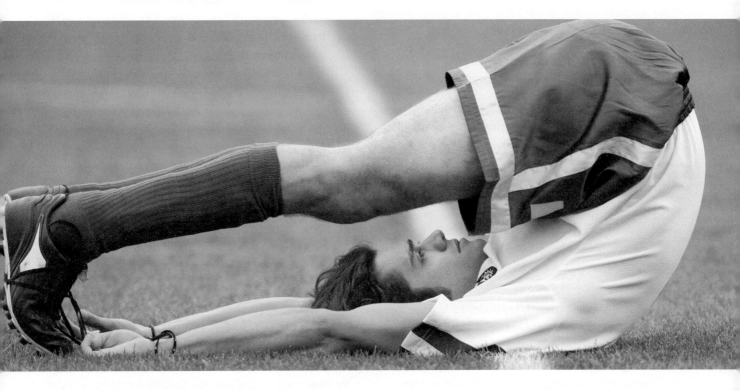

After studying this chapter, you should be able to

1. Discuss the importance of flexibility.
2. Identify the structural and physiological limits to flexibility.
3. Discuss the stretch reflex.
4. Describe the four categories of stretching techniques.
5. Identify the stretching needs of special population groups.
6. Design a flexibility exercise program.
7. Compare and contrast inappropriate stretches vs. beneficial stretches.

Flexibility is defined as the ability to move joints freely through their full range of motion. The full range of motion is determined in part by the shapes and positions of the bones that make up the joint, and in part by the composition and arrangement of muscles and tendons around the joint. For example, movement of the elbow (a hinge-type joint) is not limited solely by the arrangement of the bones themselves, because the soft connective tissues surrounding the joint also impose major limitations on the range of movement (Kubo, Kanehisa, Kawakami, Fukunaga, 2001; Hutton, 1992).

Although flexibility varies among individuals because of differences in body structure, it is important to appreciate that flexibility is not a fixed property. The range of motion of most joints can be increased with proper training techniques or can decline with disuse. This chapter introduces training designed to improve flexibility.

Benefits of Flexibility

There are many benefits to flexibility, such as increased joint mobility and efficient body movement (American College of Sports Medicine, 1998; Guissard & Duchaleau, 2004; Hutton, 1992; Kubo, Kanehisa, Kawakami, & Fukunaga, 2001; McGill, 2001). Some of the most significant benefits are

Counteracting age-related declines in flexibility. Flexibility assists the older population in maintaining mobility and decreases the risk of injury due to falls.

Decreasing aches and pains. Inflexibility can cause muscles to pull unevenly across joints. This can lead to poor posture, misalignment, and joint pain.

Enhancing daily-performance activities. Flexibility allows daily activities to be performed freely and easily, such as picking up bags of groceries, reaching high places, and turning to look over your shoulder while driving.

Reducing low back pain. A key reason to improve flexibility is its role in the prevention of low back problems. For example, most low back pain is due to misalignment of the vertebral column and pelvic girdle caused by a lack of flexibility and/or weak muscles. Low back pain is a significant problem—more than 80 percent of the population will experience back pain in their lives (Shrier, 1999). One of the reasons why back pain is so common is that people are generally inactive. Back pain can be avoided or alleviated by improving body mechanics, engaging in regular physical activity, and improving flexibility (McGill, 2001).

Enhancing sports performance. Greater range of motion and the ability to apply force can increase strength and power for sport, whether competitive or leisure.

Decreasing the risk of injury. Inflexibility is a factor in overuse injuries because of the excessive stress to less-pliable connective tissues (American College of Sports Medicine, 1998; Guissard & Duchaleau, 2004; Hutton, 1992; Kubo et al., 2001; McGill, 2001). Although it is commonly believed that stretching before physical activity reduces the incidence of muscle injury during activity, data from most research studies indicate that this is not the case. Recent research concludes that there is no good evidence that stretching reduces muscle injury and, in fact, cites evidence suggesting that stretching may contribute to injury (Witvrouw, Mahieu, Daneels, & McNair, 2004; Dec, Sparrow, & McKeag, 2000; Ingraham, 2003). The only studies suggesting that stretching offers protection from muscle injury are the ones that suggest combining the stretching with a general warm-up.

Physiological Basis for Developing Flexibility

We have already noted that the limits to flexibility are determined by the way the joint is constructed as well as by the associated muscles and tendons. Further discussion will focus on structural limitations and avoiding the complications from activating the stretch reflex.

Structural Limitations to Movement

Five primary factors contribute to the limits of movement: bone; muscle; connective tissue within the joint capsule (the joint capsule is composed of **ligaments,** which hold bones together, and **cartilage,** which cushions the ends of bones and provides protection from the friction due to joint movement); **tendons,** which connect muscle to bones and to connective tissue surrounding joints; and skin. Exercise aimed at improving flexibility does not change the structure of bone but alters the soft tissues (i.e., muscle, joint connective tissue, and tendons) that contribute to flexibility. Table 6.1 lists the contribution of the various soft tissues to total joint flexibility. Flexibility is dependent on joint structure and elasticity of the muscles and connective tissues. Because of

ligaments Connective tissue within the joint capsule that holds bones together.

cartilage A tough, connective tissue that forms a pad on the end of bones in certain joints, such as the elbow, knee, and ankle.

tendons Connective tissue that connects muscles to bones.

Structure	Resistance to Flexibility (% of total)
Joint capsule	47
Muscle	41
Tendon	10
Skin	2

TABLE 6.1 Contribution of Soft-Tissue Structures to Limiting Joint Movement

this the flexibility or range of motion for any particular joint is specific to each joint, so flexibility in one leg does not necessarily mean equal flexibility in the other leg, and flexibility in the shoulders does not guarantee flexibility in the lower back. Note that the structures associated with the joint capsule, muscles, and tendons provide most of the body's resistance to movement. Therefore, exercises aimed at improving flexibility must alter one of these three factors in order to increase the range of motion around a joint. Stretching the ligaments in the joint capsule may lead to a loose joint that would be highly susceptible to injury. However, muscle and tendon are soft tissues that can lengthen over time with stretching. Routine stretching increases the range of motion in the joint by reducing the resistance to movement from tight muscles and tendons.

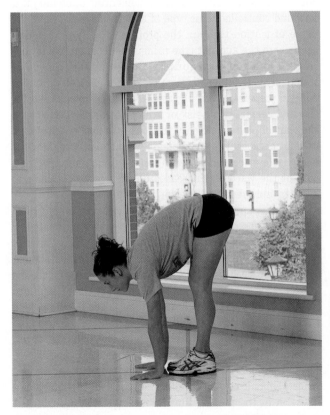

Routine stretching increases the range of motion in the joints.

Stretching and the Stretch Reflex

Before we examine specific exercises for improving flexibility, it is useful to discuss a key physiological response to stretching. Muscles contain special receptors, called *muscle spindles,* that are sensitive to stretching. When a doctor taps you on the knee with a rubber hammer, for example, the rapid stretching of muscle spindles results in a "reflex" contraction of the muscle to prevent it from stretching too far too fast. This reflex contraction, called **stretch reflex,** is counterproductive to stretching because the muscle is shortening instead of lengthening. Fortunately, the stretch reflex can be avoided when muscles and tendons are stretched very slowly. In fact, if a muscle stretch is held for several seconds, the muscle spindles allow the muscle being stretched to further relax and permit an even greater stretch (Hutton, 1992; McGill, 2001). Therefore, stretching exercises are most effective when they avoid promoting a stretch reflex.

Designing a Flexibility Training Program

Four kinds of stretching techniques are commonly used to increase flexibility: **momentum stretching** (often called ballistic stretching), **static stretching, dynamic stretching,** and *proprioceptive neuromuscular facilitation* (Deal & Muskowitz, 1999; Hutton, 1992). However, because momentum stretching (quick, bouncing movements that briefly stretch muscles) promotes the stretch reflex and increases the risk of injury to muscles and tendons, only the static, dynamic, and proprioceptive neuromuscular-facilitation methods are recommended for the average person. Elite athletes may use some forms of momentum stretching in their sport-specific training.

Momentum Stretching

Momentum stretching uses rapid or extensive bouncing in an attempt to force a joint or a limb beyond its normal range of motion. This stretching by bouncing into and out of a stretched position uses the lengthened muscle as a spring (bouncing up and down to touch your toes), which activates the stretch reflex and can lead the muscle or tendon to

stretch reflex Involuntary contraction of a muscle that occurs due to rapid stretching of that muscle.

momentum stretching Uses momentum to force a joint or limb beyond a normal range of motion.

static stretching Stretching that slowly lengthens a muscle to a point where further movement is limited.

dynamic stretching A technique that develops an active range of motion through the process of slow and controlled movements.

overstretch or tear. This form of stretching does not allow muscles to adjust and relax in a lengthened position. Momentum stretching is not considered useful for an everyday flexibility training program. However, research does support the use of momentum or "ballistic" stretching for elite athletes and sport-specific training (Newton, Kraemer, Hakkinen, 1999; Unick, Kieffer, Cheeseman, Feeney, 2005).

Static Stretching

Static stretching is effective for promoting a relaxation response, increasing blood flow to the muscle to enhance recovery after an activity, and facilitating elongation of the muscle.

Static stretching gradually lengthens a muscle to a point at which further movement is limited (slight discomfort is felt), and requires holding this position for a fixed period of time. The goal is to encourage the muscle to move to a state of increased flexibility longer than the original position. The optimal amount of time to hold the stretch for maximal improvement in flexibility is unknown. However, most investigators agree that holding the stretch position for 20 to 30 seconds (repeated three to four times) results in an improvement in flexibility. Compared with momentum stretching, the risk of injury associated with static stretching is minimal. Another benefit of static stretching is that, when performed during the cool-down period, it may reduce the muscle stiffness associated with

some exercise routines (American College of Sports Medicine, 1998; Hutton, 1992).

Dynamic Stretching

Dynamic stretching should not be confused with momentum stretching. Dynamic stretching does involve movement, but unlike the technique used in momentum stretching it is slow and controlled. This type of activity develops an active range of motion through the process of reciprocal inhibition where the **agonist** (the primary mover) muscle is contracted and the **antagonist** (the secondary mover or stabilizer) is lengthened. Most often, dynamic stretching is done in preparation for physical activity or strenuous exercise and decreases the risk of injury during the activity. At the start of physical activity the muscle is not lengthened to its limit because it is not properly warmed up; therefore it is not pliable or elastic. Engaging in dynamic stretching as a part of the warm-up increases blood flow to the moving muscles and prepares them for activity.

A warm-up with dynamic stretching begins with a small range of motion movements that are slow-paced and controlled and then gradually increases intensity and range of motion; this lubricates and warms the joint. An example of dynamic stretching would be small arm circles that gradually become bigger and quicker. It is suggested that dynamic stretches be performed in sets of 8 to 12 repetitions (Etnyre & Lee, 1987; Health Canada Physical Activity Unit, 2005; McAtee, 1999).

Dynamic stretching can also be useful in a cool-down. A slow and controlled active range of motion is performed, starting from a large arm circle and moving to a smaller range. Dynamic stretching does not lengthen the muscle but is useful in the preparation for static stretching, which is much more intense.

agonist   The muscle doing the majority of the movement, also known as the *primary mover.*

antagonist   One or more muscles assisting primary muscles in a particular movement, also known as the *secondary movers* or *stabilizers.*

Proprioceptive Neuromuscular Facilitation

A relatively new technique for improving flexibility, **proprioceptive neuromuscular facilitation (PNF)** combines stretching with alternating contraction and relaxation of muscles. There are two common types of PNF stretching: contract-relax (CR) stretching and contract-relax/antagonist contract (CRAC) stretching. The CR technique initially requires a **static contraction** of the muscle to be stretched. Then, after relaxing the muscle, the muscle is slowly stretched. The CRAC method calls for the same contract-relax routine but adds to this the contraction of the antagonist muscle, the muscle on the opposite side of the joint. The purpose of contracting the antagonist muscle is to promote a reflex relaxation of the muscle to be stretched.

How do PNF techniques compare with momentum and static stretching? First, PNF has been shown to be safer and more effective in promoting flexibility than momentum stretching (Deal & Moskowitz, 1999). Further, studies have shown PNF programs to be equal to, or in some cases superior to, static stretching for improving flexibility (McAtee, 1999). However, one disadvantage of PNF stretching is that some stretches require a partner.

The following steps illustrate how a CRAC procedure can be done with a partner:

1. After the assistant moves the limb in the direction necessary to stretch the desired muscles to the point of tightness (mild discomfort is felt), the subject statically contracts the muscle being stretched for 3 to 5 seconds and then relaxes it.

2. The subject then moves the limb in the opposite direction of the stretch by statically contracting the antagonist muscles. The subject holds this isometric contraction for approximately 5 seconds, during which time the muscles to be stretched relax. While the desired muscles are relaxed, the assistant may increase the stretch of those muscles.

3. The subject then statically contracts the antagonist muscles for another 5 seconds, which relaxes the desired muscles, and then the assistant again stretches the desired muscles to the point of mild discomfort.

This cycle of 3 steps is repeated 3 to 5 times. Figure 6.1 illustrates a partner-assisted CRAC procedure for stretching the calf muscles. Figure 6.2 shows how some PNF stretches can be done without a partner.

proprioceptive neuromuscular facilitation (PNF) A technique that combines stretching with alternating contraction and relaxation of muscles to improve flexibility.

static contraction Muscular tension is created but no movement of body parts takes place.

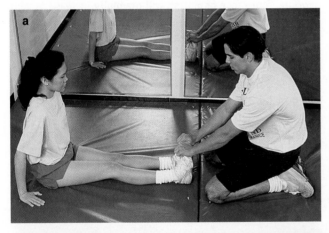

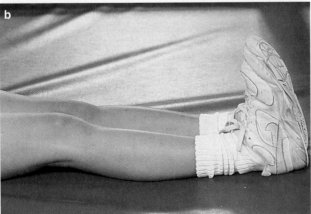

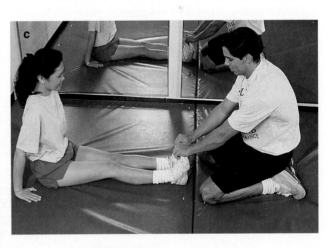

FIGURE 6.1 An example of a partner-assisted CRAC procedure for stretching the calf muscles. The subject contracts the calf muscles against resistance provided by the assistant (a). Unassisted, the subject contracts the shin (antagonist) muscles, which relaxes the calf muscles (b). While the subject continues the contraction of the shin muscles, the assistant stretches the calf muscles (c).

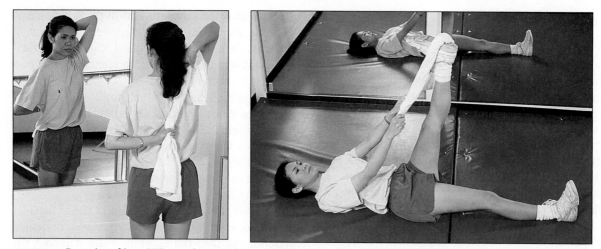

FIGURE 6.2 Examples of how PNF stretches may be done without a partner. What other creative ways can you devise to self-assist with PNF stretches?

Fitness Prescription Guidelines for Improving Flexibility

For safety reasons, all flexibility programs should consist of either PNF or static stretching exercises. The frequency and time for stretching should be 2 to 5 days per week for 10 to 30 minutes each day (Health Canada Physical Activity Guide, 2005). The first week for a stretching regimen is considered the starter phase and should consist of 2 stretching sessions; one session should be added per week during the first 4 weeks of the slow progression phase of the program. (For more details on the progression principle, see Chapter 3.) Initially, the duration of each training session should be approximately 5 minutes and should increase gradually to approximately 20 to 30 minutes following 6 to 12 weeks of stretching during the slow progression phase. The physiological rationale for increasing the time of stretching is that each stretch position is held for progressively longer durations as the program continues. For exam-

ple, begin by holding each stretched position for 15 seconds, then add 5 seconds each week, up to 30 seconds. Start by performing each of the exercises twice and progress to 4 reps. Table 6.2 illustrates a sample exercise prescription for a flexibility program.

What about the intensity of stretching? In general, a limb should not be stretched beyond a position of mild discomfort. The intensity of stretching is increased simply by extending the stretch nearer to the limits of your range of motion. Your range of motion will gradually increase as your flexibility improves during the training program.

To improve overall flexibility, all major muscle groups should be stretched. Exercises 6.1 through 6.12 illustrate the proper methods of performing 12 different stretching exercises. Integrate these exercises into the program outlined in Table 6.2.

These exercises are designed to be used in a regular program of stretching to increase flexibility. The exercises presented involve the joints and major muscle groups for which range of motion tends to decrease with age and disuse. The exercises include both static and PNF movements and may require a partner.

Week No.	Phase	Duration of Stretch Hold	Repetitions	Frequency (times/wk)
1	Starter	15 sec	2	2
2	Slow progression	20 sec	2	2
3	Slow progression	25 sec	3	3
4	Slow progression	30 sec	4	3
5	Slow progression	30 sec	4	3–4
6	Slow progression	30 sec	4	4–5
7+	Maintenance	30 sec	4	4–5

TABLE 6.2 Sample Flexibility Program with Considerations for Duration of Stretch Hold, Number of Repetitions, and Frequency of Training

Special Populations

Research shows that flexibility can be beneficial for all types of individuals. This includes special populations such as the elderly, pregnant women, and people who are physically challenged (Anderson & Spector, 2000; Orloff & Rapp, 2004; Thacker, Gilchrist, Stroup, & Kimsey, 2004). For the elderly maintaining flexibility can mean reduced risk of injury due to falls, and for pregnant women it can mean an easier labour and faster postpartum recovery (Anderson & Spector, 2000). For those who are physically challenged, flexibility can prevent the overuse injuries that are common due to physical impairment and can increase strength, which can enhance management of daily activities and maintain independence.

The Elderly

With age, unused muscles atrophy, lose elasticity, and grow weak. Ligaments and tendons shorten and tighten, which decreases range of motion and can cause aches and pains. Canada's *Physical Activity Guide to Active Living for Older Adults* suggests a physical activity program that incorporates flexibility on a daily basis (Health Canada Physical Activity Guide, 2005). The safety consideration for this group is the need for longer periods of dynamic stretching. Increase in temperature and lubrication in joints and muscles takes longer in the older population. Dynamic stretching can facilitate joint lubrication with its large range of movements, and increase temperature through the gradual increase in intensity. Some guidelines are as follows:

- Build gentle stretching and reaching into your everyday activities.

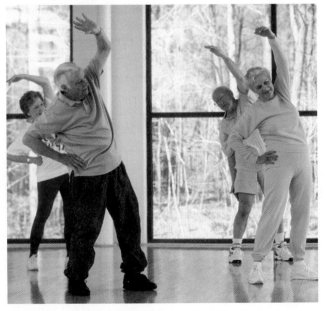

It is recommended that seniors incorporate flexibility training on a daily basis.

- Engage in reaching, bending, and stretching activities most days of the week.
- Prior to more intense physical activities, spend sufficient time engaging in dynamic stretching to ensure an increase in muscle temperature and lubrication of the joints.
- Start with large movements.
- Do not stretch to the point of extreme discomfort or pain.
- Do not hyperextend joints.
- Do not perform any stretches that cause dizziness or loss of balance.

Pregnant Women

During pregnancy a gradual weight change is desirable; however, this is likely to increase the stress on joints, ligaments, and muscles. Maintaining flexibility during this period has the benefit of assisting the body to accommodate the change in a women's centre of gravity and maintain proper posture. It can also relieve muscle soreness and tension. Increased flexibility can assist during labour and aid in a quicker postpartum recovery. Stretching while pregnant requires some modification to avoid injury. During pregnancy, joints and ligaments loosen due to the release of the hormone *relaxin*, which helps facilitate the baby's birth but can put the pregnant woman at additional risk for strains and tears. Some suggestions for safe flexibility training during pregnancy are (Anderson & Spector, 2000)

- Stretch to the point of mild tension; avoid going beyond muscle limits.
- Incorporate dynamic stretching prior to physical activity and utilize static stretching after muscles are warm.
- After the first trimester, do not perform stretches while lying flat.
- Do not hyperextend the joints.
- Do not do any stretches that cause dizziness, nausea, or shortness of breath.

People Who Are Physically Challenged

People with disabilities are less likely to engage in physical activity and flexibility training than those without disabilities (Dec et al., 2000). Individuals with physical limitations are at additional risk for developing obesity, pressure sores, infections, fatigue, and depression, which can lead to further disability and loss of independence. Many of these conditions can be minimized by incorporating regular physical activity and a safe flexibility training program. Suggestions for safe flexibility training include

- Consult a health care professional before beginning flexibility training.

- Perform stretching exercises at the beginning and end of any strenuous physical activity.
- Address the stiffness of joints for individuals who have suffered stroke, the permanent contracture of muscles in people with spinal cord injuries, and rigidity and muscle spasticity for people with Parkinson's disease or multiple sclerosis.
- Proprioceptive stretching may be more beneficial than static stretching.

There are a variety of stretches that can help maintain full range of motion around joints that have weakened, and in many cases the most useful form of stretching is proprioceptive neuromuscular facilitation (McAtee, 1999).

As applies to all exercise and flexibility programs, your health care professional should be consulted before beginning. With the physically challenged it is especially important to check with a physician to ensure that the condition will not be aggravated by certain actions or movements.

How to Avoid Hazardous Exercises

Many exercises are potentially harmful to the musculoskeletal system. For example, with PNF stretching it is easy for the assistant to push a stretch too far, which can injure tendons and muscles. The same is true of stretching muscles that have already stretched. Some stretches that are overly forceful or are over-flexed, especially for the spine, can cause compression of the vertebrae. Which exercises actually cause injury depends on how they are performed. Remember the following key points during an exercise session to help prevent injury:

- Avoid breathholding. Try to breathe as normally as possible during the exercise.
- Avoid full flexion of the knee, neck, or back.
- Do not stretch muscles that are already stretched, such as the abdominal muscles.

- Do not stretch to the point that extreme joint pain occurs.
- Use caution when using an assistant to help with passive stretches.
- Avoid forceful extension and flexion of the spine.

Many commonly practised exercises may cause injuries and are therefore inappropriate. The illustrations starting on page 145 show some of these exercises and provide alternatives to accomplish the same goals.

Motivation to Maintain Flexibility

Maintaining flexibility requires a lifetime commitment to performing regular stretching. Just as in other types of fitness training, good time management is critical if you are going to succeed. Set aside time for 3 to 5 stretching periods per week, and stick to your schedule. A key point to remember is that stretching can be performed almost anywhere because it does not require special equipment. So take advantage of windows of free time in your day and plan stretching workouts.

You are not likely to maintain a lifetime stretching program if you do not enjoy your workouts. One suggestion for making stretching more fun is to perform stretching workouts while listening to music or during a television program you enjoy. This will allow time to pass more rapidly and will make your stretching workout more pleasant.

As in other aspects of physical fitness, establishing short- and long-term flexibility goals is important in maintaining the motivation to stretch. Further, keeping a record of your workouts and improvements allows you to follow your flexibility progress and plan your future training schedule (see Laboratory 6.1 on page 151). So, establish your stretching goals today and get started toward a lifetime of flexibility.

Sample Flexibility Exercises

Exercise 6.1   Lower Leg Stretch

Purpose: To stretch the calf muscles and the Achilles' tendon.

Position: Stand on the edge of a surface that is high enough to allow the heel to be lower than the toes. Have a support nearby to hold for balance.

Movement: Rise on the toes as far as possible for several seconds (a), then lower the heels as far as possible (b). Shift your body weight from one leg to the other for added stretch of the muscles.

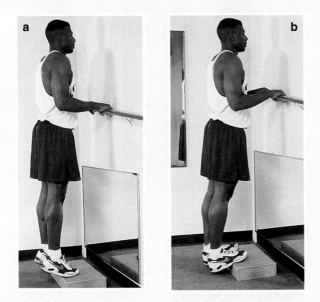

Exercise 6.2   Inside Leg Stretch

Purpose: To stretch the muscle on the inside of the thighs.

Position: Sit with bottoms of the feet together and the hands placed just above the ankle. Do not pull up on the ankles. Maintain your posture sitting upright.

Movement: Press the knees towards the floor using your leg muscles. Avoid forcing the knees down with your hands or elbows.

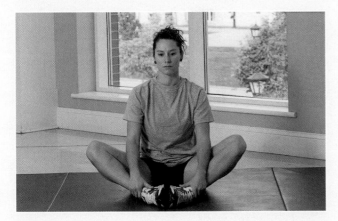

Exercise 6.3   One-Leg Stretch

Purpose: To stretch the lower back muscles and muscles in the back of the thigh.

Position: Sit with one leg straight and the other bent inwards with the sole of that foot placed against the inside of the straightened leg.

Movement: Keeping your back straight and head upright (eyes looking forward), reach both arms forward and lower body towards the straightened leg. Avoid rounding the back and pulling on the lower leg..

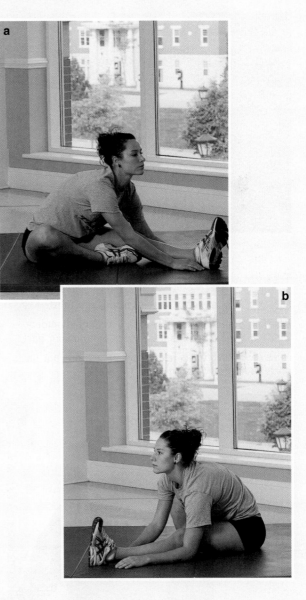

Exercise 6.4   Lower Back Stretch

Purpose: To stretch the muscles of the lower back and buttocks.

Position: Start lying on your back, knees bent and your feet flat on the floor.

Movement: Relax and place your hands behind the lower portion of the back of your thighs. Avoid pulling on the knees. Pull the knees to the chest lifting the buttocks off the ground and hold. Gently lower buttocks and legs back to the starting position.

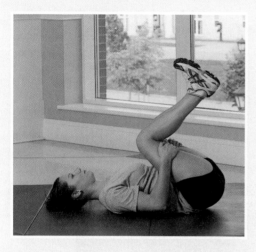

Exercise 6.5   Chest Stretch

Purpose: To stretch the muscles across the chest.

Position: Stand comfortably with your feet shoulder-width apart and your hands clasped behind your back.

Movement: With yours hands clasped behind your back, press your chest forward.

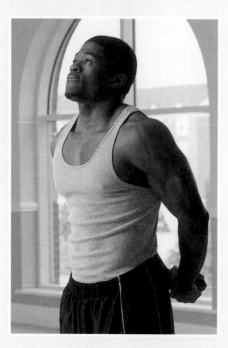

Exercise 6.6
Side Stretch

Purpose: To stretch the muscles of the upper arm and side of the trunk.

Position: Sitting on the floor with legs crossed.

Movement: Stretch one arm over the head while bending at the waist in the same direction. With the opposite arm, reach across the chest as far as possible. Hold for several seconds. Do not rotate the trunk; try to stretch the muscle on the same side of the trunk as the overhead arm. Alternate arms to stretch the other side of the trunk.

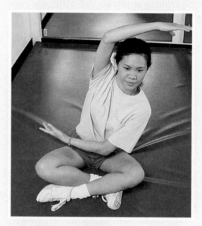

Exercise 6.7
Thigh Stretch

Purpose: To stretch the muscles in the front of the thigh of the extended (rear) leg.

Position: Kneel on one knee, resting the rear foot on the ball of the foot and placing the forward foot flat on the floor.

Movement: Lean forward and place your hands on the floor on either side of the forward foot. Lift the knee off the floor and slide the rear leg backward so that the knee is slightly behind the hips; then press the hips forward and down, and hold for several seconds. While stretching, maintain approximately a 90° angle at the knee of the front leg. Switch the positions of the legs to stretch the other thigh.

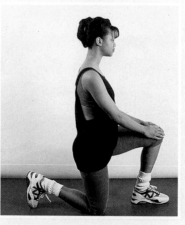

Exercise 6.8   Spine Twister

Purpose: To stretch the muscles that rotate the trunk and thighs.

Position: Lie on your back, with one leg crossed over the other and both shoulders and both arms on the floor (a).

Movement: Rotate the trunk so that the crossed-over leg stays on top and both knees approach or touch the floor (b); hold for several seconds. The shoulders and arms should remain on the floor all during the stretch. Reverse the positions of the legs and repeat the stretch.

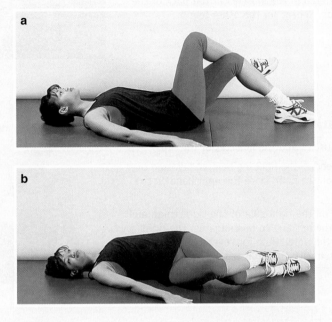

a

b

Exercise 6.9   Neck Stretch

Purpose: To stretch the muscles that rotate the neck.

Position: Stand comfortably with legs shoulder-width apart.

Movement: Tilt head down to one side—right ear to right shoulder. Do not raise shoulder or use external resistance to aid in the stretch. Gently stretch using internal muscle forces. Repeat other side.

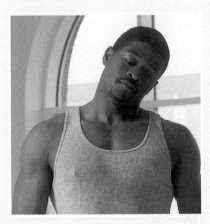

Exercise 6.10   Shin Stretch

Purpose: To stretch the muscles of the shin.

Position: Kneel on both knees, with the trunk rotated to one side and the hand on that side pressing down on the ankle.

Movement: While pressing down on the ankle, move the pelvis forward; hold for several seconds. Repeat on the other side.

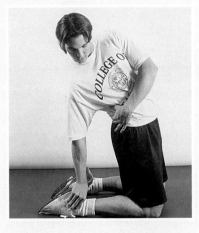

Exercise 6.11   Leg Stretch

Purpose: To stretch the muscles on the back of the hip, the back of the thigh, and the calf.

Position: Lying on your back, bring one knee toward the chest and grasp the toes with the hand on the same side. Place the opposite hand on the back of the leg just below the knee.

Movement: Pull the knee toward the chest while pushing the heel toward the ceiling and pulling the toes toward the shin. Straighten the knee until you feel sufficient stretch in the muscles of the back of the leg, and hold for several seconds. Repeat for the other leg.

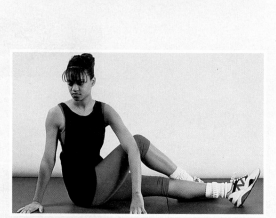

Exercise 6.12   Trunk Twister

Purpose: To stretch the trunk muscles and the muscles of the hip.

Position: Sit with the left leg extended, the right leg bent and crossed over the left knee, and the right foot on the floor. Place the right hand on the floor behind the buttocks.

Movement: Placing the left arm on the right side of the right thigh and the left hand on the floor, use the left arm to push against the right leg while twisting the trunk to the right. Hold for several seconds. Then assume the starting position with the right leg extended and so forth, and stretch the opposite side of the body.

Inappropriate Exercise

Arm Circles (Palms Down)

Purpose: To strengthen the muscles of the shoulder and upper back.

Problem: May result in irritation of the shoulder joint and, if circled forward and down, results in the use of the chest muscles instead of back muscles.

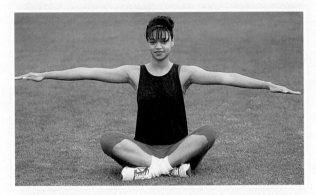

Knee Pull

Purpose: To stretch the lower back and buttocks.

Problem: Places undue stress on the knee joint.

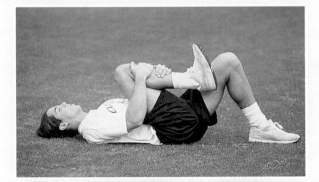

Substitute Exercise

Arm Circles (Palms Up)

In a sitting position, turn the palms up and circle the arms backward and up.

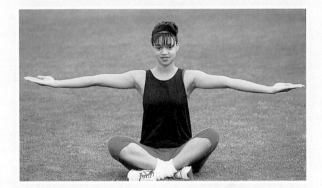

Leg Pull

Lying on your back, pull the knee toward the chest by pulling on the back of the leg just below the knee. Then, extend the knee joint and point the sole of the foot straight up. Continue to pull the leg toward your chest. Repeat several times with each leg.

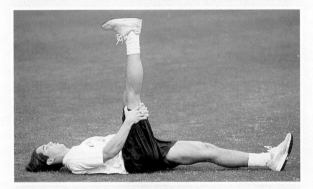

Inappropriate Exercise

Deep Knee Bends

Purpose: To strengthen the upper leg and stretch the lower leg.

Problem: This movement hyperflexes the knee and "opens" the joint while stretching the ligaments.

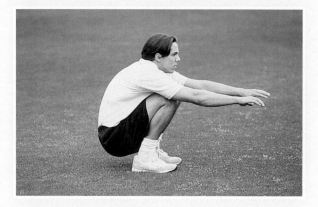

Leg Lifts

Purpose: To strengthen the abdominal muscles.

Problem: This exercise primarily recruits the hip flexor muscles and thus does not accomplish the intended purpose. These muscles are likely strong enough and do not need strengthening. In addition, this exercise produces excess compression on the vertebral disks.

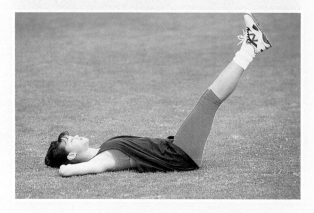

Substitute Exercise

Lunges

While standing, step forward with either foot and touch the opposite knee to the ground. Repeat with the opposite leg.

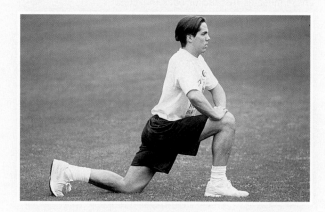

Reverse Curl

Lie on your back with the knees bent and the arms and feet flat on the ground. Maintaining about the same degree of bend at the knee joint, pull the knees up toward the chest so that the hips leave the ground. Do not allow the knees to go past the shoulders. Lower the legs back to the ground and repeat.

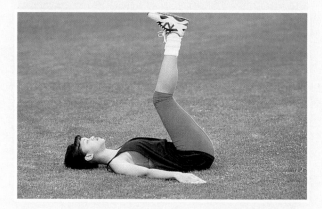

Inappropriate Exercise

Standing Toe Touch

Purpose: To stretch the lower back, buttocks, and hamstrings.

Problems: First, hyperflexion of the knee could cause damage to ligaments and, second, if performed with the back flat, damage could occur to the lower back.

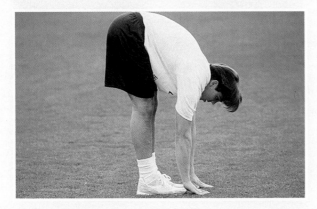

Sit-Up (Hands behind Head)

Purpose: To strengthen the abdominal muscles.

Problem: With hands behind the head, there is a tendency to jerk on the head and neck to "throw" yourself up. This could cause hyperflexion of the neck. In addition, sitting up with the back straight places undue strain on the lower back.

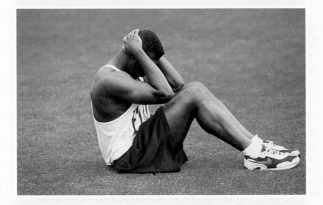

Substitute Exercise

Sitting Hamstring Stretch

Sit at leg-length from a wall. With your foot on the wall and the other knee bent with the foot between the wall and buttocks, bend forward keeping the lower back straight. The bent knee can fall to the side.

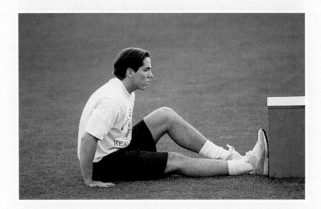

Curl-Up

Keeping the knees bent while lying on your back, cross your arms over your chest so that your fingers rest on your shoulders. Using the abdominal muscles, curl up until the upper half of the back is off the floor and then return to the starting position.

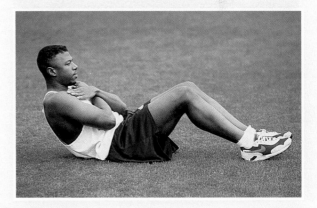

Inappropriate Exercise

Neck Circles

Purpose: To stretch the neck muscles.

Problem: Hyperextension of the neck should always be avoided. This can pinch arteries and nerves, as well as damage disks in the spine.

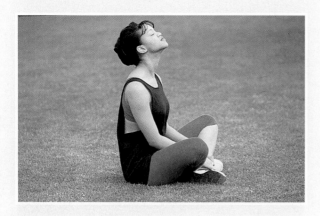

Donkey Kick

Purpose: To stretch and strengthen the buttocks.

Problem: When kicking the leg back, most people hyperextend the neck and/or back.

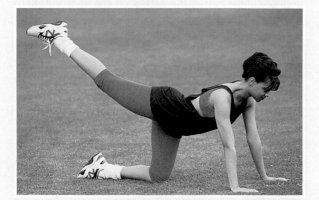

Substitute Exercise

Neck Stretches

In a sitting position, with your head and neck straight, move your head down to flex the neck, and return the head upright. Then, slowly turn your head from side to side as far as possible; attempt to point your chin at each shoulder.

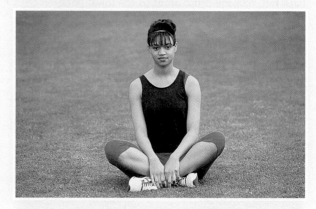

Knee-to-Nose Touch

While on your hands and knees, lift one knee toward your nose and then extend that leg to horizontal. Alternate legs. Remember: Your leg should not go higher than your hips, and your neck should remain in line with your back.

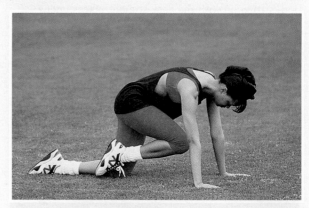

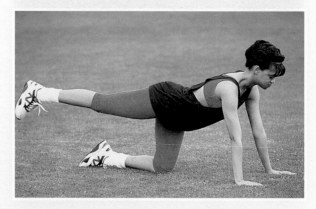

When Muscles Cramp

Muscle cramps are one of the most common problems encountered in sports and exercise. For many years the primary causes of muscle cramps were thought to be dehydration or electrolyte imbalances. Accordingly, drinking enough fluids and ensuring that the diet contains sufficient amounts of sodium (from table salt, for example) and potassium (from bananas, for example) have long been encouraged as preventive measures. Whenever muscles cramp, stretching or massage have been used to relieve the cramping until electrolyte balance can be restored.

More recent research, however, suggests that cramping may be due to abnormal spinal control of motor neuron activity, especially when a muscle contracts while shortened (Bentley, 1996). Thus, for example, the cramping that often occurs in the calf muscles of recreational swimmers when their toes are pointed may be because those calf muscles are contracting while they are shortened.

The most prevalent risk factors for cramps during exercise are muscle fatigue and poor stretching habits (failure to stretch regularly and long enough during each session). Other risk factors include older age, higher body mass index, and a family history of muscle cramps.

If cramping occurs, you should

- Passively stretch the muscle. Such stretching induces receptors that sense the stretch to initiate nerve impulses that inhibit muscle stimulation.
- Drink plenty of water to avoid dehydration or electrolyte imbalances. Sports drinks can help replenish glucose and electrolytes, but do *not* use salt tablets.
- Seek medical attention if multiple muscle groups are involved, because this could be a sign of more serious problems.

Although no strategies for preventing muscle cramping during exercise have been proven effective, regular stretching using PNF techniques, correction of muscle balance and posture, and proper training for the exercise activity involved may be beneficial.

Summary

1. *Flexibility* is defined as the range of motion of a joint.
2. Improved flexibility results in the following benefits: increased joint mobility, prevention of low back problems, efficient body movement, and improved posture and personal appearance.
3. The five structural and physiological limits to flexibility are bone, muscle, structures within the joint capsule, the tendons that connect muscle to bones and connective tissue that surrounds joints, and skin.
4. Static stretches involve stretching a muscle to the limit of movement and holding the stretch for an extended period of time.
5. Dynamic stretching uses controlled, active movements to warm up the muscles and increase blood flow.
6. Proprioceptive neuromuscular facilitation stretching is partner-assisted to achieve deep muscle tissue lengthening. It combines stretching with alternating contraction and relaxation of muscles to improve flexibility.
7. If muscle spindles are suddenly stretched, they respond by initiating a stretch reflex that causes the muscle to contract. However, if the muscles and tendons are stretched slowly, the stretch reflex can be avoided.
8. Research has shown that flexibility can be beneficial for all types of individuals. This includes special populations such as the elderly, pregnant women, and people who are physically challenged.

Study Questions

1. Define the following terms:
   agonist
   antagonist
   cartilage
   flexibility
   proprioceptive neuromuscular facilitation
   isometric contraction
   dynamic stretching
   momentum stretching

2. Describe the difference in function between ligaments and tendons.

3. Compare *static stretching* and *momentum stretching*.

4. List three primary reasons why maintaining flexibility is important.

5. List all of the factors that limit flexibility. Which factors place the greatest limitations on flexibility?

6. Compare and contrast the two recommended methods of stretching.

7. Outline the benefits of flexibility for special populations.

8. Briefly outline the guidelines for improving flexibility.

9. Describe why the stretch reflex is counterproductive to stretching, and explain how this reflex can be avoided.

Suggested Reading

DeVries, H., & Housh, T. (1994). *Physiology of exercise* (5th ed.). Dubuque, IA: Brown and Benchmark.

Fox, E., Bowers, R., & Foss, M. (1997). *The physiological basis for exercise and sports* (6th ed.). Dubuque, IA: Brown and Benchmark.

Golding, L. A. (1997). Flexibility, stretching, and flexibility testing. *ACSM's Health and Fitness Journal, 1(2),* 17–20.

Hutton, R. S. (1992). Neuromuscular basis of stretching exercises. In P. V. Komi (Ed.), *Strength and Power in Sport,* Oxford: Blackwell Scientific.

Powers, S., & Howley, E. (1997). *Exercise physiology: Theory and application to fitness and performance* (3rd ed.). Dubuque, IA: Brown and Benchmark.

Weblinks

Sports Medicine
www.sportsmedicine.com
Presents detailed information on all aspects of sports medicine.

Canadian Society for Exercise Physiology
www.csep.ca
Describes tests for aerobic power, anaerobic power, flexibility, and body composition.

TD Can, To Do Canada
www.td.ca
Canadian sports links for the disabled provides sports links to the physically disabled in Canada.

Fitness Files
http://tms.ecol.net/fitness/
Covers fitness fundamentals, flexibility, exercises to be avoided, exercise nutrition, and the treatment of exercise injuries.

Meriter Fitness
http://meriter.healthinkonline.com
Discusses injury prevention and treatment, weight training, flexibility, exercise prescriptions, and more.

The Canadian Association of Independent Living Centres
www.cailc.ca
Provides elderly Canadians with programs, services, and resources.

References

American College of Sports Medicine. (1998). The recommended quantity and quality of exercise for developing and maintaining cardiorespiratory and muscular fitness, and flexibility in healthy adults. *Medicine and Science in Sports and Exercise, 30(6),* 975–991.

Anderson, B. D., & Spector, A. (2000). Introduction to Pilates-based rehabilitation. *Orthopedic and Physical Therapy Clinics of North America, 9(3),* 396–410.

Bentley, S. (1996). Exercise-induced muscle cramp. Proposed mechanisms and management. *Sports Medicine, 21(6),* 409–420.

Deal, C. L., & Moskowitz, R. W. (1999). Neutraceuticals as therapeutic agents in osteoarthritis: The role of glucosamine, chondroitin sulfate, and collagen hydrolysate. *Rheumatic Disease Clinics of North America, 25(2),* 379–395.

Dec, K. L., Sparrow, K. J., & McKeag, D. B. (2000, April). The physically challenged athlete: Medical issues and assessment. *Sport Medicine, 29(4),* 245.

Etnyre, B. R., & Lee, E. J. (1987). Comments on proprioceptive neuromuscular facilitation stretching techniques. *Research Quarterly for Exercise and Sport, 58,* 184–188.

Guissard, N., & Duchaleau, J. (2004). Effects of static stretch training on neural and mechanical properties of the human plantar-flexor muscles. *Muscle Nerve, 29(2),* 248–255.

Health Canada Physical Activity Guide to Healthy Active Living for Older Adults, Canadian Society for Exercise Physiology. (2005, February). www.phac-aspc.qc.ca/pav-vap/paguide/.

Hutton, R. S. (1992). Neuromuscular basis of stretching exercises. In P. V. Komi (Ed.), *Strength and Power in Sport,* Oxford: Blackwell Scientific.

Ingraham, S. J. (2003). The role of flexibility in injury prevention and athletic performance: Have we stretched the truth? *Minnesota Medicine, 86(5),* 58–61.

Kubo, K., Kanehisa, H., Kawakami, Y., & Fukunaga, T. (2001). Influence of static stretching on viscoelastic properties of human tendon structures in vivo. *Journal of Applied Physiology, 90(2),* 520–526.

McAtee, R. (1999). *Facilitated stretching* (2nd ed.). Champaign, IL: Human Kinetics.

McGill, S. M. (2001). Low back stability: From formal description to issues for performance and rehabilitation. *Exercise and Sport Sciences Review, 29(1),* 26–31.

Newton, R. U., Kramer, W. J., & Hakkinen, K. (1999). Effects of ballistic training on preseason preparation of elite volleyball players. *Medicine and Science in Sports and Exercise 31(2),* 323–330.

Orloff, H. A., & Rapp, C. M. (2004). The effects of load carriage on spinal curvature and posture. *Spine, 29(12),* 1325–1329.

Shrier, I. (1999). Stretching before exercise does not reduce the risk of local muscle injury: A critical review of the clinical and basic science literature. *Clinical Journal of Sport Medicine, 9(4),* 221–227.

Thacker, S. B., Gilchrist, J., Stroup, D. F., & Kimsey, C. D. (2004). The impact of stretching on sports injury risk: A systematic review of the literature. *Medicine & Science in Sports & Exercise, 36(3),* 371–378.

Unick, J., Kieffer, H. S., Cheesman, W., & Feeney, A. (2005). The acute effects of static and ballistic stretching on vertical jump performance in trained women. *Journal of Strength and Conditioning Research, 19(1),* 206–212.

Witvrouw, E., Mahieu, N., Danneels, L., & McNair, P. (2004). Stretching and injury prevention: An obscure relationship. *Sports Medicine, 34(7),* 443–449.

LABORATORY 6.1

Flexibility Progression Log

Name_____ Age _____ Sex _____ Date _____

The purpose of this log is to provide a record of progress in increasing flexibility in selected joints.

DIRECTIONS

Record the date, sets, and hold time for each of the exercises listed in the left column.

St/Hold = Sets and hold time

Example: 2/30 = 2 sets held for 30 seconds each.

Date _____

Exercise	St/Hold	St/Hold	St/Hold	St/Hold	St/Hold	St/Hold	St/Hold
Lower leg stretch							
Inside leg stretch							
One-leg stretch							
Lower back stretch							
Chest stretch							
Side stretch							
Thigh stretch							
Spine twister							
Neck stretch							
Shin stretch							
Leg stretch							
Trunk twister							

CHAPTER 7

Nutrition, Health, and Physical Activity

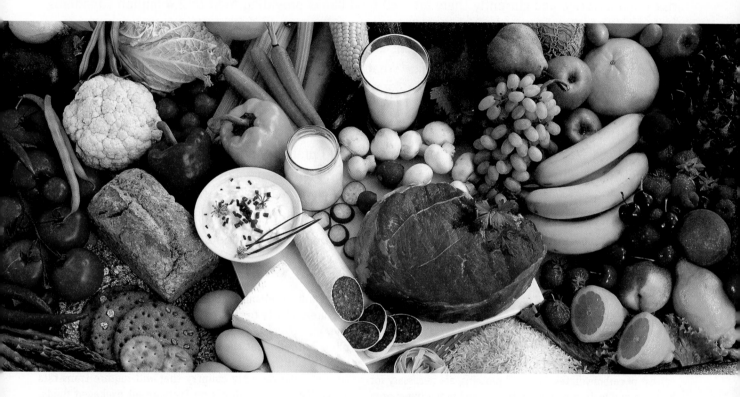

After studying this chapter, you should be able to

1. Interpret food labels and explain why Canada has implemented legislation regarding their use.

2. Describe the macronutrients and outline the primary functions of each.

3. Define the term *calorie* and differentiate the energy content of carbohydrates, fats, and proteins in the body.

4. Describe the micronutrients and outline the primary functions of each.

5. Define the term *hydrogenated*.

6. Identify the amounts of carbohydrates, proteins, and vitamins needed for physically active individuals.

7. Identify the health benefits of folic acid.

8. Define the term *natural health products,* and discuss the governmental regulations for their marketing.

9. Understand the potential benefits of irradiated foods.

10. Define the term *phytochemical*.

Nutrition can be broadly defined as the study of food and the way the body uses it to produce energy and build or repair body tissues. Good nutrition means that an individual's nutritional intake provides all the essential foodstuffs required to maintain a healthy body. Dietary deficiencies were once thought to be a thing of the past. However, disparities in nutritional well-being are evident among vulnerable populations. For example, those of lower socioeconomic status have greater incidence of low birth weight; in some inner-city areas rates are as high as 10 percent, comparable to those in developing countries (Health Canada, 2004b). The use of food banks has risen dramatically, and currently there are 460 food banks providing food to 2.4 million Canadians, including 900 000 children (Health Canada, 2004b).

In direct contrast to nutritional deficiencies, high-calorie eating and overconsumption are also problematic in Canada (see A Closer Look: "What Is a Calorie?"). Physical inactivity and increased food intake has contributed to approximately 23 percent of Canadians' being overweight, and to obesity in children rising in the last 10 years from 14 to 24 percent in girls, and 18 to 26 percent in boys (Health Canada, 2004b). Some of the consequences of obesity and poor nutrition are cardiovascular disease, diabetes, osteoporosis, cancer, and premature death. Through nutritional analysis and modification it is possible to prevent many nutrition-related diseases. An elementary understanding of nutrition is therefore important for everyone. This chapter outlines the fundamental concepts of good nutrition and provides guidelines for developing healthy eating habits. We also discuss how physical activity can modify nutritional requirements.

Basic Nutrition

Substances in food that are necessary for good health are called **nutrients**. They can be divided into two categories: macronutrients and micronutrients. **Macronutrients**, which consist of carbohydrates, fats, and proteins, are necessary for building and maintaining body tissues and providing energy for daily activities. **Micronutrients** include all other substances in food, such as vitamins and minerals that regulate the functions of the cells.

Getting the Most Out of Food Labels

In 2003, Canada revamped its food labelling system and became the country with the most comprehensive Nutrition Facts labels in the world. Prior to the changes food labelling was voluntary, and it was estimated by the Centre for Science in the Public Interest (CSPI) that only half of the foods in Canada had any printed nutritional information. Other downfalls of previous food labels were the lack of serving-size standardization and units of measure, as well as the manufacturers' ability to make misleading statements. For example, manufacturers could state that a product was full of fibre, but leave out the fat content.

In addition to tough new requirements, Canada will also become the only country that will require trans fats to be listed in the Nutrition Facts on all packaged foods. Trans fats come from oil that has been modified through a heating process, and are linked to heart disease and some cancers. There will be further discussion of trans fats later in this chapter.

Some health claims will now be allowed on labels, but only those based on scientific fact. The claims must be specifically worded so a manufacturer can't make a direct connection between its product and a health benefit. Claims like "Eating cereal A will reduce your cholesterol" will not be allowed; however, "A diet rich in vegetables and fruits reduces risk of some types of cancer" will be permitted.

Restrictions will also be placed on nutrient claims. Claims can be made regarding calories, saturated fats, salt, sugar, fibre, and protein, but each will have its own standardization requirements. For example "fat free" will be permitted only if the product has fewer than 0.5 g of fat per 100 g and contains no added fat. "Cholesterol free" will mean that there are fewer than 2 mg of cholesterol for each serving.

It is estimated that the new food labels will save the country $5 billion over 20 years in direct and indirect health care costs (Health Canada, 2004b). Margaret Cheney, chief of nutri-

nutrients Substances in food that are necessary for good health.

macronutrients Carbohydrates, fats, and proteins, which are necessary for building and maintaining body tissues and providing energy for daily activities.

micronutrients Nutrients in food, such as vitamins and minerals, that regulate the functions of the cells.

tion evaluation for Health Canada, attributes those savings to labels that make consumers aware of their choices and assist in choosing healthier foods. Indirectly, this labelling system will help the consumer prevent diabetes, heart disease, and certain cancers. Figure 7.1 lists the 13 nutrients required on Nutrition Facts labels by the Canadian government.

RNI versus DRI

Since 1995, scientists in Canada and the United States have been working to develop new recommendations for nutrient intake. The new recommendations, called the Dietary Reference Intakes (DRIs), replace Canada's Recommended Nutrient Intakes (RNI) and the U.S. Recommended Dietary Allowances (RDA) (National Academy of Science, 2003; Health Canada, 2004a).

The DRIs are based on the amounts of vitamins, minerals, carbohydrates, and fats that we need to avoid deficiencies and reduce the risk of chronic disease. The DRI is also designed to help people avoid overconsumption of nutrients that may have health consequences. For example, exceeding the upper limits of vitamin C can lead to extreme gastrointestinal distress.

Consuming a variety of foods from Canada's Food Guide to Healthy Eating provides the best opportunity to obtain the nutrient requirements set out by the DRI. In certain cases, specific vitamin or mineral supplements are recommended. For example, research has shown that supplements containing folic acid substantially reduce the risk of neural-tube birth defects. Therefore, all women who could become pregnant should take a multivitamin containing 0.4 mg of folic acid every day in addition to the folate consumed in a healthy diet (Bailey, Moyers, & Gregory, 2001; Health Canada, 2004a). Note that if you currently do not take any vitamin supplements and would like to start, it is always best to check with your health care professional (Willett & Stampfer, 2001).

Macronutrients

According to Canada's Food Guide to Healthy Eating (see Figure 7.2), a well-balanced nutritional plan comprises approximately 55 percent carbohydrates from a variety of sources; 30 percent fat, with saturated fat limited to 10 percent; and 15 percent protein. The "rainbow" shown in Figure 7.2 gives a variety of foods that can be consumed and the appropriate amounts. It is recommended that no more than 5 percent of daily calories come from alcohol (approximately two drinks daily), and that caffeine be limited to fewer than four regular cups of coffee a day. In addition, sodium levels should be kept to approximately 1.5 g per day (1500 mg).

The amount of food that you need from the Food Guide depends on your age, body size, activity level, and sex. To accommodate these variables, the Food Guide gives a lower and higher number of servings for each group. For example, young children can choose the lower number of servings in any category, while some teenagers may choose the higher value. The average

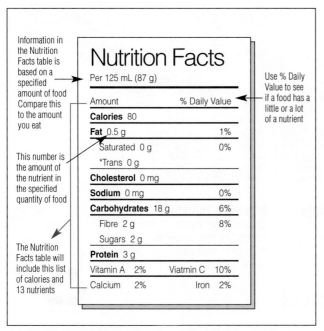

FIGURE 7.1 Canada's new Nutrition Facts label.

Source: Nutrition Facts Food Label, Health Canada, 2003. Reproduced with the permission of the Minister of Public Works and Government Services Canada, 2005.

calorie The amount of energy necessary to raise the temperature of 1 gram of water 1°C; the unit of measure used to quantify food energy or the energy expended by the body.

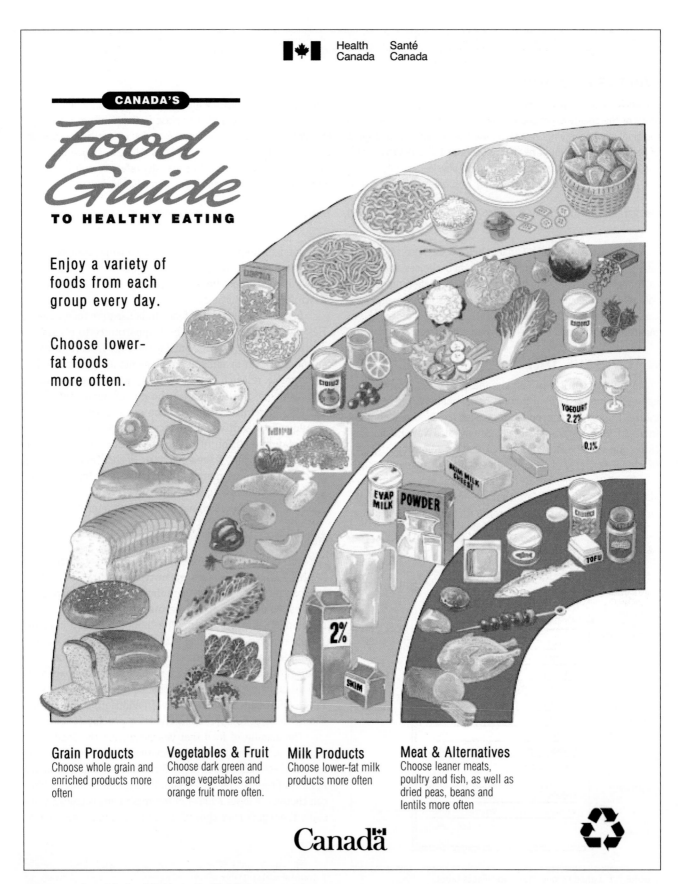

FIGURE 7.2 Canada's Food Guide to Healthy Eating.

Source: Canada's Food Guide to Healthy Eating, Health Canada, 2005. Reproduced with the permission of the Minister of Public Works and Government Services Canada, 2005.

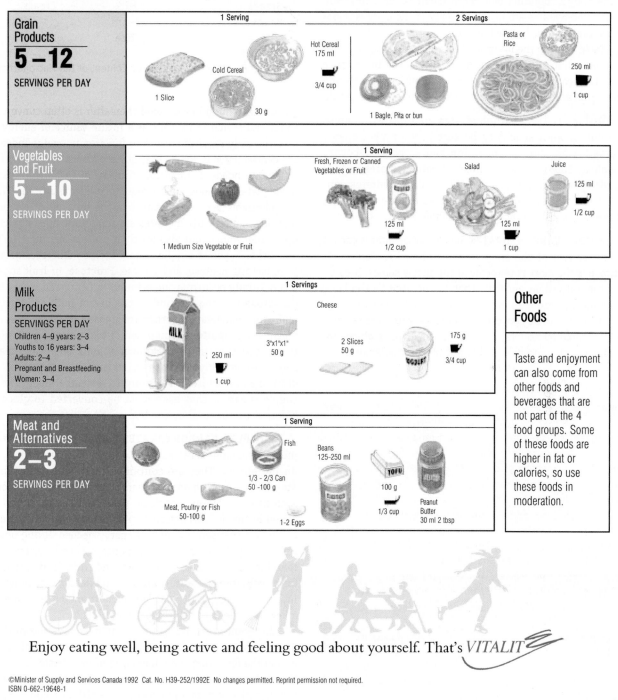

©Minister of Supply and Services Canada 1992 Cat. No. H39-252/1992E No changes permitted. Reprint permission not required.
ISBN 0-662-19648-1

FIGURE 7.2 *continued.*

Canadian wishing to maintain a healthy body weight will probably choose servings somewhere in the middle.

Macronutrients are made up of fats, proteins, and carbohydrates, and are known as "fuel nutrients" because they are the only substances that can provide the energy necessary for bodily functions. Under normal conditions, carbohydrates and fats are the primary fuels used by the body to produce energy. The primary function of protein is to serve as the body's "building blocks" to repair tissues. However, when carbohydrates are in short supply or the body is under stress, protein can be used as a fuel.

Table 7.1 lists the major food sources and energy content of carbohydrates, proteins, and fats. Given the importance of dietary carbohydrates, fats, and proteins to health and fitness, we will discuss these macronutrients in more detail.

Carbohydrates
Carbohydrates are especially important during physical activity, because they are a key energy source for muscular contraction and assist in recovery (Stephen, 2004). Dietary sources of carbohydrates include breads, grains, fruits, and vegetables. Carbohydrates contain 4 kcals of energy and can be divided into two major classes and several subclasses (see Table 7.2).

SIMPLE CARBOHYDRATES Simple carbohydrates consist of one or two of the simple sugars shown in Table 7.2. **Glucose** is the most noteworthy of the simple sugars, because it is the only sugar molecule that can be used by the body in its natural form. To be used for fuel, all other carbohydrates must first be converted to glucose. After a meal, glucose is stored by skeletal muscles and the liver as **glycogen**, a molecule composed of a chain of glucose molecules. The

Carbohydrate (4 calories/ gram)	Protein (4 calories/ gram)	Fat (9 calories/ gram)
Grains	Meats	Butter
Fruits	Fish	Margarine
Vegetables	Poultry	Oils
Concentrated sweets	Eggs	Shortening
Breads	Milk	Cream
Beans/peas	Beans	
	Rice	

TABLE 7.1 Food Sources and Energy Content of the Macronutrients

glucose remaining in the blood thereafter is often converted to fat and stored in fat cells as a future source of energy.

The body requires glucose to function normally. Indeed, the central nervous system uses glucose almost exclusively for its energy needs. If nutritional intake of carbohydrates is inadequate, the body must make glucose from protein. This is undesirable because it results in the breakdown of body protein. Dietary carbohydrates are important not only as a direct fuel source, but also for their protein-sparing effect.

Other types of simple sugars include fructose, galactose, lactose, maltose, and sucrose. **Fructose**, or fruit sugar, is a naturally occurring sugar found in fruits and in honey. **Galactose** is a sugar found in the breast milk of humans and other mammals. **Lactose** (composed of galactose and glucose) and **maltose** (composed of two glucose molecules linked together) are best known as milk sugar and malt sugar, respectively. **Sucrose** (table sugar) is composed of glucose and fructose. A key point to remember about these simple sugars is that each must be converted to glucose before it can be used by the body.

COMPLEX CARBOHYDRATES Complex carbohydrates provide micronutrients and the glucose necessary for producing energy. They are contained in starches and fibre. **Starches** are long chains of sugars commonly found in foods such as corn, grains, potatoes, peas, and beans. Starch is stored in the body as glycogen and, as previously discussed, is used for that sudden burst of energy needed during physical activity. **Fibre** is a stringy, nondigestible carbohydrate found in whole grains, vegetables, and fruits in its primary form, cellulose. Because fibre is nondigestible, it is not a fuel source; nor does it provide micronutrients. It is, however, a key ingredient in healthy eating habits.

In recent years, nutrition researchers have shown that dietary fibre provides bulk in the intestinal tract. This bulk aids in the formation and elimination of food waste products, thus reducing the time necessary for wastes to move through the digestive system and lowering the risk of colon cancer. Dietary fibre is also thought to be a factor in reducing the risk for coronary heart disease and breast cancer, and in controlling blood sugar in people with diabetes (Von Schacky,

carbohydrates A key energy source for muscular contraction. Dietary sources of carbohydrates are breads, grains, fruits, and vegetables.

glucose A sugar molecule that can be used by the body in its natural form for energy.

glycogen The storage form of glucose in the liver and skeletal muscles.

fructose Also called *fruit sugar;* a naturally occurring sugar found in fruits and in honey.

galactose A simple sugar found in the breast milk of humans and other mammals.

lactose Also called *milk sugar;* a simple sugar found in milk products; it is composed of galactose and glucose.

maltose Also called *malt sugar;* a simple sugar found in grain products; it is composed of two glucose molecules linked together.

sucrose Also called *table sugar;* a molecule composed of glucose and fructose.

complex carbohydrates Carbohydrates that provide micronutrients and the glucose necessary for producing energy. They are contained in starches and fibre.

starches Long chains of sugars commonly found in foods such as corn, grains, potatoes, peas, and beans.

fibre A stringy, nondigestible carbohydrate found in whole grains, vegetables, and fruits in its primary form, cellulose.

Major Classifications of Carbohydrates	Subclasses of Carbohydrates	Food Sources
Simple carbohydrates (simple sugars)	Fructose	Fruits and honey
	Galactose	Breast milk
	Glucose	All sugars
	Lactose	Milk sugar
	Maltose	Malt sugar
	Sucrose	Table sugar
Complex carbohydrates	Starches	Potatoes, rice, bread
	Fibre	Fruits, vegetables, bread

TABLE 7.2 Classification of Carbohydrates and the Sources of Each

Angerer, Thiesen, Kothny, & Mudra, 1999). Some types of fibre bind with cholesterol in the digestive tract and prevent its absorption into the blood, thereby reducing blood cholesterol levels.

A minimum of 25 grams of fibre is recommended on a daily basis. Excessive fibre can cause intestinal discomfort and decrease absorption of calcium and iron into the blood (Von Schacky et al., 1999). To increase the amount of fibre consumed, it is recommended that you:

- Eat a variety of foods.
- Eat at least 5 servings of fruits and vegetables and 3 to 6 servings of whole-grain breads, cereals, and legumes per day.
- Eat the skins of fruits and vegetables.
- Eat less processed food.
- Get your fibre from foods rather than pills or powders.
- Drink plenty of fluids.

Fats Fat is an efficient storage form for energy, because each gram of fat holds more than twice the energy content of either carbohydrate or protein (Table 7.1). One gram of fat contains 9 kcals of energy. Excess fat from food is stored in fat cells (called *adipose tissue*) located under the skin and around internal organs. Fat is derived not only from dietary sources, but also can be formed in the body from excess carbohydrate and protein consumption. Although fat can be synthesized in the body, fat in the diet should not be totally eliminated. Indeed, dietary fat is the only source of linoleic and linolenic acids, fatty acids that are essential for normal growth and healthy skin.

Fat also gives protection to internal organs and assists in absorbing, transporting, and storing the fat-soluble vitamins A, D, E, and K. Fats are classified as simple, compound, or derived.

SIMPLE FATS The most common of the simple fats are **triglycerides**. Triglycerides constitute approximately 95 percent of the fats in food and are the storage form of body fat. This is the form of fat that is broken down and used to

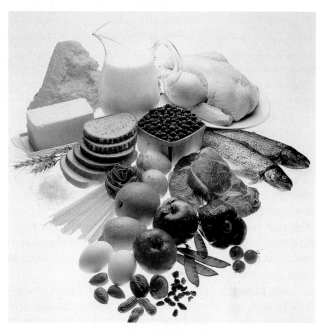

One of the main ingredients of a healthy lifestyle is well-balanced nutritional intake.

produce energy to power muscle contractions during physical activity.

Fatty acids are the basic structural unit of triglycerides. Though important nutritionally because of their energy content, fatty acids contribute to cardiovascular disease through their effects on cholesterol. Based on structure, fatty acids are classified as monounsaturated, polyunsaturated, saturated, or trans. Table 7.3 lists the dietary sources and effects on cholesterol levels of the various types of fatty acids.

fat An efficient storage form for energy, because of the energy content.

triglycerides The form of fat broken down and used to produce energy to power muscle contractions.

fatty acids The basic structural unit of triglycerides.

Type of Fatty Acid	Primary Sources	State at Room Temperature	Effect on Cholesterol
Monounsaturated	Canola* and olive oils; foods made from and prepared in them	Liquid	Lowers LDL; no effect on HDL
Polyunsaturated**	Soybean, safflower, corn, and cottonseed oils; foods made from and prepared in them	Liquid	Lowers LDL and HDL
Saturated	Animal fat from red meat, whole milk, and butter; also, coconut and palm oils	Solid	Raises LDL and total cholesterol
Trans	Partially hydrogenated vegetable oils used in cooking, margarine, shortening, baked and fried foods, and snack foods	Semisolid	Raises LDL and total cholesterol

TABLE 7.3 Classification of Fats According to Fatty Acid Type, and Their Dietary Sources and Effects on Cholesterol Levels

*Many nutritionists consider canola oil the most healthful vegetable oil because it's low in saturated fat, high in monounsaturated fat, and has a moderate level of omega-3 polyunsaturated fat.

**Contains the omega-3 and omega-6 essential fatty acids that the human body can't make on its own.

Source: Adapted from Fats: The good, the bad, the trans. *Health News*, Massachusetts Medical Society (July 25, 1999), 1–2.

Monounsaturated and polyunsaturated fatty acids are both **unsaturated fatty acids**, which are found in plants (in peas, beans, grains, and vegetable oils) and are liquid at room temperature. Because monounsaturated fatty acids seem to lower bad cholesterol levels, they are thought to be the least harmful fatty acids to the cardiovascular system. Although polyunsaturated fatty acids were favoured by nutritional researchers in the early 1980s, recent evidence suggests that polyunsaturated fatty acids may decrease levels of good cholesterol as well as bad cholesterol.

One type of polyunsaturated fatty acid, called **omega-3 fatty acid**, has recently gained widespread attention. This fatty acid, which is found primarily in fresh or frozen mackerel, herring, tuna, and salmon, is reported to be linked to lower blood cholesterol and triglycerides. However, omega-3 fatty acids are not present in canned fish because the canning process destroys the structure of these molecules. Some researchers claim that one or two servings per week of fish containing omega-3 fatty acids reduces the risk of heart disease (Von Schacky et al., 1999). Although this is an exciting possibility, more research is needed to confirm the claim.

Saturated fatty acids, which generally come from animal sources (meat and dairy products), are solid at room temperature. However, some saturated fatty acids, including coconut oil, come from plant sources (see Figure 7.3). It is well accepted that saturated fatty acids increase blood levels of cholesterol. High cholesterol levels in turn promote the buildup in the coronary arteries of fatty plaque, which can eventually lead to heart disease (Chapter 14).

Trans fatty acids, which tend to have more complex structures than the other classes of fatty acids, are responsible for raising total cholesterol in the blood. Trans fatty acids are created when polyunsaturated oils are *hydrogenated,* a heating process that changes the structure of the molecule, causing it to become semi-solid. Besides raising cholesterol levels, trans fats have been identified as the leading risk factor for coronary heart disease (Molseed, 2004). Because of their enormous health implications, trans fats will now be included on all Canadian food labels; Canada is the only country in the world that lists them (see Figure 7.1). This type of fat is found predominantly in margarine, baked goods, and fried foods and should be limited or avoided.

COMPOUND FATS For health considerations, the most important compound fats are the **lipoproteins**. These molecules are combinations of protein, triglycerides, and cholesterol. Although lipoproteins exist in several forms, the two primary types are low-density lipoproteins (LDL cholesterol) and high-density lipoproteins (HDL cholesterol). LDL cholesterol consists of a limited amount of protein and triglycerides but contains a large amount of cholesterol. It is thus associated with promoting the fatty plaque buildup in the arteries of the heart that is the primary cause of heart disease. In contrast, HDLs are primarily composed of protein, have a limited amount of cholesterol, and are associated

unsaturated fatty acid A type of fatty acid that comes primarily from plant sources and is liquid at room temperature.

omega-3 fatty acid A type of unsaturated fatty acid that lowers blood cholesterol and triglycerides and is found primarily in fresh or frozen mackerel, herring, tuna, and salmon.

saturated fatty acid A type of fatty acid that comes primarily from animal sources (meat and dairy products) and is solid at room temperature.

trans fatty acid A type of fatty acid that increases cholesterol in the blood and is a major contributor to heart disease.

lipoproteins Combinations of protein, triglycerides, and cholesterol in the blood.

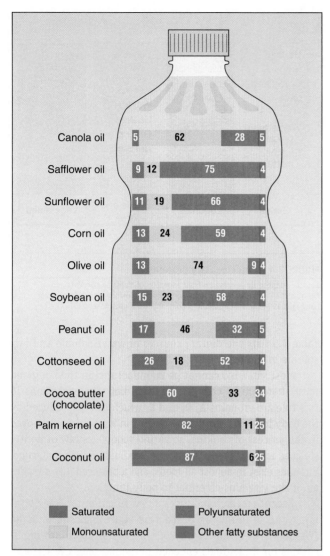

Saturated | Polyunsaturated
Monounsaturated | Other fatty substances

FIGURE 7.3 Percentages of saturated, polyunsaturated, and monounsaturated fats in common vegetable oils.

Source: Donatelle, R. J., Davis, L. G., Munroe, A. J., Munroe, A., & Casselman, M. A. (2004). *Health: The basics* (3rd ed.). Toronto: Benjamin Cummings, 186. Reprinted with permission of Pearson Education Canada Inc.

Food	Amount of Food	Cholesterol (mg)
Milk, skim	250 mL	4
Mayonnaise	15 mL	10
Butter	1 pat	11
Lard	15 mL	12
Cottage cheese	125 mL	15
Milk, low fat, 2%	250 mL	22
Half and half	60 mL	23
Hot dog*	1	29
Ice cream, ~10% fat	125 mL	30
Cheese, cheddar	30 g	30
Milk, whole*	250 mL	34
Oysters, salmon	90 g	40
Clams, halibut, tuna	90 g	55
Chicken, turkey	90 g	70
Beef,* pork,* lobster	90 g	75
Lamb, crab	90 g	85
Shrimp	90 g	125
Heart (beef)	90 g	164
Egg (yolk)*	1 each	220–275
Liver (beef)	90 g	410
Kidney	90 g	587
Brains	90 g	2637

TABLE 7.4 Cholesterol Content of Selected Foods (listed in ascending order)

Leading contributors of cholesterol to the diet.
Approximate North American Measurements.

including the synthesis of enzymes, hormones, and antibodies. These compounds regulate body metabolism and provide protection from disease.

As mentioned earlier, proteins are not usually a major fuel source. Nevertheless, under conditions of low carbohydrate intake (e.g., calorie reduction or fad diets), proteins can be converted to glucose and used as fuel. During periods of adequate dietary carbohydrate intake, excess proteins consumed are converted to fats and stored in adipose tissue as an energy reserve. One gram of protein contains 4 kcal of energy.

The basic structural units of proteins are called **amino acids**. Twenty different amino acids exist and can be linked end-to-end in various combinations to create different proteins with unique functions. The body can make 11 of these amino acids; because they are not needed in the diet, they

with a low risk of heart disease. We discuss HDL and LDL cholesterol again in Chapter 14.

DERIVED FATS Even though they do not contain fatty acids, **derived fats** are classified as fats because they are not water soluble. The best example of a derived fat is **cholesterol**, which is present in many foods from animal sources, including meats, shellfish, and dairy products (Table 7.4). Although a diet high in cholesterol increases your risk of heart disease, some cholesterol is essential for normal body function. Indeed, cholesterol is a constituent of cells and is used to manufacture certain types of hormones (e.g., male and female sex hormones).

Proteins
The primary role of dietary protein is to serve as the structural unit to build and repair body tissues. Proteins are also important for numerous other bodily functions,

derived fats A class of fats that do not contain fatty acids and are not soluble in water.

cholesterol A type of derived fat in the body that is necessary for cell and hormone synthesis.

amino acids The basic structural unit of proteins.

are referred to as **nonessential amino acids**. The remaining 9 amino acids cannot be manufactured by the body; because they must be obtained in the diet, they are called **essential amino acids.**

Most Canadians consume more protein than is necessary in the form of high-fat animal flesh. The DRI for the average man is only 63 g, while the average woman needs only 50 g. The excess is stored like any other extra calories, as fat. Protein from high-fat animal sources can lead to increased risk of heart disease, cancer, and obesity (Health Canada, 2004a). A more beneficial choice would be to reduce high-fat animal flesh with smaller portions of lean meats and fish.

Complete proteins contain all of the essential amino acids and are present only in foods of animal origin (meats and dairy products).

Incomplete proteins are missing one or more of the essential amino acids and are present in numerous vegetable sources. Therefore, vegetarians and vegans must be careful to combine a variety of foods in order to get all of the essential amino acids (see Figures 7.4 and 7.5).

Micronutrients

The category of nutrients referred to as *micronutrients* consists of vitamins and minerals. Functionally, micronutrients are as important as macronutrients and are required for sustaining life. Although they do not supply energy, they are essential to the breakdown of the macronutrients.

Vitamins **Vitamins** are small molecules that play a key role in many bodily functions, including the regulation of growth and metabolism. They are classified according to whether they are soluble in water or in fat. The class of vitamins called *water-soluble vitamins* consists of several B-complex vitamins and vitamin C. Because they are soluble in water, excess of these vitamins can be eliminated from the body by the kidneys. The *fat-soluble vitamins* are soluble in fat only and consist of vitamins A, D, E, and K. Because they are stored in body fat, it is possible for these vitamins to accumulate in the body to toxic levels.

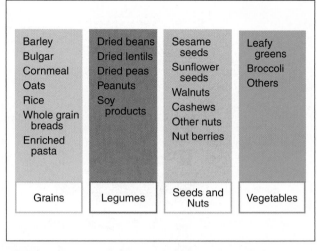

FIGURE 7.4 Complementary proteins.

Source: Adapted by permission from page 205 of *Nutrition Concepts and Controversies*, 6th ed., by Eva Hamilton, Eleanor Whitney, and Frances Sizer. Copyright 1994 by West Publishing Company. All Rights Reserved.

Table 7.5 lists the dietary sources of water-soluble and fat-soluble vitamins.

Most vitamins cannot be manufactured in the body and must therefore be consumed in the diet. The exceptions to this rule are vitamins A, D, and K, which can be produced by the body in small quantities. Vitamins in food can be destroyed in the process of cooking, so eating vegetables raw or lightly steamed is best for retaining their maximum nutritional value. Vitamins exist in almost all foods, and a balanced diet supplies all of the vitamins essential to body function.

Recent research indicates a new function for some vitamins and minerals as protectors against tissue damage (Wardlaw, 1999; Kromhout, 2001). This has important implications for individuals engaged in regular physical activity. This potential new role for micronutrients is discussed later in this chapter.

Minerals **Minerals** are chemical elements, such as sodium and calcium, that are required by the body for normal function. Like vitamins, minerals are contained in many foods and play important roles in regulating key body functions, such as the conduction of nerve impulses, muscular contraction, enzyme function, and maintenance of water balance. Minerals serve a structural function as well; calcium, phosphorus, and fluoride are important constituents of bones and teeth.

Table 7.6 illustrates the nutritionally important minerals and their functions. Three of the most widely recognized minerals are calcium, iron, and sodium. Calcium is important in its role in bone formation. A deficiency of calcium contributes to the development of the bone disease osteoporosis. Low levels of dietary iron may lead to iron-deficiency anemia, which results in chronic fatigue. High sodium intake has been associated with hypertension, a major risk factor for heart disease.

nonessential amino acids Eleven amino acids that the body can make and therefore are not necessary in the diet.

essential amino acids Amino acids that cannot be manufactured by the body and therefore must be consumed in the diet.

complete proteins Contain all the essential amino acids and are found only in foods of animal origin (meats and dairy products).

incomplete proteins Proteins that are missing one or more of the essential amino acids; can be found in numerous vegetable sources.

vitamins Small molecules that play a key role in many bodily functions.

minerals Chemical elements (e.g., sodium and calcium) required by the body for normal functioning.

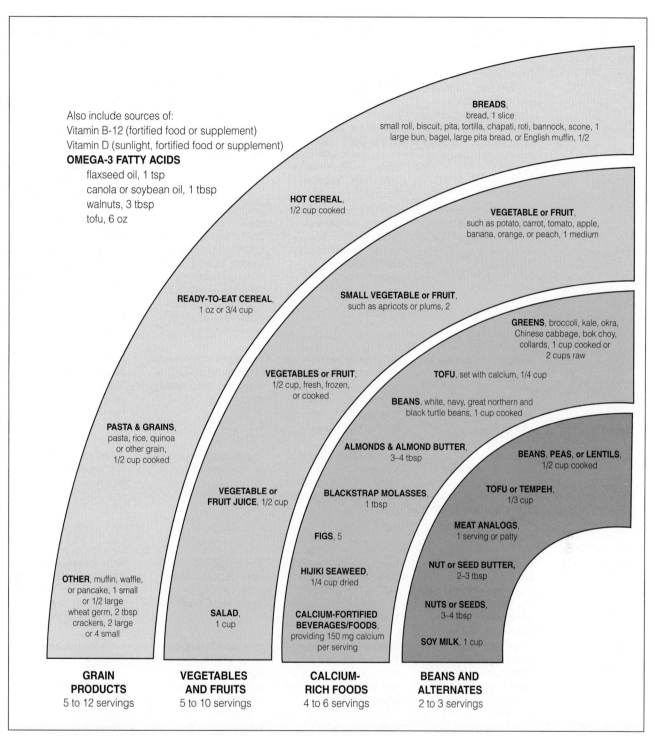

Also include sources of:
Vitamin B-12 (fortified food or supplement)
Vitamin D (sunlight, fortified food or supplement)
OMEGA-3 FATTY ACIDS
    flaxseed oil, 1 tsp
    canola or soybean oil, 1 tbsp
    walnuts, 3 tbsp
    tofu, 6 oz

BREADS,
bread, 1 slice
small roll, biscuit, pita, tortilla, chapati, roti, bannock, scone, 1
large bun, bagel, large pita bread, or English muffin, 1/2

HOT CEREAL,
1/2 cup cooked

VEGETABLE or FRUIT,
such as potato, carrot, tomato, apple,
banana, orange, or peach, 1 medium

READY-TO-EAT CEREAL,
1 oz or 3/4 cup

SMALL VEGETABLE or FRUIT,
such as apricots or plums, 2

GREENS, broccoli, kale, okra,
Chinese cabbage, bok choy,
collards, 1 cup cooked or
2 cups raw

TOFU, set with calcium, 1/4 cup

VEGETABLES or FRUIT,
1/2 cup, fresh, frozen,
or cooked

BEANS, white, navy, great northern and
black turtle beans, 1 cup cooked

PASTA & GRAINS,
pasta, rice, quinoa
or other grain,
1/2 cup cooked

ALMONDS & ALMOND BUTTER,
3–4 tbsp

BEANS, PEAS, or LENTILS,
1/2 cup cooked

**VEGETABLE or
FRUIT JUICE**, 1/2 cup

BLACKSTRAP MOLASSES,
1 tbsp

TOFU or TEMPEH,
1/3 cup

MEAT ANALOGS,
1 serving or patty

FIGS, 5

NUT or SEED BUTTER,
2–3 tbsp

OTHER, muffin, waffle,
or pancake, 1 small
or 1/2 large
wheat germ, 2 tbsp
crackers, 2 large
or 4 small

HIJIKI SEAWEED,
1/4 cup dried

NUTS or SEEDS,
3–4 tbsp

SALAD,
1 cup

**CALCIUM-FORTIFIED
BEVERAGES/FOODS**,
providing 150 mg calcium
per serving

SOY MILK, 1 cup

**GRAIN
PRODUCTS**
5 to 12 servings

**VEGETABLES
AND FRUITS**
5 to 10 servings

**CALCIUM-
RICH FOODS**
4 to 6 servings

**BEANS AND
ALTERNATES**
2 to 3 servings

FIGURE 7.5 An eating guide for healthy vegan meal planning. A healthful vegan nutritional intake requires that certain combinations of foods are consumed daily to provide all of the essential amino acids. Planning meals to conform to the proportions shown in the rainbow will result in combinations of foods that enable vegans to avoid protein deficiencies.

Source: From http://www.nutrispeak.com/veganrainbow.htm. Reprinted with permission.

Vitamin	Best Sources	Main Roles	Deficiency Symptoms	Risks of Megadoses
Fat Soluble				
A	Liver; eggs; cheese; butter; fortified margarine and milk; yellow, orange, and dark-green vegetables and fruits (e.g., carrots, broccoli, spinach, cantaloupe).	Assists in the formation and maintenance of healthy skin, hair, and mucous membranes; aids in the ability to see in dim light (night vision); needed for proper bone growth, teeth development, and reproduction.	Night blindness; rough skin and mucous membranes; infection of mucous membranes; drying of the eyes; impaired growth of bones and tooth enamel.	Blurred vision, loss of appetite, headaches, skin rashes, nausea, diarrhea, hair loss, menstrual irregularities, extreme fatigue, joint pain, liver damage, insomnia, abnormal bone growth, injury to brain and nervous system.
D	Fortified milk; egg yolk; liver; tuna, salmon; cod-liver oil. Made in skin in sunlight.	Aids in the formation and maintenance of bones and teeth; assists in the absorption and use of calcium and phosphorus.	In children, rickets, stunted bone growth, bowed legs, malformed teeth, protruding abdomen; in adults, osteomalacia, softening of the bones leading to shortening and fractures, muscle spasms, and twitching.	In infants, calcium deposits in kidneys and excessive calcium in blood; in adults, calcium deposits throughout body, deafness, nausea, loss of appetite, kidney stones, fragile bones, high blood pressure, high blood cholesterol.
E	Vegetable oils; margarine; wheat germ; whole-grain cereals and bread; liver; dried beans; green leafy vegetables.	Aids in the formation of red blood cells, muscles, and other tissues; protects vitamin A and essential fatty acids from oxidation.	Prolonged impairment of fat absorption; lysis of red blood cells; nerve destruction.	None definitely known. Reports of headache, blurred vision, extreme fatigue, muscle weakness; can destroy some vitamin K made in the gut.
K	Green leafy vegetables; cabbage; cauliflower; peas; potatoes; liver; cereals. Except in newborns, made by bacteria in human intestine.	Aids in the synthesis of substances needed for blood clotting; helps maintain normal bone metabolism.	Hemorrhage, especially in newborn infants.	Jaundice in babies; anemia in laboratory animals.
Water Soluble				
Thiamin (B$_1$)	Pork (especially ham); liver; oysters; whole-grain and enriched cereals, pasta, and bread; wheat germ; oatmeal; peas; lima beans.	Helps release energy from carbohydrates; aids in the synthesis of an important nervous system chemical.	Beriberi: mental confusion, muscular weakness, swelling of the heart, leg cramps.	None known. However, because B vitamins are interdependent, excess of one may produce deficiency of others.
Riboflavin (B$_2$)	Liver; milk; meat; dark-green vegetables; eggs; whole-grain and enriched cereals, pasta, and bread; dried beans and peas.	Helps release energy from carbohydrates, proteins, and fats; aids in the maintenance of mucous membranes.	Skin disorders, especially around nose and lips; cracks at corners of mouth; sensitivity of eyes to light.	None known. See Thiamin.
Niacin (B$_3$, nicotinamide, nicotinic acid)	Liver; poultry; meat; fish; eggs; whole-grain and enriched cereals, pasta, and bread; nuts; dried peas and beans.	Participates with thiamin and riboflavin in facilitating energy production in cells.	Pellagra, skin disorders, diarrhea, mental confusion, irritability, mouth swelling, smooth tongue.	Duodenal ulcer, abnormal liver function, elevated blood sugar, excessive uric acid in blood, possibly leading to gout, skin flushing at >100 mg.

TABLE 7.5 Vitamins: Where You Get Them and What They Do

Source: Reprinted from Jane Brody's Nutrition Book, with permission of W. W. Norton & Company, Inc. Copyright © 1981 by Jane E. Brody.

Vitamin	Best Sources	Main Roles	Deficiency Symptoms	Risks of Megadoses
Pantothenic acid	Mushrooms; liver; broccoli; eggs.	Molecule involved in energy metabolism and fat storage and breakdown.	Tingling in hands, fatigue, headache, nausea.	None.
Biotin	Cheese; egg yolks; cauliflower; peanut butter; liver.	Molecule involved in glucose production; fat storage.	Dermatitis, tongue soreness, anemia, depression.	Unknown.
Choline	Lettuce; peanuts; liver, cauliflower.	Regeneration of amino acids; nerve function	Liver malfunction.	Nausea, diarrhea, vomiting.
B_6 (pyridoxine)	Whole-grain (but not enriched) cereals and bread; liver; avocados; spinach; green beans; bananas; fish; poultry meats; nuts; potatoes; green leafy vegetables.	Aids in the absorption and metabolism of proteins; helps the body use fats; assists in the formation of red blood cells.	Skin disorders, cracks at corners of mouth, smooth tongue, convulsions, dizziness, nausea, anemia, kidney stones.	Dependency on high dose, leading to deficiency symptoms when one returns to normal amounts.
B_{12} (cobalamin)	Only in animal foods; liver; kidneys; meat; fish; eggs; milk; oysters; nutritional yeast.	Aids in the formation of red blood cells; assists in the building of genetic material; helps the functioning of the nervous system.	Pernicious anemia, anemia, pale skin and mucous membranes, numbness and tingling in fingers and toes that may progress to loss of balance and weakness and pain in arms and legs.	None known.
Folacin (folic acid)	Liver; kidneys; dark-green leafy vegetables; wheat germ; dried beans and peas. Stored in the body, so daily consumption is not crucial.	Acts with B_{12} in synthesis of genetic material; aids in the formation of hemoglobin in red blood cells.	Megaloblastic anemia; enlarged red blood cells, smooth tongue, diarrhea; during pregnancy, deficiency may cause loss of the fetus or fetal abnormalities. Women on oral contraceptives may need extra folacin.	Body stores it, so it is potentially hazardous. Can mask a B_2 deficiency. Diarrhea; insomnia.
C (ascorbic acid)	Citrus fruits; tomatoes; strawberries, melon; green peppers; potatoes; dark-green vegetables.	Aids in the formation of collagen; helps maintain capillaries, bones, and teeth; helps protect other vitamins from oxidation; may block formation of cancer-causing nitrosamines.	Scurvy; bleeding gums; degenerating muscles; wounds that don't heal; loose teeth; brown, dry, rough skin. Early symptoms include loss of appetite, irritability, weight loss.	Dependency on high doses, possibly precipitating symptoms of scurvy when withdrawn (especially in infants if megadoses taken during pregnancy); kidney and bladder stones; diarrhea; urinary tract irritation; increased tendency of blood to clot; breakdown of red blood cells in persons with certain common genetic disorders.

TABLE 7.5 *continued*

Source: Reprinted from Jane Brody's Nutrition Book, with permission of W. W. Norton & Company, Inc. Copyright © 1981 by Jane E. Brody.

Water

Approximately 60 to 70 percent of the body is water; it is important for temperature control of the body, absorption and digestion of foods, formation of blood, and elimination of wastes. Because water is involved in all vital processes in the body, it is considered the nutrient of greatest concern to the physically active individual. An individual engaging in strenuous activity in a hot, humid environment can lose 1 to 3 litres of water per hour through sweating (Powers & Howley, 2001). A loss of 5 percent of body water causes fatigue, weakness, and the inability to concentrate; a loss of 15 percent can be fatal. However, in rare cases, athletes can actually consume too much water, resulting in a low blood sodium concentration or *hyponatremia*, a condition that can also be life threatening (Murray, Stofan, & Eichner, 2003). This is most often

Best Sources	Main Roles	Deficiency Symptoms	Risks of Megadoses
Macrominerals			
Calcium			
Milk and milk products; sardines; canned salmon eaten with bones; dark-green, leafy vegetables; citrus fruits; dried beans and peas.	Building bones and teeth and maintaining bone strength; muscle contraction; maintaining cell membranes; blood clotting; absorption of B_2; activation of enzymes.	In children: distorted bone growth (rickets); in adults: loss of bone (osteoporosis) and increased susceptibility to fractures.	Drowsiness; extreme lethargy; impaired absorption of iron, zinc, and manganese; calcium deposits in tissues throughout body, mimicking cancer on X-ray.
Phosphorus			
Meat; poultry; fish; eggs, dried beans and peas; milk and milk products; phosphates in processed foods, especially soft drinks.	Building bones and teeth; release of energy from carbohydrates, proteins, and fats; formation of genetic material, cell membranes, and many enzymes.	Weakness; loss of appetite; malaise; bone pain. Dietary shortages uncommon, but prolonged use of antacids can cause deficiency.	Distortion of calcium-to-phosphorus ratio, creating relative deficiency of calcium.
Magnesium			
Green, leafy, vegetables (eaten raw); nuts (especially almonds and cashews); soybeans; seeds; whole grains.	Building bones; manufacture of proteins; release of energy from muscle glycogen; conduction of nerve impulse to muscles; adjustment to cold.	Muscular twitching and tremors; irregular heartbeat; insomnia; muscle weakness; leg and foot cramps; shaky hands.	Disturbed nervous system function because the calcium-to-magnesium ratio is unbalanced; catharsis: hazard to persons with poor kidney function.
Potassium			
Orange juice; bananas; dried fruits; meats; bran; peanut butter; dried beans and peas; potatoes; coffee; tea; cocoa.	Muscle contraction; maintenance of fluid and electrolyte balance in cells; transmission of nerve impulses; release of energy from carbohydrates, proteins, and fats.	Abnormal heart rhythm; muscular weakness; lethargy; kidney and lung failure.	Excessive potassium in blood, causing muscular paralysis and abnormal heart rhythms.
Sulphur			
Beef; wheat germ; dried beans and peas; peanuts; clams.	In every cell as part of sulphur-containing amino acids; forms bridges between molecules to create firm proteins of hair, nails, and skin.	None known in humans.	Unknown
Chlorine			
Table salt and other naturally occurring salts.	Regulation of balance of body fluids and acids and bases; activation of enzyme in saliva; part of stomach acid.	Disturbed acid–base balance in body fluids (very rare).	Disturbed acid–base balance.
Trace Minerals			
Iron			
Liver; kidneys; red meats; egg yolk; green, leafy vegetables; dried fruits; dried beans and peas; potatoes; blackstrap molasses; enriched and whole-grain cereals.	Formation of hemoglobin in blood and myoglobin in muscles, which supply oxygen to cells; part of several enzymes and proteins.	Anemia, with fatigue, weakness, pallor, and shortness of breath.	Toxic buildup in liver, pancreas, and heart.
Copper			
Oysters; nuts; cocoa powder; beef and pork liver; kidneys; dried beans; corn-oil margarine.	Formation of red blood cells; part of several respiratory enzymes.	In animals: anemia; faulty development of bone and nervous tissue; loss of elasticity in tendons and major arteries; abnormal lung development; abnormal structure and pigmentation of hair.	Violent vomiting and diarrhea. Cooking acid foods in unlined copper pots can lead to toxic accumulation of copper.

TABLE 7.6 Minerals: Where You Get Them and What They Do

Best Sources	Main Roles	Deficiency Symptoms	Risks of Megadoses
Trace Minerals, continued			
Zinc			
Meat; liver; eggs; poultry; seafood; milk; whole grains.	Constituent of about 100 enzymes.	Delayed wound healing; diminished taste sensation; loss of appetite; in children: failure to grow and mature sexually; prenatally: abnormal brain development.	Nausea, vomiting; anemia; bleeding in stomach; premature birth and stillbirth; abdominal pain; fever. Can aggravate marginal copper deficiency. May produce atherosclerosis.
Iodine			
Seafood; seaweed; iodized salt; sea salt.	Part of thyroid hormones; essential for normal reproduction.	Goitre (enlarged thyroid with low hormone production); newborns: cretinism, retarded growth, protruding abdomen, swollen features.	Not known to be a problem, but could cause iodine poisoning or sensitivity reaction.
Fluorine			
Fish; tea; most meats; fluoridated water; foods grown with or cooked in fluoridated water.	Formation of strong, decay-resistant teeth; maintenance of bone strength.	Excessive dental decay; possibly osteoporosis.	Mottling of teeth and bones; in larger doses, a deadly poison.
Manganese			
Nuts; whole grains; vegetables and fruits; tea; instant coffee; cocoa powder.	Functioning of central nervous system; normal bone structure; reproduction; part of important enzymes.	None known in human beings; in animals: poor reproduction; retarded growth; birth defects; abnormal bone development.	Masklike facial expression; blurred speech; involuntary laughing; spastic gait; hand tremors.

TABLE 7.6 *continued*

seen in endurance sports or activities such as marathons and triathlons. Chapter 11 provides more suggestions for maintaining proper hydration during training.

Most healthy Canadians meet their daily water needs by drinking a variety of beverages throughout the day. Approximately 80 percent of people's total water intake comes from water and caffeinated beverages. The other 20 percent comes from food (National Academy of Sciences, 2004). The DRIs do not establish an exact water requirement, but give some general recommendations. Women

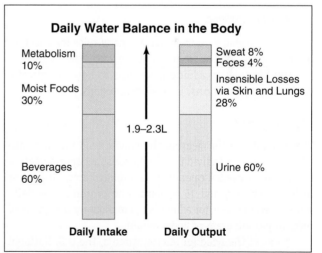

Daily Water Balance in the Body

Metabolism 10%
Moist Foods 30%
Beverages 60%

1.9–2.3L

Sweat 8%
Feces 4%
Insensible Losses via Skin and Lungs 28%
Urine 60%

Daily Intake **Daily Output**

FIGURE 7.6 Daily water intake and output by the body.

Source: Donatelle, R. J., & Davis, L. G. (1996). *Access to health.* Copyright © 1996 by Allyn & Bacon.

should consume approximately 2.7 litres from food and water each day; men should average 3.7 litres (National Academy of Sciences, 2004). Athletes or those engaging in strenuous activity will more than likely exceed the DRI recommendations. Figure 7.6 illustrates the balance between the body's sources of water intake and routes of water output.

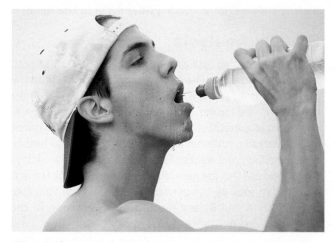

Although often overlooked nutritionally, water is a key ingredient of healthy eating.

Guidelines for Healthy Eating

Several national health agencies have suggested guidelines for healthy eating. Although they don't agree on all points, in essence they do agree on the following, as suggested by the Health Canada Office of Nutrition and Policy 2004:

Aim for fitness...
- *Aim for a healthy weight.*
- *Be physically active each day.*

Build a healthy base...
- *Choose a variety of foods from Canada's Food Guide.*
- *Choose a variety of grains daily, especially whole grains.*
- *Choose a variety of fruits and vegetables daily.*
- *Keep food safe to eat.*
- *Include essential nutrients in amounts specified by the DRI.*
- *Ensure adequate hydration.*

Choose sensibly...
- *Choose foods that are low in saturated fat and cholesterol and moderate in total fat.*
- *Choose beverages and foods to moderate your intake of sugars.*
- *Choose and prepare foods with less salt.*
- *If you choose to drink alcoholic beverages, do so in moderation.*
- *Limit caffeine.*

The following sections provide general rules for selection of the macro- and micronutrients to meet the goals of a healthy lifestyle. In addition, we discuss how to critically analyze your nutritional intake using a daily journal.

Nutrients

The general rule for meeting the body's need for macronutrients is that an individual should consume approximately 55 percent of needed calories from carbohydrates, 30 percent or less from fats, and 15 percent from proteins. The daily protein requirement for adults is approximately 0.8 grams of protein per kilogram of body weight.

To meet the need for micronutrients, the U.S. National Academy of Sciences established guidelines concerning the quantities of each micronutrient required to meet the minimum needs of most individuals (National Academy of Sciences, 2001). These DRIs are listed in Tables 7.7 to 7.9.

Once you know the recommended daily requirements for nutrients, the key question is how to choose foods to meet these goals. Previous nutritional guidelines suggested choosing foods from four basic food groups: vegetables and fruits; meats and alternatives; beans, grains, and nuts; and dairy products. Although these guidelines are still generally acceptable, they do not represent the most desirable proportions of different foods. Government health agencies responsible for setting nutritional guidelines have altered their recommendations about how we should choose foods from these groups. Refer to Figure 7.2 for an illustration of these recommendations for healthy choices using Canada's Food Guide.

The use of the Food Guide in forming good eating habits accomplishes two important goals. First, the relative proportions of foods known to promote disease are minimized. Second, "nutrient-dense" foods—that is, foods high in micronutrients per calorie—are maximized. Thus, by following the Food Guide, you are assured of getting the proper balance of macro- and micronutrients.

Until January 1, 2003, nutrition labelling was voluntary, making it difficult to follow the DRI guidelines. Further, the terms used on labels were often undefined, poorly organized, and misleading. As illustrated in Figure 7.1, the labelling system now enables consumers to choose foods based on current, accurate, and easy-to-understand information.

Calories

The number of calories regularly consumed is a key consideration for developing good eating habits. As mentioned, one problem with some nutritional intakes is excess caloric content. Therefore, monitoring total caloric intake prevents overconsumption of food.

When monitoring calories, keep in mind the following two important points. First, most people consume too many calories from simple sugars. The primary simple sugar is sucrose (i.e., table sugar). The principal nutritional problem related to simple sugars is that they contain many calories but few micronutrients. A second concern when determining caloric intake is the amount of fat consumed. Fat is high in calories, often rich in cholesterol, and contains more than twice as many calories per gram as carbohydrate or protein (1 gram of fat = 9 calories; 1 gram of carbohydrate = 4 calories; 1 gram of protein = 4 calories). Limiting fat reduces the risk of heart disease and helps avoid excess caloric intake. We discuss how to determine the optimal caloric intake for a healthy body weight in much greater detail in Chapter 8.

Dietary Analysis

From the preceding discussions, it is clear that a balanced nutritional intake is the key to good nutrition. Now the critical question is "How do I know my nutritional intake is healthy?" The answer is to keep a journal. By keeping a 3-day record of everything you eat, you will develop a snapshot of your overall nutritional habits. It is a good idea to include both weekdays and weekends in your journal (2 weekdays and 1 weekend day are generally recommended). At the end of each day, look up the nutrient content of each food (see Appendices A and B) and record this information in the tables provided in Laboratory 7.1.

TABLE 7.7 Dietary Reference Intakes (DRIs): Estimated Average Requirements for Groups

Life Stage Group	CHO (g/d)	Protein (g/d)a	Vit A (µg/d)b	Vit C (mg/d)	Vit E (mg/d)c	Thiamin (mg/d)	Riboflavin (mg/d)	Niacin (mg/d)d	Vit B6 (mg/d)	Folate (µg/d)e	Vit B12 (µg/d)e	Copper µg/d)	Iodine (µg/d)	Iron (mg/d)	Magnesium (mg/d)	Molybdenum (µg/d)	Phosphorus (mg/d)	Selenium (µg/d)	Zinc (mg/d)
Infants																			
7–12 mo		9												6.9					2.5
Children																			
1–3 y	100	11	210	13	5	0.4	0.4	5	0.4	120	0.7	260	65	3.0	65	13	380	17	2.5
4–8 y	100	15	275	22	6	0.5	0.5	6	0.5	160	1.0	340	65	4.1	110	17	405	23	4.0
Males																			
9–13 y	100	27	445	39	9	0.7	0.8	9	0.8	250	1.5	540	73	5.9	200	26	1055	35	7.0
14–18 y	100	44	630	63	12	1.0	1.1	12	1.1	330	2.0	685	95	7.7	340	33	1055	45	8.5
19–30 y	100	46	625	75	12	1.0	1.1	12	1.1	320	2.0	700	95	6	330	34	580	45	9.4
31–50 y	100	46	625	75	12	1.0	1.1	12	1.1	320	2.0	700	95	6	350	34	580	45	9.4
51–70 y	100	46	625	75	12	1.0	1.1	12	1.4	320	2.0	700	95	6	350	34	580	45	9.4
>70 y	100	46	625	75	12	1.0	1.1	12	1.4	320	2.0	700	95	6	350	34	580	45	9.4
Females																			
9–13 y	100	28	420	39	9	0.7	0.8	9	0.8	250	1.5	540	73	5.7	200	26	1055	35	7.0
14–18 y	100	38	485	56	12	0.9	0.9	11	1.0	330	2.0	685	95	7.9	300	33	1055	45	7.3
19–30 y	100	38	500	60	12	0.9	0.9	11	1.1	320	2.0	700	95	8.1	255	34	580	45	6.8
31–50 y	100	38	500	60	12	0.9	0.9	11	1.1	320	2.0	700	95	8.1	265	34	580	45	6.8
51–70 y	100	38	500	60	12	0.9	0.9	11	1.3	320	2.0	700	95	5	265	34	580	45	6.8
>70 y	100	38	500	60	12	0.9	0.9	11	1.3	320	2.0	700	95	5	265	34	580	45	6.8
Pregnancy																			
14–18 y	135	50	530	66	12	1.2	1.2	14	1.6	520	2.2	785	160	23	335	40	1055	49	10.5
19–30 y	135	50	550	70	12	1.2	1.2	14	1.6	520	2.2	800	160	22	290	40	580	49	9.5
31–50 y	135	50	550	70	12	1.2	1.2	14	1.6	520	2.2	800	160	22	300	40	580	49	9.5
Lactation																			
14–18 y	160	60	885	96	16	1.2	1.3	13	1.7	450	2.4	985	209	7	300	35	1055	59	10.9
19–30 y	160	60	900	100	16	1.2	1.3	13	1.7	450	2.4	1000	209	6.5	255	36	580	59	10.4
31–50 y	160	60	900	100	16	1.2	1.3	13	1.7	450	2.4	1000	209	6.5	265	36	580	59	10.4

Note: This table presents Estimated Average Requirements (EARs), which serve two purposes: for assessing adequacy of population intakes, and as the basis for calculating Recommended Dietary Allowances (RDAs) for individuals for those nutrients. EARs have not been established for vitamin D, vitamin K, pantothenic acid, biotin, choline, chromium, fluoride, manganese, or other nutrients not yet evaluated via the DRI process.

a   For individual at reference weight.

b   As retinol activity equivalents (RAEs), 1 RAE = 1 µg retinol, 12 µg β-carotene, 24 µg α-carotene, 24 µg β-cryptoxanthin. The RAE for dietary provitamin A carotenoids is two-fold greater than retinol equivalents (RE), whereas the RAE for preformed vitamin A is the same as RE.

c   As α-tocopherol, α–Tocpherol includes RRR–α–tocopherol, the only form of α-tocopherol that occurs naturally in foods, and the 2R–stereoisoemeric forms of α-tocopherol (RRR-β RSR-β RRS-β and RSS–α-tocopherol) that occur in fortified foods and supplements. It does not include the 2S-stereoisomeric forms of α-tocopherol (SRR-β SSR-β SRS-β and SSS-α-tocopherol), also found in fortified foods and supplements.

d   As niacin equivalents (NE), 1 mg of niacin = 60 mg of tryptophan.

e   As dietary folate equivalents (DFE), 1 DFE = 1 µg food folate = 0.6 µg of folic acid from fortified food or as a supplement consumed with food = 0.5 µg of a supplement taken on an empty stomach.

Source: From http://webhost.sun.ac.za. Reprinted with permission.

Life Stage Group	Total Water^a (L/d)	Carbohydrate (g/d)	Total Fibre (g/d)	Fat (g/d)	Linoleic Acid (g/d)	α-Linolenic Acid (g/d)	Protein^b (g/d)
Infants							
0–6 mo	0.7*	60*	ND	31*	4.4*	0.5*	9.1*
7–12 mo	0.8*	95*	ND	30*	4.6*	0.5*	**11.0**
Children							
1–3 y	1.3*	**130**	19*	ND	7*	0.7*	**13**
4–8 y	1.7*	**130**	25*	ND	10*	0.9*	**19**
Males							
9–13 y	2.4*	**130**	31*	ND	12*	1.2*	**34**
14–18 y	3.3*	**130**	38*	ND	16*	1.6*	**52**
19–30 y	3.7*	**130**	38*	ND	17*	1.6*	**56**
31–50 y	3.7*	**130**	38*	ND	17*	1.6*	**56**
51–70 y	3.7*	**130**	30*	ND	14*	1.6*	**56**
> 70 y	3.7*	**130**	30*	ND	14*	1.6*	**56**
Females							
9–13 y	2.1*	**130**	26*	ND	10*	1.0*	**34**
14–18 y	2.3*	**130**	26*	ND	11*	1.1*	**46**
19–30 y	2.7*	**130**	25*	ND	12*	1.1*	**46**
31–50 y	2.7*	**130**	25*	ND	12*	1.1*	**46**
51–70 y	2.7*	**130**	21*	ND	11*	1.1*	**46**
> 70 y	2.7*	**130**	21*	ND	11*	1.1*	**46**
Pregnancy							
14–18 y	3.0*	**175**	28*	ND	13*	1.4*	**71**
19–30 y	3.0*	**175**	28*	ND	13*	1.4*	**71**
31–50 y	3.0*	**175**	28*	ND	13*	1.4*	**71**
Lactation							
14–18 y	3.8*	**210**	29*	ND	13*	1.3*	**71**
19–30 y	3.8*	**210**	29*	ND	13*	1.3*	**71**
31–50 y	3.8*	**210**	29*	ND	13*	1.3*	**71**

TABLE 7.8 Dietary Reference Intakes (DRIs): Recommended Macronutrient Intakes for Individuals

Note: This table presents Recommended Dietary Allowances (RDAs) in **bold** type and Adequate Intakes (AIs) in ordinary type followed by an asterisk (*). RDAs and AIs may both be used as goals for individual intake. RDAs are set to meet the needs of almost all (97 to 98 percent) individuals in a group. For healthy infants fed human milk, the AI is the mean intake. The AI for other life-stage and gender groups is believed to cover the needs of all individuals in the group, but lack of data or uncertainty in the data prevent being able to specify with confidence the percentage of individuals covered by this intake.

a Total water includes all water contained in food, beverages, and drinking water.

b Based on 0.8 g/kg body weight for the reference body weight.

Source: From http://webhost.sun.ac.za. Reprinted with permission.

Macronutrient	Recommendation
Dietary cholesterol	As low as possible while consuming a nutritionally adequate diet
Trans fatty acids	As low as possible while consuming a nutritionally adequate diet
Saturated fatty acids	As low as possible while consuming a nutritionally adequate diet
Added sugars	Limit to no more than 25% of total energy

TABLE 7.9 Dietary Reference Intakes (DRIs): Additional Macronutrient Recommendations

Source: From http://webhost.sun.ac.za. Reprinted with permission.

New Dietary Reference Intakes of Nutrients

Dietary Reference Intakes (DRIs) are the daily amounts of the different food nutrients the U.S. National Academy of Sciences deems adequate for healthy individuals. Great effort has been made over the last few years to define these amounts more precisely, and an updated list of nutrients has now been published (National Academy of Sciences, 2003).

Over the past decade our increased knowledge about nutritional needs and the boom in the use of supplements have prompted the Academy to revise the way in which the values are reported. People now ask, "What are the minimal amounts of nutrients I need?" and "What are the maximal amounts that are safe?"

Even today, DRIs for some nutrients are not enough. Thus, the Academy has changed the way in which recommendations are reported. In 1997 it issued several indices to guide people in monitoring their diets. The new DRIs are divided into four categories, each of which addresses a different nutritional issue. (See the figure at right.) The new DRIs are

- **Dietary Reference Intake (DRI):** Unlike their predecessors, these DRIs are the amounts of nutrients that will meet the needs of almost every healthy person in a specific age and sex group. Also, these DRIs are meant to reduce risk, not just prevent deficiency.
- **Adequate Intake (AI):** This value is used when the DRI is not known because the scientific data aren't strong enough to produce a specific recommendation, yet there is enough evidence to give a general guideline. Thus, it is an "educated guess" at what the DRI would be if it were known.
- **Estimated Average Requirement (EAR):** This is a value that is estimated to provide one-half of the DRI for that nutrient. It is primarily used to establish the DRI. In addition, it is used for evaluating and planning the diets of large groups of people (such as the armed forces), not individuals.
- **Tolerable Upper Intake Level (UL):** This is the maximal amount that a person can take without risking adverse

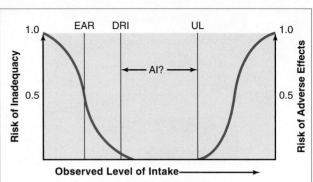

health effects. Anything above this amount might result in toxicity. In most cases this number refers to the *total* intake of the nutrient—from food, fortified foods, and nutritional supplements.

The new guidelines have changed the categorization of nutrients to group them more closely according to the functional properties of each. The following list shows the groups, the year of the latest update, and the nutrients in each.

- **Micronutrients (2001):** Vitamin A, vitamin K, arsenic, boron, chromium, copper, iodine, iron, manganese, molybdenum, nickel, silicon, vanadium, and zinc.
- **The B Vitamins and Choline (2000):** Thiamin (B_1), riboflavin (B_2), niacin (B_3), vitamin B_6, folate, vitamin B_{12}, pantothenic acid, biotin, and choline.
- **Antioxidants (2000):** Vitamin C, vitamin E, selenium, and carotenoids.
- **Calcium and Related Nutrients (1999):** Calcium, phosphorus, magnesium, vitamin D, and fluoride.

Source: National Academy of Sciences. (2003). *Dietary Reference Intakes: Applications in dietary assessment.* Washington, DC: National Academy Press.

When you have recorded the nutritive values for each day of your 3-day journal, compare your average nutrient intake with the DRI for your age and sex (Laboratory 7.1 and Table 7.7). These results will provide you with a good index of your nutritional strengths and limitations. If you find your nutritional intake deficient in any macro- or micronutrient (compared with DRI values), you should modify your intake to include foods that will provide adequate amounts of that nutrient. In contrast, if you find your nutritional intake to be excessive in any macro- or micronutrient, modify it to reduce the values.

A careful and honest analysis is a critical step in modifying poor nutrition and planning a well-balanced nutri-

tional plan. It is also an eye-opening experience, because most of us are not aware of the nutrient contents of common foods. After assessing their 3-day nutritional journal, many people are surprised by their high fat intake. The average person consumes approximately 33 to 34 percent fat (i.e., percent of total calories), which is well above the recommended 30 percent (Figure 7.2). Women should keep their fat intake under 65 g a day, and men should be under 90 g (Heart and Stroke Foundation of Canada, 2004). As mentioned earlier, a high fat intake results in an increased risk of disease and obesity.

Thus, the most likely deficiency you will encounter in your analysis is too few micronutrients. The most likely

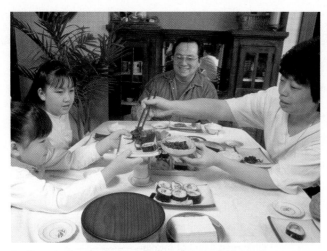

Family and cultural influences often dictate the foods we choose.

problem of excess you may encounter is overconsumption of fat, simple sugars, and calories. Remember that by following Canada's Food Guide and counting calories you can protect yourself against these common pitfalls.

Foods to Limit

Now that we have outlined the macro- and micronutrients that should be consumed on a regular basis, remember that several foods should be limited to maintain healthy eating habits. Even if you do not have the health problems that will be discussed next, determine whether close relatives have these problems. If they do, you may be a prime candidate for developing the problem later in life if you do not change your eating habits now.

First and foremost on the list of foods to limit are those with a high fat content, particularly trans fats. Both saturated and unsaturated fats are linked to heart disease, obesity, and certain cancers. In addition, it is often overlooked that dietary fat contributes more to body fat than protein or carbohydrates (Wardlaw, 1999).

Although cholesterol is a substance that the body needs to function properly, too much contributes to heart disease. Lowering blood cholesterol by dietary modifications can lower your risk of heart disease. Improvement in one's coronary heart disease risk is closely related to a decrease in dietary cholesterol, and a 1-percent reduction in cholesterol results in a 2-percent reduction in risk (Chapter 14). The new food labelling system will help identify foods high in cholesterol; however, the cholesterol content of some unlabelled foods may surprise you. Many foods that are high in cholesterol are also high in fat. Table 7.10 will help you determine your cholesterol/saturated fat index in order to rate the cardiovascular risks of certain foods.

Although salt (sodium chloride) is a necessary micronutrient, the body's daily requirement is small. For very active people who perspire a great deal, this need may increase slightly. Healthy 19- to 50-year-olds should consume approximately 1.5 g (1500 mg) of sodium per day, or 3.5 g of salt

(table salt—sodium chloride—is 40 percent sodium, so there are 3.2 to 4.8 g sodium in 8 to 12 g of salt). This amount of sodium intake is about 20 to 30 times the amount of sodium needed to replace obligatory losses from urine (~25 mg/day), skin (~100 mg/day), and feces (~25 mg/day) (National Academy of Sciences, 2003). Currently, a majority of the population consumes sodium in excess of the recommendations. The Canada Food Guide recommends an overall reduction of sodium. Reducing the amount of fast foods or packaged foods you eat can greatly reduce your intake of excess sodium.

Most people are totally unaware of the amount of salt in some foods. Figure 7.7 illustrates the "hidden" salt in an average pizza.

Ingredients

Based on medium-size combination pizza

	Amount sodium
Crust	
Pre-made from Pillsbury Hot Roll Mix (whole box)	1536 mg
Sauce	
227 g Contadina Pizza Sauce	1350 mg
Toppings	
Mozzarella (227g–283g at 150 mg/oz)	1200–1500 mg
Pork sausage (170 mg/oz) 170 g	1020 mg
Canadian bacon 57 g	1450 mg
Pepperoni 57 g	1100 mg
Black olives, 5 (sliced)	200 mg
Mushrooms (raw sliced, 125 mL)	5 mg
Onion (125 mL raw)	6 mg
Green pepper (125 mL raw)	10 mg
Seasonings/herbs/spices (1.5 mL)	500 mg
Total = 8677 mg sodium	
Extras	
Pineapple (125 mL)	2 mg
Anchovies (3.5 g)	800 mg
Cheese (125 mL)	600 mg
Tomato (1/2 med)	4 mg
Green olives (4 med sliced)	384 mg
Beef (227 g)	12 mg

FIGURE 7.7 The "hidden" salt in a typical medium pizza.

Source: Donatelle, R. J., and L. G. Davis (2002). *Access to Health*. Copyright © 2002 by Allyn & Bacon.

	Cholesterol (mg)	Saturated Fat (g)	CSI
Fish, shellfish, cooked (100 g)			
Sole	50	3	4
Salmon	74	1.5	5
Shrimp, crab, lobster	182	0.2	6
Poultry, no skin (100 g)	84.7	1	6
Beef, pork, lamb (100 g)			
15% fat (ground round)	94.6	6.3	10
30% fat (ground beef)	88.6	11.4	18
Cheeses (100 g)			
1–2% fat (low-fat, cottage cheese)	7.9	1.2	1
5–10% fat (cottage cheese)	15.1	2.8	6
32–38% fat (cheddar, cream cheese)	104.7	20.9	26
Eggs			
Whites (3)	0	0	0
Whole (1)	246	2.41	15
Fats (57.5 mL, 4 tablespoons, or 55 g)			
Most vegetable oils	0	7	8
Soft vegetable margarines	0	7.8	10
Stick margarines	0	8.5	15
Butter	124	28.7	37
Frozen desserts (1 serving)			
Frozen low-fat yogurt	*	*	2
Ice milk	13.6	2.4	6
Ice cream (10% fat)	60.6	9	13
Specialty ice cream (22% fat)	*	*	34

Varies according to brand.
Measurements are approximate values.

TABLE 7.10 The Cholesterol/Saturated Fat Index: Which Foods Promote Cardiovascular Disease?

The cholesterol/saturated fat index (CSI) compares the saturated fat in foods with the amount of cholesterol. The CSI value listed for each food indicates the relative contribution of that food to promoting cardiovascular disease. The lower the saturated fat and cholesterol, the lower the CSI. However, because saturated fat poses a greater risk than cholesterol in the diet, it is given a heavier weight in calculating CSI. For example, fruits and vegetables have a CSI of zero (the best). A food that is high in cholesterol but low in saturated fat would have an intermediate CSI value. Shrimp, for example, with 182 mg of cholesterol but virtually no saturated fat, has a CSI of 6. In contrast, lean hamburger, with approximately 95 mg of cholesterol and 6.3 grams of fat, has a CSI of 10 and carries a greater risk for promoting cardiovascular disease. For a healthy intake, the total daily CSI should range from 22 to 50, depending on the caloric content of your nutritional plan (22 for a 1200-calorie intake; 50 for a 2800-calorie intake).

Source: Adapted with permission of Simon & Schuster Inc. from *The New American Diet* by Sonja L. Connor, M.S., R.D., and William E. Connor, M.D. Copyright © 1986 by Sonja L. Connor, M.S., R.D., and William E. Connor, M.D.

An excess of salt should be avoided by individuals with high blood pressure because of the health risks. In countries where salt is not added to foods, either during cooking or at the table, high blood pressure is virtually unknown. Thus, even if you don't already have high blood pressure, you should limit salt to the minimal daily requirements.

It is generally assumed, because of the increasing availability of fast foods and the convenience of pre-packaged foods, that sugar consumption in Canada is on the rise. However, according to research by the Heart and Stroke Foundation of Canada and the Sugar Institute of Canada there is currently no accurate data on intake of sugars in Canada. Because only 43 percent of foods included in the Canadian Nutrient File (CNF) have values for total sugars, and only 31 percent for sucrose, it is impossible to know whether intake has increased, decreased, or stayed the same

(Stephen, 2004). The CNF is responsible for reporting the nutrients—for example, sugar, salt, trans fats, vitamins, and minerals—in foods commonly consumed in Canada. The Nutrient File is a comprehensive list of foods and their nutrient values (Health Canada, 2005).

It is, however, known that overconsumption of simple sugars such as sucrose or fructose, discussed earlier in this chapter, can lead to health problems. Overconsumption of these simple sugars should be avoided. The amount of sugar in sweets adds a tremendous number of calories to our daily intake. This can lead to obesity, which contributes to many health problems (e.g., type 2 diabetes). In addition, calories from sweets are considered "empty" calories because they provide few of the micronutrients the body needs to metabolize the macronutrients. Thus, complex carbohydrates are preferred because they are loaded with micronutrients. Sugar in sweets also leads to tooth decay. Although brushing your teeth after consumption can prevent this problem, it will not solve the other problems of overconsumption. One way of limiting sucrose in the diet is to use fructose as a sweetener. Fructose is twice as sweet as sucrose, so you get equal sweetness for fewer calories.

Unlike other carbohydrates, alcohol provides 7 kcal per gram and is stored not as glucose but as fat. In addition, chronic alcohol consumption tends to deplete the body's stores of some vitamins, which could lead to severe deficiencies. Thus, if for no other reason, alcohol consumption should be limited because it adds empty calories to your diet.

Your New Nutritional Plan

Now that we have presented the guidelines for healthful eating, let's put them into practice and illustrate how to construct a nutritional plan. As we discuss the steps for choosing foods, refer to Table 7.11, which presents a sample 1-day food intake for a postsecondary-age woman weighing 50 kilograms. Assuming moderate daily activities, her projected daily caloric need is approximately 1650 calories. For your use of this nutritional plan, adjust the quantities accordingly.

Because her daily intake should consist of mainly complex carbohydrates, let's start each meal with a selection of

	kcal	Fat (g)	Sat. Fat (g)	Chol. (mg)	Sod. (mg)	CHO (g)	Pro (g)	Vit A (RE)	Vit C (mg)	Ca (mg)	Iron (mg)
Breakfast											
1/2 grapefruit	38	0.1	0.02	0	0	10.7	0.8	2	41.3	14	0.1
Raisen bran (250g)	127	0	0	0	0	10.7	0.8	2	41.3	14	0.1
1 waffle (4 in. diam)	100	3	0.2	9	292	15	2	500	0	86	1.7
Lowfat milk (250 mL)	225	2.6	1.7	10	121	42	9	20	1.4	314	0.1
1 banana	105	1	0	0	1	27	1	93	10	7	0.4
Snack											
Low-fat yogurt (250 mL)	130	2.6	1.7	10	121	44	9	20	1.4	314	0.1
Lunch											
Turkey sandwich Whole wheat w/mustard	191	3.7	0.7	9	784	25	9.4	0	0	78	2.2
Baby carrots (10)	36	1	0.1	0	35	8	1	1972	8	23	0.8
Whole-wheat spaghetti (250 g)	165	1	0.2	0	4	39	8	0	0	22	1.6
w/tomato sauce (125 mL)	39	0	0	0	182	9	2	1265	8	168	1
Snack											
1 slice pizza w/ parmesan cheese	145	3	1.2	8	336	21	8	382	1	117	0.6
Dinner											
Broiled salmon (1/2 fillet)	180	5	2	83	107	0	32	189	0	21	1.8
w/mushrooms (1/2 cup)	20	0	0	0	2	4	2	0	3	5	1.4
2 whole wheat dinner rolls	150	2	0.3	0	272	27	4	0	0	60	1.4
3 spears broccoli	26	0	0	0	25	5	3	1434	87	45	0.8
Lima beans (250g)	90	0	0	0	15	21	6	332	9	29	2.2
1 peach	37	0	0	0	0	10	1	465	6	4	0.1
Totals	1669	25	8.02	129	2543	310.4	100.2	6672	177.1	1159	22.8
RDA	1690	<30%	<10%	<300	<3000	>58%	40	700	75	1000	18
% of DRI	99	45	43	43	85	128	251	953	236	116	127

TABLE 7.11 Sample Diet for a Postsecondary-Age Female Weighing 50 kilograms, Assuming Light Daily Activities

Abbreviations: Sat. Fat, saturated fat; Chol., cholesterol; Sod., sodium; CHO, carbohyrate; Pro., protein; RE, retinal equivalents; Ca., calcium

Choosing Fruits and Vegetables for High Nutrient Content

As the Food Guide suggests, a good nutritional intake includes 5 daily servings of fruits and vegetables, whether they are fresh, frozen, canned, or dried. Often, the brighter the fruit or vegetable, the higher the content of vitamins and minerals. So, to eat a healthful diet, choose fruits and vegetables of a variety of colours and kinds, especially dark green leafy vegetables, bright orange fruits and vegetables, and cooked dried peas and beans.

The following list can serve as a guide for choosing the best sources of four important nutrients:

Sources of vitamin A (carotenoids)
- Bright orange vegetables (carrots, sweet potatoes, pumpkins)
- Dark green leafy vegetables (spinach, collards, turnip greens)
- Bright orange fruits (mangoes, cantaloupes, apricots)

Sources of vitamin C
- Citrus fruits and juices, kiwis, strawberries, and cantaloupes
- Broccoli, peppers, tomatoes, cabbage, and potatoes
- Leafy greens (romaine lettuce, turnip greens, spinach)

Sources of folate
- Cooked dried beans and peas
- Oranges, orange juice
- Dark green leafy vegetables (spinach, mustard greens)

Sources of potassium
- Potatoes, sweet potatoes, spinach, winter (orange) squash
- Bananas, plantains, many dried fruits, orange juice

Source: National Academy of Sciences. (2001). *Dietary Reference Intakes: Applications in Dietary Assessment.* Washington, DC: National Academy Press.

food from the outer two layers of the rainbow in the Food Guide. This will provide mainly carbohydrates, which should be greater than 55 percent of the total caloric intake, or 930 calories. These calories may be spread out over the day in any proportion you choose. We will use foods from the inner two layers of the Food Guide rainbow to "fill in" where certain nutrients are needed.

Breakfast. Our subject first chooses grapefruit, raisin bran cereal with low-fat milk, a waffle, and a banana. This gives her 2 fruits, 2 bread/cereals, and 1 dairy product to start the day. The breakfast is low in fat, cholesterol, and sodium. A large part of the protein need is met, as well as more than 40 percent of the calcium and iron needs. The fruits alone provide almost all of the recommended vitamin A and C needs for the day.

Snack. A morning snack adds some energy and helps to suppress the appetite before lunch. Here our subject chooses a second dairy product for the day (low-fat yogurt) that provides 130 kcals of energy and lots of calcium.

Lunch. For lunch, she chooses 1 meat, 4 more servings of breads/cereals, and 2 vegetables. This lunch provides a low-calorie meal with lots of protein, vitamin A, and iron. The tomato sauce chosen was low in sodium. Be careful in choosing canned tomato sauce as it can be extremely high in sodium. The lunch also includes a turkey sandwich, which can add a considerable amount to the sodium intake, but also has the benefit of protein and other nutrients.

Snack. Our subject chooses a piece of cheese pizza for an afternoon snack to add her third dairy and seventh bread/cereal servings. Be careful in ordering pizza since some toppings (meats and additional cheese) can add lots of fat, sodium, and calories to your diet. In contrast, vegetable toppings can be added to get valuable nutrients without the fat, sodium, and calories.

Dinner. Our subject finishes the day by adding her second serving of meat and 2 more vegetables, to make a total of 5. She also adds a peach for dessert, which provides vitamin A. The salmon contains protein and plenty of omega-3 fatty acids (heart healthy). The broccoli adds vitamins A and C, and calcium, which is an important component of our subject's diet. The lima beans add vitamin A and iron.

Special Nutritional Considerations

Several conditions require special nutritional considerations, especially as they pertain to people who lead an active lifestyle. Following is a list of nutrients that may need to be supplemented, depending on your individual needs. Use these concepts to help you complete Laboratory 7.2 on page 193.

Vitamins As mentioned previously, individuals eating well-balanced meals from the food groups represented in Canada's Food Guide generally do not need vitamin supplements. Some individuals, however, may not be getting proper nutrition because of poor choices, disease, or special circumstances. Therefore, the following people may find a multivitamin supplement helpful:

- strict vegetarians
- people with chronic illnesses that depress appetite or the absorption of nutrients
- people on medications that affect appetite or digestion
- athletes engaged in a rigorous training program
- pregnant women or women who are breast-feeding infants

Choosing Your Fast Food More Wisely

As our lifestyles become faster, fast food has become a way of life. The average North American adult eats at a fast-food restaurant 6 times each month. The typical fast-food meal is high in fat and calories, factors that are major contributors to heart disease and obesity, so it is important to know how to choose foods during your next stop at the drive-through window. Keep the following guidelines in mind should you decide to grab a quick meal out:

- **Order small.** Don't "supersize" your meal. Consider these numbers: Depending on the restaurant, a double cheeseburger may contain 600 to 700 calories, 30 to 40 g fat, 120 to 140 mg cholesterol, and 1000 to 1200 mg sodium.
- **Ask for sauce on the side.** Typically, tartar sauce contains about 20 g fat and about 220 mg sodium per tablespoon. Ketchup or pickle relish are better choices.
- **Order grilled meat instead of fried.** Breaded chicken typically contains double the amount of fat than if that same piece is broiled.

- **Share fries with a friend.** A medium serving of french fries may contain more fat than a cheeseburger! Consume a cheeseburger and fries, and you've eaten more fat in one meal than you need in almost an entire day.
- **Order salads without the dressing.** Fast-food restaurants are adding more salad options. A side salad is an excellent way to include vegetables in your drive-through meal. Opting for a salad entrée will provide a meal with less fat and sodium if you choose a nonfat salad dressing. However, you must choose wisely: at one popular fast-food restaurant, one serving of reduced-calorie light Italian dressing contains 170 calories and 18 grams of fat!

On your next drive-through trip, ask for the nutrition information sheet that most restaurants offer. Then you'll be able to choose fast food that is appealing to you *and* meets your dietary goals. (See Appendix B for the nutritional content of some popular fast foods.)

- individuals on prolonged low-calorie diets
- the elderly
- individuals who are restricted to their homes (i.e., no sunlight exposure)

Iron Iron is an essential component of red blood cells, which carry oxygen to all our tissues for energy production. A deficiency of iron can result in decreased oxygen transport to tissues and thus an energy crisis. Getting enough iron is a major problem for women who are menstruating, pregnant, or nursing. Indeed, only one-half of all women of child-bearing age get the necessary 15 mg of iron per day (Wardlaw, 1999), and five percent suffer from iron-deficiency anemia. Although these individuals should not take iron supplements unless their health care professional prescribes them, they can modify their eating to ensure an adequate intake. To meet this requirement, the following nutritional modifications should be undertaken:

- Eat legumes, fresh fruits, whole-grain cereals, and broccoli, all of which are high in iron.
- Also eat foods high in vitamin C, which helps iron absorption.
- Eat lean red meats high in iron at least two or three times per week.
- Eat iron-rich organ meats, such as liver, once or twice per month.
- Don't drink tea with your meals; it interferes with iron absorption.

Calcium Calcium, the most abundant mineral in the body, is essential for building bones and teeth, as well as for normal nerve and muscle function. Adequate calcium is especially important for pregnant or nursing women. There is also some evidence that calcium may help in the prevention of colon cancer (Wardlaw, 1999).

The current calcium recommendations by Health Canada are 700 mg daily for females 19 to 49 years of age and 800 mg for females over 49 years of age. However, the current DRI recommendations for calcium intake are higher because of the tremendous health benefits such as prevention of certain cancers and osteoporosis. See Table 7.12.

Adequate calcium intake during our younger years may be a crucial factor in preventing osteoporosis in later years, which strikes one of every four women over the age of 60 (Donatelle, 2002). The following recommendations can help you get the calcium you need:

- Add dairy products to your daily intake (remember to choose those low in fat).
- Choose other calcium-rich alternatives, such as canned fish (packed in water), turnip and mustard greens, and broccoli.
- Eat foods rich in vitamin C to boost absorption of calcium.
- Use an acidic dressing, made with citrus juices or vinegar, to enhance calcium absorption from salad greens.
- Add a supplement if you can't get enough calcium in the foods you like. However, beware of supplements made

Recommendations for Calcium			
Life Stage	Age	AI (mg/d)	UL (g/d)
Infants	0–6 months	210	ND
	6–12	270	ND
Children	1–3 years	500	2.5
	4–8	800	2.5
Adolescents	9–13 years	1300	2.5
	14–18	1300	2.5
Adults	19–30 years	1000	2.5
	31–50	1000	2.5
	51–70	1200	2.5
	>70	1200	2.5
Pregnancy/Lactation	<19 years	1300	2.5
	19–50	1000	2.5

AI = adequate amount
UL = upper limit
ND = not determinable due to lack of data on adverse effects for this age group

TABLE 7.12 DRI Recommendations for Calcium

Source: National Institute of Nutrition Dietary Reference Intakes—Calcium and Related Nutrients, 2004.

with dolomite or bone meal, as they may be contaminated with lead.

Folic Acid Most people receive the DRI of folic acid by eating foods that are rich in folates, such as spinach. However, Health Canada suggests that women who are pregnant or may become pregnant take a multivitamin containing 0.4 mg of folic acid to help prevent neural tube defects (Oakley, 1993; Health Canada, 1995; Kromhout, 2001).

Folic acid may have other health benefits as well. Supplementation is effective in reducing the risk of coronary heart disease (Bailey, Moyers, & Gregory, 2001). Also, low folate levels have been associated with an increased risk of cancer, particularly colorectal cancer (Bailey, Moyers, & Gregory, 2001).

Below are some recommendations that will help you find the right supplement (Health Canada, 2004c):

- Choose a multivitamin–multimineral supplement that contains 0.4 mg folic acid in a daily dose.
- Avoid labels that say "For therapeutic use only." These supplements usually provide nutrients at a higher dose than is necessary.
- Avoid supplements containing herbs and various other extraneous non-medicinal ingredients.
- Women should not take more than one daily dose. Excessive nutrients can be harmful, particularly to an embryo in the very early stages of development.

Nutritional Aspects of Physical Fitness and Physical Activity

The number of myths about physical fitness, physical activity, and nutrition increases every year. Radio, television, newspaper, internet, and magazine advertisements are a never-ending source of fallacies. Successful athletes are often viewed as experts by the public, and their endorsement of various nutritional products are attempts to convince the public that a particular food or beverage is responsible for their success. Even though most of the claims made in commercial endorsements are not supported by research, the claims are so highly publicized that they often become accepted as fact. The truth is that there are no miracle foods to improve physical fitness or exercise performance. In the paragraphs that follow we discuss the specific needs of individuals engaging in regular physical activity.

Carbohydrates

The increased energy expenditure during physical activity creates a greater demand for fuel. Recall that the primary fuels used to provide energy for physical activity are carbohydrates and fat. Because even very lean people have a large amount of energy stored as fat, lack of fat for fuel is not a problem during physical activity. In contrast, the

How to Control Cravings for Sweets

The following guidelines can help in your quest to control your sweet tooth.

- Know how to spot sugar. When you see terms such as *sucrose, glucose, maltose, dextrose, fructose,* or *corn syrup* on food labels, beware. These are all forms of sugar.
- If sugar or its "pseudos" are in the first three ingredients on a label, avoid the product. It has a high sugar content by weight.
- Cut back on all sugars, including honey, brown sugar, and white sugar.
- Eat graham crackers, yogurt, fresh fruits, popcorn, and other healthy substitutes for high-sugar sweets when you have the munchies.

- Buy cereals that do not have sugar listed among their top ingredients. Shredded Wheat, Cheerios, and oatmeal are among the best choices.
- When baking, try cutting the sugar in recipes by one-fourth or more; you can also substitute fruit juices for sweetness or use spices such as cinnamon, anise, ginger, and nutmeg for flavouring.
- If you can't resist sweets, at least eat foods that give you some nutritional value. For example, put bananas on your oatmeal rather than brown sugar, or make oatmeal cookies rather than sugar cookies.

Source: Boyle, M., and G. Zyla. (1991). *Personal Nutrition*. St. Paul, MN: West Publishers.

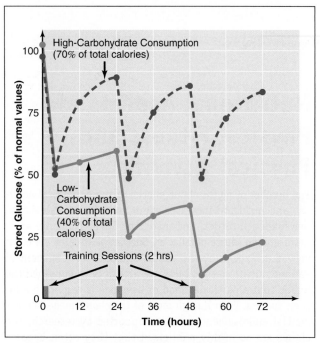

FIGURE 7.8 The importance of high-carbohydrate consumption during training. With low-carbohydrate consumption (solid line), glucose stored in muscles as glycogen is depleted by daily training sessions. With high-carbohydrate consumption (dashed line), muscle glycogen levels are maintained at near normal levels.

Source: Neiman, David C. (1995). *Fitness and sports medicine: An introduction.* Palo Alto, CA: Bull Publishing. Used with permission.

carbohydrate stores in the liver and muscles can reach critically low levels during intense or prolonged physical activity (Powers & Howley, 2001) (see Figure 7.8).

Because carbohydrates play a critical role in providing energy during physical activity, some scientists suggest that

people participating in daily physical activity should increase their intake of complex carbohydrates from 55 to 70 percent of the total calories consumed (fat is then reduced to 15 percent of total caloric intake) (Powers & Howley, 2001). If physical activity is intense, carbohydrates can be depleted from the liver and muscles, and the result is fatigue. The intensity of the physical activity dictates whether carbohydrates or fat is the predominant source of energy production (Jones & Killian, 2000; Powers & Howley, 2001).

Manufacturers of sweets have perpetuated the notion that candy can give you a quick burst of energy when needed. Does a candy bar consumed prior to physical activity provide a quick burst of energy? The answer is no. In fact, there are at least two potential problems with this type of carbohydrate consumption. First, simple sugar in the form of sweets contains only minimal amounts of the micronutrients necessary for energy production. Second, consumption of candy results in a rapid rise in blood glucose, which promotes hormonal changes that reduce blood glucose levels below normal and can create a feeling of fatigue. In this case, the effect is opposite to the one intended. Increasing the percentage of complex carbohydrates consumed and maintaining sufficient caloric intake can ensure that an adequate supply of energy from carbohydrates is stored in the muscles and the liver to meet the needs of a rigorous physical training program.

Proteins

A common myth among individuals involved in resistance-training programs is that additional protein is necessary to promote muscular growth. In fact, many bodybuilders consume large quantities of protein to supplement their normal protein consumption. Research has shown that the protein requirement for most bodybuilders is met by a normal, well-

Do Antioxidants Prevent Muscle Injury or Fatigue?

Recent research suggests that the increased muscle metabolism associated with exercise may cause an increase in free-radical production (Jenkins, 1999). Several studies have shown that this increase in free radicals may contribute to fatigue and perhaps even muscle damage. The obvious question is whether active individuals need to increase their consumption of antioxidants.

Several preliminary studies indicate a positive role for antioxidants, primarily vitamin E, in neutralizing physical activity-produced free radicals. In fact, recent reports demonstrate a reduction in muscle fatigue following administration of antioxidants (Kanter, 1995; Peterson, 2004). Several researchers suggest that an additional 400 I.U. of vitamin E be consumed daily to protect against free-radical damage. However, you should consult your pharmacist or nutritionist before consuming more than the DRI of fat-soluble vitamins. Remember that fat-soluble vitamins are stored in the body, and their accumulation may lead to toxicity.

balanced nutritional program (Lemon, 2000; Tipton & Wolfe, 2001). Therefore, the increased caloric needs of an individual engaged in a resistance-training program should come from additional food from the outer three levels of the Food Guide rainbow and not simply from additional protein. This supplies not only the extra macronutrients, but also the micronutrients necessary for energy production.

Vitamins

Some vitamin manufacturers argue that megadoses of vitamins can improve physical activity or sport performance. This belief is based on the notion that physical activity or sport increases the need for energy and, because vitamins are necessary for the breakdown of foods for energy, an extra load of vitamins should be helpful. There is no evidence to support this claim (Williams, 1989). The energy supplied for muscle contraction is not enhanced by vitamin supplements. In fact, megadoses of vitamins may interfere with the delicate balance of other micronutrients and can be toxic as well (Wardlaw, 1999).

Antioxidants

Although large doses of vitamins may be counterproductive, research has discovered a new function for some vitamins and other micronutrients (Wardlaw, 1999). These vitamins and micronutrients provide protection to cells by working as antioxidants. **Antioxidants** are chemicals that prevent a damaging form of oxygen (called *oxygen free radicals*) from causing damage to the cells. Although free radicals are constantly produced by the body, excess production of these has been implicated in cancer, lung disease, heart disease, and even the aging process (Young & Woodside, 2001).

If cellular antioxidants can combine with the free radicals as they are produced, the free radicals become neutralized before they cause damage. Therefore, increasing the level of antioxidants may be beneficial to health. Several micronutrients have been identified as potent antioxidants, including vitamins A, E, and C, beta-carotene, zinc, and selenium.

Do Health Products Provide an Edge for Health and Performance?

What are health products? Should I take them? Are they safe? Millions of people concerned about health, disease prevention, and physical performance have asked these questions. Over the past decade the use of nutritional and pharmaceutical supplements has become common in Canada. The Fraser Institute estimates that Canadians spend $1.6 billion on natural health products—vitamins, minerals, and herbs (Ramsey, 2002). In the following sections we examine what natural health products are and how they are regulated.

What Are Natural Health Products (NHPs)?

Due to the widespread use of supplements, or *natural health products* (NHP), the Canadian government has created a natural health products regulations program. Here, an NHP is defined as:

- vitamins and minerals.
- herbal remedies.
- homeopathic medicines.
- traditional Chinese medicines.
- probiotics.
- amino acids and essential fatty acids.
- a product (other than tobacco) intended to supplement their intake and contains one or more of the following ingredients: a vitamin; a mineral; an herb or other

antioxidants Chemicals that prevent a damaging form of oxygen (called *oxygen free radicals*) from causing destruction to cells.

botanical; an amino acid; a dietary substance for use by humans to supplement their intake by increasing the total daily intake; or a concentrate, metabolite, constituent, extract, or combination of these ingredients.

- a product intended for ingestion in pill, capsule, tablet, or liquid form.

Government Regulations Concerning Natural Health Products

Prior to January 2004, supplements or NHPs such as vitamins, minerals, or amino acids were regulated under the Food and Drug Act. However, largely due to their popular use by Canadians, a new classification system called the Natural Health Products Regulations has been developed to monitor the labelling and sale of NHPs (Ramsey, 2002).

In addition to supplements' prolific use, it became apparent that the classification system for them as either food or drug was not adequate. Classification of NHPs as a food or a drug would not necessarily meet the unique requirements of some of these products. For example, if an NHP such as caffeine were to be regulated as a drug then it would have to undergo reviews for safety and clinical trials for efficacy. This process could take years. If it were to be regulated as a food, caffeine labels would have limited health claims and might not provide adequate safety information.

Under the new regulatory system, before any NHP can be sold it must undergo a pre-market review and be assessed for such things as safety, quality, and effectiveness. These safety and effectiveness criteria are less stringent than for those products claiming to be drugs. These criteria are then submitted to Health Canada by means of a product-licence application. Only those products that meet the required standards will be authorized. Once authorized, licence holders are required to monitor any adverse reactions associated with their product. Serious adverse reactions must be reported to Health Canada, which then post warnings regarding particular products.

Under these regulations, manufacturers are allowed to claim effects such as diagnosis, prevention, or treatment of a disease, disorder, or abnormal physical state. The regulations disallow claims of cures. NHP can contain only those medicinal substances that do not require a prescription and are not illegal. All products must be safe for over-the-counter use, and labelled with the following information (Health Canada, 2004d):

- recommended use or purpose
- recommended dose and duration of use
- risk information including any cautions, warnings, or known adverse reactions associated with its use

- name and address of the product licence holder, and if the NHP is imported the name and address of the importer
- common name of each medicinal ingredient
- potency of the medicinal ingredients
- list of all non-medicinal ingredients
- recommended storage conditions
- lot number and expiry date
- description of the source material of the medicinal ingredients (e.g., for an herbal product the part of the plant used, such as the root; for vitamin C, the source could be sodium ascorbate).

Products requiring a prescription will continue to be regulated under the Food and Drug Act. It is also important to remember when reading labels that just because a product contains natural substances, it does not mean that it is classified as an NHP or is healthful (Health Canada, 2004d).

The Role of Supplementation in a Healthful Nutritional Plan

It is important to note that there is little scientific evidence to validate most claims that supplements improve health, physical activity, or sport performance. Table 7.13 lists and evaluates a few of the more popular supplements currently marketed for improving health and enhancing physical activity or sport performance.

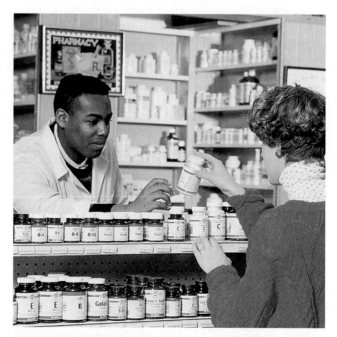

Many special considerations such as age, sex, size, and activity must be assessed in determining vitamin requirements. Consult your pharmacist or a registered dietitian when considering any dietary supplementation.

Supplement	Origin	Benefits Claimed	Evidence of Effectiveness
Androstenedione	Made by the body as part of testosterone production.	Enhances the production of testosterone and causes an increase in muscle mass.	Evidence suggests that it does not increase testosterone, and it may increase female hormones in men.
Antioxidants	Produced by cells to protect against free radical production. Some vitamins, minerals, and other chemicals in foods also have antioxidant properties.	Buffer free radical damage, which could help prevent fatigue and/or muscle damage during exercise. Also, could help protect against some diseases.	No evidence to suggest enhancement of exercise performance. Some evidence to suggest a benefit in preventing damage to tissues. Growing evidence to suggest benefits in fighting many conditions such as cancer, heart and lung disease, and aging.
Caffeine	Compound found in coffee, cola, candy, stimulants, weight-loss products.	Used to increase muscle fibre activation to increase strength, or to increase fat metabolism and endurance.	Increases endurance in events lasting greater than 20 min. No consistent effects on strength.
Carbohydrates	Component of most food. Usually found as a dietary supplement in the form of beverages or bars.	Increase of stored glucose in muscle and liver and increase in endurance.	Improves endurance in events longer than 90–120 minutes. Also helps restore glucose after exercise.
L-Carnitine	Made by the body and ingested in meat products.	Increases transport of fat in cells, reduces lactate accumulation.	Carnitine is in adequate supply in the cells, and additional amounts provide no benefit before, during, or after exercise.
Chromium picolinate	Chromium is a trace element found in several foods; picolinate is added to supplements to aid absorption in the gut.	Helps insulin action and is thought to aid glucose metabolism, blood fats, and have anabolic effects.	No good evidence for any benefits. *Side effects: Stomach upset, anemia, genetic damage, kidney damage.*
Coenzyme Q-10	Made by the body as a component of the biochemical pathway that makes ATP.	Enhances ATP production.	No evidence to suggest a benefit during or after exercise.
Creatine	Made by the body and also obtained by eating meat products.	Decreases fatigue in short, intense exercise. Increases muscle size and strength.	Increases endurance in short, intense exercise. Causes water gain in muscle but not increases in strength.
Echinacea	Herbal supplement.	Reduces duration of colds, boosts immune system, heals wounds.	Some evidence suggests it may be beneficial for these conditions. *Side effects: Uncommon, but possible GI upset, chills, nausea.*
Ginkgo Biloba	Extracts of dried leaves of *Ginkgo* plant.	Used for antioxidant properties and to improve blood flow and memory.	Does have antioxidant properties that may be beneficial in improving blood flow, improving neural function, and reducing production of stress hormones. *Side effects: nausea, headache, dizziness, skin rash, hemorrhage if used with blood thinners.*
B-Hydroxy Methyl Butyate (HMB)	Byproduct of amino acid breakdown. Also ingested in some food.	Inhibition of protein breakdown.	Scant evidence suggests some increase in muscle mass.
Ribose	Naturally occurring sugar that is now mass produced.	Used to delay fatigue during high-volume type training.	Much evidence to suggest benefits in heart muscle but very little evidence for effects on skeletal muscle.
St. John's Wort	Plant extract.	Used to treat depression and external wounds, burns, and muscle aches.	Some evidence suggests that it is beneficial for treating these conditions.

TABLE 7.13 Comparison of Dietary Supplements

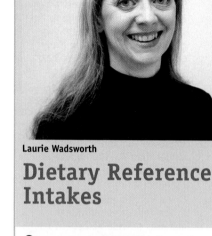

ASK AN EXPERT

Laurie Wadsworth

Dietary Reference Intakes

Q: The Dietary Reference Intake (DRI) table looks difficult to understand. Why would a moderately active postsecondary student be concerned about it?

A: The DRIs were designed for use by health professionals and researchers. These groups translated the many numbers in the tables into more usable forms for all Canadians. Canada's Food Guide to Healthy Eating is consistent with current scientific knowledge. The Food Guide provides flexibility for various energy needs through a range of servings in each food group. Nutritional quality of the foods chosen can be optimized by following the guiding statements, which emphasize whole grains, lower-fat foods, deeply coloured vegetables and fruit, and variety. Health Canada will release updated guidelines in 2006. Instead of constantly relying on a computer program to calculate average daily intakes, use the Food Guide to plan and to assess your dietary intake.

Q: I have heard a lot in the news about trans fats. Just how bad are they for my health, and what kinds of foods do I find them in?

A: Trans fat, a type of fatty acid, increases your risk of developing heart disease. While trans fats occur naturally in animal-based foods, such as beef, lamb, and dairy products, the major source of trans fats for Canadians is processed foods. These products use shortenings, margarines, and frying fats made by the process of partial hydrogenation, which turns liquid oils into semi-solid fats. The typical Canadian dietary sources of trans fats include crackers, cookies, pastries, muffins, snack foods, and fried foods such as doughnuts and french fries. The food manufacturing industry is working to reduce or remove trans fats in many processed foods. To help consumers make healthy choices, Canada was the first nation to require trans fats to be listed on the Nutrition Facts label of packaged foods. Canada is also the second country in the world trying to reduce trans fats in processed foods to the lowest possible level.

Q: I've heard that media use can affect my health. Is this true?

A: Not only does excess use of mass media require very little energy—research shows that people using mass media tend to eat more, especially when watching TV or movies. Newer research with children indicates that the advertising in commercials and programs can change the way we think about foods. This is especially true for people who watch more than 2 hours of TV daily. Viewers can become confused about which foods are the healthier choices, since most advertising emphasizes weight loss. Nutrient-content claims such as "fat free" or "diet" create a healthy sound for foods that may not be the best choices. Research by psychologists notes that people feel that they are not prone to these effects as much as other individuals and groups, which is likely a false sense of security. Health professionals have called for increased media literacy skills for people of all ages as well as limitations on some advertising strategies. With the advent of pop-up ads and push technology, even surfing the Web can affect your exposure to advertisements. Try to limit total screen time from TV and computers to 2 hours daily.

Q: I've read that physically active people need more protein. How do I know if I am getting enough protein in my diet or if I should add more to my daily intake?

A: Active bodies do require more protein than inactive bodies. The confusion comes when translating these added needs into food choices. The average Canadian adult needs about 0.8 g protein per kilogram body weight. Endurance athletes may need as much as 1.2 g/kg/day, while strength athletes may need 1.6 to 1.7 g/kg/day. Higher protein intakes will not increase muscle mass, as there is a limit to the rate of protein accrual in the body. Safety and effectiveness of individual amino acid supplements remain unclear due to inconsistent research results with human trials. Protein from food sources carries the added benefit of a variety of other needed nutrients and is the better choice. The average Canadian consumes well beyond the suggested needs, and may actually be approaching the intake suggested for strength athletes. As an example, a 70-kg weight lifter needs about 112 to 119 g/day of protein. In terms of food, three-quarters of this can be supplied by 2 cups (500 mL) of milk, a half can of tuna on a bagel, and 100 g broiled chicken breast with a baked potato and a half-cup (125 mL) of green peas. Remember, almost all foods provide some protein, since it is part of all cells. It is not necessary to increase your food intake or to use supplements to achieve the protein needs of active people.

Sources: www.hc-sc.gc.ca/fn-an/nutrition/reference/index_e.html; Health Canada. (2005). *It's your health: Trans fat.* Ottawa: Author; Innis, S. (2004). *Current issues—The inside story: An in-depth look at trans fats. What are they? Why the concern?* Toronto: Dietitians of Canada; Health Canada. (1999). Nutrient value of some common foods. Ottawa: Minister of Health; Dietitians of Canada, American Dietetic Association, and American College of Sports Medicine. (2000). Position of Dietitians of Canada, the American Dietetic Association, and the American College of Sports Medicine: Nutrition in athletic performance. *Canadian Journal of Dietetic Practice and Research, 61(4)*, 176–191; Wadsworth, L. A., & Thompson, A. M. (2005). Media literacy: A critical role for dietetic practice. *Canadian Journal of Dietetic Practice and Research, 66(1)*, 30–36; Wadsworth, L. A. (1996). Television: The media, the message and nutritional health. *Canadian Journal of Educational Communications, 25*, 137–159; Press Release from University of Illinois Urbana-Champaign on research by speech communications professor Kristen Harrison: Accessed June 8, 2005, at http://www.news.uiuc.edu/news/05/0606kidfood.html.

Detecting Supplement Fraud

Most dietary supplements on the market today are useless. Advertisements for fraudulent products are everywhere—in newspaper and magazine ads, on TV infomercials, and on the internet—and accompanying products are sold in stores and through mail-order catalogues. And consumers, in their desire to cure an ailment, improve their well-being, or improve athletic performance, respond by spending billions of dollars each year on fraudulent health products. The products they buy often do nothing more than cheat them out of their money or steer them away from products that have been proven useful. Some supplement products may do more harm than good.

How can you avoid being scammed by the maker of a worthless supplement? Marketers have sophisticated ways of making their products attractive to potential buyers, but you can protect yourself by learning about marketing ploys. Beware of the following techniques, claims, or catchphrases:

- **The product "does it all."** Be suspicious of any supplement that claims to have multiple benefits. No one product is likely to be capable of so great a range of effectiveness.

- **The product is supported by personal testimonials.** Testimonials are quite often simply stories that have been passed from person to person, and sometimes they are completely made up. Because testimonials are difficult to prove, they may be a tip-off to the possibility of fraud.

- **The product provides a "quick fix."** Be skeptical of products that claim to produce immediate results. Among the tip-offs are ambiguous language like "provides relief in days" or "you'll feel energized immediately." Unscrupulous marketers use such phrases to protect themselves against any subsequent legal action.

- **The product is "natural."** The term *natural*, which is clearly an attention-grabber, suggests that the product is safer than conventional treatments. However, *any* product—whether synthetic or natural—that is potent enough to produce a significant physiological effect is potent enough to cause side effects.

- **The product is "a new, time-tested treatment."** A product is usually one or the other, but be suspicious of any product that claims to be both a breakthrough and a decades-old treatment. If a product that claims to be an innovation, an exclusive product, or a new discovery were really so revolutionary, it would be widely reported in the media and prescribed by health professionals, not featured in obscure ads.

- **Your "satisfaction is guaranteed."** Money-back guarantees are often empty promises. To evade cheated customers, scam artists move often, rarely staying in one place for long. And the makers of this claim know most people won't go to all the trouble involved in trying to get a refund of only $9.95 or so.

- **The product's ads contain meaningless medical jargon.** The use of scientific-sounding terms such as "aerobic enzyme booster" may seem impressive and may even contain an element of truth, but these terms likely cover up a lack of scientific data concerning the product.

Always ask yourself whether a claim seems too good to be true. If it does, then the product is probably a fraud. If you're still not sure, talk to your doctor or other health professional. The Better Business Bureau can tell you whether other consumers have lodged complaints about a product or its marketers. If a product is promoted as being helpful for a specific condition, check with the appropriate professional group—for example, consult the Heart & Stroke Foundation of Canada about products that claim some effectiveness concerning heart disease.

Our knowledge of the relationship between nutrition and disease points out the importance of micronutrients and macronutrients, as well as the need to ensure adequate nutrient consumption while avoiding excesses. Individuals also need to recognize that sport and physical activity performance are enhanced by proper training and good nutrition. However, not much is known about newly discovered, unclassified, and naturally occurring micronutrient components of food and the subsequent effects on health and disease. For example, several studies have identified numerous plant compounds, called *phytochemicals,* that when ingested by humans in small amounts may protect against a variety of diseases. (See Nutritional Links to Health and Fitness, p. 184.) We still don't know whether phytochemicals, in the large amounts typically present in supplements, are safe or effective. Given our current incomplete knowledge, eating a wide variety of foods and avoiding excesses or imbalances (which can potentially result from relying too much on dietary supplements) are the best ways to obtain adequate amounts of beneficial food constituents. As previously explained, following Canada's Food Guide can help you consume a variety of foods, which reduces the risks of both inadequate and excessive dietary intake.

Current Topics in Food Safety

Many aspects of nutrition, such as food safety, have significant effects on health. In recent years there have been increased reports of illness and death due to improperly stored and prepared foods.

Do Phytochemicals Protect Against Disease?

Besides nutrients, plant foods—legumes, vegetables, fruits, and whole grains—contain a whole other "crop" of chemicals called *phytochemicals* (*phyto* means "plant"). These substances, which plants produce naturally to protect themselves against viruses, bacteria, and fungi, may help protect us from diseases as well.

Phytochemicals include hundreds of naturally occurring substances, including carotenoids, flavenoids, indoles, isoflavones, capsaicin, and protease inhibitors. Similar to vitamins and minerals, different plant foods contain different kinds and amounts of phytochemicals.

Phytochemicals fight off harmful molecules known as free radicals. These free radicals destroy living tissue just as rust destroys metal, rapidly accelerating the aging process and damaging the ability of the immune system to fight off the bacteria, viruses, and parasites that invade our bodies, leading to disease. Certain phytochemicals appear to protect against some cancers, heart disease, and other chronic health conditions. Research into their roles is ongoing, so stay tuned! Until more is known, the nutrition bottom line still applies: Eat a wide variety of fruits, vegetables, legumes, and whole grains, and count on food, not diet supplements, to get the nutrients your body needs. That way, you'll reap the potential benefits of the many phytochemicals found in all kinds of plant foods.

Sources: Dietitians of Canada; The Canadian Cancer Association; and Duyff, R. L. (1996). *The American Dietetic Association's Complete Food and Nutrition Guide.* Minnetonka, MN: Chronicle Publishing.

Foodborne Infections

According to the Institute of Food Technologists, approximately 80 million cases of foodborne bacterial disease occur worldwide each year. These illnesses produce nausea, vomiting, and diarrhea from 12 hours to 5 days after infection (Donatelle, 2002). The severity of the illness depends on the microorganism ingested and the victim's overall health. Indeed, foodborne infections can be fatal in people with compromised immune systems or those in ill health.

One of the most common types of food poisoning is caused by the bacterium *Salmonella,* found in undercooked chicken, eggs, and processed meats. *Salmonella* is in the same family of bacteria as *Enterobacteriaceae (E.coli),* which can be found in ground hamburger and has also been associated with unpasteurized apple and orange juice (Cody, Glynn, & Farrar, 1999). Because *E.coli* is associated with ground meats, it is best to cook them to a temperature of at least 71°C to avoid infection. Both *Salmonella* and *E.coli* can cause diarrhea, stomach cramps, and vomiting.

A relatively uncommon but sometimes fatal form of food poisoning is *botulism,* which usually results from improper home-canning procedures. Use the following guidelines for preventing food poisoning:

- Clean food thoroughly. Wash all produce and raw meats, and make sure cans show no sign of leaks or bulges.
- Drink only pasteurized milk.
- Don't eat raw eggs.
- Cook chicken thoroughly.

- Cook pork to an internal temperature of at least 76°C to kill parasites called *trichina.*
- Cook ground meat to an internal temperature of 71°C.
- Cook all shellfish thoroughly; steaming them open may not be sufficient.
- Be wary of raw fish; it may contain parasitic roundworms. Keep fish frozen, and cook until well done.
- Wash utensils, plates, cutting boards, knives, blenders, and other cooking equipment with soap and very hot water after preparing raw poultry.

Food Additives

Food additives are substances added to food to lengthen its storage time, change its taste or colour, or otherwise make it more appealing. Although they can provide these benefits, they may also pose a risk. One example is *nitrites,* which are found in foods such as bacon, sausages, and lunch meats. Nitrites inhibit spoilage and prevent botulism, but they also form cancer-causing agents (nitrosamines) in the body.

Organically Grown Foods

According to Agriculture and Agri-food Canada (2000), approximately 56 percent of cultivated land is treated with pesticides. Although these chemicals can save crops from disease and pests, they may also endanger human health. In recent years, many people have begun to purchase organically grown foods. **Organic** in this context refers to foods grown without the use of pesticides. Organically grown foods are more expensive than foods commonly supplied by supermarkets.

In the near future, look for new genetics techniques in biology to spawn a new world of pest- and insecticide-free foods. These new techniques combine the genetic material from various plants in an effort to produce strains of high-

organic Refers to foods that are grown without pesticides.

How to Handle Takeout Food Safely

Whether from restaurants, supermarkets, or quick-service establishments, takeout foods have become a part of our way of life. But in order to avoid foodborne illnesses, these foods must be handled with care. The next time you order takeout, keep the following recommendations in mind.

For Hot Foods

- Hot foods must be kept hot at above 60°C. First, make sure the food is hot when you pick it up or it's delivered. You can cover food with foil (to keep it moist) and keep it warm—60°C or above—in the oven (check the food's temperature with a meat thermometer). Using a crockpot is another option for some foods. It's best to eat food within 2 hours of preparation.
- If the food won't be eaten for more than 2 hours, refrigerate in shallow, covered containers. Before serving, reheat it in an oven to 74°C or until it's hot and steaming. If you

prefer, reheat food in a microwave oven—cover and rotate—and then let it stand for 2 minutes to ensure thorough, even heating.

For Cold Foods

- Cold foods must be kept cold at 4°C or below.
- If cold takeout foods are not eaten right away, refrigerate them as soon as possible. Transport and store cold foods in chilled, insulated coolers.
- Discard any foods kept at room temperature for more than 2 hours. If conditions are warmer than 32°C, toss the food after only 1 hour.
- Keep deli platters that stay out—as is the practice in buffet dining—on bowls of ice.

Source: Food and Safety Network, 2004, Guelph University; Duyff, R. L. (1996). *The American Dietetic Association's complete food and nutrition guide.* Minnetonka, MN: Chronicle Publishing.

yield crops that are resistant to diseases and pests, high in nutritional quality, and free of chemicals. Whether these new plants will live up to expectations remains to be seen.

Irradiated Foods

Irradiation is the use of radiation (high-energy waves or particles, including radioactivity and X-rays) to kill microorganisms that grow on or in food. When radioactivity is used, the food does not become radioactive; instead the irradiation serves to prolong the shelf life of the food (Canadian Food Inspection Agency, 2004; Sibbad, 2003). Indeed, irradiated food can be stored for years in sealed containers at room temperature without spoiling. In addition, irradiation can delay the sprouting of vegetables such as potatoes and onions and delay the ripening of fruits such as bananas, mangoes, tomatoes, pears, and avocados. This can result in significant cost savings.

Are these irradiated foods safe to eat? Currently, the best answer is a qualified yes. All research indicates that the foods are safe and nutritional content is maintained, but only limited data exist (Canadian Food Inspection Agency, 2002). In addition, most studies have used very low radiation levels to irradiate foods. This raises the question of what is a safe level of radiation for the treatment of foods.

Animals Treated with Antibiotics and Hormones

In recent years, consumers have grown suspicious of eating meat from animals that have been treated with antibiotics to prevent infections. Concern has developed because of the

possibility that eating such meat could lead to the development of antibiotic-resistant bacteria in humans. At present, a definitive answer to this issue is not available.

Another recent concern has been the use of hormones to increase production of meat. There are six types of growth hormones allowed for use in cattle in Canada—three natural and three synthetic. No growth hormones have been approved for use in other animals such as chicken, swine, or sheep. Some people fear that the presence of hormones in food may result in health problems that have not yet been determined. Scientific research to date has shown that food products from animals treated with these hormones do not pose a threat to human health (Health Canada, 2004e).

Summary

1. Nutrition is the study of food and its relationship to health and disease. The current primary nutrition problem in industrialized countries is overeating.
2. A well-balanced nutritional plan comprises approximately 55 percent complex carbohydrates, 30 percent fat, and 15 percent protein. These macronutrients are also called the "fuel nutrients," because they are the only substances that can be used as fuel to provide the energy (calories) necessary for bodily functions.
3. Carbohydrate is a primary fuel used by the body to provide energy. The calorie is a unit of measure of the energy value of food or the energy required for physical activity.

4. Simple carbohydrates consist of a single sugar (glucose, fructose, sucrose) or two sugars linked together (galactose, lactose, and maltose).

5. Complex carbohydrates consist of starches and fibre. Starches are composed of chains of simple sugars. Fibre is a nondigestible but essential form of complex carbohydrates contained in whole grains, vegetables, and fruits.

6. Fat is an efficient storage form for energy, because each gram contains more than twice the energy content of 1 gram of either carbohydrate or protein. Fat can be derived from dietary sources or formed from excess carbohydrate and protein consumed in the diet. Fat is stored in the body in adipose tissues located under the skin and around internal organs.

7. The primary role of protein consumption is to serve as the structural unit for building and repairing cells in all tissues of the body. Protein consists of amino acids made by the body (11 nonessential amino acids) and those available only through dietary sources (9 essential amino acids).

8. Vitamins serve many important functions in the body, including regulation of growth and metabolism. The class of water-soluble vitamins consists of several B-complex vitamins and vitamin C. The fat-soluble vitamins are A, D, E, and K.

9. Minerals are chemical elements contained in many foods. Like vitamins, minerals serve many important roles in regulating body functions.

10. Approximately 60 to 70 percent of the body is water. Water is involved in all vital processes in the body and is the nutrient of greatest concern to the physically active individual. In addition to the water contained in foods, it is recommended that 2.7 to 3.7 litres of water be consumed daily.

11. The basic goals of developing good nutritional habits are to maintain healthful body weight; eat a variety of foods following Canada's Food Guide; avoid consuming too much fat, saturated fat, and cholesterol; eat foods with adequate starch and fibre; avoid consuming too much simple sugar or too much sodium; and if you drink alcohol, do so in moderation.

12. Healthful nutritional plans decrease the intake of fats (especially saturated and trans fats), cholesterol, salt, sugar, and alcohol.

13. The intensity of physical activity dictates the relative proportions of fat and carbohydrate that are used as fuel during physical activity. In general, the lower the intensity of physical activity, the more fat is used as a fuel. Conversely, the greater the intensity of physical activity, the more carbohydrate is used as a fuel.

14. Antioxidants are nutrients that prevent oxygen free radicals from combining with cells and damaging them. The micronutrients that have been identified as potent antioxidants are vitamins E and C, beta-carotene, zinc, and selenium.

15. Food storage and preparation are key to the prevention of food poisoning. Select foods that appear clean and fresh; keep foods cold or frozen to prevent bacteria from growing; thoroughly clean fresh fruits and vegetables; and cook all meats thoroughly.

Study Questions

1. What is the role of carbohydrates in a well-balanced nutritional plan?

2. List the major food sources of carbohydrates.

3. List the various subcategories of carbohydrates.

4. Compare the three classes of fats.

5. Define *triglyceride* and discuss its use in the body.

6. Define *hydrogenated*.

7. Distinguish between saturated and unsaturated fatty acids.

8. What are omega-3 fatty acids?

9. Discuss the role of protein in a well-balanced nutritional plan.

10. What are the recommended amounts of protein for men and for women?

11. Distinguish between essential and nonessential amino acids.

12. What are the classes of vitamins, and what is the role of vitamins in body function?

13. Outline the role of minerals in body function.

14. Discuss the importance of water in a well-balanced nutritional plan.

15. What is *hyponatremia*?

16. What approximate proportions of carbohydrate, fat, and protein of the total calories consumed are recommended daily?

17. Discuss Canada's Food Guide and its role in the selection of healthy foods.

18. How many calories are contained in 1 gram of carbohydrate, fat, and protein, respectively?

19. Discuss the special need for carbohydrates in an individual who is engaging in physical activity or a sports training program.

20. Discuss the special need for protein for an individual who is engaging in physical activity or a sports training program.

21. Define *antioxidant*. Define *calorie*.

22. What is the potential role of antioxidants?

23. Discuss the impact of high-density lipoproteins (HDL cholesterol) and low-density lipoproteins (LDL cholesterol) on heart disease.

24. Define *natural health product* and give an example.
25. How does the government regulate the marketing of natural health products?
26. Compare and contrast natural health products with a good, well-rounded eating plan.

Suggested Reading

National Academy of Science, *Dietary Reference Intakes*, 2003.

Position of the American Dietetic Association, Dietitians of Canada, and the American College of Sports Medicine: Nutrition and athletic performance. *Journal of the American Dietetic Association, 100(12)*, 1543–1556, 2000.

Wardlaw, G. M. *Perspectives in Nutrition*. Dubuque, IA: McGraw-Hill, 1999.

Wood, O. B., & Bruhn, C. M. Position of American Dietetic Association: Food irradiation. *Journal of the American Dietetic Association, 100(2)*, 246–253, 2000.

Weblinks

MEDLINEplus
www.medlineplus.gov
Contains a wealth of up-to-date, quality nutrition information from the world's largest medical library, the National Library of Medicine at the U.S. National Institutes of Health. Medlineplus is for anyone with a nutrition or medical question.

Health Canada, Natural Health Products
http://herbalcollective.ca
Provides information on the regulation of NHPs.

Canadian Sugar Institute
www.sugar.ca
Presents sound nutritional advice on many diet-related questions. Includes an excellent "Health Body Calculator" for formulating diet and exercise programs.

Health Canada, Canada's Guide to Healthy Eating
www.hc-sc.gc.ca
Provides governmental guidelines for eating and use of the Food Guide.

Dietitians of Canada
www.dietitians.ca
Contains articles about all aspects of safety in food preparation, storage, and handling.

Food Safety Network
www.foodsafetynetwork.ca
Gateway to government food safety information. Includes news and safety alerts, consumer advice, national food safety programs, and foodborne pathogens.

Canadian Restaurant and Foodservices Association
www.crfa.ca
Suggestions for the safe handling and storage of food.

Health Canada Agriculture and Agri-Food
www.agr.gc.ca
Provides information on irradiation of foods and hormone use.

Health Canada Canadian Nutrient File
www.hc-sc.gc.ca/fn-an/nutrition/fiche-nutri-data/index_e.html
A comprehensive list of foods and their nutrient values.

References

Agriculture and Agri-Food Canada. (2000). *Safety of irradiated foods*. Last updated December 15, 2000. Retrieved from www.agr.gc.ca, September 2004.

Bailey, L. B., Moyers, S., & Gregory, J. F., III. (2001). Folate. In B. A. Bowman & R. M. Russell (Eds.), *Present knowledge in nutrition* (8th ed.). Washington, DC: ILSI Press.

Cody, S. H., Glynn, M. K., Farrar, J. A., et al. (1999). An outbreak of Escherichia coli 0157:H7 infection from unpasteurized commercial apple juice. *Annals of Internal Medicine, 130*, 202–209.

Donatelle, R. J. (2002). *Access to health* (7th ed.). San Francisco: Pearson Education, publishing as Benjamin Cummings.

Health Canada. (2004a). *A consumer's guide to the DRIs (Dietary Reference Intakes)*. Last updated August 31, 2004. Retrieved from www.hc-sc.gc.ca/hpfb-dgpsa/onpp-bppn/consumer_info_e.html, September 2004.

Health Canada. (2004b). *Nutrition for health: An agenda for action*. Last updated August 31, 2004. Retrieved from www.hc-sc.gc.ca, September 2004.

Health Canada. (2004c). *Folic acid and birth defects*. Last updated October 18, 2002. Retrieved from www.hc-sc.gc.ca/english/folicacid/, September 2004.

Health Canada. (2004d). *Natural Health Products Directorate: Natural health products regulations*. Last updated May 31, 2004. Retrieved from www.hc-sc.gc.ca/hpfb-dgpsa/nhpd-dpsn/nhp_regs_e.html, September 2004.

Institute of Medicine. (2003). *Dietary Reference Intakes: Water, potassium, sodium, chloride and sulfate*. Washington, DC: National Academy of Science.

Jenkins, R. R. (1999). Free radical chemistry: Relationship to exercise. *Sports Medicine, 5*, 156–170.

Jones, N. L., & Killian, K. J. (2000). Exercise limitation in health and disease. *New England Journal of Medicine, 343(9)*, 632–641.

Kanter, M. (1995). Free radicals and exercise: Effects of nutritional antioxidant supplementation. *Exercise and Sports Sciences Reviews, 23*, 375–398.

Kromhout, D. (2001). Diet and cardiovascular diseases. *Journal of Nutrition, Health and Aging, 5(3)*, 144–149.

Lemon, P. W. (2000). Beyond the zone: Protein needs of active individuals. *Journal of the American College of Nutrition, 19(5 Suppl)*, 513S–521S.

Molseed, L. (2004, June). Tracking trans fat: Cutting down on trans fat may help cut down on heart disease. *Diabetes Forecast, 57(6),* 52–55.

Murray, R., Stofan J., & Eichner, E. R. (2003). Hyponatremia and exercise. *Sport, 88(16),* 1–6. Retrieved from www.gssiweb.com/reflib/refs/667/sse_92.cfm?pid=96&CFID=722715&CFTOKEN=, September 2004.

National Academy of Sciences. (2001). *Dietary Reference Intakes: Applications in dietary assessment.* Washington, DC: National Academy Press.

National Academy of Sciences. (2003, December 11). *Dietary Reference Intakes: Guiding principles for nutrition labeling and fortification.* Washington, DC: National Academy Press.

Oakley, G. P., Jr. (1993). Folic acid preventable spina bifida and anencephaly. *Journal of American Medical Association, 269,* 1292–1293.

Peterson, J. (2004, Jan.). Aging, exercise, and phytochemicals: Promises and pitfalls. *Academy of Science, 1019,* 453–461.

Powers, S., & Howley, E. (2001). *Exercise physiology: Theory and application to fitness and performance* (4th ed.). Dubuque, IA: McGraw-Hill.

Ramsey, C. (2002). *A cure worse than the illness: Canada's proposed regulatory framework for natural health products in light of international evidence.* Vancouver: The Fraser Institute, Public Policy Sources.

Sibbad, B. (2003, March 4). Health Canada's food irradiation proposal sets off debate. *Canadian Medical Association Journal, 168(5),* 603.

Stephen, A. M. (2004). Carbohydrate intake in Canada: What we know and what we don't. *Carbohydrate News, 8.* Retrieved September 1, 2004, from www.sugar.ca.

Tipton, K. D., & Wolfe, R. R. (2001). Exercise, protein metabolism, and muscle growth. *International Journal of Sport Nutrition and Exercise Metabolism, 11(1),* 109–132.

Von Schacky, C., Angerer, P., Thiesen, K., Kothny, T., & Mudra, H. (1999). The effect of dietary omega-3 fatty acids on coronary atherosclerosis. *Annals of Internal Medicine, 130(7),* 554.

Wardlaw, G. M. (1999). *Perspectives in nutrition.* Dubuque, IA: McGraw-Hill.

Willett, W. C., & Stampfer, M. J. (2001). What vitamins should I be taking, doctor? *New England Journal of Medicine, 345,* 1819–1824.

Williams, M. H. (1989). Vitamin supplementation and athletic performance. *International Journal for Vitamin and Nutrition Research, 30 (Suppl),* 163–191.

Young, I. S., & Woodside, J. V. (2001). Antioxidants in health and disease. *Journal of Clinical Pathology, 54(3),* 176–186.

LABORATORY 7.1

Nutritional Journal

Name_____ Age _____ Sex _____ Date _____

The purpose of this laboratory is to analyze your nutritional intake for a 3-day period.

DIRECTIONS

For a 3-day period (2 weekdays and 1 weekend day), eat the foods that you typically consume. At the end of each day, record on the following chart the foods eaten for that day and the amounts of the listed nutrients contained in each. Most packaged foods now have Nutrition Facts listed on the package. See the appendices for the listings of the nutrients contained in various foods. Total the values for each nutrient at the bottom of the chart. Transfer the total to the next chart. At the end of the 3-day period, total the daily values and divide by 3 to get the average nutritional intake for each of the nutrients analyzed. Compare your average intake for each of the nutrients with those recommended at the bottom of the page for your sex and age group. Remember that this analysis is only as representative of your normal nutritional intake as the foods you eat over the 3-day period.

WRITE-UP

In the space provided on the next page, list the strengths and weaknesses in your nutritional plan and discuss the steps that can be taken to improve it.

Daily Nutrient Intake

NAME: _____ DATE: _____

Foods	Amount	kcals (total)	kcals from fat	Protein (gm)	CHO (gm)	Fiber (gm)	Fat (gm)	Fat % (kcal)	Sat. Fat (gm)	Chol. (mg)	Sodium (mg)	Vit. A (I.U.)	Vit. C (mg)	Calcium (mg)	Iron (mg)	Vit. B$_1$ (mg)	Vit. B$_2$ (mg)	Niacin (mg)
Totals																		

Three-Day Nutrient Summary

NAME: _____ DATE: _____

Day	kcals Total	kcals from Fat	Protein (gm)	CHO (gm)	Fiber (gm)	Fat (gm)	Fat % (kcal)	Sat. Fat (gm)	Chol. (mg)	Sodium (mg)	Vit. A (I.U.)	Vit. C (mg)	Calcium (mg)	Iron (mg)	Vit. B₁ (mg)	Vit. B₂ (mg)	Niacin (mg)
One																	
Two																	
Three																	
Totals																	
Average																	

DIETARY REFERENCE INTAKES*

- Kcal total (total daily energy expenditure) is body weight multiplied by kcals per pound per day:

$$\underline{\text{Body weight in lbs}} \quad \times \quad \underline{\text{kcals per lb per day}} \quad = \quad \textbf{kcal total (total daily energy expenditure)}$$
$$\text{(from Table 8.1, page 204)}$$

- Kcals from fat should be fewer than 30 percent of total calories per day:

$$\underline{30\% \ (0.3)} \quad \times \quad \underline{\text{kcals per day}} \quad = \quad \textbf{recommended MAXIMUM kcals from fat}$$

- Protein intake is 0.8 g per kg of body weight (0.36 g per lb). (Pregnant women should add 15 g, and lactating women should add 20 g):

$$\underline{0.36 \text{ gms}} \quad \times \quad \underline{\text{body weight in lb}} \quad = \quad \textbf{recommended protein intake}$$

- Carbohydrate intake should be more than 58 percent of total calories per day:

$$\underline{58\% \ (0.58)} \quad \times \quad \underline{\text{kcals per day}} \quad = \quad \textbf{recommended carbohydrate intake}$$

Fat <30 percent of nutritional intake; fibre ~30 percent of nutritional intake; saturated fat <10 percent of nutritional intake; cholesterol <300 mg; sodium <3000 mg
* See Table 7.7 on page 169 for information on vitamin and mineral DRI values.

LABORATORY 7.2

Constructing a New Nutritional Plan

Name_____ Age _____ Sex _____ Date _____

DIRECTIONS

After completing Laboratory 7.1, you should have a general idea of how your way of eating may need modification. Following the example given in Table 7.11 and the discussion in the text, choose foods to construct a new nutritional plan that meets the recommended dietary goals presented in this chapter. Fill in the blanks on the following chart with the requested information obtained from Appendices A and B or package labels. Use the totals for each column and the DRI for each nutrient in Laboratory 7.1 or Table 7.7 to determine your percentage of DRI for each nutrient.

	kcals (g)	Fat (g)	Sat. Fat (g)	Chol. (mg)	Sod. (mg)	CHO (g)	Pro (g)	Vit A (I.U.)	Vit C (mg)	Ca (mg)	Iron (mg)
Breakfast											
Lunch											
Dinner											
Totals											
DRI	*	<30%	<10%	<300	3000	>58%	**	1000	60	1200	12
% of DRI											

* See Chapter 8 for determination of kcal requirements.

** Protein intake should be 0.8 g/kg of body weight (0.36 g/lb). Pregnant women should add 15 g, and lactating women should add 20 g.

CHAPTER 8

Physical Activity, Dietary Intake, and Weight Maintenance

8

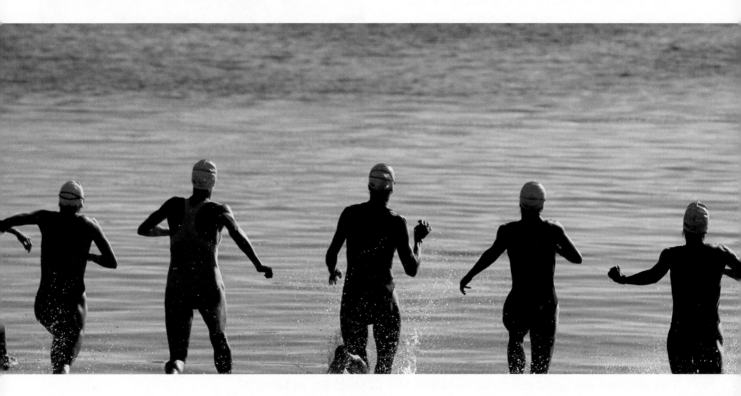

After studying this chapter, you should be able to

1. Differentiate between overweight and obesity and discuss potential causes.

2. Elaborate on four reasons why obesity should be prevented.

3. Explain the relationship between obesity and the risk of disease.

4. Outline the energy balance theory of weight maintenance.

5. Explain the roles of resting metabolic rate and exercise metabolic rate in determining daily energy expenditure.

6. List and define four basic components of a weight maintenance program.

7. Explain how to adjust one's lifestyle for a lifetime approach to weight maintenance.

8. Describe several weight loss myths.

9. Describe the eating disorders anorexia nervosa, bulimia nervosa, and binge eating disorder.

10. Describe muscle dysmorphia and explain why it has become increasingly an issue in young males.

Millions of people worldwide can be classified as overweight or obese. In Canada, the most recent Canadian Community Health Survey in 2000/2001 reported that 31.9 percent of the population aged 20 to 64 years was overweight (BMI > 27.0 kg/m^2), with another 15.6 percent with a BMI between 25.0 and 27.0 kg/m^2 (Statistics Canada, 2002). Furthermore, in this survey 14.7 percent of the adult population were classified as obese (BMI ≥ 30.0 kg/m^2). The prevalence of obesity has increased in recent years in Canada from 5.6 percent in 1985 to 14.7 percent in 2000/2001 (Statistics Canada, 2002), with no indication of levelling off.

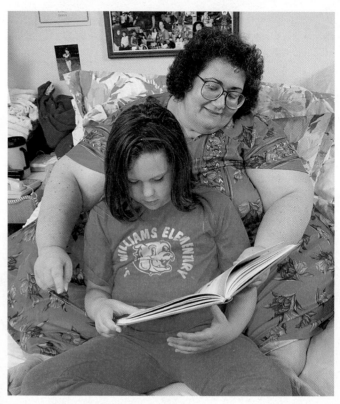

Obesity tends to run in families.

The level of fatness as well as the rate of overweight and obesity has increased in children and adolescents as well. In fact, one study comparing Canadian children from the 1960s to the 1990s noted children and adolescents of the 1990s were fatter even after controlling for maturational and size differences (Thompson, Mirwald, Baxter-Jones, & Bailey, 2002). Furthermore, Tremblay & Willms (2000, 2001) reported that from 1981 to 1997 in children ages 7 to 13 years, the rate of overweight (BMI > 85th age- and sex-specific percentile) increased from 15 to 35 percent in boys and from 15 to 29 percent in girls, while obesity (BMI 95th age- and sex-specific percentile) increased from 5 to 17 percent in boys and from 5 to 15 percent in girls. Clearly, overweight and obesity has reached epidemic proportions across the population in Canada!

One way to reverse the current trends, or at the very least prevent future cases of overweight and obesity, is to understand the causes and the three key factors in body weight management—physical activity, dietary intake, and behaviour management.

This chapter, therefore, provides a general overview of body weight maintenance. Specifically, we examine the principles of determining an ideal body weight range for health and fitness; ways to lose body fat using a combination of physical activity, dietary intake, and behaviour modification; and the principles involved in maintaining a desirable body weight throughout life.

The increasing prevalence of overweight and obesity in adults and children should alarm you for a number of reasons:

1. Overweight and obesity are difficult conditions to treat. Specifically, research shows that long-term maintenance of weight loss is rare, with a success rate of only 1 to 5 percent after 5 years (Wadden, Sternberg, Letizia, Stunkard, & Foster, 1989), regardless of the type of program used.

2. The chance of obesity's continuing from childhood or adolescence into adult years is remarkably strong. In fact, an obese child over the age of 6 years has a more than 50-percent chance of becoming an obese adult, while an obese adolescent (12 to 17 years) has a 70- to 80-percent chance of being obese in his or her adult years (Whitaker, Wright, Pepe, Seidel, & Dietz, 1997).

3. The risk of several diseases increases with obesity. More specifically, individuals who are obese tend be physically inactive and have a nutritional intake associated with atherosclerotic development. When these factors are combined, the risk increases for coronary artery disease, stroke, hypertension, colon cancer, postmenopausal breast cancer, type 2 diabetes, gallbladder disease, and osteoarthritis (Katzmarzyk, 2002).

4. The economic costs associated with obesity are prohibitive. Katzmarzyk and Janssen (2004) estimated the direct health costs and the indirect costs—which include the economic output lost as a result of illness, injury-related work disability, or premature death—to be 2.2 percent of the total health costs in Canada. These costs are and will continue to be a major burden on the Canadian health system if actions are not taken to reverse the current trends. (See also A Closer Look: "Obesity and the Risk of Disease.")

Overweight Versus Obesity

Overweight refers to a body weight greater than normal. But what is a normal weight? Normal weight is the average weight expected for a specific height. The body mass index (BMI), a ratio of weight and height derived by dividing weight in kilograms by height in metres squared, is often used to assist people in determining whether their weight is within a normal range. Thus, a normal weight refers to a BMI from 18.5 to 24.9 kg/m^2, while overweight refers to a BMI within the range of 25.0 to 29.9 kg/m^2. **Obesity** refers to an excessive accumulation of body fat at which the body fat becomes a health risk. Generally, body fat greater than 25 percent for men and 30 percent for women is considered an excessive accumulation (Bjorntorp & Brodoff, 1992; Perri, Nezu, & Viegener, 1992; Roitman, 2001; Stefanik, 1993; Stunkard & Wadden, 1993). This level of body fat is most often found in people with a BMI of 30.0 kg/m^2 or greater. As noted in Chapter 2, you must be careful in using BMI to identify body fat, since it is not a measure of body composition but a ratio of weight and height.

Differences exist in the level of risk for morbidity and mortality between overweight and obesity (Bouchard, 2000). The BMI cut-off points for overweight and obesity are justified in terms of health risks (Bouchard, 2000). Obesity is characterized by excess weight, most often in the form of adipose (fat). A second distinction is that most often the obese individual has been under a positive energy balance for a long period of time. A positive energy balance can occur when an individual either eats more than his or her body needs or expends fewer calories than he or she takes in. A third difference relates to energy expenditure: since an obese person weighs more than an overweight person, more energy is expended, on average, simply because of the energy demands needed to move a bigger body. This third difference results in an obese person's having a higher resting metabolic rate and expending more energy in physical activities than an overweight person.

What causes obesity? There is no single answer. Obesity is related to genetic traits and characteristics of a person's lifestyle (Bouchard, Shepherd, Stephens, Sutton, & McPherson, 1990; Stunkard, Sorenson, & Hanis, 1986). Studies demonstrate that children of obese parents have a greater potential to become obese than children of non-obese parents (Stunkard et al., 1986). In fact, some research suggests that a child with one obese parent has a 40-percent chance of becoming obese, while a child with two obese parents has an 80-percent chance of becoming obese (Stunkard, Harris, Pedersen, & McClearn, 1990). However, the question remains: is the increased likelihood of obesity a result of genetic factors or environmental factors? Since adopted children with low genetic potential for obesity have a greater chance of becoming obese if their adoptive parents are obese (Stunkard et al., 1986), one might suggest that environmental factors play a larger role in obesity development. In fact, this latter point clearly reflects the significant contribution of lifestyle to the development of obesity.

overweight Refers to a body weight greater than expected for a specific height.

obesity An excessive accumulation of body fat to the extent that it puts one's health at risk.

The link between genetics and obesity is not completely understood. Researchers continue to search for specific genes that could influence body fatness (see Fitness and Wellness for All: "The Search for Obesity-Related Genes"). In contrast, the tie between lifestyle and obesity is well defined. Nutritional studies demonstrate that families consuming high-fat meals have a greater risk of obesity than families who eat low-fat diets (Bjorntorp & Brodoff, 1992; Bouchard et al., 1990; Perri, Nezu, & Viegener, 1992). Similarly, children raised in households where physical activity is not encouraged have a greater potential for obesity than children reared in homes where physical activity is encouraged (Bjorntorp & Brodoff, 1992).

Many individuals gradually add fat over the years and become obese at some point in their lives. This slow increase in body fat is called **creeping obesity** because it gradually "creeps up" on us (Williams, 1996). This type of weight gain is usually attributed to poor diet (an increased food intake),

creeping obesity A slow increase in body fat over several years.

or maintained caloric intake along with a gradual decline in physical activity (Williams, 1996). Figure 8.1 illustrates the process of creeping obesity over a 5-year period. In this example, the individual gains one quarter-kilogram of fat per month (3 kg per year), resulting in a total weight gain of 15 kg over 5 years.

Regional Fat Storage

Approximately half our body fat is stored directly beneath the skin (Figure 8.2). The fact that different people can have very different regional patterns of fat storage is well known. What factor determines where body fat is stored? The answer is genetics. We inherit specific fat storage traits that determine the regional distribution of fat. This occurs due to the fact that fat cells are unequally distributed throughout the body. For example, most men have a high number of fat cells in their upper body, which results in a predominance of fat storage in the abdominal area (i.e., waist area). In contrast, most women have a high number of fat cells in the lower body, resulting in fat storage in the waist, hips, and thighs (see Figure 8.3). Excessive fat

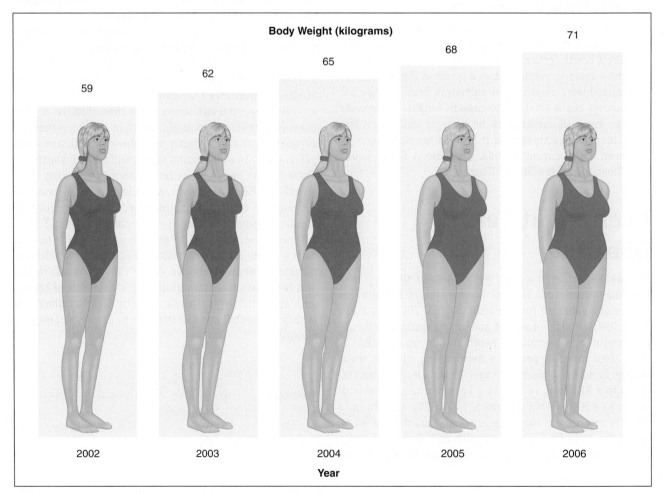

FIGURE 8.1 The concept of creeping obesity.

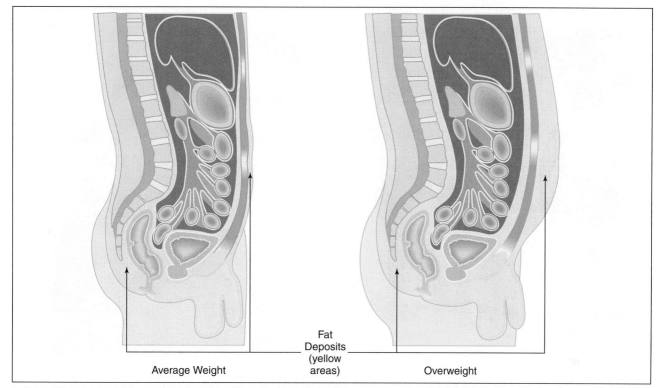

FIGURE 8.2 The sites of fat storage. Approximately 50 percent of body fat (shown in yellow) is stored directly beneath the skin.

accumulation around the middle is called "apple-shaped" obesity, whereas excessive fat accumulation primarily around the hips and thighs is called "pear-shaped" obesity. People who carry body fat primarily in the abdominal or waist area are at greater risk for developing heart disease than those who store body fat in the hips or lower part of the body (Reeder et al., 1997).

Optimal Body Weight Range

Many people are obsessed with their body weight and shape: the National Eating Disorder Information Centre reports that at any given point in time 70 percent of women

A CLOSER LOOK

Obesity and the Risk of Disease

Obesity increases the risk of developing at least 26 diseases (Katzmarzyk, 2002; Kuczmarski, 1992; Van Itallie, 1985; Williams, 1996), among the most serious of which are heart disease, colon cancer, hypertension (high blood pressure), kidney disease, arthritis, and type 2 diabetes (Williams, 1996). Obesity increases the risk of heart attack by 60 to 80 percent (Health implications of obesity: National Institutes of Health Consensus Development Conference, 1985). Further, a high correlation exists between the onset of type 2 diabetes and body fatness; more than 80 percent of individuals with type 2 diabetes are obese (Atkinson, 1992). In light of this strong link between obesity and disease, related health costs are estimated to be 2.2 percent of Canada's total health costs (Katzmarzyk & Janssen, 2004). Even though the

biological link between obesity and a specific disease is not always clear, new research has linked obesity to type 2 diabetes via a hormone called *resistin* (Steppan et al., 2001). This hormone, which is produced by fat cells and released into the blood, inhibits glucose uptake into cells. Thus it is not surprising that obese individuals, who have a large number of fat cells, also have high blood levels of resistin. The resulting inhibition of glucose uptake into cells produces high blood sugar (hyperglycemia) and type 2 diabetes.

Obesity may also contribute to emotional disorders in individuals (particularly adolescents and young adults) whose negative feelings about their body image and being obese lower their self-esteem and thus reduce their quality of life.

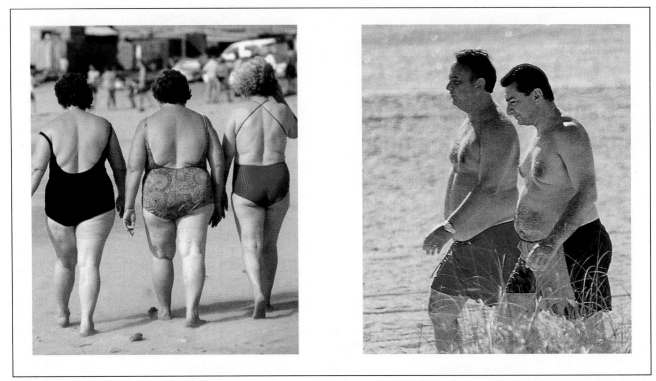

FIGURE 8.3 Typical body fat patterning for males and females. Women tend to store fat in the lower body while men tend to store it in the upper body.

and 35 percent of men are "dieting." Women are also more likely than men to be dissatisfied with their body weight and shape, with the number of dissatisfied men increasing in recent years. This obsession with body weight and shape often leads to a fixation on an ideal body weight, as well as various attempts to attain that weight. However, the body weight many people aspire to often is not a healthy body weight for them. Thus, a key question is "What is my optimal body weight for health?" Although researchers disagree on the answer to this question, some guidelines are available. In general, the body weight range that accompanies the optimal body fat level for men and women is the healthiest range. Specifically, optimal body fat for health ranges from 10 to 20 percent for men, and from 15 to 25 percent for women (Figure 8.4) (Corbin, Welk, Lindsey, & Corbin, 2003; Getchell, 1998; Hockey, 1996; Pollock & Wilmore, 1999; Powers & Howley, 2004). These ranges allow for individual differences in appearance and are associated with the lowest risk of diseases linked to body fatness. Caution is needed when determining your optimal body weight or range of body weights. The optimal body weight for you is the weight at which your body functions best. It is the weight (or range of weights) that your body comfortably fluctuates around when you are regularly physically active and eat a healthy diet. This optimal body weight range will likely differ from that of your friends, even though they may be the same age or height as you, simply because each body is built differently and has its own healthy weight range.

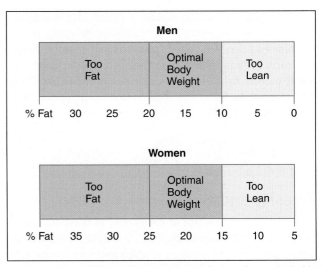

FIGURE 8.4 The concept of ideal body weight based on a desirable percentage of body fat.

Optimal Body Weight Range Based on Percentage Body Fat

A variety of methods and equipment are available for estimating body fat, including skinfold measurements as discussed in Chapter 2. (For a brief review of what is available on the market, see the Fitness–Wellness Consumer feature "Commercial Devices for Measuring Body Composition.") Once we know how to compute percentage body fat and the optimal range of body fat, how can we determine the desired range of body weight? Consider the following example of a male student who has 25 percent body fat and weighs 84 kg. What is the optimal body weight range for health in this individual? The calculations can be done in two simple steps:

Step 1. Compute *fat-free weight*—that is, the amount of total body weight contained in bones, organs, and muscles:

Total body weight − fat weight = fat-free weight

$$100\% - 25\% = 75\%$$

This means that for this student 75 percent of total body weight is fat-free weight. Therefore, his fat-free weight is

$$75\% \times 84 \text{ kg} = 63.0 \text{ kg}$$

Step 2. Calculate the optimal weight (which for men is 10 to 20 percent of total body weight). The formula to compute optimum body weight is

Optimum weight = fat-free weight ÷ (1 − optimal % fat)

Note that % fat should be expressed as a decimal. Thus, for 10 percent body fat,

Optimum weight = 63.0 ÷ (1 − 0.10) = 70.0 kg

For 20 percent body fat,

Optimum weight = 63.0 ÷ (1 − 0.20) = 78.8 kg

Hence, the optimal body weight range for this individual is between 70.0 and 78.8 kg.

Physiology of Weight Maintenance

Key physiological concepts associated with weight maintenance include the energy balance theory, the fat deficit concept, safe rates for weight loss or gain, and where fat loss occurs. Although the details of how body fat stores are reg-

ulated are beyond the scope of this text, Figure 8.5 presents a simplified overview of the processes involved. Simply stated, body fat stores are regulated by two factors: (1) the rate at which fat is synthesized and stored and (2) the rate at which energy is expended and fat is metabolized (broken down). In general, fat stores increase when energy intake exceeds energy expenditure, and decrease when energy expenditure exceeds energy intake. Note in Figure 8.5a that an increase in energy intake in response to increased appetite leads to increases in fat synthesis and storage. In contrast, fat stores are reduced when fat is broken down for use as a source of energy for the body (Figure 8.5b).

Energy expenditure and fat metabolism are discussed later in this chapter; here, the focus is on the rate of energy intake. Because the key factor determining the rate of energy

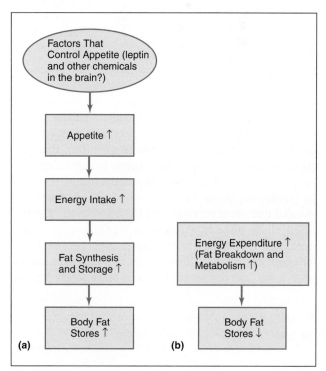

FIGURE 8.5 Regulation of body fat stores.

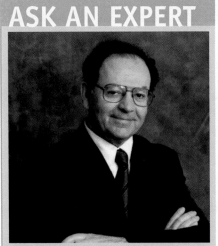
intake is appetite, the factors that regulate hunger are the subjects of intense research. Scientists have discovered in fat cells a new gene, called the obese gene (Ob), that produces the hormone leptin, which appears to depress appetite by acting on areas of the brain that control hunger (Frubeck, Gomez-Amrosi, Muruzabal, & Burrell, 2001). Research has revealed that obese mice had very low blood levels of leptin; when obese mice injected with leptin became lean, researchers became hopeful that leptin might become a cure for obesity in humans. However, those hopes were dashed when it was later discovered that many obese people produce

abnormally high levels of leptin and that leptin is but one of several interacting chemicals involved in appetite (Frubeck et al., 2001).

During the past two decades, two scientifically sound approaches to weight maintenance have emerged: the energy balance concept and the fat deficit concept.

Energy Balance Concept of Weight Maintenance

The *energy balance theory of weight maintenance* is simple and can be illustrated by the energy balance equation (Figure 8.6). To maintain your body weight, your energy intake (expressed in calories) must equal your energy expenditure, a condition called **isocaloric balance** (Figure 8.6a). If you consume more calories than you expend, you gain weight. Consuming

isocaloric balance   When energy intake equals energy expenditure.

more calories than you expend results in a **positive caloric balance** (Figure 8.6b). Finally, if you expend more calories than you consume, you lose body weight and have a **negative caloric balance** (Figure 8.6c).

From the energy balance equation presented in Figure 8.6, you should conclude that weight gain can be prevented by ensuring your energy (food) intake equals your energy (physical activity) expenditure. Further, you might conclude that weight loss is achieved either by decreasing your energy (food) intake or increasing your energy (physical activity) expenditure—in other words, by creating a negative caloric balance. In practice, weight loss programs include a reduction in caloric intake and an increase in caloric expenditure achieved through physical activity (Bailey, Barker, & Beauchene, 1993; Blair, 1993; Powers & Howley, 2004; Stunkard & Wadden, 1993).

Energy Expenditure
Estimating your daily energy expenditure is a key factor in planning a weight maintenance program when considering the energy balance equation. Your daily expenditure of energy involves your *resting metabolic rate* and *exercise metabolic rate*.

Resting metabolic rate (RMR) is the amount of energy expended during all sedentary activities. That is, RMR includes the energy required to maintain necessary bodily functions (called *basal metabolic rate*) plus the additional energy required to perform such activities as sitting, reading, typing, and digesting food. The RMR is an important component of the energy balance equation because it represents approximately 90 percent of the total daily energy expenditure in sedentary individuals (Poehlman, 1989).

Exercise metabolic rate (EMR) represents the energy expenditure during any form of physical activity (walking, climbing steps, strength training, and so on). In sedentary individuals, EMR constitutes only 10 percent of the total daily energy expenditure. By comparison, EMR can account for 20 to 40 percent of the total daily energy expenditure in active individuals (Poehlman, 1989). During heavy exercise EMR may be 10 to 20 times greater than RMR (Powers & Howley, 2004). Therefore, increased daily physical activity results in an increase in the EMR and is a key factor in weight maintenance.

Estimating Daily Energy Expenditure
Dieting is widespread in Canada as people try to reduce body fat by decreasing energy intake. The obvious goal of dieting is to consume less energy than is expended and therefore create a negative energy balance resulting in weight loss. The first step in this process is to estimate your daily caloric expenditure. One of the simplest ways to do so is presented in Table 8.1, which provides estimates of daily caloric energy

positive caloric balance   When more calories are consumed than expended.

negative caloric balance   When more calories are expended than consumed.

resting metabolic rate (RMR)   The amount of energy expended during all sedentary activities.

exercise metabolic rate (EMR)   The energy expenditure during physical activity.

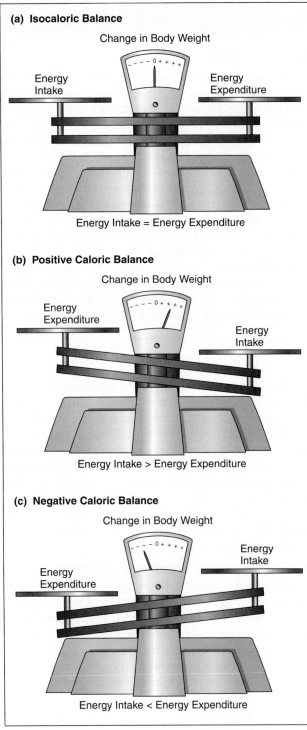

(a) Isocaloric Balance

Change in Body Weight

Energy Intake

Energy Expenditure

Energy Intake = Energy Expenditure

(b) Positive Caloric Balance

Change in Body Weight

Energy Expenditure

Energy Intake

Energy Intake > Energy Expenditure

(c) Negative Caloric Balance

Change in Body Weight

Energy Intake

Energy Expenditure

Energy Intake < Energy Expenditure

FIGURE 8.6 The concept of energy balance. (a) Isocaloric balance; (b) a positive caloric balance; and (c) a negative caloric balance.

Activity Level	Description	Calories per Kilogram of Body Weigth Expended during a 24-hour Period*
1	Very sedentary (restricted movement, such as a patient confined to a house)	29
2	Sedentary (most Canadian citizens; light work or office job)	31
3	Moderate activity (many postsecondary students; some daily activity and weekend recreation)	33
4	Very physically active (vigorous activity at least 3–4 times/week)	35
5	Competitive athlete (daily activity in high-energy sport)	37–39

TABLE 8.1 Estimation of Daily Caloric Expenditure Based on Body Weight and Physical Activity

Weight in kilograms can be converted to weight in pounds by multiplying by 2.2 lbs/kg.

the left (level 3) and estimated calories expended per kilogram of body weight (33 calories per kilogram per day) in the right-hand column. To calculate total daily energy expenditure, multiply body weight by caloric expenditure:

Daily caloric expenditure = 54.5 kilograms × 33 calories/kg/day = 1800 calories/day

Do this same calculation for your own daily caloric expenditure. To maintain your body weight, you should consume approximately that number of calories. If you need to lose weight, you should be able to create a negative energy balance by reducing your energy intake and increasing your activity level. You should recalculate your estimated caloric expenditure after losing 2.25 kg (5 lbs) of body weight; this is necessary because your weight loss results in a lowered daily energy expenditure (see Laboratory 8.1 on page 223).

Fat Deficit Concept of Weight Maintenance

The general concept that weight loss occurs due to a negative caloric balance is straightforward and easy to understand. However, another essential but often overlooked factor in weight loss is creating a fat deficit (Jequier, 1993). For instance, it is recognized that dietary fat is more easily stored as body fat than either carbohydrate or protein (Jequier, 1993). Dietary fat is more easily stored because it

expenditure based on body weight and physical activity. For example, a postsecondary-aged woman whose body weight is 54.5 kg (120 lbs) and is involved in moderate physical activity on weekends requires 1800 calories per day. This result was determined using Table 8.1, locating the activity level on

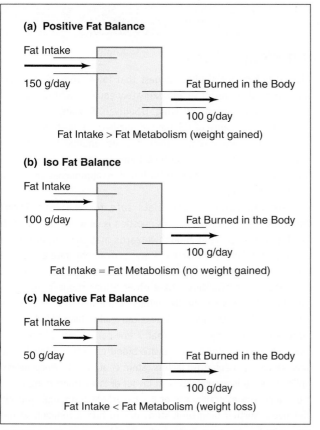

(a) Positive Fat Balance

Fat Intake

150 g/day

Fat Burned in the Body

100 g/day

Fat Intake > Fat Metabolism (weight gained)

(b) Iso Fat Balance

Fat Intake

100 g/day

Fat Burned in the Body

100 g/day

Fat Intake = Fat Metabolism (no weight gained)

(c) Negative Fat Balance

Fat Intake

50 g/day

Fat Burned in the Body

100 g/day

Fat Intake < Fat Metabolism (weight loss)

FIGURE 8.7 Importance of a low-fat caloric intake in creating a fat deficit and promoting weight loss.

is not used as a body fuel as rapidly as carbohydrate. Thus, if a positive caloric balance is created by eating excess fat, it is more likely to be stored as body fat (Jequier, 1993).

The importance of a low-fat caloric intake in weight maintenance can best be illustrated by the fact that body fat gain is a result of a continual imbalance of fat intake and fat metabolism (fat burned in the body). In other words, if you ingest more fat than you burn during the day, you gain weight (Figure 8.7a). It follows that if you consume and burn equal amounts of fat, your weight remains constant (Figure 8.7b). Finally, if you burn more fat than you consume (a fat deficit), you lose body fat and weight (Figure 8.7c). Thus, losing body fat is not as simple as creating an energy deficit; your diet must provide a caloric deficit that also results in a fat deficit.

Low-Carbohydrate Diets and Weight Loss

Almost everyone has heard about the various diet books that proclaim the secret to losing weight is a low-carbohydrate diet—indeed, several have become best-sellers. So, given the hype about low-carbohydrate diets, is there a physiological basis to support the argument that diets low in carbohydrates (and calories) provide superior weight loss compared to other diet plans?

Before we begin a discussion of the physiological basis of why low-carbohydrate diets may be effective in weight loss, it is important to appreciate that, identical to all other successful weight loss plans, low-carbohydrate diets must result in a caloric deficit for an individual to lose weight. With this fact established, is there a beneficial weight loss effect of consuming a low calorie diet that is also low in carbohydrates?

Proponents of low-carbohydrate diets argue that these diets have two major advantages over conventional diet plans (Acheson, 2004; Saris, 2003). First, eating high-carbohydrate foods promotes the use of carbohydrate as fuel and reduces the rate of fat metabolism. This argument is supported experimentally, and the physiology to explain this claim is as follows. Consuming high-carbohydrate foods promotes an increase in the hormone insulin. High insulin levels are counterproductive to weight loss because insulin stimulates fat storage and a reduction in the use of fat as a body fuel (Powers & Howley, 2004; Saris, 2003).

The second argument in favour of low-carbohydrate diets is that high-carbohydrate foods are less satiating than foods containing high levels of proteins and fats (Saris, 2003). Therefore, low-carbohydrate diets may promote satiety, reduce overall caloric intake, and assist in achieving a negative caloric balance. While evidence exists to support this argument, low-carbohydrate diets do not suppress appetite in all people.

Low-carbohydrate diets that create a caloric deficit do result in weight loss, and it is arguable that these diets may have advantages over conventional weight loss programs. Nonetheless, the long-term effectiveness and safety of low-carbohydrate diets is still in question. See A Closer Look: "More Details on Low-Carbohydrate Diets and Weight Loss."

What Is a Safe Rate of Weight Loss?

The maximum recommended rate for weight loss is 0.5 to 1 kg per week. Diets resulting in a weight loss of more than 1 kg per week are associated with a significant loss of lean body mass (i.e., muscle and body organs). The negative energy balance required to lose 0.5 kg per week is approximately 3500 calories per week. Therefore, a negative energy balance of 500 calories per day would theoretically result in a loss of 0.5 kg per week (3500 calories/week ÷ 7 days/week = 500 calories/day).

The rate of weight loss during the first several days will be greater than later in the dieting period. This happens because at the onset of a diet, there is an initial reduction in body carbohydrate and water stores, creating more weight loss (Powers & Howley, 2004). Further, some lean tissue, such as muscle, may be lost during the beginning of a diet. Therefore, more than 0.5 kg may be lost during the first 3500-calorie deficit. However, as the diet continues, weight loss will occur at a slower rate. This fact should not be discouraging, since subsequent weight loss will be primarily from body fat stores. Sticking with your

More Details on Low-Carbohydrate Diets and Weight Loss

Many different types of low-carbohydrate diets have been popularized over the years. You've probably heard of the Zone diet, Atkins New Diet Revolution, Calories Don't Count, Sugar Busters, the Scarsdale diet, or the South Beach diet. New ones continue to be introduced, but essentially they are the same diet. That is, any diet low in carbohydrates will promote physiological responses similar to other low-calorie diets.

Low-carbohydrate diets were first introduced in the 1970s and have enjoyed a recent surge in popularity. Common sales pitch for these diets include "You never feel hungry" and "You will lose weight fast." Both claims are true but can be misleading. For example, loss of appetite does occur in some people with a low-carbohydrate diet but it does not occur in everyone. Further, although it is true that most people lose body weight rapidly after beginning a low-carbohydrate diet, this initial weight loss is not fat loss. Indeed, a low-carbohydrate diet results in a reduction of body water stores and this water loss explains the rapid weight loss observed in these diets. Importantly, the water weight can be regained after a normal diet is resumed, causing some people on low-carbohydrate diets to regain weight that voids their initial weight loss (Foster et al., 2003; Powers & Howley, 2004).

Are low-carbohydrate diets superior to conventional low fat diets in promoting weight loss? This is a difficult question to answer, but recent studies suggest that low-carbohydrate diets and low fat diets result in approximately equal weight loss over a 3- to 12-month period (Meckling, O'Sullivan, & Saari, 2004; Stern et al., 2004). Because of the limited number of long-term studies, most scientists agree that more studies are required to determine which approach is superior for long-term weight loss. Nonetheless, current evidence suggests that both dietary approaches to weight loss are effective.

Are low-carbohydrate diets safe for the long term? Unfortunately, the answer to this question is currently unknown. It has been argued that health hazards may accompany low-carbohydrate diets. For example, some low-carbohydrate diets have been associated with high blood cholesterol, hypoglycemia, and other metabolic disorders. These observations suggest that low-carbohydrate diets can be dangerous. While it is true that some low-carbohydrate (and high-fat) diets can lead to high blood cholesterol, a recent study reveals that a low-carbohydrate diet with relatively low fat does not elevate blood cholesterol levels and promote cardiovascular risk factors (Stern et al., 2004). Nonetheless, while evidence is accumulating in favour of low-carbohydrate diets, the safety and effectiveness of a low-carbohydrate/high-protein diet needs further long-term study before firm recommendations can be made (Acheson, 2004; Saris, 2003).

weight loss plan for several weeks should result in significant weight loss.

Where on the Body Does Fat Reduction Occur?

A key question concerns where on the body fat loss will occur. The answer is that most fat loss occurs in areas that contain the greatest fat storage. Figure 8.8 illustrates this point in a study of obese women who completed a 14-week weight loss program that resulted in each participant's losing approximately 9 kg of fat (King & Katch, 1986). At the beginning of the study, regional fat storage was assessed using skinfold measurements, and it was determined that the largest percentage of fat was stored in the thighs, hips, and abdomen. At the completion of the study, regional fat storage was reassessed to determine where the fat loss occurred. Approximately 90 percent of the fat loss occurred in the body regions with the highest fat storage.

Lifetime Weight Maintenance

Weight loss through dieting (restricting caloric intake) in the short term is successful, relatively easy, and there are a variety of methods available. However, research clearly shows that dieting is seldom successful for the long-term maintenance of weight loss. One negative effect of dieting is the decrease experienced in resting metabolic rate. This decrease in RMR results in the body's needing fewer calories to maintain its functions. Further, this decrease in RMR may not rebound once the diet is over and caloric intake returns to previous levels. At this point weight gain often occurs—not because an individual is eating more or doing less physical activity, but because his or her physiological needs have decreased. Another reason for the lack of long-term success may be in the notion that if you go on a diet, you go off a diet. We simply do not have the cognitive control, despite our best efforts, to continuously restrict our caloric intake. This is especially true if, while "on our diet," we restrict foods that we consider bad for us. For example, when we say we won't eat chocolate on our diet, we set ourselves up for an obsession with chocolate and fixation on when we get to eat it next. This often results in our overeating chocolate when our willpower finally breaks down. We should not be so hard on ourselves in this instance, because what has happened is a normal physiological response to deprivation.

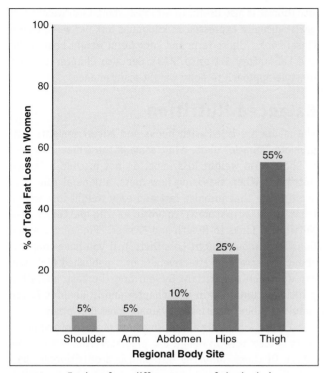

FIGURE 8.8 Fat loss from different areas of the body in women. In both sexes, fat is lost from the areas that store the most fat.

Source: Data from King, M., & Katch, F. (1986). Changes in body density, fat-folds, and girths at 2.3 kg increments of weight loss. *Human Biology, 58,* 709.

Another clear indication that dieting is seldom successful for the long-term maintenance of weight loss is the multi-billion-dollar weight loss industry. Billions of dollars are spent each year on magazines, books, diet programs, diet foods, and so on in attempts to lose weight. If there were a successful program available, there would not be a need for this industry. Rather, what is needed is a lifetime approach to body weight maintenance so that weight gain can be prevented.

Weight maintenance over the course of a lifetime is accomplished only by focusing on the combination of dietary intake, physical activity, and behaviour modification. The key factors in long-term weight maintenance are a positive attitude toward weight control, regular physical activity, and a personal commitment to maintaining a desired body composition.

Like other facets of personal or professional life, weight maintenance has its ups and downs. Be prepared for occasional setbacks. For instance, gaining weight during holiday periods is common and experienced by everyone at some time. When this type of weight gain occurs, avoid self-criticism and quickly re-establish your personal commitment to maintaining your body weight. In this case, you may want to compensate in the next few days by eating a little less at each meal and ensuring that you are obtaining adequate physical activity. You want to be careful not to

A CLOSER LOOK

Short-Term and Long-Term Weight Loss Goals

Short-term weight loss goals are designed to provide targets that can be achieved within a 2- to 4-week period. For example, an initial short-term weight loss goal might be to lose 1 kg during the first 2 weeks of your program. Achievement of each short-term goal provides the motivation to establish another short-term goal and continue the weight loss program. (See the box figure.)

Long-term weight loss goals generally focus on reaching a desired percentage of body fat within the optimal zone for health and physical fitness. For instance, a long-term goal for a male student might be to reach 15-percent body fat within the first year of his weight loss program. After reaching this long-term goal, his objective then becomes the maintenance of this desired body composition.

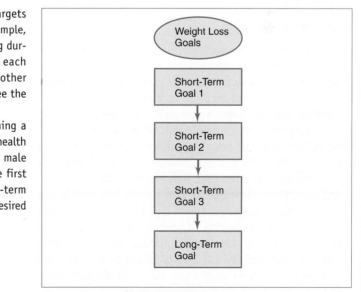

The relationship between short-term and long-term weight loss goals.

"go on a diet" and create a situation in which the short-term deprivation of food causes you to binge eat, which often results in a positive caloric balance overall. Further, you want to be careful not to fall into the yo-yo cycle of weight loss and weight gain, an unfortunate consequence of which is a lower RMR and higher "set point" body weight. In other words, people often become heavier from repeated cycles of weight loss and gain.

Finally, the importance of family and friends in lifetime weight maintenance cannot be overemphasized. Their encouragement and support can assist you in maintaining good eating habits and provide the needed support to sustain a lifetime commitment to physical activity. It is much easier to maintain your body weight if your close associates are trying to help you achieve your goals rather than tempting you to overeat or miss opportunities to be physically active. Therefore, surround yourself with friends who support you in your weight maintenance goals. See Kroll (2001) in the Suggested Reading list for more tips on lifetime weight maintenance.

Establishing a Successful Weight Maintenance Program

With knowledge and motivation, almost anyone can design a weight maintenance program. The four basic components of a comprehensive weight maintenance program are (1) the establishment of weight goals, (2) balanced nutrition, (3) a physical activity program designed to maintain or increase muscle mass, and (4) an eating management program aimed at changing eating habits that contribute to weight gain.

Weight Goals

The establishment of weight goals is a key component of any weight maintenance program. The first step is to decide where your percentage body fat should be within the optimal range (10 to 20 percent for men, 15 to 25 percent for women). Many people who begin a comprehensive weight maintenance program choose a weight that corresponds to the middle of the optimal fat range (15 percent body fat for men, 20 percent body fat for women). After choosing your long-term goal, you may find that your body weight is above or below this goal. First, determine if your weight falls within the optimal weight range determined for a healthy level of body fat for you (see page 199). If your weight falls below the optimal range, you may want to increase your body weight (see "Physical Activity and Dietary Intake to Gain Weight" on page 217). If your weight falls above the optimal range, you may want to decrease your body weight, and more particularly your body fat. Keep in mind that you must use a lifetime approach to healthy eating, physical activity, and eating management for long-term success and should not see a diet as a quick fix or short-term solution. Furthermore, in this situation it is also useful to establish short-term weight loss goals—usually expressed in kilograms lost per week (see A Closer Look: "Short-Term and Long-Term Weight Loss Goals" and Laboratory 8.1 on p. 223). See also Chapter 16 for a lifestyle approach to body weight maintenance.

Balanced Nutrition

The media are filled with books and advertisements that promote "miracle" diets. While some of these diets may lead to short-term weight loss, most do not provide balanced nutrition. When assessing new diets, a general rule is to avoid those that promise fast and easy weight loss with a temporary adjustment to your eating patterns (see Nutritional Links to Health and Fitness: "Frequently Asked Questions About Weight Loss Diets"). If you have concerns about the safety or effectiveness of a published diet, you can approach a dietitian. By learning the basic nutrition principles contained in this chapter and in Chapter 7, you should be able to critically evaluate most diet plans.

Table 8.2 presents a brief summary of some of the major types of diets used in weight loss programs (Powers & Howley, 2001). Of these, only the last plan is a nutritionally balanced, low-calorie diet; it is the only one recommended. Any safe and nutritionally sound diet should adhere to the following guidelines (AHA Dietary Guidelines, 2000; Bjorntorp & Brodoff, 1992; Perri et al., 1992; Stefanik, 1993; Stunkard & Wadden, 1993). The diet should

- Provide all the essential nutrients the body requires.
- Be low in fat (less than 30 percent of total calories) and high in carbohydrates (approximately 55 percent of total calories).
- Contain a variety of foods to appeal to your tastes and to prevent hunger between meals.
- Be compatible with your lifestyle, based on foods that are easily obtainable.
- Be a lifelong diet; that is, one that you can follow for the remainder of your life. This type of diet greatly increases your chances of maintaining your weight in the future.
- Provide foods that adhere to the principles outlined in Canada's Food Guide to Healthy Eating. Remember that a negative energy balance of 500 calories/day should result in a weight loss of approximately 0.5 kg per week, assuming caloric expenditure has not been reduced. The key to maintaining a caloric deficit of 500 calories/day is careful planning of meals, serving sizes, and accurate calorie counting.

In addition to these guidelines, some helpful reminders (some of which were covered in Chapter 7) for planning a balanced dietary intake include

- Limiting high-calorie, low-nutrient foods that are high in sugar and fat (e.g., candy bars, cookies, potato chips, etc.).

Type of Diet	Description/Comments	Recommended?
Low-carbohydrate diet	Has high fat or protein content, but is nutritionally unbalanced; not safe for long-term use.	No
Low-calorie liquid diet	Although nutritionally balanced, is monotonous and unsatisfying.	No
Very-low-calorie liquid diet	Protein/carbohydrate mixture that provides only 300–600 calories/day; is nutritionally unbalanced and not safe for long-term use.	No
Balanced low-calorie diet	Is nutritionally balanced; high in carbohydrates (approximately 60% of total caloric intake) and low in fat (less than 30% of total calories); provides a caloric deficit of 500 calories/day.	Yes

TABLE 8.2 Examples of Weight Loss Diets

- Selecting low-calorie, nutrient-dense foods such as fruits, vegetables, and whole-grain breads more often.

- Reduce the amount of fat in your diet. Eat less butter and margarine, and choose meats that are lower in fat, such as leaner cuts of beef, pork, chicken, or fish.

- Limiting fried foods; broil, bake, or microwave more often. If you use oil in your cooking, use monounsaturated oils such as olive or canola oil.

- Choosing low-fat dairy products as sources of protein (nonfat or low-fat milk, low-fat cottage cheese, and similar products).

- Selecting fresh fruits and vegetables whenever possible, and limiting fruits canned in heavy syrup.

- Limiting salt intake. Use herbs and other seasonings as substitutes for salt.

- Drinking fewer alcoholic beverages. Alcoholic beverages are low in nutrients and high in calories.

- Spreading your caloric intake throughout the day.

- Eating a variety of foods from each food group; the greater the diversity in the foods you eat, the better your chances of obtaining the daily required amounts of vitamins and minerals.

- Eating foods in moderation. All foods can fit in your dietary intake—there are some foods we simply should eat less of.

- Eating to achieve a balance from the four food groups. Balance does not mean eating the same number of servings from each food group. Rather it means eating the minimal required servings from each food group, then adding more foods as your caloric needs demand.

Keep in mind that the changes you make to your dietary intake need to be lifestyle changes. Try not to change too much all at once. Start slowly, and as you become comfortable with each new addition/change to your nutritional intake make another change. For example, start with eating healthier breakfasts (e.g., 2 pieces of whole wheat toast with 30 mL jam, ½ grapefruit, and 250 mL of skim milk; OR 175 mL high-fibre cereal with 250 mL milk and a banana; OR one pita pocket with 56 g low-fat cheese and a small bunch of grapes) for a couple of weeks; then focus on creating healthier lunches, then dinners, and so on.

Physical Activity, Muscle Mass, and Weight Maintenance

Physical activity plays a key role in weight maintenance for several reasons (Blair, 1993; Ross, Freeman, & Janssen, 2000). First, physical activity elevates your daily caloric expenditure and therefore assists you in maintaining isocaloric balance. Second, regular cardiorespiratory training improves the ability of skeletal muscles to burn fat as energy. Third, regular resistance training can reduce the loss of muscle that occurs during the aging process. Furthermore, increasing your muscle mass by resistance training results in an increased RMR, which further aids in body weight maintenance (Broeder, Burrhus, Svanevik, & Wilmore, 1992).

What if your body weight or body fat is greater than it should be? The reasons noted above also explain the importance of physical activity for long-term weight loss and maintenance. Specifically, physical activity can help you to attain a negative caloric balance. Thirty minutes of *extra* physical activity per day can increase daily caloric

Frequently Asked Questions About Weight Loss Diets

What types of weight loss diets are considered "fad diets"?

A diet is considered a fad if it gains fame but then the popularity fades quickly when consumers realize that the diet does not perform as advertised. Numerous fad diets currently exist and these diets come and go. Consumers can quickly evaluate the validity of a fad diet in the following way. In general, any diet plan that claims to provide weight loss without physical activity and/or a reduction in caloric intake will not result in the loss of body fat. An example of a fad diet is the grapefruit diet. Many myths circulated about the value of consuming large quantities of grapefruit to promote weight loss. One of these myths suggests that eating highly acidic grapefruit dissolves fat and results in a rapid loss of body weight. Although eating citrus fruits as a part of healthy eating is a good idea, there is nothing magical about grapefruit that promotes fat loss. In fact, there are no magical foods that assist in weight loss. Therefore, consumers should be wary of any fad diet that promises weight loss without providing a caloric deficit by reducing calorie intake.

What is the "glycemic index" of foods?

The "glycemic index" is a measure of how much insulin is released when a particular type of food is consumed. For example, foods that produce the highest release of insulin are assigned a high glycemic index. Since insulin release promotes fat storage in the body, proponents of low-carbohydrate diets argue that people should avoid foods with a high glycemic index.

What are high-protein diets and do they differ from low-carbohydrate diets?

High-protein diets are essentially low-carbohydrate diets that emphasize consuming high levels of proteins. Most high-protein diets that recommend consuming large quantities of protein result in a low carbohydrate intake. Therefore, any high-protein diet would also be a low-carbohydrate diet.

A health concern associated with high-protein diets is that these diets often result in the consumption of large quantities of red meat, eggs, and cheese. Therefore, high-protein diets may also be high-fat diets. A high-fat diet can result in elevated blood levels of cholesterol and an increased risk of cardiovascular disease. Moreover, a high-fat diet has been associated with an increased risk of certain cancers. For this reason, the World Cancer Research Fund recommends against the use of any high-protein diet.

Can caloric restriction slow aging and increase longevity?

The practice of caloric restriction involves consuming a balanced diet but restricting your caloric intake by approximately 20 to 40 percent below the level of energy consumed in a freely chosen diet. This practice has been shown to extend life span in a variety of animal species including rats, mice, and worms (Heilbronn & Ravussin, 2003). However, whether prolonged caloric restriction increases life span or reduces the rate of aging in humans is unknown (Heilbronn & Ravussin, 2003).

What role do dietary calcium and dairy products have on weight maintenance?

New evidence suggests that dietary calcium from dairy products may play an important role in weight maintenance. The proposed mechanism relates to the fact that calcium plays a key role in fat metabolism and fat storage (Zemel, 2004). Specifically, a diet high in calcium from dairy products has been shown to promote fat metabolism, inhibit fat synthesis, and therefore increase the loss of body fat (Zemel, 2004). These concepts have been confirmed by epidemiological data and recent clinical studies indicating that diets high in dairy products (>3 servings per day) accelerate fat loss compared with diets low in dairy products (Zemel, 2004). While these results are promising, additional studies are required to confirm the argument that increased calcium via dairy products is a useful adjunct to a weight loss program.

expenditure by 250 calories. Furthermore, as previously noted, engaging in activities that promote cardiorespiratory endurance enhances the body's ability to burn fat, and strength training increases RMR (due to increased muscle mass), both of which enhance fat loss. Thus, a sound recommendation for weight loss is to engage in cardiorespiratory training (running, cycling, swimming, and so on) and strength training. (See A Closer Look: "What Intensity of Aerobic Activity Is Best for Burning Fat?" for some details about the relationship between physical activity and fat metabolism.) The combination of these two types of training will maintain cardiorespiratory endurance and reduce the loss of muscle that typically occurs during a negative caloric balance.

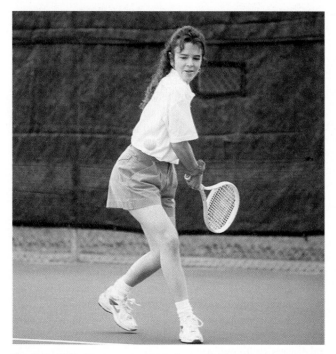

Physical activity is a key component of any weight maintenance program.

How much physical activity must be performed during a weight loss program? In general, the physical activity should expend at least 250 calories. Further, it is recommended that the negative caloric balance be shared equally by physical activity and diet. For instance, if an individual wishes to achieve a 500-calorie/day deficit, this should be done by increasing energy expenditure (physical activity) by 250 calories/day and by decreasing caloric intake by 250 calories/day.

Although intensity of physical activity is an important factor in improving cardiorespiratory endurance, it is the total amount of energy expended that is important in weight loss. Some authors have argued that low-intensity prolonged activity is better than short-term, high-intensity activity (e.g., sprinting 50 metres) in burning fat calories and promoting weight loss (Bailey, 1991; Romijn et al., 1993). However, recent evidence clearly demonstrates that high- and low-intensity physical activities can promote fat loss (Powers & Howley, 2004), and that fat is oxidized (burned) at high rates over a large range of intensities (Achten, Gleeson, & Jeukendrup, 2002). Nonetheless, for sedentary or obese individuals, low-intensity activity is the better choice because it can be performed for longer time periods and results in an increase in the ability of skeletal muscle to metabolize fat as an energy source (Powers & Howley, 2004; Tremblay, Coveney, Despres, Nadeau, & Prud'homme, 1992).

Table 8.3 contains estimates of the caloric costs of several types of physical activities. To compute your caloric expenditure (per minute) during an activity, simply multiply your body weight in kilograms by the values in the cal/min/kg column in Table 8.3 and by the physical activity time. For example, if a 70-kg individual plays 20 minutes of handball, how many calories did he or she expend? The total estimated caloric expenditure is computed as follows:

Caloric expenditure = 70 kg × 0.1603 cal/min/kg × 20 min
= 224 calories

	Cal/min/kg	Cal/min*	METs**
Archery (American Round)	0.0412	2.8	2.3
Bowling (with three other bowlers)	0.0471	3.2	2.7
Golf (playing in a foursome)	0.0559	3.8	3.2
Walking (10.5 min km on a grass surface)	0.0794	5.4	4.5
Cycling (4-min km)	0.0985	6.7	5.6
Canoeing (9.3-min km)	0.1029	7.0	5.8
Swimming (55-min km)	0.1333	9.1	7.6
Running (6.2-min km)	0.1471	10.0	8.0
Cycling (3.1-min km)	0.1559	10.6	8.5
Handball (singles)	0.1603	10.9	9.1
Skipping rope (80 turns/min)	0.1655	11.3	9.5
Running (5-min km)	0.1856	12.6	10.0
Running (3.7-min km)	0.2350	16.0	12.8

*These values are for a 68-kg person.
**1 MET equals your resting metabolic rate.

TABLE 8.3 Energy Costs for Selected Sporting Activities

Source: From Getchell, B. (1992). *Physical Fitness: A Way of Life.* Copyright © 1992. Reprinted with permission from Benjamin Cummings.

Physical Activity and Appetite

A common question is whether physical activity increases appetite. Although the high-intensity training programs used by many athletes may increase appetite, a moderate physical activity program in individuals who are sedentary or obese does not increase appetite (Mayer et al. 1954). In fact, engaging in moderate physical activity may diminish appetite (Mayer et al., 1954).

Eating Management

The fourth and perhaps most important component of long-term body weight maintenance is eating management. To effectively manage your body weight, you must understand what, when, where, why, how, and with whom you eat. Most people eat in response to a variety of triggers. Seldom do we eat only in response to hunger; we are more likely to be responding to other triggers. You must learn what triggers eating for you. Are you likely to eat because you are angry? Or sad? Do you consume a lot of food at one time in an attempt to feel better? Do you eat simply because it is noon and you are accustomed to eating at noon? Do you eat when you are watching TV or a movie just because you are conditioned to do so rather than because you are hungry and need a snack? Do you want to eat pizza or fried chicken simply because you walked by a fast-food restaurant that emits these cooking odours? These are only some of the questions you need to ask yourself about your eating attitudes and behaviours. You may find it useful to keep a journal of what, when, where, why, how, and with whom you eat for a week or two to better understand your eating. You could use a format like the example at the bottom of the page.

Eating management may be the most important component of body weight maintenance, since there may be eating behaviours or attitudes you've acquired over time that need changing. (See also Laboratory 8.2.)

behaviour modification   A technique used in psychological therapy to promote desirable changes in behaviour.

overeating   The consumption of excessive calories that leads to a positive caloric balance.

Research demonstrates that behaviour modification plays a key role in achieving long-term weight loss and weight maintenance (Bjorntorp & Brodoff, 1992; Perri et al., 1992; Stefanik, 1993; Stunkard & Wadden, 1993). **Behaviour modification** is a technique used in psychological therapy to promote desirable changes in behaviour. The rationale behind it is that many behaviours are learned. For example, attending movies at the theatre elicits, in many people, a response of eating popcorn and candy. Because these types of responses are learned, they can also be eliminated (unlearned). In regard to weight maintenance, behaviour modification is used primarily to reduce or (ideally) eliminate social or environmental stimuli that promote overeating.

Overeating is defined as the consumption of excessive calories that leads to a positive caloric balance. The first step in an eating management program is to identify the social or environmental factors that promote overeating. This can also be done by keeping a written record of daily activities for 1 or 2 weeks to identify factors associated with consumption of excessive calories. In recording your daily eating habits, consider the following social or environmental factors (Williams, 1996):

- *Activities.* What activities are associated with eating? You may find a correlation between specific types of activities, such as watching TV and eating snacks.
- *Emotional behaviour before or during eating.* What emotions are associated with eating? For instance, do you overeat when you are depressed or under stress?
- *Location of meals.* Where do you eat? Are specific rooms associated with snacks?
- *Time of day and level of hunger.* Do you eat at specific times of the day? When you eat, are you hungry?
- *People involved.* With whom do you eat? Are specific people associated with periods of overeating?

After identifying the factors that influence your eating attitudes and behaviour, start a program aimed at correcting those behaviours that contribute to eating excessive calories. The following weight maintenance techniques have been used successfully for many years. Although it is not essential to use each of them, adhering to several will make weight maintenance easier (Williams, 1996).

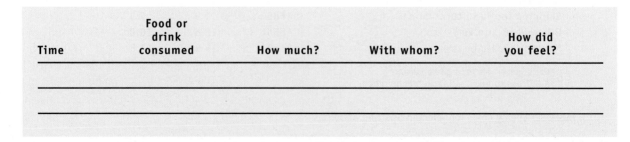

Time	Food or drink consumed	How much?	With whom?	How did you feel?

What Intensity of Aerobic Activity Is Best for Burning Fat?

Many people assume that the intensity of aerobic exercise (running, cycling, and so on) must be maintained at a low level for fat to be burned as fuel. It is true that fat is a primary fuel source during low-intensity exercise. But as the figure in this box shows, the total amount of fat burned during physical activity varies with the intensity of the activity, and for a given exercise duration more total fat is metabolized during moderate-intensity physical activity. Therefore, moderate-intensity physical activity (that is, approximately 50 percent VO_2max) is typically the optimal intensity of physical activity for burning the most fat during an endurance exercise workout. For more details on this topic, see Coyle (1995) in the Suggested Reading list at the end of this chapter.

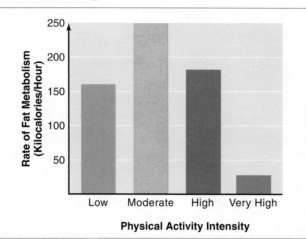

The rates of fat metabolism at low intensity (20 percent VO_2max), moderate intensity (50 percent VO_2max), high intensity (80 percent VO_2max), and very high intensity (100 percent VO_2max) physical activity. While this figure is not intended to reveal any "ideal" physical activity intensity for all individuals, it indicates that moderate-intensity physical activity is often optimal for maximizing the amount of fat metabolized during physical activity.

Source: Coyle, E. (1995). Fat metabolism during exercise. *Sports Science Exchange* (Gatorade Sports Science Institute), *8*, 6.

- *Make a personal commitment to maintaining your weight.* This is the first step toward behaviour modification and weight maintenance. The establishment of realistic short- and long-term weight loss goals, if needed, assists in maintaining a lifelong commitment to weight maintenance.

- *Develop healthy eating patterns.* Avoid eating when you are not hungry. Learn to eat slowly and only while sitting at the table. Finally, keep food portions to the minimum amount within your caloric guidelines.

- *Have a plan when you attend social settings where overeating is encouraged.* If you go to parties where excessive foods are served, don't go to these functions hungry. Eat a low-calorie snack before going.

- *Limit snacking.* Snack only when you are hungry, choosing low-calorie foods such as carrots, celery, apples, grapes, and so on.

- *Engage in daily physical activity.* Regular physical activity that uses large-muscle groups can play an important role in maintaining isocaloric balance and thereby assisting in weight maintenance.

- *If applicable, reward yourself for successful weight loss with nonfood rewards.* Rewards or positive feedback are an important part of behaviour modification. For example, after reaching your short-term weight loss goal reward yourself by doing something you like (going to the beach, going hiking, or buying a new CD).

- *Think positively.* Limit negative thinking about how difficult weight maintenance can be. Positive thinking promotes confidence and maintains the enthusiasm necessary for a lifetime of successful weight maintenance.

- *Give up the concept of "dieting."* When you limit or restrict your caloric intake, you are likely to feel as if you are depriving yourself. This often results in bingeing or overeating. Remember, this is a lifetime approach to eating, not "going on a diet" for the short term without altering negative eating attitudes and behaviours.

- *Eliminate the notion of forbidden foods (chips, cookies, candies).* All foods can fit in your plan for healthy eating. Some foods you will eat in smaller amounts and not so frequently. Consult Chapter 7 and Canada's Food Guide to Healthy Eating for more details on variety, balance, and moderation.

- *Normalize your eating through hunger and satiety.* Learn to listen to your body, eat when you are hungry, and stop eating when you are full.

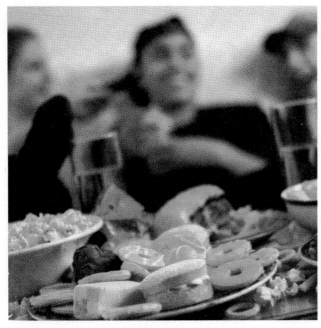

Have a plan to limit caloric intake when you attend parties or social gatherings that encourage overeating.

- *Remember, you must make this a lifetime approach to eating well.* You are not altering your eating attitudes and behaviours for a short term, but for your lifetime. View these changes positively and as better ways to eat for optimal health.
- *View setbacks as temporary.* Do not give up when setbacks occur, simply adjust your eating attitudes and behaviours to reflect your long-term goal of weight maintenance.

Weight Loss Myths

Since there is a multi-billion-dollar weight loss industry, numerous myths exist. Below, we debunk some of the myths that cause confusion among people attempting to control or lose weight.

Diet Pills Work

A number of over-the-counter diet pills are available on the market, and most contain caffeine and other mild stimulants (see Fitness–Wellness Consumer: "Are Diet Pills Safe and Effective?"). Unfortunately, these products have not

spot reduction The false notion that exercise applied to a specific region of the body will result in fat loss in that region.

cellulite The "lumpy," hard fat that often gives skin a dimpled look.

been scientifically proven to assist in achieving safe and permanent weight loss. One study of individuals using commercially available diet pills reported that fewer than 3 percent of users lost weight and they retained this weight loss longer than 12 months (Wadden et al., 1989).

Spot Reduction Works

The notion that exercise applied to a specific region of the body will result in fat loss in that region is called **spot reduction**. Will performing curl-ups, for example, result in a reduction in abdominal fat? The answer is no. There is no scientific evidence to show that exercise promotes fat loss in local regions of the body (Gwinup, Chelvam, & Steinberg, 1971). Rather, when a caloric deficit exists, fat loss occurs from the largest sites of fat stores rather than from the areas exercised (King & Katch, 1986).

Eating Before Bedtime Makes You Fatter

Some people believe that eating immediately prior to going to bed at night results in a greater fat gain than if the same meal were consumed during the day. These ideas are probably unfounded. Although eating a late-night meal or snack might not be a good dietary habit, this practice does not result in a greater weight gain than if the same meal had been consumed at another time during the day. Remember, it is the combination of daily caloric intake and energy expenditure that determines positive energy balance, not the timing of the meal (Bjorntorp & Brodoff, 1992; Perri et al., 1992).

Cellulite Is a Special Type of Fat

It is commonly believed that two kinds of body fat exist: cellulite and regular fat (Corbin et al., 2003). The term **cellulite** refers to the "lumpy," hard fat that often gives skin a dimpled look. In reality, cellulite is just plain fat, not a special type of fat. The dimpled appearance comes from fat accumulating in small clusters beneath the skin.

Some health spas advertise that vigorous massages provided by machines can remove cellulite and improve the appearance of your skin. However, no scientific evidence exists that massage techniques are effective in promoting body fat loss or altering skin appearance.

Fat-Dissolving Creams Are Effective

Over the years, numerous companies have marketed "weight loss creams" that claim to cause spot reduction of fat when applied to the skin. This is an attractive idea, as evidenced by the fact that companies have made millions of dollars from selling these products. Despite the boastful claims made by manufacturers, there is limited scientific evidence to suggest these creams are effective.

Saunas, Steambaths, and Rubber Suits Can Aid in Weight Loss

Another myth related to the loss of body fat is the notion that sitting in saunas or steambaths or running in a rubber suit melts body fat. Although saunas and steambaths do temporarily increase your metabolic rate, they do not melt away fat, nor do they significantly contribute to weight loss (Stunkard & Wadden, 1993). For similar reasons, exercising in a rubber suit does not promote greater fat loss than would be achieved by performing the same exercise in comfortable clothes.

However, these three methods do cause a decrease in body weight from the loss of body water due to sweating. This body weight loss has been believed by some to be a loss of fat, but this is not the case. Body weight lost in this way is regained as soon as body water is restored to normal levels.

Caution is necessary when using saunas or steambaths (or exercising while wearing a rubber suit) because your body temperature may increase well above normal. In fact, hyperthermia (abnormally high body temperature) may result. This puts additional stress on the heart and circulatory system and increases the risk of cardiac problems for older individuals or anyone with heart problems.

Eating Disorders

The low social acceptance of individuals with a high percentage of body fat (Chambliss, Finley, & Blair, 2004) and an emphasis on having the "perfect" body have increased the risk for and incidence of eating disorders (Thompson & Chad, 2002).

The term **eating disorders** is used to describe a range of unhealthy eating and body weight issues. The most common eating disorders are anorexia and bulimia nervosa. Some estimates are that as many as 5 to 10 percent of the

population are living with an eating disorder. Although eating disorders affect people of every age, socioeconomic class, and ethnic background, girls and women account for 90 to 95 percent of all cases. However, the incidence of eating disorders is rising in boys and men.

Common features of eating disorders include:

- abnormal eating habits
- preoccupation with food
- distorted body image
- intense fear of gaining fat
- excessive and compulsive exercise
- feelings of ineffectiveness
- low self-esteem
- depression
- conforming or overachieving
- abnormal menstruation

(*adapted from the National Eating Disorder Information Centre*).

It should be noted that not all the characteristics listed above are present in every individual with an eating disorder. There are also distinctions between anorexia and bulimia nervosa, as noted below.

Anorexia Nervosa

Anorexia nervosa is a common eating disorder characterized by attempts at thinness through regimented dieting, which

eating disorders   A range of unhealthy eating and body weight issues.

anorexia nervosa   An eating disorder characterized by a dramatic weight loss achieved through strict dieting.

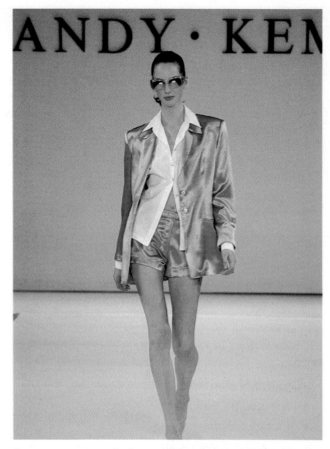

There are enormous societal pressures for young women to be thin.

leads to a dramatic weight loss. The end result of anorexia nervosa is a state of starvation as the individual becomes emaciated through an intense fear of fat resulting in a refusal to eat. The psychological causes of anorexia nervosa are unclear, but they seem to be linked to an unfounded fear of fatness that may be related to familial or societal pressures to be thin (Williams, 1996).

The incidence of anorexia nervosa has grown in recent years. Individuals with the highest probability of developing this eating disorder are upper-middle-class young women who are extremely self-critical. It is estimated that the incidence of anorexia nervosa is as high as one in every 200 adolescent girls (Andersen, 1983; Borgen & Corbin, 1987).

Individuals with anorexia nervosa may use a variety of techniques to remain thin, including starvation, excessive exercise, and laxatives. The effects of anorexia nervosa

include excessive weight loss, cessation of menstruation, and, in extreme cases, death. Because anorexia nervosa is a serious mental and physical disorder, medical treatment by a team of professionals (physician, psychologist, dietitian) is needed. A person may require years of psychological counselling and nutritional guidance. The first step in seeking treatment is recognizing a problem exists. The following are common symptoms of anorexia nervosa:

- an intense fear of gaining weight or becoming obese
- feeling fat even at normal or below-normal body fatness because of a highly distorted body image
- in women, the absence of three or more consecutive menstrual cycles
- the possible development of odd behaviours concerning food: for example, the preparation of elaborate meals for others but of only a few low-calorie foods for their own consumption

Bulimia Nervosa

About 50 percent of individuals with anorexia nervosa eventually develop **bulimia nervosa**. Individuals with bulimia nervosa are characterized by a strong desire to be thin interrupted by binge eating, followed by efforts to avoid calorie absorption and feelings of guilt and lack of control. In essence, individuals with bulimia nervosa repeatedly ingest large quantities of food and then force themselves to vomit or use laxatives to prevent weight gain. Frequent vomiting may result in damage to the teeth and the esophagus from stomach acids. Like anorexia nervosa, bulimia nervosa is also most common in young women, is psychological in origin, and requires professional treatment when diagnosed. Several authors indicate that the prevalence of bulimia may be as low as 1 percent or as high as 20 percent among girls and women aged 13 to 23 years (Andersen, 1983; Borgen & Corbin, 1987).

Most individuals with bulimia nervosa look "normal" and are of normal weight. However, even when their bodies are slender, their stomachs may protrude due to being stretched by frequent eating binges. Other common symptoms of bulimia nervosa include the following (Leeds, 1998):

- recurrent binge eating
- a lack of control over eating
- regular self-induced vomiting and use of diuretics or laxatives
- strict fasting or use of vigorous exercise to prevent weight gain
- averaging two or more binge-eating episodes a week during a 2- to 3-month period
- obsession with body shape and weight

bulimia nervosa   An eating disorder characterized by a strong desire to be thin interrupted by binge eating followed by efforts to avoid calorie absorption and feelings of guilt and lack of control.

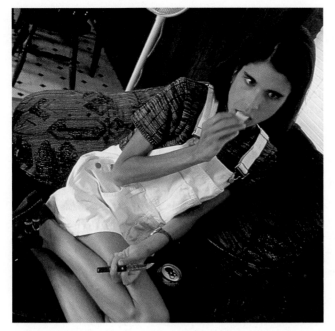

People with anorexia nervosa often have distorted body images.

Binge Eating Disorder

The **binge eating disorder** is similar to bulimia nervosa in that it involves frequent sessions of binge eating with a feeling of lack of control over what is eaten, how much is eaten, and the way it is eaten. The difference is that individuals with a binge eating disorder do not take measures to avoid calorie absorption (Donatelle, 2005). Unlike individuals with anorexia or bulimia nervosa, the individuals who have a binge eating disorder are most often obese. Common characteristics of binge eating disorder include one or more of the following:

- eating rapidly
- eating until uncomfortably full
- eating large amounts of food even when not hungry
- eating alone
- disgust, depression, or guilt over what was eaten

Physical Activity and Dietary Intake to Gain Weight

A small number of people consider themselves too thin and want to gain body weight. Men and women can suffer from self-image problems if they believe they are too skinny. However, men are more likely than women to want to gain weight. In fact, most men desire an increase in muscle mass.

Although current social attitudes stress leanness in women, many women agree that some degree of body curvature is desirable. Also, many men want muscular bodies because of the improved self-image that comes with increased muscularity (Williams, 1996). A new disorder, termed *muscle dysmorphia* (discussed later), may develop in males who become obsessed with their body image and muscularity.

Body weight gain can be achieved in two ways. First, you can create a positive caloric balance and gain additional body fat. Second, you can increase your body weight by increasing your muscle mass through a resistance-training program.

Gaining Body Fat

Before deciding to gain body fat, you should determine whether your current body composition is within the desired range. If your percentage body fat is below the recommended range (fewer than 8 percent of people fall into this category), you may wish to add body fat to reach the optimal percentage body fat. Nonetheless, before looking at a dietary means for gaining fat, you should examine the cause of your being too lean (Williams, 1996).

Several lifestyle problems could contribute to a low percentage of body fatness (Williams, 1996). For example, are you getting enough sleep? If not, you may be burning large amounts of energy and creating a negative caloric balance. Do you drink a lot of coffee? Coffee can influence body weight in two ways. First, more than three to five cups of coffee per day can reduce your appetite. Second, consumption of coffee or other caffeine-containing beverages increases your resting metabolism for several hours. Do you skip meals? Failing to eat regularly may result in a negative caloric balance, fat loss, and the inability to maintain an optimal level of body fat or body weight.

If lifestyle is not the problem, consult your physician to rule out the possibility that the cause of your low body fat is a hormonal imbalance or other disease that influences body weight. After discussing with your physician your desire to gain fat and obtaining medical clearance to do so, consider the following recommendations:

1. Establish a weight gain goal that will place you at the low end of the recommended percentage body fat range.
2. Create a positive caloric balance. This is accomplished by increasing your total caloric intake to exceed your daily expenditure. A positive caloric balance of 500 calories per day will generally result in a weight gain of about 0.5 kg per week, a reasonable goal.

binge eating disorder An eating disorder that involves frequent sessions of consuming large amounts of food without attempting to avoid calorie absorption.

3. To create a positive caloric balance, compute your daily caloric expenditure and increase your caloric intake to exceed expenditure. When creating a positive caloric diet, use the basic principles of nutrition discussed in Chapter 7 and in Canada's Food Guide so that you adhere to the recommended guidelines for fat, carbohydrate, and protein intake.

4. Consult a registered dietitian or physician. Although anyone can gain weight while eating a positive caloric diet, the safest means is with the assistance of these professionals.

Gaining Muscle Mass

If your percentage of body fat is within the recommended range and you still wish to increase your body weight, your goal should be to gain muscle weight, not fat. Unfortunately, there are no over-the-counter products or shortcuts for gaining muscle (see Nutritional Links to Health and Fitness). The key to gaining muscle mass is a program of rigorous strength training combined with an increase in caloric intake to meet the increased energy expenditure and energy required to synthesize muscle. Physical activity programs designed to improve muscular strength and size are discussed in Chapter 5. The focus here is on the dietary adjustments needed to optimize gains in muscle mass. Again, in order to gain muscle mass you need to create a small positive caloric balance to provide the energy required to synthesize new muscle protein and to cover the energy expended during resistance training.

How much energy is expended during routine resistance training? The amount is surprisingly small. For instance, a 70-kg man performing a 30-minute resistance workout probably burns fewer than 70 calories (Williams, 1996). The reason for this low caloric expenditure is that during 30 minutes in the weight room the average person spends only 8 to 10 minutes actually lifting weights; more time is spent in recovery periods between sets.

How much energy is required to synthesize 0.5 kg of muscle mass? Current estimates are approximately 2500 calo-

ries, of which about 400 calories (100 grams) must be protein (Williams, 1996). To compute the additional calories required to produce an increase in muscle mass, you must first estimate your rate of muscular growth. This is difficult because the rate of muscular growth during resistance training varies among people. While relatively large muscle mass gains are possible in some individuals, studies have shown that most men and women rarely gain more than 0.11 kg of muscle per week during a 20-week resistance training program (3 days/week, 30 minutes/day). If we assume that the average muscle gain is 0.11 kg per week and that 2500 calories are required to synthesize 0.5 kg of muscle, a positive caloric balance of fewer than 100 calories per day is needed to promote muscle growth (0.11 kg/week × 2500 calories/0.5 kg = 550 calories/week; therefore, 550 calories/week ÷ 7 days/week = 79 calories/day).

What are the dietary guidelines for gaining muscle mass? The major adjustments in dietary intake are an increased caloric intake and assurance that you are obtaining adequate amounts of dietary protein. If you follow the dietary guidelines discussed in Chapter 7 and in Canada's Food Guide for Healthy Eating while producing a positive caloric balance, your diet will contain enough protein to support an increase in muscle mass. When planning your diet, consider the following points:

- To increase your caloric intake, use Canada's Food Guide for Healthy Eating (presented in Chapter 7). This will ensure that your diet meets the criteria for healthy living and provides adequate protein for building muscle.

- Limit intake of high-fat foods and your positive caloric balance to approximately 80 calories per day. Increasing your positive caloric balance above this level will promote not a faster rate of muscular growth but an increase in body fat.

- If you discontinue your resistance-training program, lower your caloric intake to match your daily energy expenditure.

Do Protein Supplements Have a Role in Promoting Muscle Growth?

Many of the numerous nutritional products advertised as "wonder drugs" for promoting muscle growth are high-protein (and often high-calorie) drinks. Are they effective? There is no scientific evidence to support the notion that these products result in increases in muscular size or strength. The only proven and safe method of building muscle mass is regular resistance training coupled with a nutritionally sound diet. (See Powers & Howley [2004] for a review of this topic.)

Do you need higher intakes of protein to promote muscle growth? Although consumption of small quantities of high-

protein drinks may not be harmful, if you are eating a typical North American diet you don't need to increase your protein intake to achieve muscle growth (Williams, 1996; Powers & Howley, 2004). Here's why: to achieve normal growth and development, the DRI for protein is 0.8 grams per kilogram (kg) of body weight, which means that a 70-kg man needs 56 g of protein per day (70 kg × 0.8 g/kg/day = 56 g/day). Since the average daily Canadian diet contains about 100 g of protein, which is well above the DRI, no protein supplementation is needed to promote muscle growth.

Muscle Dysmorphia

Muscle dysmorphia, a form of body dysmorphia (an unhealthy preoccupation with physical appearance), describes an unhealthy preoccupation with body size and muscularity (Graves & Welsh, 2004). The prevalence of muscle dysmorphia has increased in recent years. It occurs almost exclusively in males and is characterized by a preoccupation with being lean and muscular, negative beliefs about one's body resulting in body avoidance or anxiety, and interference in everyday life roles (Hildebrandt, Langenbucher, & Schundt, 2004).

Summary

1. Millions of people in Canada carry too much body fat for optimal health.
2. *Overweight* is defined as a weight greater than what is considered normal for a specific height.
3. *Obesity* is defined as an excessive accumulation of body fat—that is, more than 25 percent for men and more than 30 percent for women, at which the body fat places one at health risk.
4. Obesity is linked to many diseases, including heart disease, type 2 diabetes, and hypertension.
5. The optimal percentage body fat for health is believed to be 10 to 20 percent for men and 15 to 25 percent for women.
6. The energy balance theory of weight maintenance states that to maintain your body weight, your energy intake must equal your energy expenditure.
7. Evidence suggests that creating a fat deficit is an essential factor in weight loss. This is because dietary fat is more easily stored as body fat than carbohydrate or protein.
8. Total daily energy expenditure is the sum of resting metabolic rate and exercise metabolic rate.
9. The four basic components of a comprehensive weight maintenance program are weight goals, balanced nutrition, a physical activity program designed to increase caloric expenditure and maintain muscle mass, and an eating management program designed to modify the behaviours that contribute to weight gain.
10. Weight loss goals should include short- and long-term goals.
11. Numerous weight loss myths exist. This chapter discredits weight loss myths concerning diet pills, spot reduction, eating before bedtime, cellulite reduction, fat-dissolving creams, and the use of saunas, steam baths, and rubber exercise suits.
12. Resistance training and a positive caloric balance are required to produce increases in muscle mass.
13. Two relatively common eating disorders, anorexia nervosa and bulimia nervosa, are serious medical conditions that require professional treatment.
14. Muscle dysmorphia is an unhealthy preoccupation with body size and muscle mass.

Study Questions

1. What is obesity? What diseases are linked to obesity?
2. What is overweight? How does it differ from obesity?
3. Discuss the potential causes of obesity.
4. Discuss the concept of optimal body weight. How is optimal body weight computed?
5. Explain the roles of resting metabolic rate and exercise metabolic rate in determining total caloric expenditure. Which is more important in total daily caloric expenditure in a sedentary individual?
6. Outline a simple method for computing your daily caloric expenditure. Give an example.
7. List the four major components of a weight maintenance program.
8. Why is eating management perhaps the most important component of a weight maintenance program?
9. Discuss the weight loss myths concerning diet pills, spot reduction, eating before bedtime, cellulite reduction, fat-dissolving creams, and the use of saunas, steam baths, and rubber exercise suits.
10. Define *anorexia nervosa, bulimia nervosa,* and *binge eating disorder.*
11. What are common symptoms of eating disorders?
12. Define the following:

    energy balance theory of weight maintenance

    isocaloric balance

    negative caloric balance

    positive caloric balance
13. Explain the fat deficit concept of weight maintenance.
14. What is cellulite? Can it be "massaged" away?
15. How does creeping obesity occur? Can it be prevented?
16. Discuss the process of combining nutritional intake and physical activity to increase muscle mass.

Suggested Reading

Coyle, E. (1995). Fat metabolism during exercise. *Sports Science Exchange* (Gatorade Sports Science Institute), 8.

Going, S., & R. Davis. (2001). Body composition. In J. Roitman (Ed.), *ACSM's Resource Manual for Guidelines for Exercise Testing and Prescription.* Philadelphia: Lippincott, Williams & Wilkins.

Kroll, S. (2001). Three tips to help your clients combat creeping obesity. *ACSM's Health and Fitness Journal, 5(3),* 22–24.

Manore, M. (1999). Low-carbohydrate diets for weight loss are back. *ACSM's Health and Fitness Journal, 3(5),* 41–43.

Manore, M. M. (2003). Dietary supplements for weight loss: Do they work? Are they safe? *American College of Sports Medicine's Health & Fitness Journal, 7(4)*, 17-21.

McInnis, K. (2000). Exercise for obese clients: Benefits, limitations, and guidelines. *ACSM's Health and Fitness Journal, 4(1)*, 25-31.

Ross, R., Freeman, J. A., & Janssen, I. (2000). Exercise alone is an effective strategy for reducing obesity and related co-morbidities. *Exercise and Sport Sciences Reviews, 28(4)*, 165-170.

Weblinks

National Eating Disorder Information Centre

www.nedic.ca

A website developed by a Toronto-based, non-profit organization, established in 1985 to provide information and resources on eating disorders and weight preoccupation.

Health Canada, Office of Nutrition Policy and Promotion

www.hc-sc.gc.ca/hpfb-dgpsa/onpp-bppn/index_e.html

A website that promotes the nutritional health and well-being of Canadians by collaboratively defining, promoting, and implementing evidence-based nutrition policies.

The Center for Weight and Health

www.nature.berkeley.edu/cwh/

A website that facilitates interaction among researchers, policy makers, and community-based providers from various disciplines and institutions concerned about weight, health, and food security.

Health Canada, Food Program

www.hc-sc.gc.ca/food-aliment/dg/e_about_us.html

A website intended to help Canadians maintain and improve their health through established policies and standards related to food safety and nutrition.

References

Acheson, K. (2004). Carbohydrate and weight control: Where do we stand? *Current Opinion in Clinical Nutrition and Metabolic Care, 7*, 485-492.

Achten, J., Gleeson, M., & Jeukendrup, A. E. (2002). Determination of the exercise intensity that elicits maximal fat oxidation. *Medicine and Science in Sports and Exercise, 34(1)*, 92-97.

AHA Dietary Guidelines. (2000). Revision 2000: A statement for healthcare professionals from the nutrition committee of the American Heart Association. *Circulation, 102*, 2284-2299.

Andersen, A. (1983). Anorexia nervosa and bulimia. *Journal of Adolescent Health Care, 4*, 15-21.

Atkinson, R. (1992). Treatment of obesity. *Nutritional Reviews, 50*, 338-345.

Bailey, C. (1991). *The new fit or fat.* Boston: Houghton Mifflin.

Bailey, J., Barker, R., & Beauchene, R. (1993). Age-related changes in rat adipose tissue cellularity are altered by dietary restriction and exercise. *Journal of Nutrition, 123*, 52-58.

Bjorntorp, P., & Brodoff, B. (Eds.). (1992). *Obesity.* Philadelphia: Lippincott.

Blair, S. (1993). Evidence for success of exercise in weight loss control. *Annals of Internal Medicine, 119*, 702-706.

Borgen, J., & Corbin, C. (1987). Eating disorders among female athletes. *Physician and Sports Medicine, 15*, 89-95.

Bouchard, C. (2000). Introduction. In C. Bouchard (Ed.), *Physical activity and obesity* (pp. 3-20). Champaign, IL: Human Kinetics.

Bouchard, C., Shepherd, R., Stephens, T., Sutton, J., & McPherson, B. (Eds.). (1990). *Exercise, fitness, and health: A consensus of current knowledge.* Champaign, IL: Human Kinetics.

Bouchard, C., Tremblay, A., Despres, J., Nadeau, A., Lupien, P. J., Theriault, G., Dussault, J., Moorjani, S., Pinault, S., & Fournier, G. (1990). The response to long-term overfeeding in identical twins. *New England Journal of Medicine, 322*, 1477-1482.

Broeder, C., Burrhus, K., Svanevik, L., & Wilmore, J. (1992). The effects of either high intensity resistance or endurance training on resting metabolic rate. *American Journal of Clinical Nutrition, 55*, 802-810.

Chagnon, Y. C., Rice, T., Perusse, L., Borecki, I. B., Ho-Kim, M. A., Lacaille, M., Pare, C., Bouchard, L., Gagnon, J., Leon, A. S., Skinner, J. S., Wilmore, J. H., Rao, D. C., & Bouchard, C. (2001). Genomic scan for genes affecting body composition before and after training in Caucasions from HERITAGE. *Journal of Applied Physiology, 90*, 1777- 1787.

Chambliss, H. O., Finley, C. E., & Blair, S. N. (2004). Attitudes toward obese individuals among exercise science students. *Medicine and Science in Sports and Exercise, 36(3)*, 468-474.

Corbin, C., Welk, G., Lindsey, R., & Corbin, W. (2003). *Concepts of physical fitness.* St. Louis: McGraw-Hill.

Coyle, E. (1995). Fat metabolism during exercise. *Sports Science Exchange* (Gatorade Sports Science Institute), *8*, 6.

Donatelle, R. J. (2005). *Health: The basics* (6th ed.). San Francisco: Pearson Education.

Foster, G., Wyatt, H. R., Hill, J. O., McGuckin, B. G., Brill, C., Mohammed, B. S., Szapary, P. O., Rader, D. J., Edman, J. S., & Klein, S. (2003). A randomized trial of low-carbohydrate diet for obesity. *New England Journal of Medicine, 348*, 2082-2090.

Frubeck, G., Gomez-Amrosi, J., Muruzabal, F., & Burrell, M. (2001). The adipocyte: A model for integration of endocrine and metabolic signaling in energy metabolism regulation. *American Journal of Physiology, 280,* E827–E847.

Getchell, B. (1998). *Physical fitness: A way of life* (5th ed.). Needham Heights, MA: Allyn and Bacon.

Graves, B. S., & Welsh, R. L. (2004). Recognizing the signs of body dysmorphic disorder and muscle dysmorphia. *American College of Sports Medicine's Health & Fitness Journal, 8(1),* 11–13.

Gwinup, G., Chelvam, R., & Steinberg, T. (1971). Thickness of subcutaneous fat and activity of underlying muscles. *Annals of Internal Medicine, 74,* 408–411.

Health implications of obesity: National Institutes of Health Consensus Development Conference. (1985). *Annals of Internal Medicine, 103,* 977–1077.

Heilbronn, L., & Ravussin, E. (2003). Calorie restriction and aging: Review of the literature and implications for studies in humans. *American Journal of Clinical Nutrition,* 78: 361-369.

Hildebrandt, T., Langenbucher, J., & Schundt, D. G. (2004). Muscularity concerns among men: Development of attitudinal and perceptual measures. *Body Image, 1(2),* 169–181.

Hockey, R. (1996). *Physical fitness: The pathway to healthful living* (8th ed.). St. Louis: Times Mirror/Mosby.

Jequier, E. (1993). Body weight regulation in humans: The importance of nutrient balance. *News in Physiological Sciences, 8,* 273–276.

Katzmarzyk, P. T. (2002). The Canadian obesity epidemic, 1985–1998. *Canadian Medical Association Journal, 166(8),* 1039–1040.

Katzmarzyk, P. T., & Janssen, I. (2004). The economic costs associated with physical inactivity and obesity in Canada: An Update. *Canadian Journal of Applied Sciences 29(1),* 90–115.

King, M., & Katch, F. (1986). Changes in body density, fat-folds, and girths at 2.3 kg increments of weight loss. *Human Biology, 58,* 709.

Kuczmarski, R. (1992). Prevalence of overweight and weight gain in the United States. *American Journal of Clinical Nutrition, 55,* 495s–502s.

Leeds, M. (1998). *Nutrition for healthy living.* Boston: WCB-McGraw-Hill.

Mayer, J., Marshall, N., Vitale, J., Christensen, J., Mashayekhi, M., & Stare, F. (1954). Exercise, food intake, and body weight in normal rats and genetically obese adult mice. *American Journal of Physiology, 177,* 544–548.

Meckling, K., O'Sullivan, C., & Saari, D. (2004). Comparison of a low-fat to a low-carbohydrate diet on weight loss, body composition, and risk factors for diabetes and cardiovascular disease in free-living, overweight men and women. *Journal of Clinical Endocrinology and Metabolism, 89,* 2717–2723.

Perri, M., Nezu, A., & Viegener, B. (1992). *Improving the long-term management and treatment of obesity.* New York: John Wiley and Sons.

Poehlman, E. (1989). A review: Exercise and its influence on resting energy metabolism in man. *Medicine and Science in Sports and Exercise, 21,* 515–525.

Pollock, M., & Wilmore, J. (1999). *Exercise in health and disease* (3rd ed.). Philadelphia: W. B. Saunders.

Powers, S., & Howley, E. (2004). Exercise physiology: Theory and application to fitness performance (5th ed.). St. Louis: McGraw-Hill.

Reeder, B. A., Senthilselvan, A., Depres, J. P., Angel, A., Liu, L., Wang, H., & Rabkin, S. W. (1997). The association of cardiovascular disease risk factors with abdominal obesity in Canada. *Canadian Medical Association Journal, 157(1 suppl),* S39–S45.

Roitman, J. (Ed.). (2001). *ACSM'S resource manual for guidelines for exercise testing and prescription.* Philadelphia: Lippincott.

Romijn, J., Coyle, E., Sidossis, L., Gastaldelli, A., Horowitz, J. F., Endert, E., & Wolfe, R. R. (1993). Regulation of endogenous fat and carbohydrate metabolism in relation to exercise and duration. *American Journal of Physiology, 265,* E380–E391.

Ross, R., Freeman, J., & Janssen, I. (2000). Exercise alone is an effective strategy for reducing obesity and related comorbidities. *Exercise and Sport Sciences Reviews, 28(4),* 165–170.

Saris, W. (2003). Sugars, energy metabolism, and body weight control. *American Journal of Nutrition, 78,* 850S–857S.

Statistics Canada. (2002). *Health indicators, May 2002.* Catalogue No. 82-221-XIE.

Stefanik, M. (1993). Exercise and weight control. In J. Holloszy (Ed.), *Exercise and sport science reviews,* Baltimore: Williams and Wilkins.

Steppan, C. M., Bailey, S. T., Bhat, S., Brown, E. J., Banerjee, R. R., Wright, C. M., Patel, H. R., Ahima, R. S., & Lazar, M. A. (2001). The hormone resistin links obesity to diabetes. *Nature, 409,* 307–312.

Stern, L., Labal, N., Seshadri, P., Chicano, K. L., Daily, D. A., McGrory, J., Williams, M., Gracely, E. J., & Samaha, F. F. (2004). The effects of low-carbohydrate versus conventional weight loss diets in severely obese adults: One-year follow-up of a randomized trial. *Annals of Internal Medicine, 140,* 778–785.

Stunkard, A., Sorensen, T., & Hanis, C. (1986). An adoption study of human obesity. *New England Journal of Medicine, 314,* 193–198.

Stunkard, A., & Wadden, T. (Eds.). (1993). *Obesity: Theory and therapy.* New York: Raven Press.

Stunkard, A. J., Harris, J. R., Pedersen, N. L., & McClearn, G. E. (1990). The body mass index of twins who have been reared apart. *The New England Journal of Medicine, 322(21),* 1483–1487.

Thompson, A. M., & Chad, K. E. (2002). The relationship of social physique anxiety to risk for developing an eating disorder in young females. *Journal of Adolescent Health, 31(2),* 183–189.

Thompson, A. M., Mirwald, R. L., Baxter-Jones, A. D., & Bailey, D. A. (2002). Secular trend in the development of fatness during childhood and adolescence. *American Journal of Human Biology, 14,* 669–679.

Tremblay, A., Coveney, S., Despres, J., Nadeau, A., & Prud'homme, D. (1992). Increased resting metabolic rate and lipid oxidation in exercise-trained individuals: Evidence for a role of beta-oxidation. *Canadian Journal of Physiology and Pharmacology, 70,* 1342–1347.

Tremblay, M. S., & Willms, J. D. (2000, 2001). Secular trends in the body mass index of Canadian children. *Canadian Medical Association Journal, 163,* 1429–1433.

Van Itallie, T. (1985). Health implications of overweight and obesity in the United States. *Annals of Internal Medicine, 103,* 983–988.

Wadden, T., Sternberg, J., Letizia, K., Stunkard, A., & Foster, G. (1989). Treatment for obesity by very low calorie diet, behavior therapy, and their combination: A five-year prospective. *International Journal of Obesity, 13(Suppl. 2),* 39–46.

Whitaker, R. C., Wright, A., Pepe, M. S., Seidel, K. D., & Dietz, W. H. (1997). Predicting obesity in young adulthood from childhood and parental obesity. *The New England Journal of Medicine, 337(13),* 869–873.

Williams, M. (1996). *Lifetime fitness and wellness.* Dubuque, IA: Wm. C. Brown.

Zemel, M. B. (2004). Role of calcium and dairy products in energy partitioning and weight management. *American Journal of Clinical Nutrition, 79,* 907S–912S.

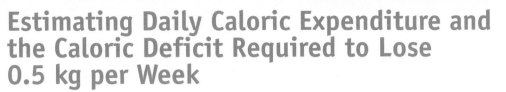

LABORATORY 8.1

Estimating Daily Caloric Expenditure and the Caloric Deficit Required to Lose 0.5 kg per Week

Name_____ Age _____ Sex _____ Date _____

PART A. ESTIMATION OF YOUR DAILY CALORIC EXPENDITURE

Using Table 8.1 (page 204), compute your estimated daily caloric expenditure.

    Estimated daily caloric expenditure = _____ calories/day.

PART B. CALCULATION OF CALORIC INTAKE REQUIRED TO PROMOTE 0.5 KG PER WEEK OF WEIGHT LOSS

Recall that 0.5 kg of fat contains approximately 3500 calories. Therefore, a negative caloric balance of 500 calories per day should result in a weight loss of 0.5 kg per week. Use the following formula to compute your daily caloric intake to result in a daily caloric deficit of 500 calories.

    estimated daily caloric expenditure – 500 calories (deficit) = daily caloric intake needed to produce a 500-calorie deficit

In the space provided, compute your daily caloric intake needed to produce 0.5 kg per week of weight loss.

_____ (estimated caloric expenditure) –

_____ – 500 _____ (caloric deficit)

= _____ target daily caloric intake

PART C. CALCULATION OF CALORIC INTAKE AND DAILY CALORIC EXPENDITURE REQUIRED TO PROMOTE 0.5 KG PER WEEK OF WEIGHT LOSS

A negative caloric balance of 500 calories per day can also be obtained by a combination of increasing daily caloric expenditure and decreasing caloric intake.

    In the spaces below, compute the caloric expenditure and caloric intake needed to produce 0.5 kg per week of weight loss.

_____ (estimated caloric expenditure) + 250* (caloric deficit) = _____

    – 250 = _____ target daily caloric intake.

*Remember that to create a greater caloric expenditure you have to increase your physical activity level beyond what you currently do.

LABORATORY 8.2

What Triggers Your Eating?

Name_____ Age _____ Sex _____ Date _____

Many things cause us to eat. Usually, just by identifying the triggers that cause you to eat, you can develop a strategy to counter those habits. Use the questions below to determine your motivation for eating.

For each question, record Yes or No in the blank.

EMOTIONAL

1. I cannot lose weight and keep it off. _____
2. My eating is out of control. _____
3. Even if I'm not hungry, I eat. _____
4. I eat when stressed or upset. _____
5. Food gives me great pleasure and I use it as a reward. _____
6. Eating is usually on my mind. _____
7. My eating causes problems with weight management. _____
8. I go on eating "binges" or find myself eating constantly. _____
9. My eating habits cause me embarrassment. _____
10. I use food to help me cope with feelings. _____

SOCIAL

11. I eat whenever others around me are eating. _____
12. If anyone offers food, I take it. _____
13. Whenever I am in a stressful social situation, I want to eat. _____
14. Whenever I am in a relaxed social situation, I want to eat. _____
15. I eat more in a social setting than I do at home. _____
16. I eat less when others are around to see me. _____
17. In a social setting, the amount of food I eat depends on the group of people. _____
18. I eat different foods in a social setting than I do at home. _____

ENVIRONMENTAL

19. I eat more at restaurants than I do at home. _____
20. I eat less at restaurants than I do at home. _____
21. If I smell food I can't resist the urge to eat. _____
22. If I walk by a restaurant or bakery I can't resist the urge to eat. _____
23. I like to eat while reading or watching TV. _____
24. I find food comforting in different environmental conditions, such as on a rainy day or in cold weather. _____
25. I find food comforting when I am in unfamiliar surroundings. _____
26. If I am outdoors, I feel as if I can eat more. _____

INTERPRETATION

Insignificant influence: If you answered Yes to 1 question within a section or fewer than 6 questions total, weight management is probably relatively easy for you.

Some influence: If you answered Yes to 2 questions within a section or 6 to 9 questions total, there are issues that are complicating your weight management. It might help to talk with a health care professional while developing a weight management plan.

Signficant influence: If you answered Yes to 3 questions within a section or 10 to 13 questions total, there are several issues affecting your weight management plan. Speaking with a health care professional or counsellor can help you deal with issues that trigger your eating.

Severe influence: If you answered Yes to 4 or more questions within a section or 14 or more questions total, there are many issues that complicate your weight management. Counselling and speaking with a health care professional will help you to develop a weight management plan.

CHAPTER 9

Stress Management and Modifying Unhealthy Behaviour

9

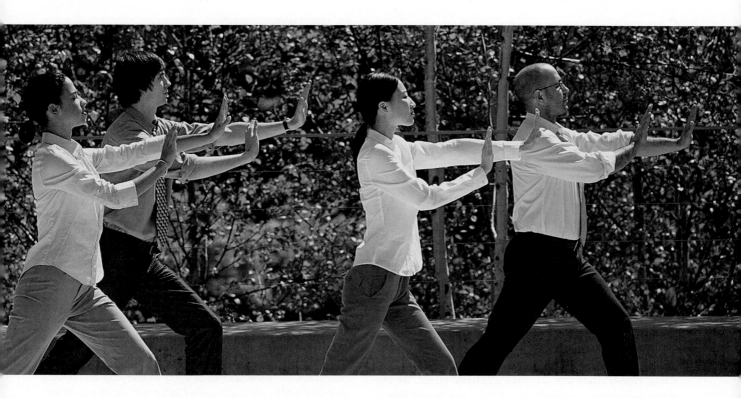

After studying this chapter, you should be able to

1. Describe *stress* and *stressors*.
2. Outline the steps involved in stress management.
3. Describe the three phases of the general adaptation syndrome.
4. Identify sources of psychosocial stress.
5. Describe several relaxation techniques used to manage stress.
6. Outline the general model for behaviour modification.
7. Provide an example of how to modify an unhealthy behaviour.
8. Identify the most common types of accidents.
9. Outline steps to reduce your risk of accidents.

Although many behaviours affect your health, the five most important are regular physical activity, good nutrition, weight maintenance, stress management, and modification of unhealthful behaviours that increase your risk of getting a disease or having an accident (Brooks, 2003; Donatelle & Davis, 2000; Perna, Schneiderman, & LaPerriere, 1997). Other chapters focus on improving health through physical activity, eating well, weight maintenance, and actively reducing the risk of cancer and heart disease. This chapter expands on these strategies by introducing the concepts of stress reduction and behaviour modification aimed at reducing your risk of disease and accidents.

Stress Management

Studies suggest that 10 to 15 percent of Canadian adults may be functioning at less than optimal levels because of stress-related anxiety and depression (Brooks, 2003). Indeed, millions of people take medication for stress-related illnesses, resulting in billions of dollars lost annually to businesses and government through employee absenteeism and health care costs. Therefore, stress is a major health concern in Canada that affects not only individual lives but also the economy as a whole.

Stress: An Overview

Stress is a physiological and psychological response to a change in our environment that may have a positive or negative effect on us. It is our reaction to the **stressor** that determines the amount of impact. Many of our daily activities cause one form of stress or another. Positive stress, or something that presents an opportunity for personal growth, is called **eustress**. For example, getting married, starting a new job, or even making new friends can cause nervousness or excitement, effects of eustress. **Distress**, or negative stress, causes strain and can have a harmful effect. We regularly face distress with divorce, death, and severe illness. **Adaptation** is an attempt to cope with any given stressor. While adjusting to distress, however, strain and anxiety can result. **Strain** is the wear and tear on our bodies and minds while trying to adjust to a stressor.

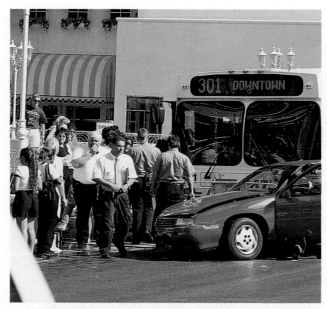
Automobile accidents are one of the many causes of stress in our society.

There are many sources of stress in everyday life. Driving in heavy traffic, being involved in an automobile accident, moving to a new home, encountering emotional conflicts at work or school, or experiencing personal financial problems are just a few.

Stress and Disease

From a medical standpoint, stress can affect emotional and physical health. Chronic (persistent) stress has been linked to elevated blood pressure, heart disease, hormonal imbalances, reduced resistance to disease, and emotional disorders (Brooks, 2003; Donatelle & Davis, 2000; Perna, Schneiderman, & LaPerriere, 1997). The biologist Hans Selye was one of the first scientists to develop a scientific theory to explain the relationship between stress and disease. Selye proposed that humans adapt to stress in a response he termed the **general adaptation syndrome**, which involves three stages: an alarm stage, a resistance stage, and an exhaustion stage (Selye, 1978).

stress   The way your mind and body react when you are forced to adapt to the persons and/or situations around you.

stressor   A factor that produces distress or eustress.

eustress   Good stress.

distress   Stress that may negatively affect health.

adaptation   An attempt to cope with any given stressor.

strain   Wear and tear on the mind and body while trying to adapt to a stressor.

general adaptation syndrome   A pattern of responses to stress that consists of an alarm stage, a resistance stage, and an exhaustion stage.

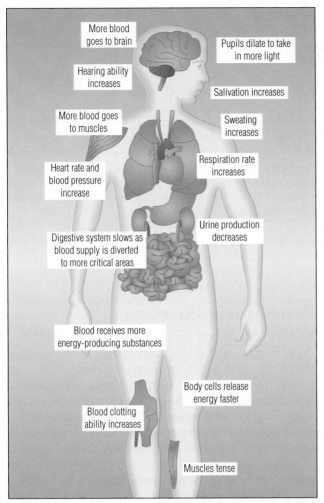

FIGURE 9.1 The immediate physiological effects of stress.

Source: Donatelle, R. J., Davis, L. G., Munroe, A. J., Munroe, A., & Casselman, M. A. (2004). *Health: The basics* (3rd ed.). Toronto: Benjamin Cummings, 62. Reprinted with permission of Pearson Education Canada Inc.

In the *alarm stage,* the body responds to stress by activating the sympathetic nervous system (Figure 9.1). This activation prompts many physiological changes, including the release of stress hormones (e.g., ephinephrine, norepinephrine, and cortisol), increased muscle tension, and elevations in heart rate and blood pressure (Selye, 1978). During the alarm stage, an individual often experiences anxiety, headaches, disrupted eating and sleeping patterns, and the body becomes susceptible to disease and more prone to accidents.

With continued exposure to stress, the individual reaches the *resistance stage,* during which the body opposes the stress by activating mechanisms that resist disease effectively. In short, the resistance stage represents an improved ability to cope with stress (Selye, 1978).

If the stressor persists, the individual reaches the *exhaustion stage.* Selye suggested that in this stage the body becomes very vulnerable to disease because it loses the ability to respond to the stressor due to the depletion of its resources. Note that "exhaustion" in this sense is not the fatigue associated with the conclusion of a hard exercise

session or the end of a long day, but instead a life-threatening type of physical and psychological depletion that occurs after days or weeks of exposure to stressors.

Although Selye's model of adaptation to stressors is still viewed as an important contribution to our understanding of the response to stressors, many newer research findings discount some aspects of the model. For example, it is no longer thought that the increased susceptibility to disease in the exhaustion stage is due to the body's *failure* to respond to the stressors; instead, current evidence indicates that the underlying cause of many stressor-related diseases *is* the body's prolonged response to the stressors. Research into the relationships among the nervous system, the endocrine system (which produces hormones), and the immune system (which protects against disease) has shown that prolonged exposure to stressors results in a continual release of stressor hormones, including cortisol. High levels of cortisol in the blood impair the immune system's ability to fight infections, which increases the risk of contracting disease (Anderson et al., 1998; Brooks, 2003; Holroyd et al., 2001; Sewitch, 2001).

As previously mentioned, prolonged distress increases not only the chances of infection, but also the risk for many other problems. As a result, stress management skills are important tools in preventing stress-related conditions. Before we discuss stress management skills, let's begin with a discussion on identifying sources of distress and eustress.

Assessment of Stress

Stressors can be acute (such as the death of a loved one), cumulative (such as a series of events leading to a divorce), or chronic (such as daily job-related pressures). Although it is clear that chronic or extreme stressors are unhealthy, some degree of stress is required to maximize performance. For instance, athletes and business professionals often perform better when faced with mild to moderate stressors. As noted above, *eustress,* or positive stress, results in improved performance. Although some level of stress is desirable, each of us has a breaking point in terms of stress. This idea is illustrated in Figure 9.2. When we surpass the stress level needed to optimize performance (optimal stressor) we reach our stress "break point," and *distress* (negative stress) results. Distress leads to a decline in performance, and chronic distress can increase the risk of disease.

Different people may react differently to the same stressful situation. For example, a violent movie may evoke anger in one person and no emotion in another. This difference in "stress perception" is due to personality differences. When it comes to stress, individuals can be classified into one of three personality categories: type A, type B, and type C (Figure 9.3). Type A individuals are highly motivated, time-conscious, hard driving, impatient, and sometimes hostile. They have a heightened response to stress. Because stress is a risk factor for heart disease, type A people exhibit this risk (Williams, 1996). In contrast, type B individuals are easygoing,

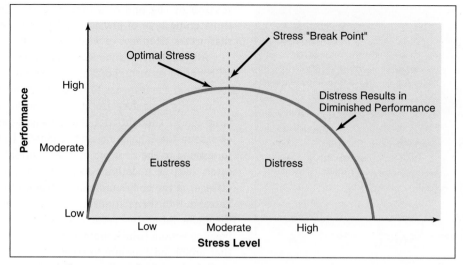

FIGURE 9.2 The concepts of eustress and distress.

nonaggressive, and patient. Type B personalities do not generally respond greatly to stress and are considered to be at low risk (from a stress perspective) for heart disease. People with type C personalities have many of the qualities of type A people. They are confident, highly motivated, and competitive. However, these unique individuals use their personality traits to their advantage by maintaining a constant level of emotional control and channelling their ambition in creative directions. Interestingly, although type C personalities are highly driven, they experience the same low stress-related risk for heart disease as type B personalities.

psychosocial stressors The many events in daily life that can cause good or bad stress.

Psychosocial Stressors

As discussed in Chapter 1, an individual's wellness is based on the interactions among his or her physical, emotional, intellectual, spiritual, social, environmental, and occupational health. These components are the variables of psychosocial health. They can also be the sources of various types of stressors, or **psychosocial stressors**. These are the many events in our daily lives that can cause some sort of stress, good or bad. They can be simple things, such as the social adjustments and readjustments we make as we move from work, to play, to family all in one day. Others can come from change, new jobs, or new homes.

We can all relate to the major stressors in life: the constantly rising cost of tuition, job loss, and family breakup. But psychologist Richard Lazarus (Lazarus, 1985) suggests that it's the daily hassles—life's little annoyances—that

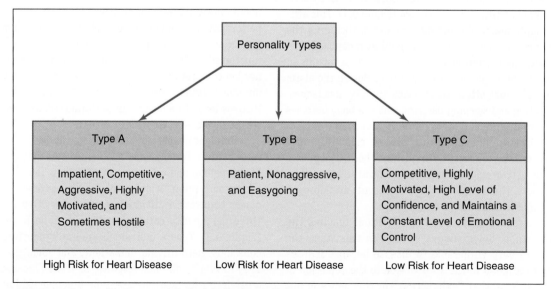

FIGURE 9.3 Personality types and their risks for heart disease.

have a cumulative effect on our psychosocial well-being. Minor inconveniences such as losing your keys, having a flat tire, discovering a stain on your shirt, or forgetting your wallet may seem inconsequential individually. Put all of these irritations into one day and you can see how they add up to a harmful amount of stress.

Goal setting is another area that can be a source of negative stress. We are faced with relentless demands to succeed—whether as a parent, a professional, or a student, expectations are high. Consequently, we often set goals for ourselves that put us under an enormous amount of pressure. For example, you may equate being a successful student with maintaining an A average in all courses, being involved in several extracurricular activities, and having an active social life. Striving to achieve all of this may result in your being overscheduled and therefore losing focus in one or more areas, causing schoolwork or friendships to suffer. We compound stress by setting goals and then behaving in a completely contradictory manner—consider the student who wants to maintain an A average, but instead of studying spends the majority of her time out late partying with friends. The frustration associated with this sort of goal setting and inconsistent behaviour can be overwhelming and result in a significant amount of distress.

In Chapter 1, environmental health was referred to as awareness and protection of our surroundings. Conversely, environmental distress occurs when we encounter events like the B.C. wildfires of 2003, or the devastating effects of the Indian Ocean tsunami in 2004. Our physical environment is uncontrollable, and individuals who live through natural or industrial disasters experience a prolonged state of the alarm stage, with heightened physiological changes that may last for days or weeks. This constant distress can have damaging effects on the body, as discussed above regarding the exhaustion stage. However, most of us live with environmental stressors that we may be unaware of, things like noise or air pollution. Even though we may be unaware of these stressors, our bodies are still making the required adjustments through the general adaptation syndrome to deal with them. Unable to get away from these stressors, our bodies may exist in a constant resistance phase that over time may result in stress-related disorders.

Other forms of psychosocial stressors can come from a variety of situations, such as overcrowding; discrimination; prejudice concerning sex, race, social status, or lifestyle; poverty; and unemployment. However, none may be as powerful as self-imposed distress. How we feel about ourselves has a tremendous effect on how we deal with the other sources of psychosocial stress in our lives.

Individuals who lack **self-efficacy**—a sense of personal power to cope with stressful situations—doubt their skills or ability to successfully master difficult problems. This often leads to a person having a low opinion of himself or herself, or low self-esteem. People with low self-esteem often give in to anger, frustration, and ultimately defeat. This reinforces the belief that they are somehow incompetent or ineffectual.

Some research indicates that **self-esteem**, a sense of satisfaction with oneself, and a sense of self-efficacy can greatly alter the effect that various diseases have on a person. Low self-esteem may impair the immune system and its ability to combat disease, and in some cases can even increase the symptoms of chronic illnesses such as HIV and AIDS (Perna, Schneiderman, & LaPerriere, 1997). Those with a higher sense of self-esteem and self-efficacy, such as the Type C personality referred to in Figure 9.3, may be able to minimize their risk for certain diseases. People who believe in their own effectiveness may also be able to lessen symptoms of more chronic disorders or illnesses. They may see life's challenges as an opportunity for personal growth, and know from past experience that they can successfully deal with the ultimate outcome of events.

The first step in learning to deal with stress is to examine your stress level; a convenient way to do this is to complete the questionnaire provided in Laboratory 9.1. If the results suggest that you are under stress, you should begin implementing stress reduction techniques like the ones discussed later in this chapter.

Steps in Stress Management

Now that you have identified the difference between distress and eustress and evaluated your level of stress using Laboratory 9.1, you can begin to manage your stress levels using stress management techniques. Although there are no magic formulas or nutritional supplements capable of eliminating distress, there are two general steps to managing everyday stressors (Williams, 1996; Howley & Franks, 1997): reduce the overall number of stressors in your life, and learn to cope with life's daily hassles by improving your ability to relax.

Stress Reduction   Reducing sources of distress is the ideal means of reducing the effects of stress in your life. The first step in stress reduction is to recognize those factors that promote daily stress. After identifying these factors, you should eliminate activities that result in daily distress. While it may not be possible to avoid all stressors, many "unnecessary" forms can be eliminated.

A classic stressor that can often be avoided is overcommitment, a frequent cause of distress in postsecondary students. Plan your time carefully and prioritize your activities. It may not be possible to do everything that you want to do during a given day or week. Plan a daily schedule that allows you to do the things you need to accomplish without being overwhelmed by less important activities. A Closer Look: "Time-Management Guidelines" discusses some key elements of time management.

self-efficacy The belief in one's ability to accomplish the task at hand.

self-esteem A sense of satisfaction with oneself.

Time-Management Guidelines

Use the following guidelines to improve your time-management skills and increase your productivity:

Establish goals. Establish a list of goals that you hope to accomplish. Identify your immediate and long-term goals, and rank your goals according to priority. By establishing and prioritizing goals, you can focus your efforts on those projects most important to you.

Use a daily planner. Plan your day using a daily planner. Chart your schedule hour by hour, and prioritize your most important goals.

Evaluate your time-management skills regularly. At the completion of your day, take 5 to 10 minutes to evaluate your time management. Note time wasted and make plans to correct these mistakes for the following day.

Learn to say no to activities that prevent you from achieving your goals. Before you accept a new responsibility, complete your current task or eliminate an unnecessary project. Although saying no is often difficult, it is critical to manage your time well.

Delegate responsibility. Most of us like to feel in control, and this makes delegation of responsibilities to others dif-

ficult. Nonetheless, if you become overloaded when working on a group project don't be afraid to ask for assistance. Delegating responsibility to others is an easy way to reduce your workload and lower stress.

Eliminate distractions. Interruptions and distractions can steal precious time from your day. Identify those factors that distract you and eliminate them if possible.

Schedule time for you. Find time each day to relax and do something you enjoy. Remember that taking an occasional break from your work is not wasting time and will improve your overall productivity by helping to energize yourself.

Reward yourself when you complete a goal. One of the simple pleasures in life is to reward yourself after you complete a goal. The reward can come in many forms: a new pair of shoes, a movie, a few days of relaxation, and so on. The importance of rewarding yourself cannot be overemphasized. People perform better when rewarded for a job well done, and a reward is an excellent means of providing encouragement (even for yourself) for future good work.

Coping with Stress: Relaxation Techniques

Because it is impossible to eliminate all stressors from daily life, it is necessary to use stress management techniques to reduce the potentially harmful effects of stress. Most of these techniques are designed to produce relaxation, which reduces the stress level. The following are some of the more common approaches used.

PROGRESSIVE RELAXATION Progressive relaxation is a stress-reduction technique for reducing muscular tension using exercises designed to promote relaxation. In essence, the technique is practised as follows. While sitting quietly or lying down, contract and then relax various muscle groups one at a time, beginning with the feet and then moving up the body to the hands and neck, until a complete state of muscle relaxation is achieved. The details of this technique are outlined in A Closer Look: "Progressive Relaxation Training."

Proponents of progressive relaxation techniques argue that relaxing the muscles in this manner will also relax the mind and therefore relieve stress. The theory behind this concept is that an anxious (stressed) mind cannot exist in a relaxed body.

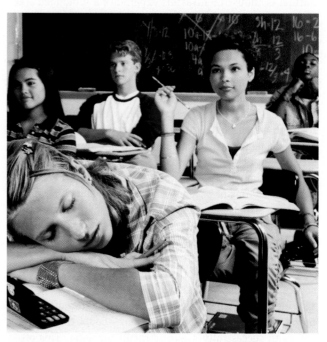

Obtaining adequate sleep is one of the best ways to reduce stress.

Progressive Relaxation Training

There are many types of progressive relaxation training methods, and more than 200 different exercises have been described. In essence, the technique involves contracting and relaxing muscle groups, starting in your lower body and moving toward your upper body. The following technique is one of many that are easy to learn and use (Donatelle & Davis, 2000):

1. The first step is to assume a relaxed position (either sitting or lying down). Extend your legs, put your arms at your sides, and close your eyes. Let your muscles relax and your body go limp.
2. Take a few slow, deep breaths and concentrate on relaxing muscular tension.
3. Contract the following muscle groups in the order they are presented. For each muscle group, contract the muscle as hard as possible for 5 seconds. Release the contraction and take a deep breath. Repeat this procedure two or more times until the muscle group is relaxed. Try to limit your contraction to the isolated body parts described here:
   a. Curl the toes on your right foot. Repeat this action with your left foot.
   b. Bend your right foot toward your head as far as possible. Repeat this action with your left foot.
   c. Extend your right foot downward (point your toes) as far as possible. Repeat this action with your left foot.
   d. Contract your right upper leg (thigh). Repeat this action with your left leg.
   e. Contract your stomach muscles by attempting to curl your upper body (like a curl-up without performing the curl-up).
   f. Contract your shoulders by moving your shoulders as far forward as possible (keep your head and arms in place).
   g. Contract your shoulders by moving your shoulders as far backward as possible (keep your head and arms in place).
   h. Spread the fingers on your right hand as far as possible. Repeat this action with the left hand.
   i. Contract the muscles in your forearm by making a fist with your right hand. Repeat this action with your left hand.
   j. Contract the muscles in the front of your neck by bringing your head forward (chin to chest) as far as possible.
   k. Open your mouth as wide as possible.
   l. Wrinkle your forehead.

With practice you will improve your ability to isolate the muscle groups described, and your ability to relax using this technique will also improve. As you become more comfortable with progressive relaxation, feel free to incorporate your own exercises into this routine.

BREATHING EXERCISES A simple way of achieving relaxation is by performing **breathing exercises**:

1. Assume a comfortable position, sitting or lying down, with eyes closed.
2. Begin inhaling and exhaling slowly. Count from 1 to 3 during each inhalation and each exhalation to maintain a slow and regular breathing pattern.
3. Now combine stretching and breathing to provide greater relaxation and stress reduction. For example, stretch your arms toward the ceiling as you inhale, then lower your arms during exhalation.

Try this exercise for 5 to 15 minutes in a quiet room. Although breathing exercises may not reduce all stress, they have been shown to be a simple means of stress reduction.

REST AND SLEEP One of the most effective means of reducing stress and tension is to get adequate rest and sleep. How much sleep do you need? It appears that individual needs vary greatly; however, a good guideline is 7 to 9 hours of restful sleep per night (see A Closer Look: "How Much Sleep Is Enough?"). Further, because of the body's natural hormonal rhythms, it is recommended that you go to bed at approximately the same time every night.

In addition to a good night's sleep, 15 to 30 minutes of rest per day is useful in stress reduction. This can be achieved as simply as putting your feet up on a desk or table and closing your eyes. A well-rested body is the best protection against distress and fatigue.

PHYSICAL ACTIVITY Although prolonged or high-intensity exercise can impose mental and physical stress, research has shown that light to moderate physical activity can reduce many types of stress. The recommended types of physical activities for optimal stress reduction are low- to moderate-intensity aerobic exercises such as running, swimming, and cycling. The guidelines for these types of exercises prescription are presented in Chapter 3. Other popular types of activities for reducing distress and achieving relaxation are yoga, tai-chi, and Pilates. Many gyms and health clubs offer classes in these forms of exercise.

How good is physical activity at reducing stress? Studies have shown that physical activity is a very effective form of stress reduction (Berger & Owen, 1988; Brooks, 2003;

breathing exercises A simple way of achieving relaxation by regulating the speed and depth of breathing.

How Much Sleep Is Enough?

To determine your sleep needs, perform the following simple experiment. Continue to get up at the same time every day, but vary your bedtime over a period of 2 weeks. Keep records of how you feel each day. Do you feel groggy after 6 hours of sleep? Do you feel refreshed after an 8-hour sleep? How do you feel if you sleep 10 hours? Because either too little sleep or too much sleep often makes you feel sluggish, the objective is to find the optimum amount of sleep for you. This can be done by "listening" to your body and adjusting your sleep schedule accordingly.

Assuming a relaxed position is important in progressive relaxation techniques.

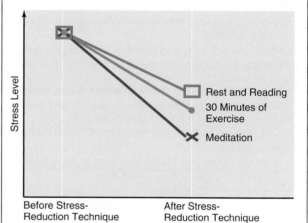

FIGURE 9.4 The effects of exercise and other activities on stress reduction.

Raglin & Morgan, 1987). Figure 9.4 compares the effects of a 30-minute session of light to moderate exercise (running) to three other common forms of stress reduction: rest, reading, and meditation. In this study, meditation provided the greatest stress reduction, with physical activity finishing a close second (Perna, Schneiderman, & LaPerriere, 1997).

Why does regular physical activity reduce stress? Several possibilities exist. One theory is that physical activity causes the brain to release several naturally produced tranquilizers, called *endorphins*, that reduce stress levels (Farrell, 1987). Endorphins work by blocking the effects of stress-related chemicals in the brain. Another theory is that physical activity may be a diversion that frees your mind from worry or other stressful thoughts. Another possibility is that regular physical activity results in an improvement in physical fitness and self-image, which increases your resistance to distress. A final possibility is that all of these factors may be involved in the beneficial

effects of physical activity on stress management. The next time you feel stressed, do some physical activity; you will feel and look better as a result.

MEDITATION Meditation has been practised for centuries in an effort to produce relaxation and achieve inner peace. There are many types of meditation, and there is no scientific evidence that one form is superior to another. Most types of meditation have the same common elements: sitting quietly for 15 to 20 minutes twice a day, concentrating on a single word or image, and breathing slowly and regularly. The goal of meditation is to reduce distress by achieving a complete state of physical and mental relaxation. The following is a brief overview of how meditation is practised (note that beginning a successful program of meditation may require initial instruction from an experienced individual):

1. First, choose a word or sound, called a *mantra,* to be repeated during the meditation. The idea is that this word or sound should become your symbol of complete relaxation. Choose a mantra that has little emotional significance for you, such as the word *red.*
2. To begin meditation, find a quiet area and sit comfortably with your eyes closed. Take several deep breaths and concentrate on relaxation; let your body go limp.

meditation An ancient method that aims to produce relaxation and achieve inner peace.

Can Nutritional Supplements Reduce Emotional Stress?

Because vitamins are good for us, many people mistakenly believe that the more they take, the better they'll feel. Unfortunately, many manufacturers have taken advantage of this belief by marketing products they advertise as "magic bullets" for reducing stress. In truth, no nutritional products have been proven to reduce psychosocial stressors. And because taking large amounts of *any* vitamin could pose health risks, consult your physician first. (For a complete review of vitamins and minerals, see Clarkson, 1991.)

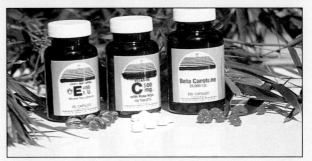

Although the advertisements for numerous nutritional products claim the products reduce stress, none of these products have been proven effective for stress reduction.

3. Concentrate on your mantra. This means that you should not hear or think about anything but your mantra. Repeat your mantra over and over again in your mind and relax. Avoid distracting thoughts and focus only on the mantra.

4. After 15 to 20 minutes of concentration on the mantra, open your eyes and begin to move your thoughts away from the mantra. End the session by making a fist with both hands and saying to yourself that you are alert and refreshed.

VISUALIZATION Sometimes called *imagery*, **visualization** uses mental pictures to reduce stress. The idea is to create an appealing mental image (such as a quiet mountain setting) that promotes relaxation and reduces stress. Visualization is similar to meditation except that instead of using a mantra, you substitute a relaxing scene. If you fail to reach a complete state of relaxation, don't be discouraged. Achieving complete relaxation with this technique may require numerous practice sessions.

In summary, there are many ways to successfully manage many stressors. The key is to find the technique that is best for you and stick with it. Regular physical activity may be the only type of stress management you require. However, if physical activity alone is not sufficient, try one of the other forms of stress management as well. Remember, regardless of your personality type or your lifestyle, you can successfully manage stress by applying one or more of the previously discussed techniques.

Stress Management: Closing Remarks

For the millions of Canadians who experience significant stress, the first step in preventing or treating the problem is recognizing that a problem exists. The way to begin is to assess your level of stress using an appropriate stress-identification questionnaire, such as the one in Laboratory 9.1 on page 243. The next step is to select a stress management technique that

is right for you—one that you enjoy, and, perhaps most importantly, one that you will practise regularly. Read on for answers to some questions about stress management.

Modifying Unhealthy Behaviour

A healthy lifestyle is achieved by eliminating unhealthy behaviour; this requires behaviour modification. Behaviour modification is the process of changing an undesirable behaviour to a more desirable behaviour. In the next two sections we discuss behaviour modification and provide specific examples of how unhealthy behaviours can be eliminated.

Model for Changing Behaviour

The general plan for modifying behaviour is similar for all types of behaviour modification (Table 9.1). A logical starting point in eliminating unhealthy behaviours is to analyze your current behaviour and identify problem areas. Laboratory 9.1 on page 243 is designed to assist you.

The desire to change is the key point in any behaviour modification plan. Without a genuine desire to make lifestyle changes, any behaviour modification plan is doomed to fail.

After identifying the problem and establishing a desire to change a specific behaviour, you next move to analyze the history of the problem. The objective here is to learn what factors contribute to the development of the behaviour to be modified. Learning the cause is useful when developing a strategy for change.

visualization A relaxation technique that uses appealing mental images to promote relaxation and reduce stress; also called *imagery*.

Step No.	Action
1	Identify the problem.
2	Desire change.
3	Analyze the past and current history of the problem.
4	Establish short-term written goals.
5	Establish long-term written goals.
6	Sign a contract (with friends).
7	Develop a strategy for change.
8	Implement the strategy and learn new coping skills to deal with the problem.
9	Evaluate your progress. Provide friends with progress reports.
10	Plan a long-term strategy for maintaining behaviour changes.

TABLE 9.1 General Steps in Behaviour Modification

The next two steps in the behaviour modification plan (steps 4 and 5 in Table 9.1) are the development of short- and long-term goals for behaviour change. Short-term goals establish the need for a rapid change in behaviour. Long-term goals provide the incentive required to maintain behaviour changes. The importance of goal setting in behaviour modification cannot be overemphasized. A behaviour modification plan without goals is like a race without a finish line.

The sixth stage in the behaviour modification plan is to sign a behaviour modification contract in the presence of friends (Laboratory 9.2). The purpose of signing a formal contract is to confirm in writing your commitment to a behaviour change. Having friends present during the signing of the contract is important. They provide moral support and encouragement during the difficult early period of behaviour change.

The final four steps (steps 7 to 10) incorporate the development of a strategy for behaviour change, the learning of new coping skills, evaluation of your progress, and the planning of long-term maintenance for behaviour change.

Many people who have had previous difficulty in changing behaviour develop the attitude that some bad habits cannot be changed. This is not true! Unhealthy behaviours are learned; therefore, they can be unlearned.

Specific Behaviour Modification Goals

Let's fill in the details of our behaviour modification model by illustrating how these plans can be applied specifically to smoking cessation and weight loss.

Smoking Cessation   As previously mentioned, cigarette smoking is a serious health concern that increases the risk of cancer and heart disease. According to Health Canada (2004), an estimated 21 percent of the population aged 15 and older are smokers. This is a slight decease from the 22 percent rate of 2001. An increased effort to keep individuals from smoking has resulted in 120 000 fewer teenagers, and 300 000 fewer adults, smoking. If this rate remains the same, by 2050 there will be more than 150 000 fewer smoking-related deaths. Currently, Health Canada estimates that 22 percent of all deaths in Canada are attributable to smoking. It is expected that current tobacco-control efforts will help to reverse this trend, but smoking cessation begins with the individual.

The first step in smoking cessation is having the desire to stop. After expressing this desire and analyzing smoking behaviour (see A Closer Look: "Causes of Smoking Behaviour"), each individual can develop a three-phase plan to stop smoking that incorporates steps 4 through 10 of the general steps of the behaviour modification model. Phase 1

A CLOSER LOOK

Causes of Smoking Behaviour

Before beginning a smoking cessation effort, it is useful to ask the question "Why do I smoke?" Three explanations have been proposed to explain smoking behaviour:

1. social learning theory
2. nicotine addiction theory
3. opponent process theory

The social learning theory of smoking argues that smokers develop the habit of smoking from peers and continue the habit because of social reinforcement. Positive support from friends who smoke and the social interaction that centres around smoking make this habit difficult to break.

A second potential explanation for smoking behaviour is that the smoker develops an addiction to nicotine. The evidence for

this theory comes from smokers themselves, who attest to the sensation of a "smoker's high" and report that smoking cessation often leaves them with withdrawal symptoms and a physical craving for nicotine.

The theory of the opponent process argues that smoking results from two opposing processes, one pleasant and one unpleasant. Social reinforcement and the "smoker's high" interact to cause a pleasant emotion, whereas attempts to stop smoking result in unpleasant withdrawal symptoms that can be eliminated by smoking. Therefore, the pleasant sensation of smoking and the unpleasant sensation of not smoking combine to encourage regular smoking behaviour.

Managing Stress Behaviours

Stress is not something that you can run from or wish into nonexistence. To control stress, you must meet it head-on and use as many resources as you can to ensure that your coping skills are fine-tuned and ready to help you. In planning your personal strategy for success, you should consider the following:

Making Decisions for You

Following a few simple guidelines may help you not only to enjoy more guilt-free time but also to become more productive during work hours.

Plan life, not time. Determining what you want from life rather than what you can get done may help change the way you use time. Evaluate all your activities, even the most trivial, to determine whether they add to your life. If they don't, get rid of them.

Decelerate. Rushing is part of the Canadian work ethic and mindset that says "Busy is better." It can be addictive. When rushed, ask yourself if you really need to be. What's the worst that could happen if you slowed down? Tell yourself at least once a day that failure seldom results from doing a job slowly or too well. Failures happen when rushing causes a lack of attention to detail.

Learn to delegate and share. The need to feel in control is powerful. If you are unusually busy, leave details to someone else. Don't be afraid to ask others to help or share the workload and responsibilities.

Learn to say no. Give priority to what is most critical to your life, your job, or your current situation. Decide what things you can do, what things you must do, and what things you want to do, and delegate the rest to someone else either permanently or until you complete some of your priority tasks. Before you take on a new responsibility, finish or drop an old one.

Schedule time alone. Find time each day for quiet thinking, reading, exercising, or other enjoyable activities.

Checklist for Change: Assessing Your Life Stressors

Have you assessed the major stressors in your life? Are they people, events, or specific activities?

Have you thought about what you may be doing to worsen your stress levels? Do you often worry about things that never happen? Are you often anxious about nothing?

Have you thought about what you could change to reduce your stress levels?

Do you have a network of friends and family members who can help you reduce your stress levels? Do you know where you could go to get professional advice about how to start reducing them?

Have you thought about what changes you'd like to work on first? Have you developed a plan of action? When do you want to start?

Checklist for Change: Assessing Community Stressors

Have you considered what in your environment may cause stress for you and the people around you?

Could these stressors be changed? How could they be changed? Why would changing them make a difference?

What on your campus or in your living situation causes undue stress for you or your friends? What could you do to change these stressors?

What advice might you give to your school administrators to help them reduce unnecessary stress among students?

Critical Thinking

You just scraped by to pay your tuition bill in January, then your university announced a large tuition hike for next year. You already work a part-time job and seem to spend all your "free time" studying. The stress you've got now is beginning to get to you, and you realize that you will have to work another 5 to 10 hours per week just to pay your bills next year. And tuition is likely to go up in your final year as well. How can you manage your time and finances so you can complete your degree?

Begin with your own current situation: How can you make better use of your time? Could you prioritize your week in such a way that you could find the extra time to work? Finally, even if you make enough money, you will need to deal with the increased stress. What will you do to keep the stress in check?

Source: Donatelle, R. J., Davis, L. G., Munroe, A. J., Munroe, A., & Casselman, M. A. (2004). *Health: The basics* (3rd ed.). Toronto: Benjamin Cummings, 76. Reprinted with permission of Pearson Education Canada Inc.

is often termed the *preparation phase.* In this phase, smokers develop the confidence to stop smoking by establishing short-term and long-term goals, signing a written contract, and developing a plan to stop smoking.

The second phase of smoking cessation is commonly termed *cessation.* On the cessation date established in the *stop smoking contract,* the individual stops smoking. Quitting smoking "cold turkey" has been shown to be more effective than a gradual slowdown (Hales, 1998). After a smoking cessation program has begun, it is important that the individual receive strong peer support, especially during the first few days and weeks.

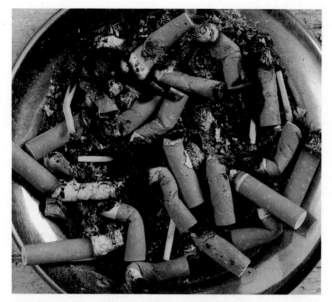

Cigarette smoking increases the risk of cancer and heart disease. The importance of cessation cannot be overemphasized.

The final phase of smoking cessation is termed the *maintenance phase*. The obvious objective of the maintenance phase is to ensure that the individual does not start smoking again. Several strategies can assist in this process. Continued peer and family support for the individual's decision to stop smoking is critical, and its importance cannot be overemphasized. A second strategy is to avoid social circumstances that accept or encourage smoking. For example, if going to a bar encourages smoking, then the individual should avoid bars. Finally, self-education about the health hazards of smoking provides a continual incentive to maintain a smokeless life.

Weight Maintenance In Chapter 8 we discussed the general principles of weight maintenance. Unfortunately, maintaining a healthy weight is difficult for many people. Clearly, the application of behaviour modification principles is essential in weight management. Although no single weight maintenance program works for all people, the following 8 components are common ingredients in most successful efforts:

1. The individual desires to lose weight or to prevent future weight gain.
2. The program begins with a 2-week nutritional intake diary that includes the kinds and amounts of food eaten and the environmental and social circumstances involved.
3. Short- and long-term weight loss goals are established in regard to healthy eating, physical activity, and managing eating behaviours.
4. If the goal is to lose weight, the individual signs a weight loss contract with friends.
5. If the goal is to lose weight, the new nutritional plan includes a balanced nutritional intake that results in a negative caloric balance. Further, the addition of a regular physical activity program is a key factor in any successful weight loss plan. (See Chapter 8 for details.)
6. New coping skills for overeating include limiting exposure to those environments or social settings (such as parties) that promote it.
7. If the goal is weight loss, the individual evaluates weight loss progress on a weekly basis and gets positive feedback from a support group (such as a spouse, friends, or relatives).
8. After achieving weight loss goals, the individual makes a plan for long-term maintenance of the behavioural changes made so that he or she remains at the desired weight (e.g., a balanced nutritional intake, a physically active lifestyle, and various eating management techniques).

In summary, weight maintenance is a specific application of general behaviour-modification principles. Indeed, these 8 components incorporate most of the general behaviour-modification principles outlined in Table 9.1. Remember: the key elements in a weight maintenance program are the desire to lose or to maintain weight; establishment of goals; development of a plan; and positive feedback from peer and family support.

Accident Prevention

Accidents are among the top 10 causes of death for Canadians. Although accidents come in many forms, the most common types are automobile accidents, falls, poisonings, drownings, and fires. While most accidents may seem to be a matter of chance, this is not the case! By using behaviour modification, you can reduce your risk of accidents by gaining control over many risk factors. Let's examine the most common risk factors for accidents.

Risk Factors for Accidents One of the most important accident risk factors is an unsafe attitude, which promotes risk-taking behaviours. For example, people who are overly confident in their driving skills may speed on a winding or wet road and increase their chances of having an automobile accident. Similarly, people who are overconfident in their job skills may take unnecessary risks at work.

Some people crave excitement or the sensation of danger (Hales, 1998). This type of thrill-seeking attitude increases the risk of accidents. These people often engage in high-risk physical activities such as skydiving, auto racing, or rock climbing, which increase their risk of injury due to accidents.

Stress also increases your risk of accidents (Donatelle & Davis, 2000; Hales, 1998). During periods of emotional or physical stress, people tend to be less careful. If you find yourself having a series of small mishaps or "near misses" when performing routine activities such as yardwork, housecleaning, or sports activities, this may be an indication that you should reduce your stress level by resting and using stress management techniques.

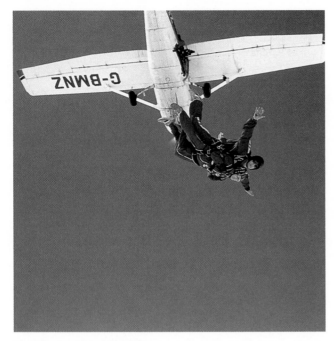

Skydiving is a high-risk activity.

As we have seen, alcohol and other drugs may increase your risk of accidents by altering your judgment and by decreasing reaction speed and motor coordination. Alcohol is involved in nearly one-half of all auto accidents and plays a major role in many boating accidents. Similarly, cocaine and marijuana use are associated with a wide range of accidents, including automobile accidents, falls, drownings, and fires.

A number of environmental factors can increase your risk of accidents. For example, storing combustible materials close to a heater and failing to have properly operating smoke detectors increase your risk of injury by fire. Other factors, such as failing to properly maintain ladders or steps around your home or workplace, may also increase your risk of accidental injury.

Reducing Your Risk of Accidents A number of steps can be taken to reduce your risk of injury. The key is to increase your awareness of the risk factors. Table 9.2 summarizes key steps that can reduce your risk of injury from vehicular accidents, falls, poisoning, drowning, and fire. Take time to study each of these recommendations and alter your lifestyle to reduce your injury risk.

Bicycle or motorcycle accidents

- Always wear a helmet and use reflectors and protective clothing when riding.
- Ride with the traffic.
- Obey the rules of the road (e.g., use turn signals) and ride defensively.

Automobile accidents

- Never drive while or after using drugs or alcohol.
- Do not drive when you are overly tired or sleepy.
- Maintain your motor vehicle in good mechanical condition.
- Obey the rules of the road and drive defensively.
- If you need assistance, stay in your car and wait for help.
- Always wear your seat belt.
- Always drive within the legal speed limit.
- Do not drive when emotionally upset.

Falls

- Use handrails when going up and down stairs.
- Do not attempt to climb ladders or stairs when ill or physically impaired due to drug use.
- Maintain ladders and steps in good working condition.
- Never run up or down stairs.
- Make sure stairways are well lit.

Poisoning

- Properly label all drugs.
- Never take more of any drug than is recommended.
- Keep all drugs out of the reach of children.
- Use only nontoxic cleaning materials.
- Increase your knowledge of poisons.
- Do not take medication in the dark.
- Discard old or expired prescriptions.
- Do not combine drugs.
- Keep the poison control centre's telephone number near your phone.

Fire

- Reduce the risk of fire in your home or workplace by storing combustible materials in a safe place.
- Maintain smoke detectors, fire extinguishers, and sprinkler systems in proper working condition.
- Know how to use a fire extinguisher properly.
- Practise safe evacuation procedures from your home and workplace.

Drowning

- Learn to swim and learn proper water safety procedures.
- Do not swim alone or in the dark.
- Dive only in designated areas.
- Do not swim immediately after eating or when tired.
- Do not swim when using drugs of any kind.
- Avoid swimming in dangerous waters, such as rivers or oceans with strong currents.
- Learn cardiopulmonary resuscitation.

TABLE 9.2 Reducing Your Risk of Injury

Summary

1. The five key behaviours that promote a healthy lifestyle are health-related physical activity, good nutrition, weight maintenance, stress management, and modification of unhealthy behaviours.
2. *Stress* is defined as a physiological and psychological response to things in our environment that make us feel uncomfortable. Any factor that produces stress is called a *stressor*.
3. Psychosocial stressors can result from a broad range of events, from dealing with life's daily aggravations and setting hard-to-reach goals to coping with environmental disasters and world discord.
4. *Eustress* is a positive form (or good form) of stress that can result in personal growth and satisfaction. *Distress* is a negative form of stress that can cause negative physical and emotional outcomes.
5. Two steps in stress management are to reduce stress in your life and to learn to cope with stress by improving your ability to relax.
6. Common relaxation techniques to reduce stress include progressive relaxation, visualization, meditation, breathing exercises, rest and sleep, and physical activity.
7. Behaviour modification is the process of changing an undesirable behaviour to a more desirable behaviour. The general model of behaviour modification can be applied to achieve any desired health-related behaviour.
8. The five most common types of accidents are automobile accidents, falls, poisonings, drownings, and fires.
9. Risk factors for accidents include unsafe attitudes, stress, drug use, and an unsafe environment.

Study Questions

1. Define *stress*. What is a *stressor*?
2. What is *eustress*? What is *distress*?
3. Why is stress management important to health?
4. List the steps in stress management. Identify some common stress management (relaxation) techniques.
5. Give examples of psychosocial stressors.
6. How can the environment affect the body?
7. How can self-esteem and self-efficacy affect health?
8. Define *behaviour modification*. What are the steps involved in behaviour modification?
9. Outline a plan to use behaviour modification to eliminate a specific unhealthy behaviour.
10. Explain how physical activity is useful in reducing stress.
11. List the key guidelines for the development of a time-management program.
12. List the steps to reduce your risks of injury due to automobile accidents, falls, poisonings, drownings, and fires.

Suggested Reading

Benson, H. (2000). *The relaxation response.* New York: Avon, Wholecare.

Cowley, G. (1999, June 14). Stress-busters: What works. *Newsweek, 60–62.*

Donatelle, R., & Davis, L. (2000). *Access to health.* Needham Heights, MA: Allyn & Bacon.

Greenberg, J. (1999). *Comprehensive stress management* (6th ed.). Dubuque, IA: Brown and Benchmark.

Weblinks

MEDline
www.ncbi.nim.nih.gov
National Library of Medicine's search service providing access more than 10 million citations.

Canadian Medical Association
www.cma.ca
Includes many sources of information about a wide variety of medical problems, including stress-related disorders.

WebMD
www.webmd.com
A leading source for medical news and information.

References

Anderson, B. L., et al. (1998). Stress and immune responses after surgical treatment for regional breast cancer. *Journal of the National Cancer Institute, 90,* 30–36.

Berger, B., & Owen, D. (1988). Stress reduction and mood enhancement in four exercise modes: Swimming, body conditioning, hatha yoga, and fencing. *Research Quarterly for Exercise and Sport, 59,* 148–159.

Brooks, M. V. (2003, July–September). Health-related hardiness and chronic illness: A synthesis of current research. *Nurses Forum, 38(3),* 11–20.

Clarkson, P. (1991). Vitamins and trace minerals. In D. Lamb and M. Williams (Eds.), *Ergonomics* (pp. 123–175). Madison, WI: Brown and Benchmark.

Donatelle, R., & Davis, L. (2000). *Access to health.* Needham Heights, MA: Allyn & Bacon.

Farrell, P. (1987). Enkephalins, catecholamines, and psychological mood alterations: Effects of prolonged exercise. *Medicine and Science in Sports and Exercise, 19,* 347–353.

Hales, D. (1998). *An invitation to health* (8th ed.). San Francisco: Benjamin Cummings.

Health Canada. (2004, Sept. 12). Research increase in deaths in Canada due to smoking. Retrieved from www.hc-sc.gc.ca, September 2004.

Holroyd, K. A., et al. (2001). Management of chronic tension-type headache with tricyclic antidepressant medication, stress management therapy, and their combination: A randomized trial. *Journal of the American Medical Association, 285(17),* 2208–2215.

Howley, E., & Franks, B. D. (1997). *Health fitness instructor's handbook* (3rd ed.). Champaign, IL: Human Kinetics.

Lazarus, R. (1985). The trivialization of distress: Preventing health risks behaviors and promoting coping with illness. In Rosen, J. C., & Solomon, L. J. (Eds.), *Prevention in Health Psychology* (pp. 279–298). Hanover, NH: University Press of New England.

Perna, F. M., Schneiderman, N., & LaPerriere, A. (1997, March). Psychological stress, exercise and immunity. *International Journal of Sports Medicine, 18(Supp. 1),* S78–S83.

Raglin, J., & Morgan, W. (1987). Influence of exercise and quiet rest on state anxiety and blood pressure. *Medicine and Science in Sports and Exercise, 19,* 456–463.

Selye, H. (1978). *The stress of life* (rev. ed.). New York: McGraw-Hill.

Serido, J., Almeida, D. M., & Wethington, E. (2004, March). Chronic stressors and daily hassles: Unique and interactive relationships with psychological distress. *Journal of Health and Social Behaviour, 45(1),* 17–33.

Sewitch, M., et al. (2001). Psychological distress, social support, and disease activity in patients with inflammatory bowel disease. *American Journal of Gastroenterology, 96(5),* 1470–1479.

Williams, M. (1996). *Lifetime fitness and wellness.* Dubuque, IA: Wm. C. Brown.

Stress Index Questionnaire

Name_____ Age _____ Sex _____ Date _____

DIRECTIONS

The purpose of this stress index questionnaire is to increase your awareness of stress in your life. Circle either Yes or No to answer each of the following questions.

Yes	No	1. I have frequent arguments.
Yes	No	2. I often get upset at work.
Yes	No	3. I often have neck and/or shoulder pains due to anxiety/stress.
Yes	No	4. I often get upset when I stand in long lines.
Yes	No	5. I often get angry when I listen to the local, national, or world news or read the newspaper.
Yes	No	6. I do not have a sufficient amount of money for my needs.
Yes	No	7. I often get upset when driving.
Yes	No	8. At the end of a workday I often feel stress-related fatigue.
Yes	No	9. I have at least one constant source of stress/anxiety in my life (e.g., conflict with boss, neighbour, mother-in-law).
Yes	No	10. I often have stress-related headaches.
Yes	No	11. I do not practise stress management techniques.
Yes	No	12. I rarely take time for myself.
Yes	No	13. I have difficulty keeping my feelings of anger and hostility under control.
Yes	No	14. I have difficulty managing time wisely.
Yes	No	15. I often have difficulty sleeping.
Yes	No	16. I am generally in a hurry.
Yes	No	17. I usually feel that there is not enough time in the day to accomplish what I need to do.
Yes	No	18. I often feel that I am being mistreated by friends or associates.
Yes	No	19. I do not regularly perform physical activity.
Yes	No	20. I rarely get 7 to 9 hours of sleep per night.

SCORING AND INTERPRETATION

Answering Yes to any of the questions means that you need to use some form of stress management techniques (see the text for details). Total your Yes answers and use the following scale to evaluate the level of stress in your life.

Number of Yes Answers	Stress Category
6–20	High stress
3–5	Average stress
0–2	Low stress

LABORATORY 9.2

Behaviour Modification Contract

Name_____ Age _____ Sex _____ Date _____

DIRECTIONS

Complete the following behaviour modification contract, using friends or peers as witnesses. See the reverse of this sheet for an example of a completed contract.

BEHAVIOUR MODIFICATION CONTRACT

1. I _____ (name) agree to make the following behavioural change(s):

_____

_____

_____

_____

beginning on _____ (date).

2. My short-term goal(s) are to

_____

_____

by _____ (date).

3. My long-term goal(s) are to

_____

_____

_____

_____

4. I will assess my progress on the desired behavioural change on a regular basis:
_____ (note how often).

Further, I will report my progress to at least two friends and/or peers on a regular basis.

Signed: _____   Date: _____

Witness: _____   Witness: _____

BEHAVIOUR MODIFICATION CONTRACT

1. I _____John Doe_____ agree to make the following behavioural change(s):

Stop smoking _____

_____

_____

_____

beginning on ___May 20, 2007___ (date).

2. My short-term goal(s) are to

Stop smoking _____

_____

by ___by 5/20/2007___ (date).

3. My long-term goal(s) are to

Remain smoke free during the rest of my life _____

_____

4. I will assess my progress on the desired behavioural change on a regular basis:

weekly _____ (note how often).

Further, I will report my progress to at least two friends and/or peers on a regular basis.

Signed: ___John Doe_____   Date: ___April 1, 2007_____

Witness: ___Roberto Jimenez_____   Witness: ___William Jones_____

CHAPTER 10

Sexual Health and Drug Use

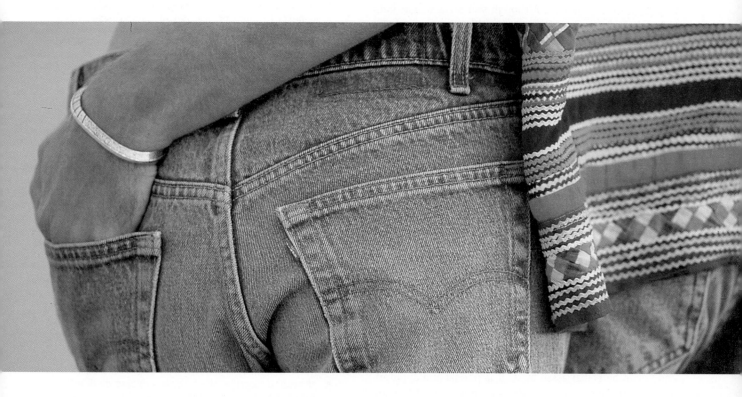

After studying this chapter, you should be able to

1. Describe a sexually healthy adult.

2. List the most common sexually transmitted infections in Canada.

3. Outline the incidence of sexually transmitted infections in Canada.

4. Identify the guidelines to reduce the risk of sexually transmitted infections.

5. Differentiate between the terms *use, misuse,* and *abuse* with specific reference to alcohol, marijuana, and cocaine.

6. Outline the acute physiological effects of alcohol, marijuana, and cocaine use.

7. Describe the long-term health consequences of alcohol, marijuana, and cocaine use.

8. List several guidelines that can be used to maintain control when consuming alcohol and to avoid drug abuse.

Throughout this book we have discussed factors that influence your health and well-being. Two important factors that influence health and wellness are sexuality and drug use. This chapter discusses these health issues, with an emphasis on preventing sexually transmitted infections and drug abuse.

Sexual Health

An often overlooked (or ignored) component of health and wellness is sexual health. Although you are a sexual individual from birth, sexuality is something you must learn (anatomy, desires, pleasures, etc.). Discovering your sexuality should be a lifelong process, whether you are 40, 60, or 80 years old, or you recently had a baby, or you have lost a breast or testicle to cancer.

You learn about sexuality from a variety of sources, including

- yourself (as you grow and adapt to the societal and cultural expectations placed upon you)
- your family, in particular your parents ("birds and bees" talk, what is considered acceptable and appropriate behaviours)
- your friends (tall tales and real-life experiences; what they have seen or read)
- the media (TV, video, print, internet, etc.)
- music (sexual references and innuendos in song lyrics)
- your religion (rules, expectations, moral development)
- school, college, university (actual teachings and societal expectations)

The key is to keep an open mind about your sexuality and not to be embarrassed by it. It is normal and appropriate to be curious about your sexuality and to want to learn more. A recent national survey found that Canadian students' sexual knowledge was less in 2002 than what it was in 1989 (Garmaise, 2003). Despite this reduced knowledge, evidence from a series of surveys conducted in British Columbia in 1980, 1990, and 2000 noted safer sexual practices in 2000, including more questioning of potential partners about their past, condom use, and maintenance of long-term monogamous relationships (Netting & Burnett, 2004). Often there is a misguided impression that "everyone is doing it." This is not the case, with 30 percent of the respondents in the survey from the year 2000 reporting a celibate lifestyle.

Being open to learning more about your sexuality is one characteristic of a sexually healthy adult. Other characteristics are listed in Table 10.1.

- appreciates own body
- interacts with both sexes (family, friends, others) in appropriate and respectful ways
- expresses love and intimacy appropriately
- avoids exploitive relationships
- takes responsibility for sexual behaviours (and understands the consequences)
- seeks information when needed from appropriate sources
- enjoys sexual feelings without necessarily acting on them
- decides what is personally "right" and acts on those values
- communicates the desire or lack of desire to engage in sexual activity
- accepts refusals from partner to engage in sexual activity
- is able to communicate about limits, contraceptive and STI protection, and the meaning of sex in the relationship prior to engaging in sexual activity
- demonstrates tolerance and acceptance of people with different sexual values regarding their sexuality
- understands the impact of the media on thoughts, feelings, values, and behaviours related to sexuality
- if sexually active, uses contraceptive devices to prevent unwanted pregnancy and condoms to prevent the spread of STIs

TABLE 10.1 Characteristics of a Sexually Healthy Adult

Source: Adapted from Debra W. Haffner. (Dec. 1992–Jan. 1993). Toward a new paradigm on sexual health. *SIECUS Report*, 21(2), 29. With permission of SIECUS (www.siecus.org).

Sexually Transmitted Infections

Every year many people in Canada are infected by one or more **sexually transmitted infections (STIs)**. The term STI replaces STD (sexually transmitted disease) since it is a term encompassing more infections that may be asymptomatic (Health Canada, 2004b). After years of lower rates of infection, the number of bacterial STIs has been increasing in Canada since 1997 (Wong & Sutherland, 2002). STIs are generally spread through vaginal, anal, or oral sexual contact. More than 20 different STIs have been identified. Current

sexually transmitted infections (STIs)   A group of more than 20 diseases generally spread through sexual contact.

estimates are that one in four people in Canada will contract at least one STI in their lifetime. The most common STIs include AIDS, chlamydia, gonorrhoea, venereal warts, genital herpes, and syphilis (Daniels, Hillman, Barton, & Goldmeir, 1993).

AIDS

AIDS is a fatal disease that develops from infection by the human immunodeficiency virus (HIV), which was discovered in the mid-1980s. A virus is a tiny infectious agent that cannot live independently and must invade a host cell to survive. The explanation for the choice of AIDS as a name for this disorder is as follows (Strong, DeVault, Sayad, & Yarber, 2005):

A—The disease is not inherited but must be *acquired*

I—*Immuno,* because the virus affects the immune system (your immune system is responsible for protection against infectious diseases and cancer)

D—*Deficiency,* because the body's immune system is deficient

S—*Syndrome,* because the symptoms of AIDS occur together

When HIV enters the bloodstream, immune cells rush to the virus in an attempt to destroy this invading agent. However, upon entry into the bloodstream, HIV enters circulating immune cells and uses these cells as a host to replicate itself. Importantly, the entry of HIV into immune cells eventually disarms those cells and impairs the body's ability to fight infections. Over time, the level of HIV in the blood increases and the immune system gradually becomes weaker and weaker, resulting in immunodeficiency and the development of AIDS. Later in this chapter, we will discuss the difference between HIV and full-blown AIDS.

Current estimates are that more than 57 000 people in Canada have tested positive for HIV, with an estimated 2500 new cases identified each year (Public Health Agency of Canada, 2004). The Fitness and Wellness for All box provides a quick look at the race and sex distributions of positive HIV test reports in Canada for 2004.

AIDS/HIV is a major health problem around the world, with more than 57 million individuals infected (Health Canada, 2004a). Of these 57 million people, 21 million have

AIDS Acquired Immune Deficiency Syndrome: a fatal disease that develops from infection by the human immunodeficiency virus (HIV).

FITNESS AND WELLNESS FOR ALL

Who's Testing Positive for HIV in Canada?

In 2004, 2529 Canadians tested positive for HIV (Public Health Agency of Canada, 2004). Since 1985 (when reporting of positive HIV test was initiated), there have been 57 674 positive HIV tests in Canada. It should be noted that not all individuals infected with HIV are tested for the virus and that these numbers reflect the number of Canadians with positive test results (the actual number of individuals living with HIV is higher). The pie charts in this box have been created using data from the Public Health Agency of Canada (2004). They indicate that certain groups of Canadians who test positive for HIV are disproportionate compared to their proportion of the Canadian population.

Sex Even though men make up about half of the population, almost 75 percent of new positive HIV tests each year occur in men. Note, however, that a disproportionate rise in the number of women testing positive for HIV occurred since 1995, where less than 10 percent of the positive results were found in women.

Race The proportion of new positive cases for 2004 in white Canadians has decreased from 84.6 percent in 1979–1998 to 60.6 percent. At the same time, the proportion of positive reports has increased among Black

Canadians from 8.6 percent to 15.5 percent and in Aboriginal Canadians from 2.8 percent to 14.8 percent. However, it should be pointed out that ethnic status is only available on approximately one-third of all positive test reports.

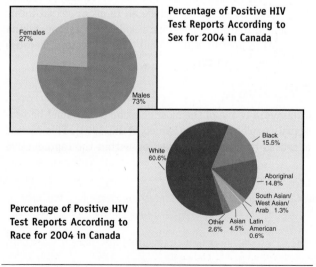

Percentage of Positive HIV Test Reports According to Sex for 2004 in Canada

Percentage of Positive HIV Test Reports According to Race for 2004 in Canada

Source: Public Health Agency (2004). *HIV and AIDS in Canada. Surveillance Report to Surveillance and Risk Assessment December 2004.* Division, Centre for Infections Prevention Control, Public Health Agency of Canada.

died. There are approximately 15 000 new infections world-wide on a daily basis. According to Health Canada (2004a), the virus is

- outstripping the efforts to contain it
- reversing hard-won development gains
- increasing mortality among children under 5
- reducing life expectancy
- burdening health systems
- exacerbating poverty and inequality
- afflicting education systems
- striking business and economies
- eroding human rights
- diminishing political stability and national security

Clearly, AIDS/HIV is a global problem.

Many people infected with HIV are unaware they carry the virus because symptoms may not appear for months or even years after infection. Evidence now suggests that in many cases the virus may remain dormant in the body for 5 to 10 years before creating health problems (Daniels et al., 1993; Watanabe, 2001). After this incubation period, the virus begins to multiply and eventually damages certain cells of the immune system. Because an impaired immune system is incapable of preventing infections and cancer, the body becomes vulnerable to a variety of diseases. When disease symptoms appear through HIV infection, the individual has developed AIDS.

Early symptoms of AIDS include constant fatigue, fever, weight loss, swollen lymph nodes, and sore throat. Symptoms that develop later include night sweats, chronic infections, skin disorders, and ulcers of the membranes lining the nose, mouth, and other body cavities.

HIV can be transmitted by any exchange of body fluids (such as blood, semen, and vaginal secretions). Common methods of transmission include all forms of sexual inter-course and sharing hypodermic needles. At present, taking measures to prevent AIDS is your only protection, because there is no known cure.

Chlamydia

Chlamydia is one of the most common STIs among hetero-sexual people worldwide (Daniels et al., 1993). This disease is caused by a bacterial infection within the reproductive organs and is spread through vaginal, anal, and oral sex. Health Canada in 2003 reported almost 57 000 new cases of chlamydia (2004b).

Symptoms of chlamydia vary among individuals. More than 70 percent of women infected do not develop symptoms and are unaware they carry the bacteria. Symptoms in women include a yellowish vaginal discharge and occasional bleeding between menstrual periods. In men, early symptoms include painful urination and a watery discharge from the penis.

Fortunately, chlamydia can be cured by administration of antibiotics. If untreated, however, chlamydia can result in infertility in men and women. Further, untreated chlamydia in women can lead to pelvic inflammatory disease, an infec-tion of the lining of the abdominal and pelvic cavity. Common symptoms of pelvic inflammatory disease include pain in the lower abdominal cavity, fever, and menstrual irregularities. If you suspect that you have been infected by chlamydia or any other STI, seek STI testing immediately at your local health clinic.

Gonorrhoea

Gonorrhoea is another common STI, with approximately 7400 new cases reported in Canada in 2003 (Health Canada, 2004b). The infection can be transmitted through vaginal, anal, and oral contact. Similar to chlamydia, gonorrhoea is caused by a bacterial infection and is curable with antibiotic treatment. Untreated gonorrhoea may spread to the prostate, testicles, kidney, and bladder and can result in sterility in men and women (Daniels et al., 1993; Robbins & Angell, 1997).

More than 80 percent of men develop symptoms within 2 to 10 days after sexual contact with an infected person. Typical symptoms include a milky discharge from the penis and painful urination (Robbins & Angell, 1997). In contrast, only 20 percent of women infected with gonorrhoea develop symptoms. When symptoms are present, they include painful urination and an occasional fever (Robbins & Angell, 1997). The lack of symptoms in women poses a serious problem because they are unaware that they have been infected and may unknowingly spread the disease.

It should be noted that after reaching an all-time low in 1997, the rate of infection for gonorrhoea has risen (Hansen, Wong, & Perrin, 2003). In fact, there was a 45-percent increase in the rate of gonorrhoea from 1997 to 2001, with the most dramatic increase (68 percent) found among men aged 30 to 39.

Venereal Warts

Venereal warts (also known as *genital warts*) are caused by a small group of viruses called *human papilloma viruses* (Daniels et al., 1993; Robbins & Angell, 1997). Infection generally occurs through sexual contact with an infected individual; after exposure, the virus penetrates the skin or mucous membranes of the genitals or anus, and warts appear within 6 to 8 weeks (Daniels et al., 1993; Robbins & Angell, 1997).

chlamydia A sexually transmitted infection caused by a bacterial infection within the reproductive organs and spread through vaginal, anal, and oral sex.

gonorrhoea A common sexually transmitted infection, transmitted through vaginal, anal, and oral contact.

venereal warts Warts caused by a small group of viruses called *human papilloma viruses;* spread through sexual contact.

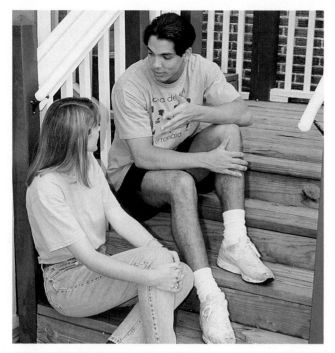
Maintaining a monogamous relationship is a good strategy for reducing your risk of sexually transmitted infections.

Warts may develop as a series of small itchy bumps on the skin and range in size from that of a pinhead to that of a pencil eraser on portions of the external genitals that are dry (such as the penis). Men can detect these warts by routinely examining their genitals for suspicious growths. If, however, the warts are inside the reproductive tract, symptoms may be absent. In women, these warts are often first detected by a physician during a routine Pap smear. Similarly, venereal warts on the rectum must be diagnosed by a physician.

Treatment for venereal warts may take several forms. Warts can be painted with several different types of medication, which dries up the warts within a few days. Also, the warts can be removed by cryosurgery (freezing them), laser surgery, or excision surgery.

Do venereal warts present a serious health threat? Not always. Many venereal warts will disappear on their own without treatment. The greatest risk is that, left untreated in women, venereal warts increase the risk of uterine and cervical cancer. Exactly how venereal warts result in cancer is unclear. What is known is that within 5 years after infection, about 30 percent of all untreated warts result in a precancerous growth. If this precancerous growth remains untreated, 70 percent will lead to cancer (Daniels et al., 1993; Robbins & Angell, 1997).

Genital Herpes

Genital herpes is a general term for a family of diseases caused by viral infections. The same family of viruses also cause what are commonly called "cold sores" around the mouth (Health Canada, 2003a). Genital herpes is highly con-

tagious and is most commonly transmitted by direct contact with open sores during any form of sexual activity (such as hand-to-genital contact, oral, anal, or vaginal sex). Symptoms of herpes vary from sores (blisters) on the mouth, rectum, and genitals to fever and swollen glands. Interestingly, symptoms may disappear and reappear without warning.

At present, there is no cure for herpes, but newly developed drugs show promise. Although treatment with cold-sore medication reduces the pain and irritation of the sore, remember that rubbing anything on the herpes blister increases the chance of spreading herpes-laden fluids to other body parts or to other people. Keep the infected area clean and dry. Always wash your towels after each use. Loose fitting clothing made of natural materials, such as cotton, may ease your discomfort (Health Canada, 2003a).

Syphilis

Syphilis is a well-known STI that can be transmitted through direct sexual contact. In 2003, more than 800 new cases of syphilis were reported in Canada (Health Canada, 2004b). The rate of infection is increasing in males and females (Health Canada, 2002). Like chlamydia and gonorrhoea, syphilis is caused by a bacterial infection and can be cured by antibiotics (Health Canada, 2004b).

The symptoms of untreated syphilis vary because the disease generally progresses through several distinct stages. Early symptoms of syphilis generally include a painless sore (called a *chancre*) located at the initial site of infection (such as on the penis, vaginal walls, or mouth). The size of the chancre may vary, but it is often about the size of a dime. In men and women, this chancre will completely disappear in 3 to 6 weeks.

One month to one year after the disappearance of the chancre, secondary symptoms appear. These include a skin rash or white patches on the mucous membranes of the mouth, throat, or genitals. Hair loss may occur, lymph glands may become swollen, and infectious sores may develop around the mouth or genitals. After the appearance of these secondary symptoms, the disease may once again "go into hiding," and all symptoms may disappear.

Although an individual may be without symptoms for several years, the syphilis infection slowly spreads to organs throughout the body. Late stages of untreated syphilis may result in heart damage, blindness, deafness, paralysis, and mental disorders.

genital herpes   A general term for a family of diseases caused by viral infections; highly contagious and transmitted through hand-to-genital contact, oral, anal, or vaginal sex.

syphilis   A sexually transmitted infection transmitted through direct sexual contact; caused by a bacterial infection and cured by antibiotics.

Reducing Your Risk for Sexually Transmitted Infections

There is no cure for AIDS or genital herpes, and although treatment methods exist for many other STIs, prevention is clearly the best approach. Laboratory 10.1 will help you to evaluate your risk of STIs. The keys to preventing STIs are education and responsible action. Although most individuals agree education about sexuality is important, the timing of when it should occur is a contentious issue. Regardless of the timing, a key point to include is how to make responsible decisions based upon personal values and beliefs. It is also critical to consider ethnic differences in terminology, awareness of STIs, non-exclusive sexual relationships, and experiences with the sexual health services available (Connell, McKevitt, & Low, 2004). Further, peer education programs have been shown to be effective in delaying first sexual intercourse and promoting increased condom use in adolescent men and women (Caron, Godin, Otis, & Lambert, 2004).

---

drug use Consuming a drug in the way it was intended to be used.

drug misuse Taking a drug for a purpose other than for which it was intended.

drug abuse Excessive use of a drug leading to negative personal, family, social, or professional consequences.

Complete abstinence from sexual activity is the only certain way to prevent STIs; however, if you do engage in sexual activity, following the guidelines presented in A Closer Look below will greatly reduce your risk of developing one of these diseases. See A Closer Look on page 253 for answers to additional questions about STIs.

Drug Use, Misuse, and Abuse

Any substance that causes a chemical reaction in the body is called a drug. **Drug use** refers to consuming a drug in the way it was intended to be used. An example of drug use is taking a pain reliever to provide relief from a headache. **Drug misuse** refers to taking a drug for a purpose other than that for which it was intended. Drug misuse includes using someone else's prescription, not completing a prescription, not following the directions when taking your medication, as well as using a drug for a different purpose. An example of drug misuse is taking someone else's prescription when you think you have the same infection. **Drug abuse** refers to the excessive use of a drug. Excessive use is difficult to quantify since it differs for each person. Consider excessive use to be the amount at which negative personal, family, social, or professional consequences occur.

Since drugs cause a chemical reaction in the body, there is the potential for addiction to or a physiological or psychological dependence on the drug. Even without addiction, the use of alcohol or recreational drugs increases your risk of

---

A CLOSER LOOK

Reducing Your Risk for Sexually Transmitted Infections

Sexually transmitted infections (STIs) are most often spread through sexual contact, which includes sexual intercourse (vaginal–penile contact), oral–genital contact, hand-to-genital contact, and anal intercourse. Remember, no one is immune to STIs. Adhering to the following will reduce your risk of contracting STIs (Donatelle & Davis, 2006; Hales, 1998):

- Understand that abstinence is the only absolute way of preventing STIs. Short of abstinence, maintaining a monogamous relationship with an uninfected partner is the best way of avoiding STIs.
- Always practise safe sex (including vaginal, anal, and oral sex), which means properly using a good-quality latex condom each and every time you engage in any sexual activity.
- Avoid casual sexual contact. If you have more than one sexual partner, do not be afraid to ask intimate questions about each partner's sexual history. Avoid sexual encounters with anyone who is at high risk for STIs (such as intravenous drug users and prostitutes).
- Never share with others hypodermic needles or syringes, or any other devices through which exchange of blood can occur. HIV can also be spread by sharing razors, ear-piercing instruments, and tattoo instruments.
- Limit drug and alcohol use, because they may dull your senses and reduce your ability to make sound decisions concerning sexual activity.
- Whenever possible, wash your hands and genitals before and after sexual encounters, and urinate after sexual intercourse.

Collectively, these practices can reduce your risk of developing an STI. If you become concerned about the possibility that you have contracted an STI, immediately stop all sexual activity. Make an appointment with the most appropriate health practitioner at once, because STIs can be detected only by blood tests or examinations of genital fluids.

accidents and may damage your health either in the short or long term. Over the past 10 years, several new substances have arrived on the drug scene, and some drugs that have been popular for years are still in vogue (A Closer Look, p. 254). Nonetheless, the most commonly used and abused drugs in Canada continue to be alcohol, marijuana, and cocaine.

Alcohol

Alcohol is the most widely used recreational drug in Canada, and the most popular drug on college and university campuses. Alcohol use has declined in Canada from the mid-1970s to the mid-1990s (Ramstedt, 2004), with more than 70 percent of Canadians aged 15 or older reporting alcohol consumption in the past year (Drug & Alcohol Information Line, 2004). Consumption is highest in young adults (particularly college and university students), males, and those with higher incomes. Approximately one-third of university students report consuming more than 15 drinks per week, a level considered "at greater risk of health problems." Furthermore, 18 percent of students reported missing classes because of a hangover. It should also be noted that consumption of alcohol since 1996 has begun to increase once again (Ramstedt, 2004).

Although many people drink to "get high," in reality alcohol is a central nervous system depressant that slows the functioning of the brain, resulting in impaired vision, reduced reaction time, and impaired motor coordination.

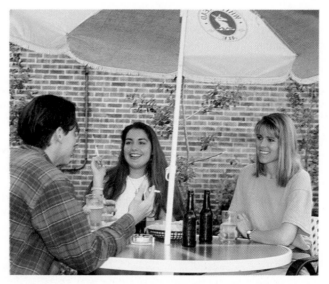

Social drinking is popular among college and university students.

Overconsumption of alcohol further impairs your judgment. As a central nervous system depressant, alcohol decreases your inhibitions. One inhibition may be a fear of danger. By decreasing the fear of danger, it can encourage risk-taking behaviours (such as driving too fast), which increases the likelihood of accidents. Drinking too much can also increase your risk of using poor judgment in social situations and in making decisions concerning sexual behaviour.

Sexual Health and Drug Use **253**

What's Fashionable on the Drug Scene Today?

Among the numerous new prescription and nonprescription drugs that have become popular for recreational use among Canadians during the past several years is the prescription painkiller OxyContin. The illegal use of this habit-forming drug, which was developed to ease the suffering of patients with painful diseases such as cancer, has grown markedly across Canada in recent years. Its addictive qualities have led to abuse among some recreational users; many have overdosed on the powerful painkiller, and others have turned to crime to feed their habits.

Another group of drugs that have widespread popularity—the so-called club drugs—includes some new drugs and some drugs that have been in recreational use for decades. Among the most common club drugs, used by young adults at all-night dance parties such as "raves" or "trances," are Ecstasy, GHB, ketamine, Rohypnol, methamphetamine, and LSD. The use of these drugs can cause serious health problems (see the table below), and in some cases their use can be fatal (Liska, 2000). Moreover, when taken in combination with alcohol, the dangers associated with using club drugs are multiplied.

Drug (chemical name)	Slang or street names	Route of administration	Acute effects on body	Long- or short-term health effects
Methylene-dioxymethamphetamine (MDMA)	Ecstasy, XTC, X, Adam, Clarity, Lover's Speed	Orally; tablet or capsule	Acts as a stimulant; increases heart rate and blood pressure	Because it is neurotoxic, use results in permanent damage to neurons (nerve cells).
Gammahydroxybutyrate (GHB)	Grievous Bodily Harm, G, Liquid ecstasy, Georgia Home Body	Orally; can be in liquid, white powder, tablet, or capsule forms	Acts as an intoxicating sedative (central nervous system depressant); increases release of growth hormone, so is sometimes used by body builders to build muscle	Overdose can occur quickly; symptoms include nausea, vomiting, and loss of consciousness; large overdoses can be fatal.
Ketamine	Special K, K, Vitamin K, Cat valliums	Orally or smoked with marijuana or tobacco; produced in liquid form or as white powder	Acts as an anaesthetic that produces dreamlike states and hallucinations	High doses can cause amnesia, impaired motor function, depression, and fatal respiratory problems.
Rohypnol	Roofies, Rophies, Roche, Forget-me Pill Date Rape Drug	Orally; produced in tablet form that easily dissolves in water	Acts as a sedative; produces drowsiness	Acute adverse effects include decreased blood pressure, confusion, and loss of memory.
Methamphetamine	Speed, Ice, Chalk, Meth, Crystal, Crank, Fire, Glass	Orally; produced as a white powder	Can produce excited speech, increased physical activity levels, and agitation	Chronic use can lead to memory loss, aggression, psychotic behaviour, and cardiac and nervous system damage.
Lysergic Acid Diethylamide (LSD)	Acid, Boomers, Yellow Sunshine	Orally; produced in tablet, capsule, or liquid form	Acute effects include dilated pupils, increased heart rate and body temperature, sweating, dry mouth, and loss of appetite	Long-term use can result in psychotic behaviour and hallucinations.

Alcohol Abuse and Undernutrition

Undernutrition is commonly associated with chronic alcohol abuse because the presence of alcohol repeatedly irritates the gastrointestinal system. Over time, the continued irritation of the gastric lining resulting from the consumption of alcohol often reduces appetite, and the ensuing lowered food intake forces the body to function on a diet deficient in calories and essential nutrients. The resulting undernutrition can, in extreme cases, promote a loss of muscle mass and abnormal functioning of many body organs.

The best approach to dealing with this problem is to seek professional help for alcoholism. In many cases the cessation of alcohol use eliminates the alcohol-induced reduction in appetite, and the individual's return to normal eating habits provides the calories and nutrients needed for improved health. In severe cases of alcohol-related undernutrition, the advice of a physician or a dietitian is required.

In fact, approximately 10 percent of students reported drinking and driving, and 25 percent reported being physically assaulted by a person who had been drinking (Drug & Alcohol Information Line, 2004).

Chronic abuse of alcohol over a period of years can result in liver disease (cirrhosis), damage to the nervous system, and an increased risk of certain cancers (Robbins & Angell, 1997). Development of liver disease due to years of drinking may eventually result in total liver failure and death. The damage to the nervous system that results from alcohol abuse is localized to the left side of the brain, which is responsible for written and spoken language, logic, and mathematical skills. The degree of brain damage that occurs appears to be directly related to the amount of alcohol consumed. Further, repeated irritation of the gastrointestinal system by alcohol has been linked to cancers of the esophagus, stomach, mouth, tongue, and liver. Another—and often overlooked—problem linked to chronic consumption of alcohol is undernutrition (see above, Nutritional Links to Health and Fitness).

Addiction to alcohol is usually a slowly developing condition that can happen to anyone. Research into the causes of alcoholism has revealed that addiction to alcohol may have hereditary, psychological, and environmental components. Unfortunately, the details of how and why alcoholism begins are still somewhat a mystery.

You can assess your drinking habits by answering the questions in Laboratory 10.2. If you feel that you might be drinking too much, seek professional help from Alcoholics Anonymous. The following guidelines may assist you in maintaining control over your drinking habits (Donatelle & Davis, 2006; Hales, 1998):

- Set limits and stick to them. If you are at a party and feel that you are drinking too much, learn to say no and switch to a nonalcoholic beverage.
- When drinking, stick to the rule of 1 drink per hour (1 drink = 1 beer, 1 glass of wine, or 1.5 oz of hard liquor). This will reduce the likelihood that you will become physically or mentally impaired by alcohol.
- Wine, beer, and mixed drinks are less intoxicating than straight liquor. Stick to more dilute drinks instead of the higher-alcohol beverages.
- Eating and drinking at the same time will slow the rate of alcohol absorption and reduce your chance of becoming impaired. Never drink on an empty stomach.
- When leaving a party or bar after drinking, don't drive; call a cab or have someone who hasn't been drinking drive you home.

Marijuana

Use of marijuana became popular in Canada in the 1960s, and it remains one of the most popular illegal drugs among college and university students (Liska, 2000). The percentage of Canadians aged 15 or older who admit to using marijuana nearly doubled from 1989 to 2002 (Statistics Canada, 2002). Specifically, 6.5 percent of Canadians indicated marijuana use in 1989, and 12.2 percent in 2002. Almost half of marijuana

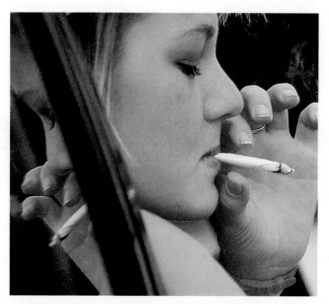

Smoking marijuana may increase your risk of accidents and health damage.

users do so less than once a month, with 10 percent reporting weekly use and another 10 percent reporting daily use. Men are more likely to use marijuana than women, and younger individuals (15 to 24 years) are more likely to use than older persons (>25 years). **Marijuana** is a plant mixture (stems, leaves, or seeds) from either the *Cannabis sativa* or *Cannabis indica* (hemp) plants that is either ingested or smoked. The active chemical in marijuana that produces physical effects is tetrahydrocannabinol (THC); the higher the THC concentration in the marijuana, the greater the effect. The THC concentration in the marijuana currently available is 2 to 4 times greater than what was available in the 1960s, ranging between 0.5 and 3.0 percent.

Marijuana can be used in many forms. It can be brewed and drunk as a tea, or it can be baked into cookies or brownies. However, marijuana is most often smoked in pipes or by rolling the marijuana into cigarettes. Effects are generally felt within 15 to 30 minutes and disappear within 2 to 3 hours.

Since marijuana depresses the central nervous system, it induces a sense of relaxation in its users. However, the immediate effects are increased heart rate and blood pressure, bloodshot eyes, and dry mouth and throat. Use of marijuana impairs motor coordination and may increase your risk of accidents. Further, acute use of marijuana alters the normal function of memory centres in the brain. This memory loss resembles that observed in normal aging. However, whether these changes in function put long-term marijuana users at risk for early mental disorders is not clear.

Long-term use of marijuana presents several dangers. First, consistent users of marijuana may become psychologically dependent on its use. Further, regular smoking of marijuana causes lung damage similar to that caused by smoking tobacco (Liska, 2000). The effect of long-term marijuana use on the heart is not well known; however, many investi-

gators believe that marijuana increases the workload on the heart, which may eventually result in damage.

Cocaine

The use of **cocaine** (coke) or crack in Canada has increased since 1994, with current estimates of more than 300 000 Canadians (Statistics Canada, 2002) having used the drug in the past year.

Cocaine is a powerful stimulant derived from the leaves of the South American coca shrub, which grows primarily in the Andes Mountains. Cocaine, which is extracted from the coca leaves using a multi-step process, produces a white powder (similar to sugar in appearance). Varying the extraction process can produce several different forms of cocaine, such as crack cocaine, rock cocaine, or freebase cocaine.

Cocaine can be used in several ways. Common uses include snorting (sniffing cocaine into the nose), smoking, and intravenous injection. All routes of administration result in a rapid and short-lived high that generally lasts from 5 to 20 minutes. Cocaine is a highly addictive drug; when the cocaine high disappears, the user wants more. Spending over $1000 per day for cocaine is not uncommon for an addict. As a result of their addiction, cocaine addicts often suffer psychological damage, which eventually contributes to loss of jobs and financial ruin.

The immediate physiological effects of cocaine are varied. The drug is an anaesthetic and a central nervous system stimulant. Cocaine use increases heart rate and blood pressure. Other effects include a feeling of euphoria and heightened self-confidence. In large doses, cocaine is extremely dangerous, and numerous deaths have resulted from overdoses. Further, long-term cocaine use may damage the heart, the brain, and the respiratory system.

Treatment for cocaine addiction requires professional help. If you or anyone you know uses cocaine, seek professional help at once. Cocaine addiction is a serious problem that requires immediate attention.

Say No to Drugs

Drug abuse cuts across all segments of the population (see Fitness and Wellness for All, below). Avoiding drug use

marijuana   A plant mixture (stems, leaves, or seeds) containing the active chemical tetrahydrocannabinol.

cocaine   A powerful stimulant derived from the leaves of the South American coca shrub, which grows primarily in the Andes Mountains.

FITNESS AND WELLNESS FOR ALL

The Pervasiveness of Drug Abuse in Canada

Drug use, misuse, and abuse occurs in people of all ages, education and income levels, and ethnic groups. Still, research shows that some people are more likely to use illegal drugs and are consequently at greater risk for drug use. For example, young males with risk-taking personalities and a strong antipathy toward school are at high risk for experimenting with drugs (*Tracking the Hidden Epidemics*, 2001). Social factors that increase an indi-

vidual's risk for drug use include frequent exposure to drug users, easy access to drugs, and poverty. In contrast, drug use is less common in individuals who are independent thinkers and are not easily influenced by their peers. Further, compared to individuals who are uninterested in schoolwork, individuals who attend school regularly and earn good grades are less likely to try illegal drugs.

requires self-discipline and control. Several steps can help protect you from the temptation to use drugs (Donatelle & Davis, 2006; Hales, 1998):

1. *Increase your self-esteem.* Take pride in yourself and your achievements; this will boost your confidence and improve your ability to say no to drugs.
2. *Learn how to cope with stress.* When stressed, use one or more of the stress management techniques discussed in Chapter 9 (such as physical activity or progressive relaxation).
3. *Develop numerous interests.* Develop interest in hobbies or sports that give you pleasure.
4. *Practise assertiveness.* Becoming assertive is an important key to learning to say no to drugs.

Summary

1. Sexual health is a component of health and wellness often overlooked. Sexually healthy adults are self-responsible and take actions to protect their physical and mental health.
2. Some of the most common sexually transmitted infections include AIDS, chlamydia, gonorrhoea, venereal warts, genital herpes, and syphilis.
3. All sexually transmitted infections require medical treatment. Successful treatments for chlamydia, gonorrhoea, venereal warts, and syphilis are available. At present, there is no cure for AIDS or genital herpes.
4. Most sexually transmitted infections can be avoided by following "safe sex" guidelines.
5. Alcohol, marijuana, and cocaine are the most widely used and abused drugs in Canada.
6. Use of alcohol, marijuana, and cocaine increases your risk of accidents, and prolonged use of these substances may result in addiction and damaged health.
7. Alcohol is the most common recreational drug used in Canada.
8. Chronic abuse of alcohol can result in liver disease, damage to the nervous system, and increased risk of certain cancers.
9. Long-term use of marijuana may result in dependence and may increase your risk of cardiopulmonary diseases (similar to tobacco smoking).
10. Cocaine is a highly addictive drug that, when taken in large doses, can be lethal.

Study Questions

1. List 10 characteristics of a sexually healthy adult.
2. When and where do we learn about our sexuality?
3. Outline the guidelines for reducing your risk of contracting a sexually transmitted infection.
4. Name the six most common STIs in Canada.
5. Which of the most common STIs are currently incurable?
6. Discuss the relationship between venereal warts and uterine or cervical cancer.
7. Define *drug use, misuse,* and *abuse.* Give an example of each.
8. Discuss the short-term and long-term effects of alcohol use.
9. List four steps that can help you feel less tempted to use drugs.
10. Discuss the short-term and long-term effects of marijuana and cocaine use.

Suggested Reading

Black, A., Francouer, D., Rowe, T., Collins, J., Miller, D., Brown, T., David, M., Dunn, S., Fisher, W. A., Fleming, N., Fortin, C. A., Guilbert, E., Hanvey, L., Lalonde, A., Miller, R., Morris, M., O'Grady, T., Pymar, H., Smith, T., & Henneberg, E. (2004). Canadian contraception consensus. *Journal of Obstetrics and Gynaecology Canada, 26(4),* 347–387, 389–436.

HIV/AIDS Update. (2001). Atlanta: Centers for Disease Control and Prevention.

Liska, K. (2000). *Drugs and the Human Body* (6th ed.). Englewood Cliffs, NJ: Prentice Hall.

Netting, N. S., & Burnett, M. L. (2004). Twenty years of student sexual behaviour: Subcultural adaptations to a changing environment. *Adolescence, 39(153),* 19–38.

Ramstedt, M. (2004). Alcohol consumption and alcohol-related mortality in Canada, 1950–2000. *Canadian Journal of Public Health, 95(2),* 121–126.

Watanabe, M. (2001). AIDS: 20 years later. *The Scientist, 15,*1.

Weblinks

Canadian Centre on Substance Abuse
www.ccsa.ca

The Canadian Centre on Substance Abuse is Canada's national addictions agency. Their mission is to provide objective, evidence-based information and advice that will help reduce the health, social, and economic harm associated with substance abuse and addictions.

The Centre for Addiction and Mental Health
www.camh.net

The Centre for Addiction and Mental Health is Canada's leading addiction and mental health teaching hospital. Using the latest in scientific advances, through integrated and compassionate clinical practice, health promotion, education, and research, this centre is successful in transforming the lives of people affected by addiction and mental illness.

Health Canada

www.hc-sc.gc.ca

Health Canada's website can be used to obtain the most updated information on STIs and drug use.

Statistics Canada

www.statcan.ca

Statistics Canada's website can be used to obtain the most recent statistics (prevalence, risk ratios, etc.) on STIs and drug use.

References

Caron, F., Godin, G., Otis, J., & Lambert, L. D. (2004). Evaluation of a theoretically based AIDS/STD peer education program on postponing sexual intercourse and on condom use among adolescents attending high school. *Health Education Research, (19)2*, 185–197.

Connell, P., McKevitt, C., & Low, N. (2004). Investigating ethnic differences in sexual health: Focus groups with young people. *Sexually Transmitted Infections, 80(4)*, 300–305.

Daniels, D., Hillman, R., Barton, S., & Goldmeir, D. (1993). *Sexually transmitted disease and AIDS*. London: Springer-Verlag.

Donatelle, R., & Davis, L. (2006). *Access to health* (9th ed.). San Francisco: Benjamin Cummings.

Drug & Alcohol Information Line. (2004). Alcohol—Patterns and Trends. Retrieved from http://sano.camh.net/info-line/tp13.htm on August 19, 2004.

Garmaise, D. (2003). National school survey reveals gaps in knowledge of HIV/AIDS. *Canadian HIV/AIDS Policy & Law Review/Canadian HIV/AIDS Legal Network, 8(3)*, 32–33.

Hales, D. (1998). *An invitation to health* (8th ed.). Redwood City, CA: Benjamin Cummings.

Hansen, L., Wong, T., & Perrin, M. (2003). Gonorrhoea resurgence in Canada. *International Journal of STD & AIDS, 14(11)*, 727–731.

Health Canada. (2002). Infectious syphilis in Canada. Retrieved from www.hc-sc.gc.ca/pphb-dgspsp/publicat/epiu-aepi/std-mts/infsyph_e.html on August 18, 2004.

Health Canada. (2003a). Genital herpes. Retrieved from www.hc-sc.gc.ca/pphb-dgspsp/publicat/std-mts/sti_k.html on August 18, 2004.

Health Canada. (2003b). HIV and AIDS in Canada. Surveillance Report to December 31, 2003. Retrieved from www.hc-sc.gc.ca/pphb-dgspsp/publicat/aids-sida/haic-vsac1203/index.html on August 18, 2004.

Health Canada. (2004a). HIV/AIDS. Retrieved from www.hc-sc.gc.ca/datapcb/iad/ih_hivadis-e.htm on August 18, 2004.

Health Canada. (2004b). Reported cases and rates of notifiable STI from January 1 to December 31, 2003, and January 1 to December 31, 2002. Retrieved from www.hc-sc.gc.ca/pphb-dgspsp/std-mts/stdcases-casmts/index/html on August 18, 2004.

Liska, K. (2000). *Drugs and the human body,* Englewood Cliffs, NJ: Prentice Hall.

Netting, N. S., & Burnett, M. L. (2004). Twenty years of student sexual behaviour: Subcultural adaptations to a changing environment. *Adolescence, 39(153)*, 19–38.

Public Health Agency of Canada. (2004). HIV and AIDS in Canada. Surveillance Report to December 31, 2004. Surveillance and Risk Assessment Division, Centre for Infectious Prevention and Control, Public Health Agency of Canada.

Ramstedt, M. (2004). Alcohol consumption and alcohol-related mortality in Canada, 1950–2000. *Canadian Journal of Public Health, 95(2)*, 121–126.

Robbins, S., & Angell, M. (1997). *Basic pathology*. Philadelphia: W. B. Saunders.

Statistics Canada. (2002). Health reports: Use of cannabis and other illicit drugs. *The Daily*, Wednesday, July 21, 2004. Retrieved from www.statcan.ca/Daily/English/040721/d040721a.htm on August 18, 2004.

Strong, B., DeVault, C., Sayad, B., & Yarber, W. (2005). *Human sexuality*. St. Louis: McGraw-Hill, 2005.

Tracking the hidden epidemics: Trends in STIs in the United States, 2000. (2001). Atlanta: Centers for Disease Control and Prevention.

Watanabe, M. (2001). AIDS: 20 years later. *The Scientist, 15, 1*.

Wong, T., & Sutherland, D. (2002). Canadian STI national goals and phase-specific strategies. *Sexually Transmitted Infections, 78(Suppl I)*, i189–i190.

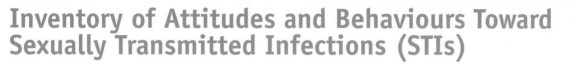

LABORATORY 10.1

Inventory of Attitudes and Behaviours Toward Sexually Transmitted Infections (STIs)

Name_____ Age _____ Sex _____ Date _____

This laboratory is designed to assist you in identifying attitudes and behaviours that increase your risk of contracting an STI. Remember, all STIs are preventable and your attitude and behaviour determines your risk of being infected. Please read the following statements about sexual attitudes and behaviours and identify whether each statement is true or false for you. After completion of this exercise, go to the key at the bottom of the page and compute your level of risk for contracting an STI.

TRUE OR FALSE

_____ 1. I maintain a monogamous sexual relationship with a trusted partner.

_____ 2. I never engage in sexual activities without the use of a condom.

_____ 3. I never use alcohol or other drugs prior to sexual activities.

_____ 4. I am knowledgeable about the health risks associated with STIs.

_____ 5. I have a thorough knowledge about how all STIs are transmitted.

_____ 6. I do not share needles or syringes to inject drugs.

_____ 7. I am concerned about the risk of contracting an STI.

_____ 8. I always discuss STIs and "safe sex" with new partners prior to having sexual relations.

_____ 9. I always avoid sexual contact if I believe there is any risk of contracting an STI.

_____ 10. I believe that responsible "safe sex" is one of the best ways to reduce the chances of getting an STI.

SCORING AND INTERPRETATION

Count the number of False answers to all 10 statements and calculate your risk level for contracting an STI as follows:

  0 False answers = low risk for infection with STI
  1–3 False answers = high risk for infection with STI
  4 or more False answers = very high risk for infection with STI

After calculating your risk for contracting STIs, please review all of the statements that you answered with a False answer and take action to correct this attitude or behaviour so that you can respond to these statements with a True answer in the future. Answer the following questions to help you evaluate your sexual practices and think about STI prevention.

1. List three ways to bring up the subject of STIs with a new partner. How would you ask whether he or she has been exposed to any STIs or engaged in any risky behaviours?

2. List three ways to bring up the subject of condom use with your partner. How might you convince someone who does not want to use a condom?

3. If you had an STI that is possible to pass on (e.g., herpes), how would you tell your partner(s), and what precautions would you take during each act of sexual activity?

Alcohol Use Inventory

Name_____ Age _____ Sex _____ Date _____

This laboratory is designed to increase your awareness of your drinking habits. For this inventory to provide a valid assessment of your drinking behaviours, you must answer each question honestly.

DIRECTIONS

Please check under Yes or No for each of the following questions regarding your use of alcohol.

	Yes	No
1. Do you often drink alone?	_____	_____
2. When drinking, do you often worry about running out of alcoholic beverages?	_____	_____
3. Do you drink alcohol on a daily basis?	_____	_____
4. When stressed, do you immediately drink alcohol to reduce your stress levels?	_____	_____
5. Do you crave alcohol during all parts of the day?	_____	_____
6. Do you have trouble saying no to drinking at a party?	_____	_____
7. Do you sometimes have trouble remembering what you did the night before?	_____	_____
8. Does your drinking impair your school or job performance?	_____	_____
9. Does your drinking impair your ability to use good judgment or cause you to have accidents?	_____	_____
10. Do you ever lie about how much you drink to friends or family?	_____	_____

Answering Yes to only one of the questions above suggests that you may be drinking too much. Answering Yes to two questions is a clear warning sign that you may have or are developing an alcohol abuse problem. Answering Yes to three or more questions indicates that you have a serious alcohol abuse problem and that you should seek professional help.

CHAPTER 11

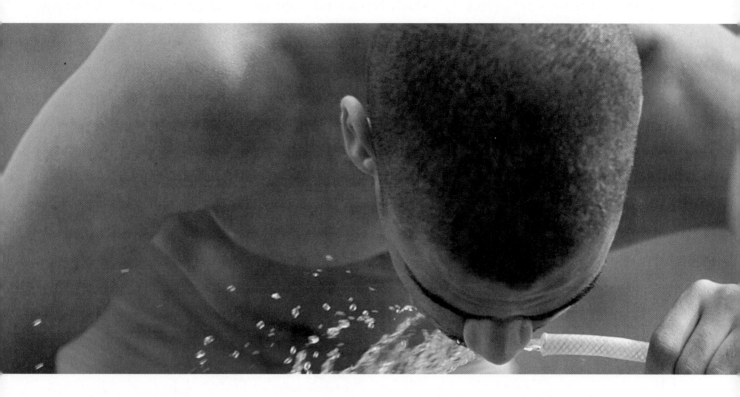

Physical Activity and the Environment

11

After studying this chapter, you should be able to

1. Describe how to prevent heat loss during physical activity.
2. List several guidelines for physical activity in a hot environment.
3. Differentiate among the various types of heat injury.
4. Identify how heat acclimatization reduces the risk of heat injury.
5. Describe the appropriate clothing for physical activity in a cold environment.
6. Explain why physical activity at a high altitude results in a higher heart rate and increased ventilation.
7. List two major forms of air pollution that affect physical activity performance.
8. Outline a strategy for coping with air pollution during physical activity.

Most of us know from personal experience that environmental factors can affect our physical performance. For example, hot environments, high altitude, and air pollution can elevate exercising heart rates, promote laboured breathing, and impair tolerance to physical activity. A general understanding of how environmental factors can influence physical activity performance is important for the active individual. In this chapter, we discuss common environmental hazards that should be considered when planning workouts, and outline ways to cope with environmental stress. In particular, we focus on heat and humidity, cold, altitude, and air pollution.

Before we turn to a discussion of physical activity in a hot environment, it's important to know a bit about body temperature regulation in humans. Humans are **homeotherms** (*homeo,* "same," and *therm,* "temperature"), which means our internal body temperature is regulated to remain close to a set point—37°C (98.6°F). If body temperature falls too far below or rises too far above this "normal" temperature, serious injury can result (Figure 11.1), so the body must maintain precise control over its temperature to avoid life-threatening situations.

homeotherms   Animals that regulate their body temperatures to remain close to a set point. Humans regulate their body temperatures around the set point of 37°C (98.6°F).

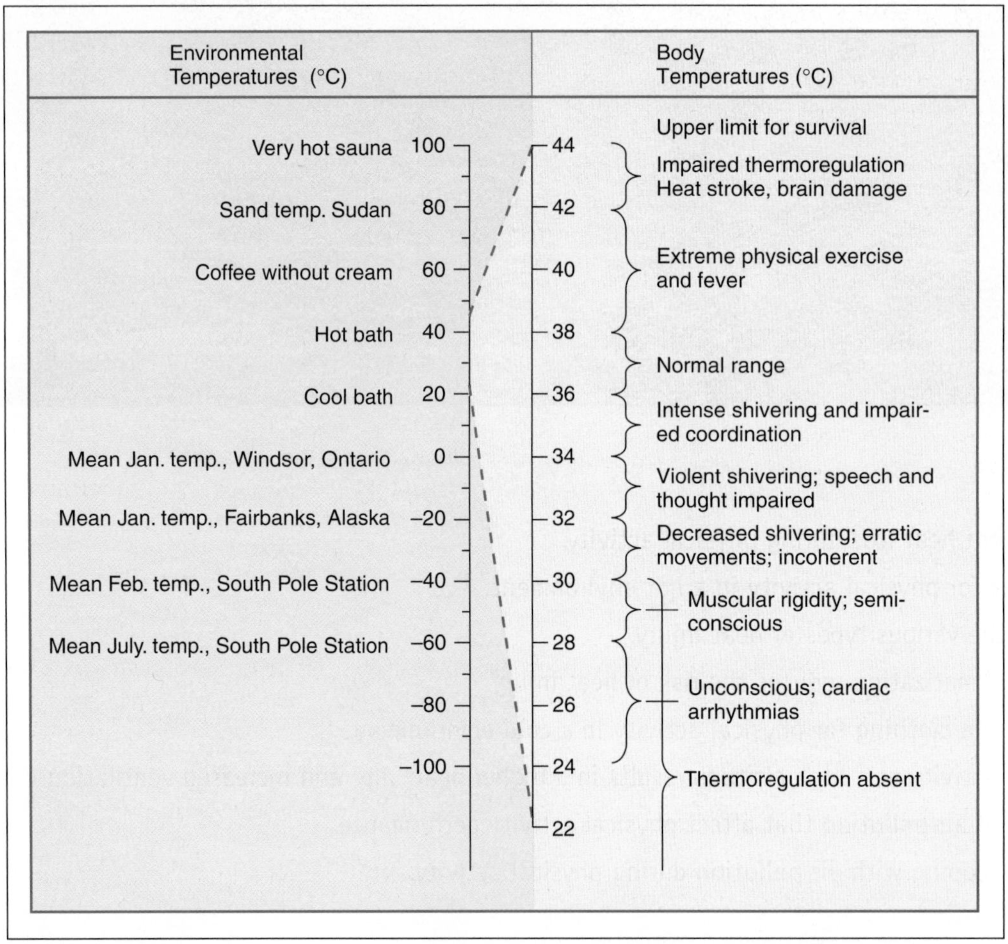

FIGURE 11.1 A comparison of temperature extremes: the environment (at left) and the body (at right). Note that even relatively small changes in body temperature can have serious consequences.

Source: Adapted from Brooks, G., Fahey, T., & White, T. (1996). *Exercise physiology: Human bioenergetics and its application.* New York: Macmillan.

Physical Activity in the Heat

When physically active, humans produce heat as a byproduct of muscular contractions. High-intensity activities using large muscle groups produce more body heat than low-intensity activities involving small muscle groups. Thus, when large muscle groups are used vigorously in hot conditions, the body must eliminate excess heat in order to prevent a dangerous rise in body temperature. If the body cannot eliminate enough heat to keep from exceeding 41°C (105°F), then heat injury can ensue (Brooks, Fahey, & White, 2000). The signs of impending heat injury are cramps, dizziness, nausea, lack of sweat production, and dry, hot skin.

In the next section we discuss how heat is lost from the body during physical activity and outline key factors to consider when active in a hot environment.

Heat Loss During Physical Activity

The primary means of heat loss during physical activity are convection and evaporation. **Convection** is heat loss by the movement of air (or water) around the body. During **evaporation**, heat loss occurs due to the conversion of sweat (water) to a gas (water vapour).

Convective heat loss occurs only when the air or water molecules moving over the surface of the body are cooler than skin temperature; the faster the flow of cool air or water around the body, the greater the heat loss. Minimal convective cooling occurs during physical activity in a hot environment where there is limited air movement (riding a stationary bicycle, for example). In contrast, bicycling outdoors on a cold day or swimming in cool water results in a lot of convective cooling.

On a warm day with limited air movement around the body, evaporation is the most important means of body heat loss (Brooks et al., 2000). The evaporation of sweat on the skin's surface removes heat from the body, even if the air temperature is higher than body temperature, as long as the air is dry. However, if the air temperature is high and the **humidity** is also high (i.e., the air is relatively saturated with water), then evaporation is retarded and body heat loss is decreased. Under these conditions, heat produced by the contracting muscles is retained, and body temperature increases gradually throughout the duration of the activity. Prolonged activity in a hot and humid environment can result in a dangerously high increase in body temperature. Figure 11.2 illustrates the differences in body temperature rise during activity in a high-temperature/high-humidity environment, a high-temperature/low-humidity environment, and a low-temperature/low-humidity environment.

Guidelines for Physical Activity in the Heat

Short-term exposure (30 to 60 minutes) to an extremely hot environment is sufficient heat stress to cause heat injury in some people (Neiman, 1995), especially those at high risk for heat injury. (The elderly and those with low cardiovascular endurance levels are most susceptible.) Even individuals who are physically fit and accustomed to the heat are at risk in a hot environment.

Heat stress on the body is not simply a function of the air temperature; both the temperature and the humidity must be considered. As indicated in Figure 11.3, the higher the humidity, the higher the "effective" temperature—that is, the temperature that the body senses. At high levels of humidity, evaporation is retarded and the body cannot get rid of the heat normally lost through evaporative processes. This causes body temperature to increase above what it would be on a less humid day at the same ambient temperature.

Although it is obvious that many activities are extremely dangerous at high air temperatures (55°C, 130°F), it may not be obvious to most people that the body undergoes the same heat stress at only 29°C (84°F) when the relative humidity approaches 100 percent. In other words, the effective temperature remains at 55°C. Thus, high humidity causes a moderately high ambient temperature to be sensed by the body as extremely hot (Figure 11.3).

The best way to determine whether environmental conditions are imposing a heat load on your body is to monitor your heart rate. An increase in body temperature during physical activity in a hot environment will result in great increases in heart rate compared with physical activity in a cooler environment. This point is illustrated in Figure 11.4, which shows the large differences in heart rate in responses to three different conditions. A temperature-induced increase in heart rate is significant because it increases the difficulty of training within your target heart rate zone (Chapter 4).

Suggested Clothing for Hot Environments

Although it may be impossible to prevent body heat gain during physical activity in a hot environment, there are ways to reduce the risks of heat injury. Wearing the appro-

---

convection   Heat loss by the movement of air (or water) over the surface of the body.

evaporation   The conversion of water (or sweat) to a gas (water vapour); the most important means of removing heat from the body during physical activity.

humidity   The amount of water vapour in the air.

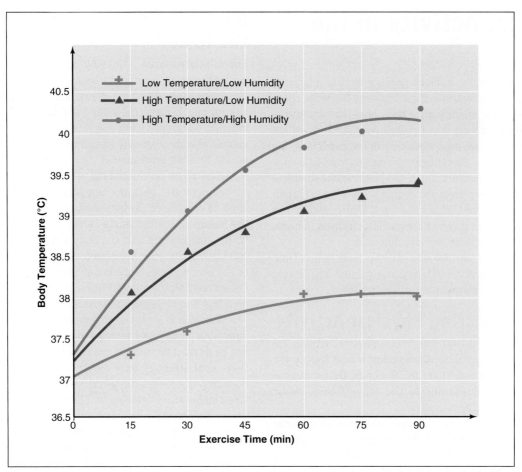

FIGURE 11.2 Body temperature responses to prolonged physical activity in a high-temperature/high-humidity environment, a high-temperature/low-humidity environment, and a low-temperature/low-humidity environment.

priate clothing is essential to minimizing the possibility of overheating (Foss & Keteyian, 2000). Clothing should be minimal to maximize the body surface area exposed for evaporation. It should be lightweight and made from materials that readily absorb moisture and allow air to move freely through them, features that promote evaporative and convective cooling. Cottons and linens are best for these purposes. Because dry clothing retards heat exchange compared to the same clothing when wet, switching to dry clothing when your clothes become saturated with sweat delays the resumption of evaporative cooling, and thus makes little sense when you want to stay cool. Heavy clothing and clothing made of rubber or plastic retard evaporative heat loss by trapping humid air next to the skin. In addition, because dark colours absorb radiant heat from the sun, light-coloured clothing should be worn during outdoor activities.

acclimatization The physiological adaptations that occur to assist the body in adjusting to environmental extremes.

heat injury Bodily injury that can occur when the heat load exceeds the body's ability to regulate body temperature.

Heat Acclimatization

Physical activity in a hot, or even a moderately hot, environment will cause the body to adapt or *acclimatize* to this condition. **Acclimatization** refers to the physiological adaptations that occur to assist the body in adjusting to environmental extremes. When the body needs to dissipate heat, these changes include an earlier onset of sweating, a higher sweat rate (i.e., more evaporative cooling), and an increase in blood volume (Foss & Keteyian, 2000). Interestingly, heat acclimatization occurs rapidly. Within 10 to 12 days of heat exposure, the physiological responses to physical activity in the heat are drastically altered (McArdle, Katch, & Katch, 2001). The end result is that heat acclimatization promotes a decreased heart rate and lower body temperature. A key point here is that heat acclimatization decreases the likelihood of experiencing heat injury during physical activity.

Heat injury can occur when the activity heat load exceeds the body's ability to regulate body temperature. It is a serious condition and can result in damage to the nervous system, and in extreme cases death. The following are the most common types of heat injury:

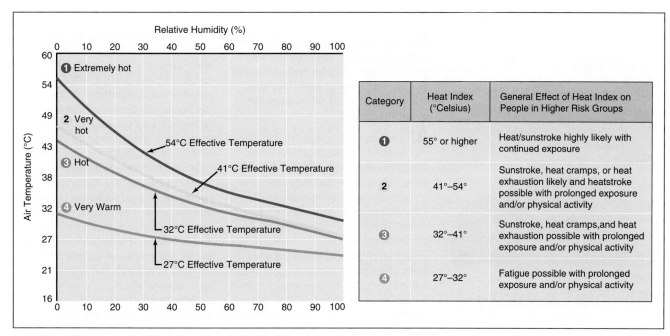

FIGURE 11.3 The concept of "heat index," or "effective" temperature.

Source: Donatelle, R. J., and Davis, L. G. (1996). *Access to health*. Englewood Cliffs, NJ: Prentice Hall.

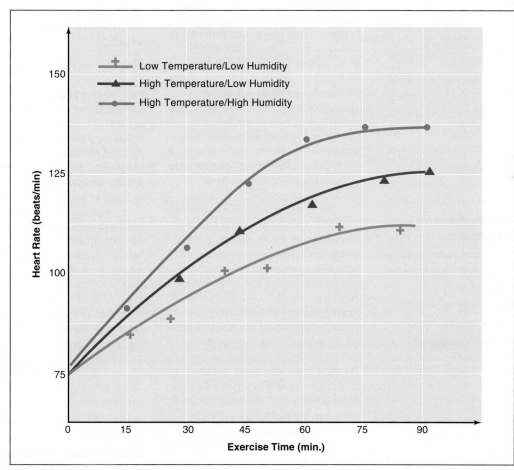

FIGURE 11.4 Changes in heart rate during prolonged activity under three different environmental conditions.

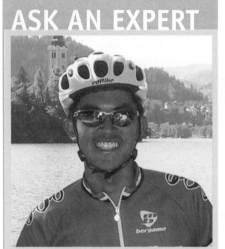

Stephen S. Cheung, Ph.D.

Physical Activity in Extreme Conditions

Stephen S. Cheung, Ph.D., is an Associate Professor in the School of Health and Human Performance at Dalhousie University in Halifax. He is the Director of the Environmental Ergonomics Lab (http://myweb.dal.ca/ scheung), where his primary research concerns the impact of thermal stress on human physiology and performance. His recent work involves the mechanisms of fatigue during exercise in the heat, and also the physiological responses and protection of the hands during cold exposure. Stephen's career choice as an exercise physiologist was prompted by his passion for cycling, which began with watching Steve Bauer win the silver medal at the 1984 Olympics. Stephen commutes by bike, takes part in road races, and enjoys riding tandem with his wife Debbie and towing his boys Zachary and Jacob in their trailer. Since 2002, Stephen has merged his scientific and cycling backgrounds as the Sport Science and Training Editor for the bicycling website www.pezcyclingnews.com.

Q: There is great debate around the best drink (water, electrolyte drink, glucose drink, etc.) for replenishment of fluid lost through sweating. What drink, if any, would you suggest for physical activity?

A: The threat of dehydration on exercise performance and health is absolutely unequivocal. Water comprises 40 to 65 percent of our body mass, and is the most important nutrient for the maintenance of health and even life. Hunger strikers who consume water can survive nearly 100 days. However, remove water from the equation and death often occurs within a week! Sweat is excreted by the body to maximize heat dissipation via evaporation, and humans typically lose 1 to 1.5 litres of water an hour during moderate exercise in warm environments through sweating. Higher levels of fitness and adaptation to heat generally result in greater sweating rates. Dehydration by even 1 to 2 percent of body weight can dramatically impair physical and mental performance. This is worsened by the fact that our thirst sensors are not very sensitive, such that we usually do not feel thirsty until we have already lost about 2 percent of our body weight. Therefore, scientific bodies such as the American College of Sports Medicine repeatedly emphasize the importance of drinking as much and as often as comfortable, especially in the heat. What to drink, though, is not as clear.

The "ideal" sports drink is the Holy Grail of a multi-billion-dollar industry. Every company claims that its formulation is scientifically proven to be the most effective concoction of carbohydrates, electrolytes, and other ingredients (e.g., proteins, vitamins), and, indeed, studies can be found to demonstrate the efficacy of almost every possible ingredient. There is consensus on certain general parameters. For example, the ideal concentration of carbohydrate is in the range of 6 to 8 percent (most sodas are about 10 percent in comparison), and the addition of moderate amounts of electrolytes (e.g., sodium) also appears to increase the absorption of the drink. Beyond that, questions such as the ideal carbohydrate, electrolyte, and possibly protein composition remain very much open to debate.

I take a much more pragmatic approach to the question of what is the ideal sports drink. To me, whatever tastes good and that you will drink consistently and in significant volumes is the best sports drink! Just like shoe fit, taste preference is such an individual thing that a sports drink may be scientifically perfect, but if you don't like the taste it's absolutely worthless.

With that in mind, a sports drink is not always required for moderate exercise, especially if your purpose for exercise includes weight loss. If you are doing moderate exercise to burn excess calories and the exercise is not too long, then it's pointless to add back the calories that you're burning off. If you're exercising at a moderate pace for fewer than 60 to 90 minutes, carbohydrates and electrolytes are not essential to performance, and water is the primary consideration.

Q: Is it possible to become dehydrated when exercising in extreme cold, and if so how should we monitor our hydration to maintain normal body water?

A: Just because it is cold does not mean that you stop sweating or losing fluid, so it is just as important to keep thinking about hydration. Much of the sweat that you are producing gets evaporated very quickly, so you may be losing fluid but not really feeling hot and sweaty. You are also breathing in cold and dry air, and the first question might be whether breathing cold air can harm your lungs. Fortunately, your mouth and nasal passages are extremely efficient at warming up and humidifying the air before it reaches your lungs, even at high rates of ventilation such as those seen in Nordic skiers. However, most of the fluid used to humidify that incoming air is then lost when you exhale. Therefore, respiratory losses and sweating can still account for a significant amount of fluid loss during exercise in the cold. Therefore, the basic rule of "drink before you are thirsty" applies to both hot and cold environments. Besides, you might as well drink the water in your bottle before it freezes!

Q: Often there are warnings about exercising in the heat. Is it just as dangerous to exercise in extremely cold weather?

continued

A: The dangers of exercising in cold weather are slightly different than in the heat. There is some risk of dehydration, but the main concern is maintaining body heat and preventing the threat of hypothermia. The other threats are cold injuries such as frostnip and frostbite. Exposed skin can freeze very quickly in extremely cold and windy weather. Therefore, it is important to cover up as much of the skin as possible when exercising in the cold and to heed warnings about wind chill, which combines temperature and wind speed into a single temperature value. As your mom always said, the best way to keep warm in the cold is to wear a hat. That is because the skin around your face, neck, and head does not really close (vasoconstrict) in response to cold, and your head can be responsible for up to 40 percent of the total heat loss from your body.

If you are exercising heavily and stopping frequently, the sweat you produce can get your clothing very wet when you stop because the water vapour gets trapped in your clothing and then condenses back to water. This decreases the insulation of your clothing and increases your rate of heat loss. Therefore, I would recommend minimizing the number of rest stops you take. For example, rather than exercising hard and then stopping to rest, it would be better to keep exercising continuously at a more moderate rate.

Remember that water is an excellent conductor of heat, removing heat from the body 25 times faster than air. Therefore, it becomes essential to keep dry in the cold, and to really beware of the threat posed by water. That means taking extreme care when crossing streams, engaging in water sports (even on a warm summer day), and especially when going onto frozen bodies of water. If you fall into water, the sudden cold shock can cause you to gasp and take very quick breaths (hyperventilate) and rapidly elevate your heart rate, making it almost impossible to hold your breath and potentially causing drowning.

Q: Being physically active in high altitudes can cause some people to experience fatigue and shortness of breath. How can we acclimatize to improve our tolerance for high-altitude activities?

A: There has certainly been a boom in the popularity of high-altitude sports like mountain climbing, along with high-altitude trekking trips. If anything, disasters like the deaths on Everest in 1996 have only fuelled interest. The primary problem with high altitude is that the decrease in atmospheric pressure means a decrease in the partial pressure of oxygen. This leads to a condition of hypoxia in our bodies, as our respiratory system has great difficulty in bringing enough oxygen into our bodies. Ultimately, this results in impaired physical performance, fatigue, and three specific clinical problems: acute mountain sickness (fatigue, headache, nausea), high altitude cerebral edema (HACE, fluid buildup in your skull), and high altitude pulmonary edema (HAPE, fluid buildup in your lungs). If you ascend to altitude too quickly, these problems can ultimately prove fatal. Therefore, gradual adaptation to altitude and effort is absolutely critical from both a performance and a safety perspective.

It is very difficult and often expensive to adapt to high altitudes and hypoxic environments while at lower altitudes. There are possibilities such as the hypoxic tents and houses used by some athletes, where they sleep in tents/rooms that have a lower concentration of oxygen to simulate high altitude. However, these systems are usually out of reach logistically and financially to most individuals.

The best way to adapt to altitude is to take a very gradual approach. If you are going up to moderate altitude—for example, Whistler Mountain, B.C., at 2182 m—the first thing you will typically notice is an increase in breathing rate as the body tries to bring in more oxygen. You will likely feel fatigued the first few days, partly due to this sensation of increased breathing. Therefore, it is best if you take the first 2 to 3 days really easy, and either rest completely or do only light exercise before gradually increasing your exercise duration and intensity. At these altitudes, there is almost no risk of major medical problems.

If you are ascending to high altitude—greater than 3000 m—the same process of adaptation must be applied. Generally, the higher the altitude, the longer the adaptation period required.

Heat Cramps: Heat cramps are characterized by muscle spasms or twitching of limbs. This usually occurs in people who are not acclimatized to the heat. Anyone with these symptoms should be moved to a cool place, made to lie down, and given 250 to 500 mL of water.

Heat Exhaustion: Heat exhaustion results in general weakness, fatigue, a possible drop in blood pressure, blurred vision, occasionally a loss of consciousness, and profuse sweating from pale, clammy skin. Heat exhaustion can occur in an acclimatized individual. First aid should consist of moving the victim to a cool place, removing the clothing, applying cold water or ice, and administering 250 mL of water.

Heat Stroke: Heat stroke is a life-threatening emergency. A person experiencing heat stroke stops sweating, and the skin is hot and red. Muscles are limp. There is involuntary limb movement, seizures, diarrhea, vomiting, and a rapid, strong heartbeat. The individual may hallucinate and eventually lapse into a coma. Any of these signs should be taken very seriously. Seek emergency medical assistance immediately and administer first aid by moving the victim to a cool place, removing clothing, and lowering body temperature as rapidly as possible (immersing in water or ice, and/or fanning).

Adverse Effects of Dehydration

Physical activity in the heat can be extremely dangerous depending on intensity, ambient temperature, relative humidity, clothing, and state of hydration (water content of the body). Although some forms of heat injury can occur prior to significant weight loss due to sweating, the table in this box shows how weight loss during physical activity can be a predictor of some of the dangers associated with physical activity in the heat. The loss of body weight during activity in the heat is simply due to water loss through sweating. Thus, prolonged, profuse sweating is the first warning signal of impending dehydration.

% Body Weight Loss	Symptoms	% Body Weight Loss	Symptoms
0.5	Thirst	6.0	Impaired temperature regulation, increased heart rate
2.0	Stronger thirst, vague discomfort, loss of appetite	8.0	Dizziness, laboured breathing during exercise, confusion
3.0	Concentrated blood, dry mouth, reduced urine output	10.0	Spastic muscles, loss of balance, delirium
4.0	Increased effort required during activity, flushed skin, apathy	11.0	Circulatory insufficiency, decreased blood volume, kidney failure
5.0	Difficulty in concentrating		

These conditions have several similarities: they are initiated by heat exposure; they involve significant loss of water and electrolytes; and in them the body undergoes an increase in heat storage, as indicated by a high core temperature. The most important of these is the loss of water, a factor that can be prevented by drinking plenty of fluids

Guidelines for Fluid Intake during Physical Activity in a Hot Environment

Because the sweat you lose during physical activity is replaced with water from the blood, the ultimate danger during prolonged activity in the heat is the loss of blood volume. The best strategy for preventing a decrease in blood volume is maintaining a regular schedule of fluid intake during physical activity. Thirst for fluid lags behind fluid loss, because your body does not recognize a need for fluid until the composition of the blood has changed. Therefore, you should begin to drink within 10 to 20 minutes after beginning activity, before a fluid deficit accumulates. The following fluid replacement schedule will help in meeting your body's need for water (Maughan & Shirreffs, 1997):

Contents of Fluid

The drink should:

- be low in sugar (generally less than 8 grams per 100 mL of water)
- be low in electrolytes (sodium and potassium)
- be cold (approximately 8–13°C, or 45–55°F)

Fluid Intake Before Workout

Drink approximately 200 mL (6 oz) of the fluid 20 to 30 minutes prior to any physical activity.

Fluid Intake During Workout

Thirst is a poor gauge of the amount of fluid needed. Drink approximately 100 to 200 mL (3 to 6.6 oz) every 10 to 20 minutes during the activity, regardless of whether you feel thirsty.

Fluid Replacement After Workout

In general, you should consume 30 mL (~1 oz) of fluid for every minute of activity performed. Another means of estimating how much fluid you need is to weigh yourself before your activity and immediately after your cool-down period. The difference in body weight is a measure of how much fluid was lost via sweating, and more than that amount should be replaced. In fact, each ounce of body weight lost due to sweating is equivalent to 1 fluid ounce. For example, a pre-/post-activity body weight difference of 1 kg (2.2 lb) indicates that 1 L (32 oz) of sweat was lost during exercise. Therefore, consumption of more than 1 L of fluid is required to replenish body fluid stores.

whenever it's hot. Inattention to any of the signs of heat injury can lead to heat stroke and ultimately to death. Do not take these symptoms lightly!

Given the dangers of combined high heat and humidity, should you even consider physical activity under these conditions? The answer is yes, but when doing so in the heat keep the following in mind:

- Start slowly, and keep your activity relatively short (15 to 20 minutes).
- Monitor your heart rate often, and keep the intensity low so that you maintain your target heart rate zone.
- Wear appropriate clothing (see the section on proper clothing in the next column).
- Drink plenty of cold fluids before, during, and after the activity (see Nutritional Links to Health and Fitness, p. 270).
- Do not use salt tablets. Although it was once thought that salt tablets replaced the salt lost from the body in sweat during physical activity, recent research indicates that no supplemental salt is necessary. As discussed in Chapter 7, many people consume too much salt, and supplemental salt is actually counterproductive to coping with heat stress. The crucial element in staying hydrated is not taking supplemental salt, but instead replacing lost body water. See A Closer Look on page 270 for a brief discussion of the adverse effects of dehydration.
- Schedule physical activity for the coolest part of the day. Mornings are best because much of the radiant heat from the ground has been lost overnight and the air temperature is most likely the lowest of the day. After sunset is the second best time, because the radiant heat from the sun is not a factor. If you must be physically active during the heat of the day, try to find a shaded area. This might mean choosing an indoor facility or hiking/jogging in a wooded area.

Physical Activity in the Cold

Physical activity at temperatures below 15.5°C (60°F) dictates that some combination of warm clothing and production of muscle heat is required to prevent too much body heat loss. Failure to adequately combine warm clothing with muscle heat in extremely cold temperatures increases the likelihood of experiencing a large decline in body temperature (*hypothermia*), which can be life threatening (Brooks et al., 2000). Indeed, physical activity in the cold for long periods (e.g., 1 to 4 hours) or swimming in cold water may overwhelm the body's ability to prevent heat loss, resulting in hypothermia. Severe hypothermia can result in a loss of judgment, which increases the risk of further cold injury. Hypothermia can be avoided by following some simple guidelines.

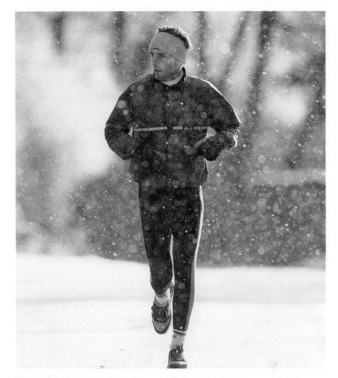

Physical activities in the cold can be enjoyable if the proper clothing is worn.

- Limit the duration of physical activity in cold weather.
- Wear layers of clothing.
- Wear clothing appropriate for cold temperatures (e.g., polypropylene, Gore-Tex, hat and gloves).
- Be active with friends; use the buddy system and never go out in extreme temperatures alone.
- Never become dehydrated; cold-weather sports and activities require hydration.

A question that is often asked is "Can you damage your lungs by breathing cold air during physical activity?" Research suggests that activity in temperatures between 0°C and −10°C does not present a major risk to lung tissues (Irlbeck, 1998). Indeed, inhaled cold air is rapidly warmed by the nasal passages and airways, so that by the time the gas reaches the lungs, it is close to body temperature.

Appropriate Clothing for Cold Environments

The key to physical activity in the cold is wearing appropriate clothing—that is, clothing that traps just enough of the heat produced so that normal body temperature is maintained, but not enough to produce overheating. The ideal clothing permits sweat to be transferred from the skin to the outer surface of the clothing, so that it does not evaporate from your skin and cause too much heat loss.

Trapping heat is best accomplished by *layering*—wearing multiple layers of clothing so that air, an excellent insulator, is trapped between the layers. The thicker the zone of trapped air between the body and the outside of the clothing, the more effective the insulation; thus, several layers of lightweight clothing provide much greater insulation than a single bulky coat. The transfer of moisture away from the skin is important because wet clothing can lose its insulating properties and can even facilitate the loss of body heat (A Closer Look, p. 273). Good materials for transporting moisture away from the skin are wool or synthetics such as polypropylene. For some information on advances in cold-weather clothing, see the box below.

The amount of clothing needed to provide comfort during activity varies with the temperature, the wind speed, and the intensity and duration of the activity. Wearing too little clothing obviously allows the loss of too much heat. It's often important to cover your head, because 30 to 40 percent of body heat is lost through the head. Too much clothing, in contrast, can limit your freedom of movement, but more importantly it can result in an accumulation of body heat and sweating. During extreme cold, the loss of body heat that results from sweating can lead to hypothermia, which can be fatal (McArdle et al., 2001).

The major complicating factor in the cold is wind. The greater the wind speed in a cold environment, the colder it feels. In other words, the wind makes the "effective" temperature colder than the actual air temperature. The effect by which wind makes you feel colder than the air temperature is referred to as *wind chill* (Figure 11.5).

Wind Speed, (km/h)	Ambient Temperature, °C														
	4	2	−1	−4	−7	−9	−12	−15	−18	−21	−23	−26	−29	−32	−34
	Effective Temperature, °C														
Calm	4	2	−1	−4	−7	−9	−12	−15	−18	−21	−23	−26	−29	−32	−34
8	2	−1	−4	−7	−11	−14	−17	−21	−24	−27	−30	−33	−37	−40	−43
16	1	−3	−6	−9	−13	−16	−20	−23	−27	−30	−33	−37	−41	−44	−47
24	0	−4	−7	−11	−14	−18	−22	−25	−28	−32	−36	−39	−43	−46	−50
32	−1	−4	−8	−12	−15	−19	−23	−26	−30	−34	−37	−41	−44	−48	−52
40	−1	−5	−9	−13	−16	−20	−24	−27	−31	−35	−38	−42	−46	−50	−53
48	−2	−6	−9	−13	−17	−21	−24	−28	−32	−36	−39	−43	−47	−51	−55
56	−2	−6	−10	−14	−18	−22	−26	−29	−33	−37	−41	−44	−48	−52	−56
64	−3	−7	−11	−14	−18	−22	−26	−30	−34	−38	−42	−46	−49	−53	−57

Little Danger   **Danger**   **Great Danger**

Convective heat loss at wind speeds above 64 kmph have little additional effect on body cooling.

FIGURE 11.5 The wind chill index.

Source: McArdle, W. D., Katch, F. I., & Katch, V. L. (2001). *Exercise physiology: Energy, nutrition, and human performance* (5th ed.). Philadelphia: Lippincott Williams & Wilkins.

FITNESS–WELLNESS CONSUMER

Advances in Cold-Weather Clothing

Even though wearing several layers of clothing is beneficial for cold-weather activity (because the air trapped between layers provides great insulation), physical activity in the cold can be extremely dangerous if the clothing becomes wet from perspiration. Thus, materials that help remove moisture from the skin (a process called "wicking") are better when worn next to the skin than are materials that absorb moisture, such as cotton.

DuPont has designed a fabric called CoolMax that, according to comparison tests, wicks moisture away from the skin better than wool, polypropylene, cotton, and other fibres. CoolMax contains specially engineered fibres that transport perspiration away from the body and to the surface of the garment, where it can evaporate quickly while providing great breathability—even when wet.

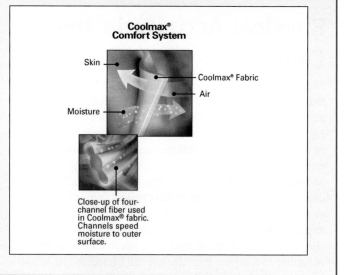

Coolmax® Comfort System

Skin

Coolmax® Fabric

Air

Moisture

Close-up of four-channel fiber used in Coolmax® fabric. Channels speed moisture to outer surface.

Physical Activity in the Cold

Physical activities in a cool or cold environment can be safe as well as pleasurable if the appropriate clothing is worn. If the intensity of the activity causes you to sweat or if you get wet in the rain, a dangerous condition could occur. One study (Thompson & Hayward, 1996) examined the effects of cold, rain, and wind on performance tolerance and hypothermia. Subjects were asked to attempt a 5-hour walk at 5°C (41°F) at a brisk pace. At the end of 1 hour the subjects were exposed to constant rain and wind in addition to the cold. These conditions were severe enough that only 5 of 16 subjects could complete the 5-hour walk.

During the first hour of walking, body temperature actually rose 1 degree! However, with the onset of wind and rain, body temperature started to decrease, even when some subjects began shivering. The shivering produced weakness and loss of manual dexterity. Over the last 2 hours, body temperature was variable in those completing the walk. Of the five subjects who completed the walk, two experienced a severe decrease in body temperature because they were not able to maintain the walking pace due to fatigue from shivering.

This study illustrates the importance of air temperature, wind, and water interaction. If clothing gets wet, it conducts heat from the body so fast that heat production during activity may not be sufficient to maintain body temperature. It is important to note that the subjects in this study were not wearing protective rainwear. Any type of waterproof clothing would have given them significant additional time to be active in the wind and rain. In contrast, a very fit individual who was capable of increasing intensity in the conditions of this study might have been able to complete the 5 hours without rainwear.

Physical Activity and Altitude

Each year, more and more people go to high altitudes to participate in recreational activities such as skiing, hiking, and camping. How does the body respond to physical activity at high altitudes, and how can you adjust your fitness prescription?

The primary concern with activity at high altitudes (i.e., altitudes above 1500 m) is that the lower barometric pressure limits the amount of oxygen transported in arterial blood (Brooks et al., 2000). This results in a reduction in oxygen transported to the working muscles, and therefore both physical tolerance and VO_2max are reduced. As shown in Figure 11.6, at altitudes above about 1500 m (the approximate elevation of the village of Lake Louise, Alberta), the reduction increases as a function of increasing altitude: the higher the altitude, the greater the reduction in VO_2max and physical tolerance.

To cope with this lowered oxygen delivery to the working muscles, the body makes several physiological adjustments (see Figure 11.7). Breathing becomes deeper and faster in an attempt to maximize oxygen transfer from the lungs to the blood. Heart rate rises to increase blood flow and

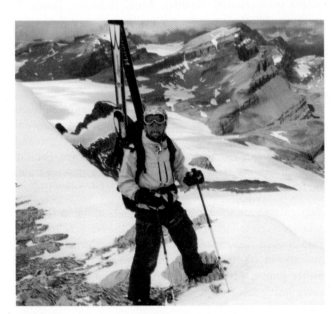

Altitude presents a significant challenge to the body.

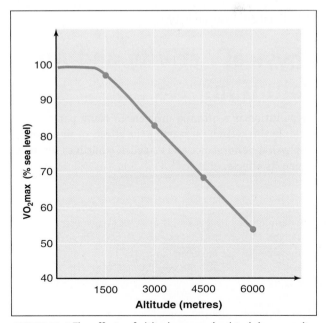

FIGURE 11.6 The effects of altitude on maximal training capacity.

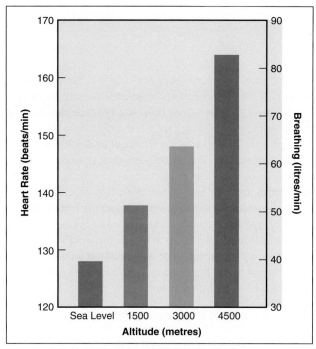

FIGURE 11.7 The effect of elevation on heart rate and ventilation during moderate physical activity.

oxygen delivery to the working muscles. To stay within your target heart rate zone during physical activity at high altitude, it is necessary to lower your activity intensity to a level below your normal intensity. In general, there is little need to alter the time or frequency of your training during a brief stay at high altitude. However, the air is very dry at high altitudes, which results in increased water loss during breathing (Brooks et al., 2000). In addition, the body decreases its water content as a way of coping with the stress of altitude exposure. Be sure to drink plenty of fluids during and after the activity.

Physical Activity and Air Pollution

Air pollution is a growing problem in many parts of the world. In this section we examine the effects of air pollution on physical performance and establish guidelines for minimizing its effects.

ozone A gas produced by a chemical reaction between sunlight and the hydrocarbons emitted from car exhausts.

carbon monoxide A gas produced during the burning of fossil fuels such as gasoline and coal; also present in cigarette smoke.

sulphur dioxide A yellowish-brown gas that is a byproduct of burning fossil fuels.

particulates Tiny solid particles or liquid droplets that are suspended in the air.

Major Forms of Air Pollution

Two major pollutants that affect physical performance are ozone and carbon monoxide (Carlisle & Sharp, 2001; Pierson, 1989). **Ozone** is a gas produced primarily by a chemical reaction between sunlight and the hydrocarbons emitted from car exhausts. This form of pollution is extremely irritating to the lungs and airways. It causes tightness in the chest, coughing, headaches, nausea, throat and eye irritation, and, worst of all, bronchoconstriction (Paz, 1997). In fact, exposure to ozone can trigger an asthma attack.

In an effort to protect citizens from air pollution, Environment Canada monitors air quality and issues health alerts when it is poor. Stage 1 health alerts are issued when ozone reaches 0.2 ppm (parts per million), and stage 2 alerts are issued at 0.35 ppm. These alerts suggest that anyone with lung problems such as asthma should not engage in physical activities outdoors.

Many large metropolitan areas now have stage 1 alerts on more than 100 days out of the year. Although the long-term effects of ozone exposure are not clear, recent research suggests that chronic exposure to ozone results in diminished lung function (Paz, 1997).

Carbon monoxide is a gas produced during the burning of fossil fuels, such as gasoline and coal, and it is also present in cigarette smoke. This pollutant binds to hemoglobin in the blood and reduces the blood's oxygen-carrying capacity. High levels of carbon monoxide can impair physical performance by reducing oxygen delivery to the working muscles (Adir et al., 1999). In cities where traffic is heavy and congested, carbon monoxide can be a serious deterrent to physical activity. For example, research suggests that runners in large metropolitan areas exhibit carbon monoxide levels in the blood that are twice the level necessary to negatively affect performance (Tikuisis, Kane, McLellan, Buick, & Fairburn, 1992).

There are several major air pollutants that can affect sport and physical activity performance. This section will discuss a few of those pollutants and their effects on the body.

Sulphur dioxide is a gaseous byproduct of burning fossil fuels often produced by smelters, refineries, and industrial boilers. The gas itself takes on a yellowish-brown colour and in humans can aggravate heart and lung disease. For the outdoor athlete it can obstruct breathing passages and increase the incidence of colds, asthma, and bronchitis.

Particulates are solid or minute droplets of liquid that are small enough to remain suspended in the air. Fine particles may remain suspended in the air for days or even weeks and may be transported long distances. An example is cigarette smoke. Particulates can irritate the lungs and can carry heavy metals and carcinogenic agents deep into the lungs.

Into Thin Air: Simulating High-Altitude Exposure without Compromising Athletes' Training

Using the latest in mountaineering hardware—a tent that is supplied with reduced amounts of oxygen and can be placed on top of a bed—two University of Calgary exercise physiologists are developing training programs that will allow athletes and mountain climbers to gain the benefits of high-altitude exposure while sleeping in the comfort of their own homes.

"The essential rationale of any altitude exposure is to evoke a response from the kidney to produce erythropoeitin," explains David Smith who, with Stephen Norris, works with Canada's elite athletes and their coaches at the National Sport Centre.

Erythropoeitin, or EPO, is a hormone that stimulates the production of red blood cells, which carry oxygen to the working muscles. Oxygen is vital for muscle cells to produce energy.

The increased ability to carry oxygen is also triggered—to a lesser degree—by physical activity, in turn providing athletes with greater endurance. For athletes normally living at sea level, high-altitude exposure may boost endurance up to an additional 4 to 7 percent. "At the elite level, that's huge," says Smith.

There are approximately 25 altitude training centres around the world at a height of between 1600 and 2500 metres, a range considered best for living and training at altitude for between 12 to 28 days at a time. However, a pitfall of high-altitude training is that it limits how much and how intensely athletes can train, thereby negating the purpose of actual physical training.

"To combat this, a training method has evolved whereby athletes live at high altitude but train at low altitudes," says Smith. "The 'live high–train low' method provides the best of both worlds: an increase of red blood cell production without compromising physical fitness."

Training and high altitude exposure aren't the only way athletes boost their performance. Unfortunately, illegal methods such as "blood doping" (infusing additional blood prior to an athletic event) and "hormonal blood boosting" (injecting synthetic forms of EPO) also enhance performance by increasing the number of red blood cells.

"There has been a lot of controversy in the last years because of the Tour de France scandal [in 1999] where cyclists were injecting EPO," says Smith. "There is not only a move in the international sporting circles to curtail the rampant use of EPO injections because it is unfair and unethical, but also to put in place safe practices that will naturally increase red blood cell production to provide athletes with an alternative."

In 2000, after spending more than 10 years studying how exercise and altitude affect athletic performance, Smith and Norris received generous funding from the Calgary Olympic Development Association that allowed them to purchase an altitude tent and embark on a long-term research project.

Currently, the researchers are working to identify individual response procedures using the altitude tent. "Not everyone responds the same way to altitude and we are trying to understand the reasons for this," says Smith. While genetics may play a role in determining who responds faster, Smith hypothesizes that the training status prior to altitude exposure is also very important; "but we really have no idea at this point, nor do other scientists around the world."

While these programs will certainly benefit some of the elite winter athletes Smith and Norris work with, they are also hoping that high-altitude mountain climbers can use this technology. "By actually acclimatizing in advance in a tent in your own home, you could go straight [to a mountain] and do a climb."

Smith and Norris, who are both professors at the University of Calgary's Faculty of Kinesiology, collaborate with Jon Kolb and sports medicine physician Victor Lund. They also receive technical assistance from Rosie Neil, Jennifer Henderson, Maura Hooper, and Flora Hillis. Their research is funded by the National Sports Centre, the Sports Sciences Association of Alberta, and the Calgary Olympic Development Association.

Source: Diana Rucker, SPARK writer. Rucker is a medical sciences masters student and writer in the University of Calgary's SPARK program (Students Promoting Awareness of Research Knowledge). Courtesy of the University of Calgary. *Gazette 30(24)*, March 19, 2001.

Nitrogen dioxide is an amber-coloured gas that is emitted by coal-powered electrical boilers and automobiles. Low levels can increase a person's susceptibility to colds and flu. It is a precursor of ozone.

Hydrocarbons are multiple chemical compounds that contain different combinations of carbon and hydrogen. Most cars emit hundreds of different types of hydrocarbon compounds. For the individual who likes to engage in outdoor physical activity, hydrocarbons can cause respiratory irritation making it difficult to breathe.

Photochemical smog, a brown, hazy mix of particulates and gases, is a common sight in many urban cities. The haze comes from nitrogen and hydrocarbons reacting to the presence of sunlight. This type of smog is most likely to develop

nitrogen dioxide An amber-coloured gas found in smog.
hydrocarbons Chemical compounds that contain carbon and hydrogen.
photochemical smog The brownish-yellow haze resulting from the combination of hydrocarbons and nitrogen oxides.

on days when there is little wind and high traffic congestion. Most often it occurs in areas that experience a **temperature inversion**, where a cool layer of air is trapped under a layer of warmer air, preventing circulation.

The most noticeable adverse effects are difficulty breathing, burning eyes, headaches, and nausea. It is not recommended that you be active in areas of dense traffic congestion.

Coping with Air Pollution

The best way to minimize the effects of air pollution during physical activity is to limit outdoor activities when ozone or carbon monoxide levels are highest (Figure 11.8). On hot summer days, ozone levels are highest around midday (11 a.m. to 3 p.m.), when the sun's ultraviolet rays are strongest. Limit outdoor activities during this time and also when automobile traffic is heavy. Carbon monoxide levels reach approximately 35 ppm in moving traffic and can exceed 100 ppm in slow and congested conditions (Neiman, 1995). Because these levels can extend 20 to 30 metres away from traffic, the outdoor enthusiast should avoid heavily travelled roads and/or stay at least 30 metres away from the road if possible. Exposure to carbon monoxide (from sitting in traffic with the windows down or being in a smoke-filled room) can be detrimental before physical activity, too, because carbon monoxide leaves the blood so slowly. In fact, the body may require more than 6 hours to remove significant amounts of carbon monoxide from the blood (Neiman, 1995). When in doubt, consult Environment Canada's air quality forecast at **www.msc-smc.cc.qc.ca**.

Remember that air pollution is not always visible. Therefore, you must be aware of the times of day at which various pollutants are in highest concentrations and limit outdoor activities during these times. Pollutants not only affect physical performance; chronic exposure to them is also hazardous to your health. So, don't simply try to avoid pollution; do what you can to reduce pollution in order to have a cleaner environment in which to be active. Walk or take the bus when possible, recycle waste, don't burn leaves or garbage; these are just a few things that we can do to make a better environment in which to live.

Summary

1. Evaporation is the most important means of heat loss during physical activity in a hot environment.
2. Although it is generally safe to be active in a hot environment, consider these guidelines:
   - Start slowly and reduce your total activity time.
   - Adjust your intensity to avoid exceeding your target heart rate.
   - Wear loose, light-coloured clothing.
   - Drink plenty of fluids before, during, and after physical activity.
3. Heat acclimatization occurs after several days of exposure to a hot environment. It results in a greater ability to lose body heat and reduces the likelihood of heat injury.
4. Although long-term physical activity in a cold environment could result in hypothermia, short-term physical activity in a cold environment does not generally pose a serious threat to heat balance.
5. Sport or activity at high altitude results in a reduced amount of oxygen in the arterial blood, which reduces oxygen transport to the working muscles and lowers both VO_2max and physical tolerance.
6. At high altitude, it is necessary to reduce the intensity of physical activity below normal in order to stay within your target heart rate range. However, there is little need to reduce the time or frequency of your training during brief stays at moderate altitudes.
7. There are several major air pollutants that can affect physical activity performance. The best way to minimize effects is to avoid being active during times of the day when pollutants are at their highest.
8. Ozone is produced by a chemical reaction between sunlight and automobile exhaust. Carbon monoxide is produced by the burning of fossil fuels. Both forms of air pollution can impair physical tolerance.
9. The best way to minimize the effects of air pollution during physical activity is to avoid activity when ozone or carbon monoxide levels are highest. Ozone levels are highest during hot summer days. Carbon monoxide levels are highest when automobile traffic is heavy.

temperature inversion A weather condition occurring when a layer of cool air is trapped under a layer of warmer air.

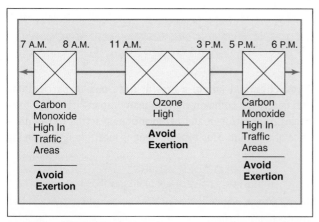

FIGURE 11.8 Times of day to limit outdoor physical activity due to high levels of ozone and carbon monoxide.

Study Questions

1. Define the term *homeotherm*.
2. How is body heat lost during swimming?
3. What is the most important means of heat loss during physical activity in a hot environment?
4. List guidelines for fluid intake during and after physical activity in hot environments.
5. Describe the appropriate clothing for physical activity in hot and cold environments.
6. Outline the major types of heat injury, and list the symptoms of each.
7. Why does physical activity at high altitude result in higher heart rates and increased ventilation compared to the same physical activity performed at sea level?
8. Discuss the effects of air pollution on physical tolerance.
9. What guidelines should you follow to minimize your exposure to air pollution?
10. Define the term *acclimatize*.
11. Distinguish among the terms *ozone, carbon monoxide,* and *particulates*.
12. Describe the difference between *convection* and *evaporation*.
13. Define *temperature inversion*.

Suggested Reading

Burke, L. M. (2001). Nutritional needs for exercise in the heat. *Comparative Biochemistry and Physiology, 128(4),* 735–748.

Fox, E., Bowers, R., & Foss, M. (1997). *The physiological basis for exercise and sport* (6th ed.). Dubuque, IA: Brown and Benchmark.

Maughan, R. J., & Shirreffs, S. M. (1997). Recovery from prolonged exercise: Restoration of water and electrolyte balance. *Journal of Sports Science, 15(3),* 297–303.

Nieman, D. C. (1996). *Fitness and sports medicine: An introduction* (3rd ed.). Palo Alto, CA: Bull Publishing.

Noakes, T. D. (2000). Exercise and the cold. *Ergonomics, 43(10),* 1461– 1479.

Powers, S. K., & Howley, S. M. (2001). *Exercise physiology: Theory and application to fitness and performance* (4th ed.). Dubuque, IA: Brown and Benchmark.

Sawka, M. N., & Montain, S. M. (2000). Fluid and electrolyte supplementation for exercise heat stress. *American Journal of Clinical Nutrition, 72(Suppl),* 564S–572S.

Terrados, N., & Maughan, R. J. (1995). Exercise in the heat: Strategies to minimize the adverse effects on performance. *Journal of Sports Science, 13,* S55–S62.

Weblinks

Environment Canada
www.ns.ec.qc.ca
Lists weather and atmosphere conditions.

Gatorade Sports Science Institute
www.qssiweb.com
Contains many articles related to fluid replacement during exercise; enables visitors to add their names to a mailing list and receive new articles.

Cold Weather Exercise Safety
www.sportsmedicine.com
Presents guidelines for exercise, the treatment of injuries, and cold-weather clothing.

Northern Outfitters
www.northernoutfitters.com
Links to sites for several cold-weather clothing outfitters.

Canadian Medical Association
www.cma.ca
Highlights the latest information for the medical professional.

References

Adir, Y., Merdler, A., Ben Haim, S., Front, A., Harduf, R., & Bitterman, H. (1999). Effects of exposure to low concentrations of carbon monoxide on exercise performance and myocardial perfusion in young healthy men. *Occupational and Environmental Medicine, 56(8),* 535–538.

Brooks, G. A., Fahey, T. D., & White, T. (2000). *Exercise physiology: Human bioenergetics and its applications* (4th ed.). New York: Macmillan, 2000.

Carlisle, A. J., & Sharp, N. C. (2001). Exercise and outdoor ambient air pollution. *British Journal of Sports Medicine, 35(4),* 214–222.

Foss, M. L., & Keteyian, S. J. (2000). *Physiological bases for exercise and sport* (6th ed.). Dubuque, IA: McGraw-Hill.

Irlbeck, D. (1998). Normal mechanisms of heat and moisture exchange in the respiratory tract. *Respiratory Care Clinics of North America, 4(2),* 189–198.

McArdle, W. D., Katch, F. I., & Katch, V. L. (2001). *Exercise physiology: Energy, nutrition, and human performance* (5th ed.). Philadelphia: Lippincott, Williams & Wilkins.

Maughan, R. J., & Shirreffs, S. M. (1997). Recovery from prolonged exercise: Restoration of water and electrolyte balance. *Journal of Sports Science, 15(3),* 297–303.

Nieman, D. C. (1995). *Fitness and sports medicine: An introduction* (3rd ed.). Palo Alto, CA: Bull Publishing.

Paz, C. (1997). Some consequences of ozone exposure on health. *Archives of Medical Research, 28(2),* 163–170.

Pierson, W. E. (1989). Impact of air pollution on athletic performance. *Allergy Proceedings, 10(3),* 209–214.

Thompson, R. L., & Hayward, J. S. (1996). Wet–cold exposure and hypothermia: Thermal and metabolic responses to prolonged exercise in the rain. *Journal of Applied Physiology, 81(3),* 1128–1137.

Tikuisis, P., Kane, D. M., McLellan, T. M., Buick, F., & Fairburn, S. M. (1992). Rate of formation of carboxy-hemoglobin in exercising humans exposed to carbon monoxide. *Journal of Applied Physiology, 72(4),* 1311–1319.

LABORATORY 11.1

Physical Activity in Harsh Environments

Name_____ Age _____ Sex _____ Date _____

DIRECTIONS

Answer the following True-or-False questions related to exercise and the environment. If a statement is false, change it to make it true. You can check your answers against those provided on the next page.

TRUE OR FALSE

_____ 1. Evaporation is the primary means of heat loss during physical activity in a hot environment.

_____ 2. When physically active in a hot, humid environment, you should wear loose, dark-coloured clothing.

_____ 3. Exercise at high altitude results in an increased amount of oxygen in the arterial blood.

_____ 4. At high altitude, it is necessary to reduce the intensity of physical activity to maintain a heart rate within your target heart rate range.

_____ 5. Ozone levels are highest during cool, winter days.

_____ 6. Humans regulate their body temperatures around the set point of 37°C.

_____ 7. Low-intensity physical activity using small muscle groups produces more body heat than high-intensity activities incorporating large muscle groups.

_____ 8. An increase in body temperature during physical activity in a hot environment will result in large increases in heart rate compared with activity in a cool environment.

_____ 9. The strategy for physical activity in the cold is to wear enough clothing to trap just enough heat to maintain body temperature but not overheat.

_____10. Heat injuries are nonfatal conditions that result in cramps and fatigue.

ANSWERS

1. True

2. False: When physically active in a hot, humid environment, you should wear loose, *light-coloured* clothing.

3. False: Physical activity at high altitude results in a *reduced* amount of oxygen in the arterial blood.

4. True

5. False: Ozone levels are highest during *hot, summer* days.

6. True

7. False: *High-intensity physical activities using large muscle groups produces more body heat than low-intensity physical activities incorporating small muscle groups.*

8. True

9. True

10. False: Heat injuries are *serious and can result in damage to the nervous system and, in extreme cases, death.*

SHORT ANSWER

1. If a friend planned to do some physical activity in a warm, high-humidity environment, what advice would you give to him/her to remain safe?

   _____

   _____

   _____

2. What advice would you give to a friend who wanted to do physical activities in a cold climate?

   _____

   _____

   _____

CHAPTER 12

Physical Activity for Special Populations

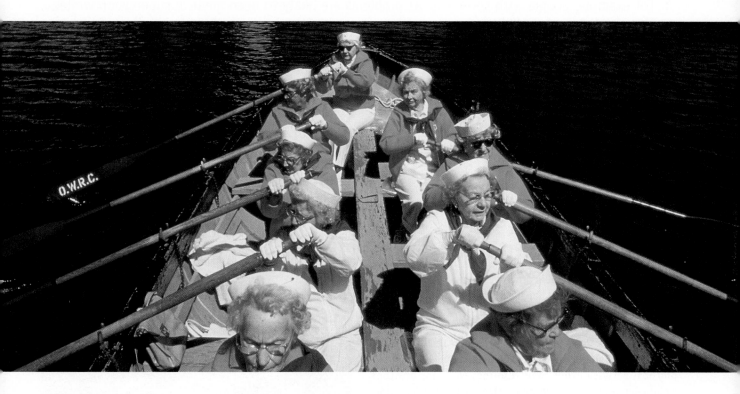

After studying this chapter, you should be able to

1. Describe the factors that should be considered when developing a physical activity program for an individual with orthopedic problems.

2. Outline the physical activity guidelines for an individual who is obese.

3. Describe the physical activity guidelines for individuals with coronary heart disease.

4. Outline the physical activity recommendations for individuals with hypertension.

5. Describe physical activity programs for individuals with type 1 or type 2 diabetes.

6. List the benefits of physical activity for people with asthma.

7. Outline the considerations for starting or maintaining a physical activity program during pregnancy.

8. Describe the physiological changes that accompany aging, and list the general guidelines for maintaining a physically active lifestyle.

Many people with special medical concerns want and need to participate in physical activity. For most of these individuals, it is safe and healthy to be physically active. Although engaging in physical activity may or may not be of direct benefit to the condition in question, in most cases engaging in physical activity benefits the individual by increasing energy levels, increasing stamina, enhancing quality of life, and improving overall wellness.

People with special medical concerns may need to use certain precautions when beginning an exercise or training program. A few conditions necessitate medical supervision during physical activity, and in some conditions exercise may be ill advised. In most instances, the decision to start a program should be made in consultation with a physician.

For example, people with serious heart problems are likely to need medical supervision while exercising. Usually, exercise is performed under the direct supervision of nurses and exercise specialists in a hospital or other institutional setting. In contrast, after consulting with their physicians, individuals with an orthopedic problem (e.g., joint problems) or diabetes often need only modify the "standard" exercise prescription (discussed in Chapter 4).

In this chapter we provide physical activity and exercise guidelines for individuals with some of the more common health concerns. Certainly, a huge variety of special concerns may dictate modification of a physical activity program. If you have special health concerns that are not discussed here, consult your physician before beginning a physical activity or exercise program.

Orthopedic Problems

Individuals with orthopedic problems, such as bone or joint disorders, often need to take special care when designing a physical activity program. The objective is to find a mode of physical activity that uses large muscle groups not associated with the problem area. For example, if the orthopedic problem is in the lower leg, this would mean undertaking physical activity other than running, walking, or other weight-bearing activity. Riding a stationary bicycle, swimming, and using a rowing machine are non–weight-bearing activities that use large muscle groups and are considered excellent for developing aerobic fitness. In addition, the muscles of the upper body and the uninjured leg could undergo resistance training.

Making accommodations to the physical activity program is somewhat easier if the problem is in the arm. In this instance, the individual could incorporate physical activities using the legs as well as the uninjured arm. Because arm movement provides balance in many whole-body activities, it would be wise to select physical activities in which maintenance of balance is not a requirement (e.g., stationary cycling, walking, and stair-climbing).

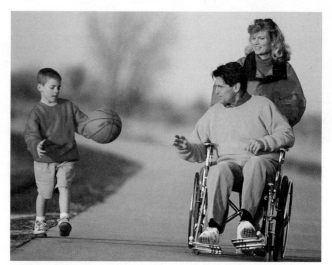

By using alternative modes of physical activity, fitness levels can be maintained even when injury or disability makes physical activity difficult.

Osteoporosis refers to a disease characterized by low bone-mineral density and a deterioration of bone tissue in which bones become fragile or brittle and individuals are at risk of bone fractures (American College of Sports Medicine, 1995). Although men and women are both at risk of osteoporosis and osteoporotic fractures, the prevalence is much greater in women. Thus, in specific regard to prevention of osteoporosis or prevention of osteoporotic fractures, the American College of Sports Medicine Position Stand on Osteoporosis and Exercise (1995) is as follows:

osteoporosis A disease characterized by low bone-mineral density and a deterioration of bone tissue in which bones become fragile or brittle and individuals are at risk of bone fractures.

1. Weight-bearing physical activity is essential for the normal development and maintenance of the human skeleton. Activities that focus on increasing strength may also be beneficial, particularly for non–weight-bearing bones.
2. Sedentary women may increase bone mass slightly by becoming more active but the primary benefit of the increased activity may be in avoiding the further loss of bone that occurs with inactivity.
3. Physical activity cannot be recommended as a substitute for hormone replacement therapy at the time of menopause.
4. The optimal program for older women includes activities that improve strength, flexibility, and coordination, which may indirectly but effectively decrease the incidence of osteoporotic fractures by lessening the likelihood of falling.

Obesity

Exercise prescriptions for individuals who are obese require special attention. For example, in individuals who are obese, limitations are produced by the following conditions: heat intolerance, shortness of breath during heavy physical activity, lack of flexibility, frequent musculoskeletal injuries, and a lack of balance during weight-bearing activities such as walking or running (Fransen, 2004).

Physical activity programs for individuals who are obese should emphasize activities that can be sustained for a longer period of time (30+ minutes), such as walking, swimming, or bicycling. It is important that the type of physical activity chosen is one the individual enjoys (McInnis, 2000). People who are obese should limit physical activities in hot or humid environments. The initial goal should be to increase voluntary energy expenditure and to establish a physically active lifestyle. Therefore, the beginning physical activity intensity should be below the typical target heart rate range for improving cardiorespiratory endurance, and the initial time of activity should be short (about 5 to 10 minutes/day) to reduce the risk of soreness and injury (American College of Sports Medicine, 1998). Time should be gradually increased in 1-minute increments to achieve an energy expenditure of approximately 200 to 300 kcals per workout. As the musculoskeletal system adapts to the activity, the intensity, too, can gradually be increased. Thus, according to the FITT prescription, healthy adults who are overweight or obese are advised to be active at least 3 days per week, preferably on alternating days to permit joint and muscle recuperation and adaptation. The intensity of physical activity should reach 55 to 65 percent of maximal heart rate. Time should start at 5 to 10 minutes and be gradually increased to 30 minutes or more. Finally, the type of physical activity engaged in should be low-impact, enjoyable, and convenient.

Due to decreased stability and mobility in individuals who are overweight and obese, it is important to improve the strength of postural muscles and engage in balance training to reduce their risk of falls (Clark, 2004). A complete overview of balance and strength training for individuals who are obese is presented by Clark (2004) in the Suggested Readings included at the end of the chapter.

Coronary Heart Disease

Coronary heart disease is the major disease of the cardiovascular system. It is discussed in detail in Chapter 14. In brief, **coronary heart disease** is the result of plaque causing a blockage or reduction in blood flow in the blood vessels supplying the heart. Physical activity and, more specifically, exercise training can improve functional capacity and reduce the clinical symptoms in individuals with coronary heart disease (American College of Sports Medicine, 1994). Given the variation in individuals with coronary heart disease, it is not possible to provide a generic exercise prescription. Thus, it is the position of the American College of Sports Medicine that individuals with coronary heart disease should consult their physicians for individually designed physical activity programs (American College of Sports Medicine, 1994).

Hypertension

Hypertension refers to abnormally high blood pressure. It is discussed in detail in Chapter 14. Physical activity is an integral component of the prevention, treatment, and control of hypertension (Pescatello et al., 2004). Using the FITT prescription, healthy individuals with hypertension should engage in moderate-intensity (40 to 60 percent of aerobic capacity) endurance physical activities for 30 minutes or more on most, preferably all, days of the week (Pescatello et al., 2004). It is also recommended that individuals who are hypertensive supplement their endurance activities with resistance training.

Diabetes

Diabetes is a metabolic disorder characterized by high blood-glucose levels. Diabetes is often associated with complications of the cardiovascular, renal, neurologic, and ophthalmologic systems (James, Young, Mustard, & Blanchard, 1997). In fact, diabetes is one of the leading causes of death in Canada, and its incidence is increasing (Chen & Millar, 2000).

coronary heart disease   The result of plaque forming a blockage in one or more coronary arteries.

hypertension   Abnormally high blood pressure.

There are two types of diabetes. **Type 1 diabetes** usually occurs in the young and is due to abnormally low levels of the hormone insulin; it is also called *insulin-dependent diabetes*. The cause of this type of diabetes is thought to be the immune system's destruction of the cells in the pancreas that produce insulin. **Type 2 diabetes** often occurs in obese, sedentary, middle-aged adults due to a reduction in the ability of insulin to transport glucose from the blood into cells. This form of diabetes generally is due to the lack of sensitivity of the cells to the action of insulin. Although the specific cause is not known, it is clear that obesity increases the severity of the disease (Steyn et al., 2004). Because individuals with type 2 diabetes generally do not have problems producing insulin, they generally do not require insulin treatment and so their condition is also referred to as *non–insulin-dependent diabetes*. This type of diabetes also has been referred to as *adult-onset diabetes* because it primarily affected adults. However, this is no longer the case, as many adolescents who are obese are now being diagnosed.

The three most important tools for managing diabetes are dietary intake, physical activity, and insulin (Ryan, 2000; Steyn et al., 2004). It is estimated that 90 percent of type 2 diabetes cases can be prevented by eating well and engaging in physical activity (Ryan, 2000; Tudor-Locke, Bell, & Meyers, 2000). There is great motivation to use dietary intake and physical activity to control blood glucose because of the considerable trouble, expense, and even danger associated with taking insulin. The danger is associated with the possibility of taking too much, which could result in a coma. Moreover, individuals with diabetes who take oral medication to control blood glucose are at increased risk of cardiovascular disease (Ruderman, Devlin, & Schneider, 2001).

Physical activity benefits individuals with diabetes in four major ways. First, engaging in physical activity may help control blood glucose in individuals with type 2 diabetes by improving the transport of glucose into cells, which also reduces insulin requirements. Although this effect has been thought to last only a short time after physical activity, mounting evidence suggests that the effect may be long-lasting for individuals with type 2 diabetes (Kelley & Goodpaster, 2001). The roles of dietary intake and physical activity in controlling blood glucose are briefly discussed in the Nutritional Links to Health and Fitness box opposite.

Second, the greatest benefit of physical activity to individuals with diabetes may be that it helps in controlling body weight (Tudor-Locke et al., 2000; Steyn et al., 2004). One of the single most important objectives for individuals with diabetes is not to become obese, because this leads to higher blood glucose levels, increased blood lipids, and elevated blood pressure. If an obese person with diabetes loses weight, glucose levels may return to normal without taking insulin or oral hypoglycemic drugs (Steyn et al., 2004). Obviously, physical activity can play an important role in weight management for individuals with diabetes.

Third, individuals with diabetes are at high risk for heart disease. A lack of physical activity is considered a primary risk factor for heart disease, as noted in Chapter 14. Because regular physical activity leads to reduced blood pressure, total cholesterol, LDLs, and triglycerides, and to increased HDLs in individuals with diabetes who are obese (McGavock et al., 2004), the importance of physical activity in lowering their risk of heart disease cannot be overlooked.

Last, but certainly not least, regular physical activity results in many psychological and social benefits that enhance the daily lives of individuals with diabetes (Wing et al., 2001). Improvements in self-confidence, self-control, self-esteem, vigour, and wellness in general are especially important.

The guidelines for developing exercise prescriptions differ for the two categories of diabetes. Each is examined separately.

Physical Activity for Individuals with Type 1 Diabetes

Before engaging in physical activity, individuals with type 1 diabetes must work with a physician to learn to manage resting blood glucose levels. This is important because physical activity, like insulin, acts to lower blood glucose (Kelley & Goodpaster, 2001). Indeed, the combination of physical activity and insulin can produce low blood glucose levels, which can lead to seizures or loss of consciousness.

Generally, individuals with type 1 diabetes can participate in the same activities as individuals without diabetes. The recommended training intensity for individuals with type 1 diabetes is identical to the recommended values for healthy individuals (Chapters 4 to 6). However, physical activity should be performed daily so a regular pattern can be established for glucose control. The daily physical activity time should be only 20 to 30 minutes. The following guidelines should be considered when becoming physically active:

- Get a thorough medical examination, and tell your physician about your plans to engage in physical activity.
- Be active with a partner.
- Use footwear designed for the planned activity, and maintain good foot hygiene.
- Consume a meal 1 to 3 hours prior to the activity.

type 1 diabetes   Also called *insulin-dependent diabetes*; a result of abnormally low levels of insulin.

type 2 diabetes   Also called *non–insulin-dependent diabetes* or *adult-onset diabetes*; a result of a reduced ability of insulin to transport glucose from the blood to the cells.

- Consume a snack composed of complex carbohydrates after the activity.
- If so advised by your physician, reduce your insulin dose before the activity. (The amount will depend on the type of insulin you take and the amount of physical activity you do.)
- Avoid using the muscle in which a short-acting insulin injection was given.
- Avoid late-evening physical activities, because while you are asleep you cannot monitor any physical activity-induced changes in blood glucose.
- Monitor blood glucose before, during, and after physical activity.
- Carefully monitor how your blood glucose responds to different forms of physical activity.

Physical Activity for Individuals with Type 2 Diabetes

The most important factor for individuals with type 2 diabetes is the length or time of the activities. Because one of the major objectives of physical activity for those with type 2 diabetes is assisting in the reduction of body fat, the recommended physical activity time is longer than that for individuals with type 1 diabetes. It is generally short initially (5 to 10 minutes/day) and gradually increases over a period of weeks, reaching a total workout time of 60 minutes/session (Albright et al., 2000). The frequency of physical activity should be increased gradually from 3 to 5 days per week in an effort to maximize energy expenditure and promote weight loss. Because of the long duration and relatively high frequency of physical activity, individuals with type 2 diabetes should maintain a physical activity intensity near the lower end of the target range (40 to 60 percent of aerobic capacity) to reduce the risk of injury (Ruderman et al., 2001; Tudor-Locke et al., 2000).

Asthma

Asthma is a condition that reduces the size of the airways leading to the lungs and often results in sudden difficulty in breathing. It is triggered by a number of factors, including air pollution, pollen, and physical activity. The incidence of asthma is on the rise (especially in children). Although solid evidence is lacking, this increased incidence may result from the presence of mould, mildew, and pollutants in indoor air. Fortunately, asthma can be controlled by proper medication.

It is generally agreed that individuals with asthma can safely participate in all types of physical activity. However, a prerequisite for physical activity is a proper medication program to control it (Storms, 2003). Once the asthma is under control, the exercise prescription is identical to those for individuals without asthma. However, a wise precaution is to be physically active with others and keep medication (an inhaler) handy when active in case of a sudden asthma attack.

The following guidelines should be followed by individuals with asthma who are beginning a physical activity program.

- Work with your personal physician to develop the proper medical protocol to control your asthma.
- Be physically active with a partner or a group, not on your own.
- Limit physical activity in cold weather.
- Carry your inhaler when you are physically active.

asthma   A condition that reduces the size of the airways leading to the lungs; it can result in a sudden difficulty in breathing.

NUTRITIONAL LINKS TO HEALTH AND FITNESS

The Roles of Dietary Intake and Physical Activity in Controlling Blood Glucose

The interaction between the types and amounts of macronutrients in the diet and the type and amount of physical activity greatly influences the level of glucose in the blood. Both physical activity and the hormone insulin have the effect of removing glucose from the blood and getting it into working muscle cells.

Whereas individuals without diabetes on a normal diet need not be concerned about blood glucose levels during physical activity, individuals with diabetes about to be physically active must be concerned with the amount and type of micronutrients they have eaten. Among the three major macronutrients, carbohydrates affect blood glucose levels most dramatically. Moreover, because physi-

cal activity reinforces the action of insulin in clearing the blood of glucose (Ryan, 2000), individuals with diabetes must learn how different types of physical activity affect blood glucose levels. Individuals with diabetes who fail to recognize the effects of various types of physical activity on their blood glucose levels run the risk of lowering those levels so much that they become lethargic and disoriented and appear drunk. Thus, the primary goal of a physical activity program for the person with diabetes is to try different types of physical activity and determine the effects on blood glucose. In this way, the individual can learn to manage blood glucose levels and keep blood glucose in a safe range.

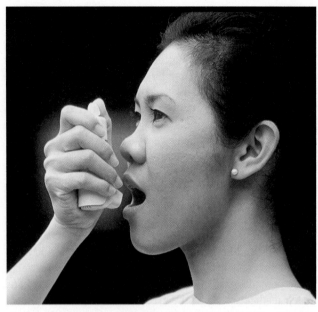

Physical activity can be safe and healthy for individuals with asthma if they take the proper precautions.

- Limit physical activity in polluted environments; properly filtered indoor air may be preferable to outdoor air.

Pregnancy

Can women safely engage in physical activity during a normal pregnancy? The answer is generally yes, but the decision to be physically active during pregnancy must be made by each woman after consultation with her physician. To date, most evidence suggests that physical activity does not pose a serious risk to the health of the fetus or the mother (Davies, Wolfe, Mottola, & MacKinnon, 2003). It is recommended that the Physical Activity Readiness Medical Examination for Pregnancy (PARmed-X for Pregnancy), a questionnaire developed by the Canadian Society for Exercise Physiology and endorsed by the Society of Obstetricians and Gynaecologists of Canada and Health Canada, be used by pregnant women and their practitioners as a screening tool (Physical Activity Readiness Medical Examination for Pregnancy, 2002). Included in the PARmed-X for Pregnancy are practical prescriptions for engaging in cardiovascular and strength training activities.

The guidelines listed below should be followed by women engaging in physical activity during pregnancy. See also Chapter 16 for more suggestions.

- Consult your physician and complete the PARmed-X for pregnancy.
- Do not increase the amount of physical activity you typically performed before your pregnancy.
- Do not participate in sports that have a high risk of injury (e.g., contact sports).

- Limit physical activities that require lying on the back to 5 minutes. The weight of the fetus may reduce blood flow through vessels supplying blood to the lower extremities.
- Limit physical activities that place major importance on balance, such as dancing or treadmill walking.
- In the final 3 months of the pregnancy, limit activities that use quick, jerking movements because they may cause joint strains.
- Wear good supportive footwear and adequate breast support.
- Limit physical activity in the heat. Remember: the primary dangers of physical activity during pregnancy are elevated body temperature and lack of blood flow to the baby. Because water removes heat from the body better than air, aquatic activities are an excellent means of preventing large gains in body heat.
- Monitor your pulse and remain at the low end of your target heart rate zone. Don't exceed 140 beats/minute.
- Concentrate on non–weight-bearing physical activities such as cycling or swimming.
- Drink plenty of fluids.
- Stop immediately and call your doctor if you experience any of the following: shortness of breath, dizziness, numbness, tingling, abdominal pain, or vaginal bleeding.

Aging

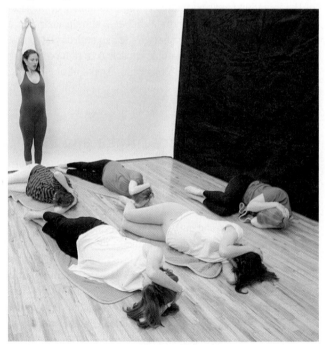

Physical activity can be beneficial for the mother and the developing fetus.

Throughout this text we have focused on young individuals (about 18 to 25 years of age). In this section we shift our focus to considering physical activity for older individuals. Who are the elderly? Usually, the defining age for elderly is considered to be 65, because this is the age when retirement and old age pension benefits begin. However, when considering physiological capacity, we cannot equate ability with age. Many individuals above 65 years of age have the physical capacity of people one-third their age, and their number is growing.

Everyone experiences a significant decline in VO_2max with age (Figure 12.1). However, recent research has shown that older individuals engaging in a regular program of vigorous physical activity can maintain the aerobic capacity of someone one-third their age (Spirduso & Cronin, 2001). Note in Figure 12.1 that a 75-year-old individual may have the aerobic capacity of a 25-year-old!

Although this may seem like a new idea, the adaptability of the human body has been known for centuries. About 400 B.C., Hippocrates said,

> All parts of the body which have a function, if used in moderation and exercised in labours in which each is accustomed, become thereby healthy, well-developed and age more slowly, but if unused and left idle they become liable to disease, defective in growth, and age quickly.

Obviously, the normal biological changes that take place during aging are inevitable. However, recent scientific evidence suggests that an active lifestyle can delay the aging process and result in a longer, healthier, and happier life (Vandervoot & Symons, 2001).

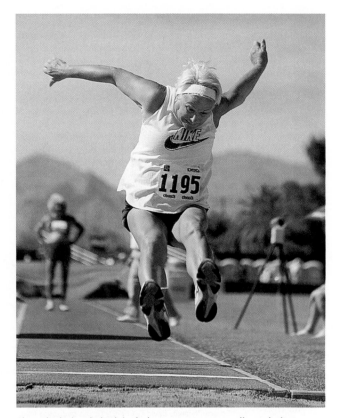

Chronological and physiological age are not necessarily equivalent.

Physiological Changes with Aging

Aging results in a gradual decline in biological function. Many of the age-related changes in the body begin to appear between the ages of 30 and 40 (Vandervoot & Symons, 2001). As illustrated in Figure 12.2, the physiological changes that accompany aging are similar to those seen with inactivity or the prolonged weightlessness experienced by astronauts.

The most common functional changes with aging are decreased cardiorespiratory function, increased body fat, and elevated musculoskeletal fragility (Vandervoot & Symons, 2001). What causes these age-related changes? Interestingly, approximately one-half of the decline in functional capacity is due to a decrease in physical activity (Vandervoot & Symons, 2001). Physical activity decreases with age through the adult years, to the extent that the majority of older adults are not obtaining sufficient physical activity to obtain health benefits. Therefore, regular physical activity including cardiovascular and strength training activities may improve cardiorespiratory function (Mazzeo et al., 1998), delay the age-related degradation of lean body mass (Tarpenning, Hamilton-Wessler, Wiswell, & Hawkins, 2004), assist in maintaining a favourable percentage body fat (Chilibeck et al., 2002), maintain the mineral content of bone during the aging process, and assist in managing the symptoms associated with menopause (O'Brien, Cousins, & Edwards, 2002).

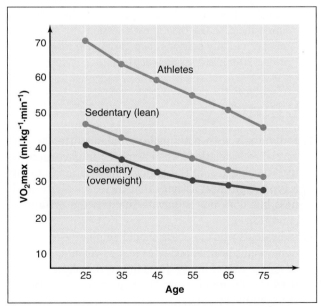

FIGURE 12.1 Changes in VO_2max with advancing age. A decline of approximately 10 percent per decade occurs after age 25.

Source: Neiman, David C. (1995). *Fitness and sports medicine: A health-related approach.* Palo Alto, CA: Bull Publishing Co. Reprinted with permission.

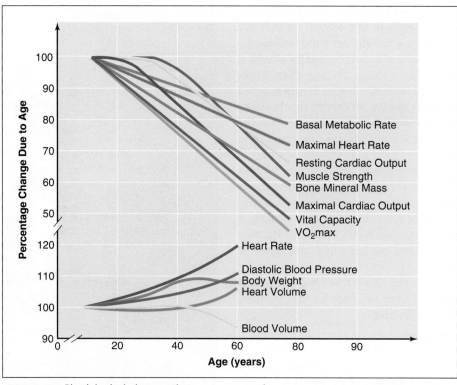

FIGURE 12.2 Physiological changes that accompany aging.

Source: Neiman, David C. (1995). *Fitness and sports medicine: A health-related approach.* Palo Alto, CA: Bull Publishing Co. Reprinted with permission.

Guidelines for Physical Activity

It is important for everyone to remain physically active. However, older individuals should seek advice from their physicians and limit physical activities that present a high risk of orthopedic problems. Activities such as walking, cycling, swimming, and light resistance training are generally recommended. When designing an exercise prescription for older individuals, the basic principles for the development of fitness apply (Chapter 3). The following guidelines outline some specific considerations for men older than 40 years and women older than 50 years.

- Due to the risks of heart disease associated with age, a physician-supervised, graded exercise stress test is recommended before engaging in any vigorous physical activity program.

- Non–weight-bearing activities are recommended to reduce the risk of musculoskeletal problems. Weight-bearing activities are beneficial, particularly for maintaining bone–mineral density, but should be performed with balance support to avoid falls.

- Physical activity intensity should be at the lower end of the target heart rate range.

- The time of physical activities should be modified to meet the needs (and abilities) of each individual. For example, in the beginning stages it is likely that many

unconditioned elderly individuals cannot engage in physical activity for more than 5 to 10 minutes per session. In this case, individuals may exercise several times per day for short durations (three 10-minute sessions/day). As the individual progresses, he or she can slowly increase the time of each session and reduce the number of daily sessions (two 15-minute sessions/day or one 30-minute session/day).

Summary

1. Individuals with orthopedic problems often require special considerations when engaging in physical activity. The objective of the exercise prescription is to find a type of physical activity that increases physical fitness but does not aggravate the existing orthopedic condition.

2. Individuals who are obese should emphasize the use of non–weight-bearing activities (e.g., swimming, cycling) to reduce risk of injury. In addition, the physical activities should be of lower than normal intensity and engaged in for 30+ minutes.

3. Given the variation in severity and prognosis in individuals with coronary heart disease, these individuals require an individualized prescription for their physical activities.

4. Individuals with hypertension are recommended to do moderate-intensity physical activities for 30 or more minutes on a daily basis.

5. Type 1 diabetes is a result of a deficiency in the amount of insulin in the body. Type 2 diabetes is a result of the ineffectiveness of insulin in the body. The role of insulin in the body is to transfer glucose from the blood into the cells.

6. The key to developing a sound program for individuals with type 1 diabetes is learning how to manage blood glucose levels during physical activity. If blood glucose can be managed, individuals with diabetes can participate in the same physical activities as individuals without.

7. Only minor differences exist between the exercise guidelines for individuals with type 1 or type 2 diabetes. The most important difference is that individuals with type 2 diabetes can generally participate in longer physical activity sessions.

8. Asthma is a condition that results in a sudden reduction in the size of the airways. If their asthma is medically controlled, individuals can safely participate in physical activities.

9. Pregnancy need not prevent women from being physically active. Physical activity can be beneficial for the mother and poses little risk for the fetus.

10. Aging is a slow, gradual decline in biological function. The most common functional changes seen with aging and inactivity are decreased cardiorespiratory function, reduced lean body mass, increased body fat, and musculoskeletal fragility. Approximately one-half the decline in functional capacity observed with aging is due to a decrease in physical activity.

Study Questions

1. What type of physical activities may be prescribed for an individual with an orthopedic problem in the lower extremity? The upper extremities? The back?

2. List the problems likely to be encountered by an individual who is obese and becomes physically active.

3. How does physical activity benefit someone with coronary heart disease?

4. Compare and contrast the FITT principles for an individual with hypertension to a healthy adult.

5. Distinguish between type 1 and type 2 diabetes.

6. Contrast the special guidelines to be followed by individuals with type 1 and type 2 diabetes who wish to become physically active.

7. What special considerations should be taken by an individual with asthma who is physically active?

8. List the guidelines to be followed for starting or maintaining physical activity during pregnancy.

9. List the primary physiological changes seen with aging.

10. List the guidelines for establishing a fitness program for an older individual.

Suggested Reading

American College of Sports Medicine. (1994). Position stand: Exercise for patients with coronary heart disease. *Medicine and Science in Sports and Exercise, 26(3),* i–v.

American College of Sports Medicine. (1995). Position stand: Osteoporosis and exercise. *Medicine and Science in Sports and Exercise, 27(4),* i– ii.

American College of Sports Medicine. (1998). Position stand: Exercise and physical activity for older adults. *Medicine and Science in Sports and Exercise, 30(6),* 992–1008.

American College of Sports Medicine. (2000). Position stand: Exercise and type II diabetes. *Medicine and Science in Sports and Exercise, 32(7),* 1345–1360.

American College of Sports Medicine. (2004). Position stand: Exercise and hypertension. *Medicine and Science in Sports and Exercise, 36(3),* 533–553.

Bouchard, C. (2000). *Physical activity and obesity.* Champaign, IL: Human Kinetics.

Clark, C. J., & Cochrane, L. M. (1999). Physical activity and asthma. *Current Opinion in Pulmonary Medicine, 5(1),* 68–75.

Clark, K. N. (2004). Balance and strength training for obese individuals. *ACSM's Health & Fitness Journal, 8(1),* 14–20.

Davies, G. A. L., Wolfe, L. A., Mottola, M. F., & MacKinnon, C. (2003). Joint SOGC/CSEP clinical practice guideline: Exercise in pregnancy and the postpartum period. *Canadian Journal of Applied Physiology, 28(3),* 329–341.

Physical Activity Readiness Medical Examination for Pregnancy [PARmed-X for Pregnancy]. (2002). Ottawa: Canadian Society for Exercise Physiology. Available online at www.csep.ca/forms.asp.

Sato, Y. (2000). Diabetes and life-styles: Role of physical exercise for primary prevention. *British Journal of Nutrition, 84 (Suppl 2),* S187–S190.

Spirduso, W. W., & Cronin, D. L. (2001). Exercise dose–response effects on quality of life and independent living in older adults. *Medicine and Science in Sports and Exercise, 33 (Suppl 6),* S598–S608.

Weblinks

Canadian Association for the Advancement of Women in Sport and Physical Activity

www.caaws.ca

Includes information on physical activity and exercise for women of all ages.

Canadian Society for Exercise Physiology

www.csep.ca

Includes information on physical activity and exercise for various special populations.

Health Canada
Includes information on specific health conditions (e.g. type 1 and 2 diabetes, coronary heart disease, hypertension, and asthma).

References

Albright, A., Franz, M., Hornsby, G., Kriska, A., Marrero, D., Ullrich, I., & Verity, L. S. (2000). American College of Sports Medicine position stand on exercise and type II diabetes. *Medicine and Science in Sports and Exercise, 32(7)*, 1345–1360.

American College of Sports Medicine. (1994). Position stand: Exercise for patients with coronary heart disease. *Medicine and Science in Sports and Exercise, 26(3)*, i–v.

American College of Sports Medicine. (1995). Position stand: Osteoporosis and exercise. *Medicine and Science in Sports and Exercise, 27(4)*, i–vii.

American College of Sports Medicine. (1998). Position stand: The recommended quantity and quality of exercise for developing and maintaining cardiorespiratory and muscular fitness, and flexibility in healthy adults. *Medicine and Science in Sports and Exercise, 30*, 975–991.

Chen, J., & Millar, W. J. (2000). Are recent cohorts healthier than their predecessors? *Health Reports, 11(4)*, 9–23. Catalogue No. 82-003.

Chilibeck, P. D., Davison, K. S., Whiting, S. J., Suzuki, Y., Janzen, C. L., & Peloso, P. (2002). The effect of strength training combined with bisphosphonate (etidronate) therapy on bone mineral, lean tissue, and fat mass in postmenopausal women. *Canadian Journal of Physiology and Pharmacology, 80(10)*, 941–950.

Clark, K. N. (2004). Balance and strength training for obese individuals. *ACSM's Health & Fitness Journal, 8(1)*, 14–20.

Davies, G. A. L., Wolfe, L. A., Mottola, M. F., & MacKinnon, C. (2003). Joint SOGC/CSEP clinical practice guideline: Exercise in pregnancy and the postpartum period. *Canadian Journal of Applied Physiology, 28(3)*, 329–341.

Fransen, M. (2004). Dietary weight loss and exercise for obese adults with knee osteoarthritis: Modest weight loss targets, mild exercise, modest effects. *Arthritis and Rheumatology, 50(5)*, 1366–1369.

James, R., Young, T. K., Mustard, C. A., & Blanchard, J. (1997). The health of Canadians with diabetes. *Health Reports, 9(3)*, 47–52. Catalogue No. 82-003-XPB.

Kelley, D. E., & Goodpaster, B. H. (2001). Effects of exercise on glucose homeostasis in type II diabetes mellitus. *Medicine and Science in Sports and Exercise, 33(6 Suppl)*, S495–S501.

Mazzeo, R. S., Cavanagh, P., Evans, W. J., Fiatarone, M., Hegberg, J., McAuley, E., & Startzell, J. (1998). American College of Sports Medicine position stand on exercise and physical activity for the older adult. *Medicine and Science in Sports and Exercise, 30(3)*, 992–1008.

McGavock, J. M., Eves, N. D., Mandic, S., Glenn, N. M., Quinney, H. A., and Haykowsky, M. J. (2004). The role of exercise in the treatment of cardiovascular disease associated with type 2 diabetes mellitus. *Sports Medicine, 34(1)*, 27–48.

McInnis, K. J. (2000). Exercise for obese clients: Benefits, limitations, guidelines. *ACSM's Health & Fitness Journal, 4(1)*, 25–31.

O'Brien Cousins, S., & Edwards, K. (2002). Alice in menopauseland: The jabberwocky of a medicalized middle age. *Health Care Women International, 23(4)*, 325–343.

Pescatello, L. S., Franklin, B. A., Fagard, R., Farquhar, W. B., Kelley, G. A., & Ray, C. A. (2004). American College of Sports Medicine position stand: Exercise and hypertension. *Medicine and Science in Sports and Exercise, 36(3)*, 533–553.

Physical Activity Readiness Medical Examination for Pregnancy [PARmed-X for Pregnancy]. (2002). Ottawa: Canadian Society for Exercise Physiology. Available online at www.csep.ca/forms.asp.

Ruderman, N. D., Devlin, J., & Schneider, S. (2001). *Handbook of exercise in diabetes*. Alexandria, VA: American Diabetes Association.

Ryan, A. S. (2000). Insulin resistance with aging: Effects of diet and exercise. *Sports Medicine, 30(5)*, 327–346.

Spirduso, W. W., & Cronin, D. L. (2001). Exercise dose–response effects on quality of life and independent living in older adults. *Medicine and Science in Sports and Exercise, 33(6 Suppl)*, S598–S608.

Steyn, N. P., Mann, J., Bennett, P. H., Temple, N., Zimmet, P., Tuomilehto, J., Lindstrom, J., & Louheranta, A. (2004). Diet, nutrition and the prevention of type 2 diabetes. *Public Health and Nutrition, 7(1A)*, 147–165.

Storms, W. W. (2003). Review of exercise-induced asthma. *Medicine and Science in Sports Exercise, 35(9)*, 1464–1470.

Tarpenning, K. M., Hamilton-Wessler, M., Wiswell, R. A., & Hawkins, S. A. (2004). Endurance training delays age of decline in muscle strength and muscle morphology. *Medicine and Science in Sports and Exercise, 36(1)*, 74–78.

Tudor-Locke, C. E., Bell, R. C., & Meyers, A. M. (2000). Revisiting the role of physical activity and exercise in the treatment of type II diabetes. *Canadian Journal of Applied Physiology, 25(6)*, 466–492.

Vandervoot, A. A., & Symons, T. B. (2001). Functional and metabolic consequences of sacropenia. *Canadian Journal of Applied Physiology, 26(1)*, 90–101.

Wing, R. R., Goldstein, M. G., Acton, K. J., Birch, L. L., Jakicic, J. M., Sallis, J. F., Smith-West, D., Jeffery, R. W., & Surwit, R. S. (2001). Behavior science research in diabetes: Lifestyle changes related to obesity, eating behavior, and physical activity. *Diabetes Care, 24(1)*, 117–123.

Prevention and Rehabilitation of Physical Activity–Related Injuries

13

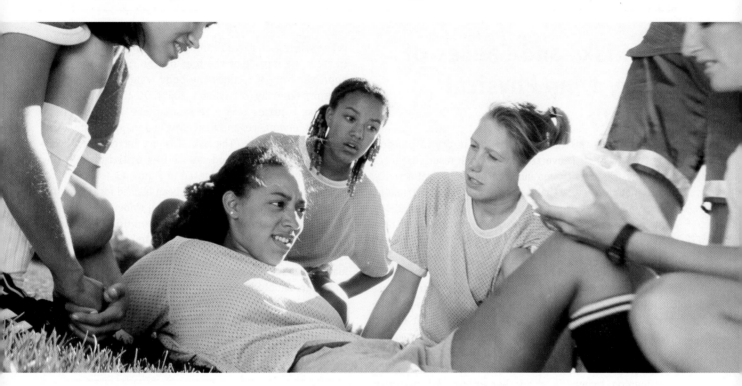

After studying this chapter, you should be able to

1. Identify the role of overtraining in increasing the risk of physical activity–related injury.

2. List the signs and symptoms of overtraining.

3. Outline the major reasons why high-impact activities result in injury and suggest methods to reduce the risk of injury when engaging in high-impact activities.

4. Explain acute and delayed-onset muscle soreness.

5. Outline possible causes of muscle strains and ways in which they can be avoided.

6. Define *tendonitis,* and discuss how it should be treated.

7. Describe ligament sprains and how to avoid them.

8. Describe the most common injuries to the lower extremities.

9. Outline the general guidelines for the treatment of injuries.

10. Define *cryokinetics,* and discuss its use in the rehabilitation process.

In the quest for physical fitness many people abide by the old adage "No pain, no gain." The problem with this approach is that excessive or improper physical activity increases the risk of injury to joints, muscles, tendons, and ligaments. Bone and soft-tissue injuries are painful and result in lost activity time. Many people begin a physical activity program with unrealistic expectations, do too much too quickly, and as a result suffer with sore muscles and joints.

Although most physical activity–related injuries can be prevented, almost everyone who engages in regular physical activity is going to experience one or more injuries during his or her lifetime. In this chapter we discuss the causes, prevention, and treatment of physical activity–related injuries.

The Risks and Causes of Injury from Physical Activity

There are many risk factors related to injury in physical activity. One factor is **overtraining**, which results from too much physical activity, too much intense physical activity, or not enough recovery time between workouts. Overtraining results in a deterioration in performance (Lac & Maso, 2004). Signs of overtraining include increased resting heart rate, reduced appetite, weight loss, irritability, disturbed sleep, elevated blood pressure, frequent injuries, increased incidence of colds and flu, and chronic fatigue (Lac & Maso, 2004).

To prevent overtraining, a good guideline is to increase the intensity or time of your training no more than 10 to 15 percent each week (Dufek, 2002). In addition, it is suggested that you vary the type of physical activities you do (called *cross training*). For example, if you normally cycle 3 to 4 days per week, you could replace one day of cycling with jogging, swimming, or another activity. Alternatively, you could incorporate within-activity cross training (Dufek, 2002). In the case of swimming, you could vary the stroke you use; in running, you could use different terrains (hills, flat surface, beach, etc.). Listen to your body, and if you notice any overtraining signs or symptoms reduce the intensity or time of your physical activities and increase your rest time. Avoidance of overtraining can greatly reduce your chance of injury and help you maintain a positive attitude about physical activity and physical fitness.

It is estimated that between 27 and 70 percent of individuals who run sustain at least one injury per year from running (Hreljac, Marshall, & Hume, 2000). Many of those injuries involve the hip, back, foot, and knee. One of the major factors responsible for this type and number of injuries

is the severity of stress running places on the legs and feet. In fact, the impact of the foot on the running surface is approximately 2.5 times the body weight of the runner (Murphy, Connolly, & Beynnon, 2003). Other potential causes of these injuries relate to inadequate development of strength, endurance, and flexibility, and inappropriate warm-ups and cool-downs. The risk of injury increases with distance, frequency, speed, as well as utilizing improper stretching techniques, as noted in Figure 13.1.

Although many factors have been blamed for the injuries runners encounter, there is convincing evidence that only a few play a significant role in causing injuries. The factors most closely correlated with running injuries are improper training techniques, inadequate shoes, and alignment abnormalities in the legs and feet (Hreljac et al., 2000). Although all factors should be considered, the most important factor seems to be improper training techniques; they account for two-thirds of all injuries (Duffey, Martin, Cannon, Craven, & Messier, 2000).

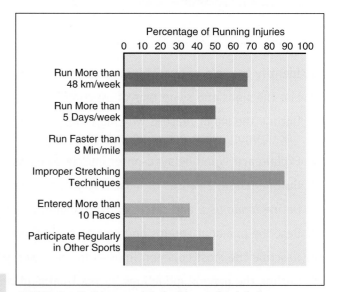

FIGURE 13.1 Factors associated with running injuries.

Source: Neiman, D. C. (1995). *Fitness and sports medicine: An introduction*, 3rd ed. Palo Alto, CA: Bull Publishing Co., 1995. Reprinted with permission.

overtraining A phenomenon in which too much physical activity and not enough recovery time results in injuries.

The Role of Nutrition in Repair of Physical Activity–Induced Injuries

Nutrition may be important to the repair of physical activity–induced injuries in at least two ways. First, repair of damaged muscle involves synthesizing new muscle fibres (to replace damaged fibres removed by the body's repair systems), and this growth process requires an individual's dietary intake of protein to contain sufficient amino acids to act as the building blocks for the new fibres. This does *not* mean that supplemental dietary protein is required to repair damaged muscle adequately. You will have enough protein for repairing damaged muscle by simply following the dietary guidelines discussed in Chapter 7.

The second way that nutrition may affect the repair of injury involves the role of antioxidants in minimizing the extent of injury-induced damage. Immediately after an injury, a variety of chemicals are released in the injured area. Among them are free radicals and various substances that cause inflammation—which, in preparing the area for eventual rebuilding, causes additional tissue destruction. Antioxidants may play a role in limiting the extent of injury by acting as a scavenger of the free radicals released during the injury and the early stages of the repair process.

Although much more research is needed in this area to understand the role of nutrition in the repair of injury, one thing is clear: it is obviously wise to ensure that you consume the DRI of vitamins and minerals each and every day.

Although little can be done about some alignment abnormalities in the legs and feet, a change in shoes can help prevent injury in many cases. A decrease in injuries is often noted after changing to shoes that increase the cushioning and support for the arch of the foot. The use of shoes specially designed for running also reduces injuries.

Since aerobics became popular in the early 1970s, fitness classes have been associated with high rates of injury. From its original form consisting of routines combining dance and calisthenic-type exercises, aerobics has evolved into specialized programs such as water aerobics, low-impact aerobics, step aerobics, and specific dance aerobics. Approximately one-half of all participants in traditional aerobic fitness classes report injuries (Macintyre & Joy, 2000), which occur at a rate of approximately one injury per 100 hours of activity. Further, aerobic fitness class instructors experience approximately twice the rate of injuries of their in-class participants (Francis, Francis, & Welshone-Smith, 1985). One study found that more than three sessions per week, improper shoes, and nonresilient surfaces were the primary causes of injury (Macintyre & Joy, 2000).

Thus, improper training techniques (e.g., excessive distance or duration) are the major causes of injuries. High-volume training such as excessive distance or duration may cause wear to tissues, such as connective tissue in joints. For a brief discussion of the role of nutrition in repair of physical activity–induced injuries, see the Nutritional Links to Health and Fitness box above.

Common Injuries: Cause and Prevention

Although many injuries can occur as a result of physical activity, some are more common than others. This section discusses the cause and prevention of many general types of injuries associated with physical activity, exercise, or sport.

Back Pain

Cause One of the most important health concerns in Canada is back pain. In fact, back pain is the second most common reason for needing to see a physician. Further, most people who experience back pain will experience that pain again. Among the many causes of back pain are improper lifting techniques, weak muscles, poor posture, and bone disorders (Table 13.1). Treatments include painkillers, muscle relaxants, anti-inflammatory drugs, bracing, traction, bed rest, surgery, and therapeutic exercises. Even without any form of treatment, approximately 80 percent of back patients recover spontaneously (Devereaux, 2004). Thus, it is not clear whether the treatments for back pain only serve to lessen the pain or are in fact beneficial in speeding recovery.

In most cases, back pain is preventable. A knowledge of the following factors, which lead to a higher-than-normal risk of recurring back pain, may help in alleviating back pain or preventing future back problems.

Poor posture	Lack of flexibility in hamstring muscles
Improper lifting of heavy loads	Quick, jerking movements of the spine
Frequent bending from the waist	Osteoporosis
Weak lower back muscles	Increasing age
Being overweight	Sitting/standing in the same position for a long time
Lack of flexibility in lower back	

TABLE 13.1 Risk Factors for Back Pain

Back problems are of critical concern when engaging in physical activity. Depending on the exact nature of the problem, physical activity may be helpful or harmful. You should attempt to find the cause of back problems before engaging in physical activity. It is possible that certain types of activity may compound the problem and thus should be avoided.

Exercise has been effectively used in pain clinics for treating back pain (Maher, 2004). In addition, exercise can be used to prevent or correct some back problems by strengthening weak muscles and stretching the stronger ones. If you have a problem with your back, consult your physician before beginning a training program in order to determine what complications or benefits may result from your physical activity.

Prevention Physical activity can play a key role in preventing back pain. Physical activities that increase flexibility and strength, reduce body fat, improve balance between the abdominal and back muscles, and prevent osteoporosis reduce your risk of developing back problems (Maher, 2004). In addition, in consultation with your physician, chiropractor, or physiotherapist, you may find specific physical activities or exercises that help alleviate back pain that you may be experiencing.

If muscles on one side of a joint are stronger than those on the other side, the resulting imbalance of forces can pull the associated body parts out of alignment. You should do activities that strengthen the longer, weaker muscles and stretch the short, stronger ones. For example, individuals with an exaggerated curvature in the lower back should strengthen the abdominal muscles and stretch the muscles of the lower back and hips (Figure 13.2).

The following guidelines should help you prevent the onset of back pain:

- Maintain a healthy body weight and body composition. Obesity, particularly abdominal obesity, puts great strain on the lower back.
- Warm up before engaging in physical activity.
- Strengthen the abdominal muscles.
- Stretch the lower back and hamstring muscles.
- When lying down, lie on your side with your knees and hips bent. Limit lying on your back, and when you do, place a pillow under your knees.
- During prolonged standing, reduce the strain on the lower back by propping one foot on an object such as a rail or box, which bends the leg at the hip and knee. Adjust your position frequently.
- Avoid quick, jerking movements of the spine.
- Do not overextend the neck or lower back. Do not overflex the neck.
- Avoid stretching the long/weak muscles, especially the abdominal muscles.

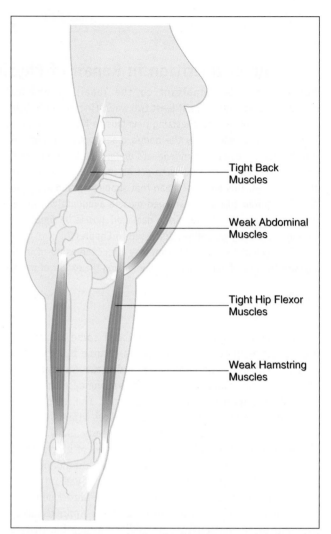

FIGURE 13.2 Major muscles involved in posture and their typical conditions during poor posture. The muscle imbalances shown here lead to poor posture, which can result in back pain.

- Avoid passive back or neck stretches or any ballistic passive stretches (Chapter 6).
- Avoid movements that place force on spinal disks, such as extending and rotating the spine simultaneously, trunk and neck circling, and double leg lifts.
- During prolonged sitting, adjust your position frequently.
- If possible, use an ergonomically correct chair and desk when doing office work.
- When studying for prolonged periods, take frequent breaks in which you engage in brief bouts (5 to 10 minutes) of physical activity.
- Listen to your body; when it is uncomfortable, adjust its position.
- Avoid forceful hyperextension and flexion of the spine.
- Avoid improper lifting. Squat to lift an object (bend at the knees) rather than bending at the waist.

Acute Muscle Soreness

Cause **Acute muscle soreness** may develop during or immediately following physical activity that has been too long or too intense for your level of physical fitness. Even though popular belief has linked the buildup of lactic acid to acute muscle soreness, lactic acid is not the cause of this type of soreness (Powers & Howley, 2004). Instead, it is more likely caused by other alterations in the chemical balance within muscle, increased fluid accumulation in muscle, or injury to muscle tissue.

Prevention Physical activities that are more strenuous or prolonged than normal are likely to cause the aforementioned changes that result in acute muscle soreness. Novice exercisers should be particularly cautious in this regard when beginning a training program. These changes can be further prevented by gradually beginning and ending each physical activity session. Begin slowly with a warm-up period of 5 to 15 minutes (Chapter 3) to allow muscles to raise their internal temperature slowly to avoid damage during the more stressful activities. Finally, a cool-down regimen is important in allowing the muscles to return to their normal, pre-exercise physiological condition.

Delayed-Onset Muscle Soreness

Cause **Delayed-onset muscle soreness (DOMS)** develops 24 to 48 hours after a bout of exercise that was excessive in duration or intensity (Connolly, Sayers, & McHugh, 2003). DOMS is also common following new or unique physical activities that use muscle groups unaccustomed to the workload. For example, it is not unusual for a runner to experience soreness in the upper body following the initiation of a strength-training program.

The cause of soreness in DOMS is likely microscopic tears in the muscle (Connolly et al., 2003), which cause swelling and pain. Many investigators believe this type of injury occurs primarily during the lengthening phase of muscular contraction (eccentric phase; Chapter 5). The damage is due to the greater force placed on the muscle during this phase of the contraction. For example, downhill running (which emphasizes such contractions) by an individual unaccustomed to this activity will generally produce soreness in the leg muscles within 24 to 48 hours. Similarly, in people unaccustomed to walking up and down steps, DOMS also occurs 24 to 48 hours after stair climbing.

Prevention As with acute muscle soreness, DOMS can be prevented by refraining from activities that are more strenuous or prolonged than usual. Start with a warm-up and limit the intensity and duration of the first several workouts. Remember that eccentric contractions are more likely to result in muscle damage than concentric (shortening) contractions. Therefore, in the beginning stages of an exercise program, try to limit activities that involve large numbers of eccentric contractions (e.g., walking down steps, running downhill, and performing certain movements during strength training). Build tolerance to these activities if they are to be part of your training regime.

Muscle Strains

Cause If a muscle is overstretched or forced to shorten against an extremely heavy weight (as when lifting a heavy box), muscle fibres may be damaged. This damage, which is referred to as a **strain**, can range from a minor separation of fibres to a complete tearing of fibres (Prentice, 2004). The following classification system has been developed for categorizing the degree of muscle damage due to strain:

1st-Degree Strain: Only a few muscle fibres are stretched or torn (Figure 13.3a). Movement is painful, but a full range of motion is still possible.

2nd-Degree Strain: Many muscle fibres are torn (Figure 13.3b), and movement is extremely painful and limited. The torn area may be apparent as a soft, sunken area in the muscle. Swelling may occur around the tear due to hemorrhage (bleeding).

3rd-Degree Strain: The muscle is torn completely (Figure 13.3c). The tear can be in the belly of the muscle, in the tendon, or at the point where the tendon attaches to the bone. Movement is generally impossible. Initial pain is intense but quickly subsides because nerve fibres are also damaged. Surgery is usually necessary for repair.

Prevention Since strains occur when muscles generate excessive force, it is logical that strains can be prevented by limiting the amount of stress placed on muscles. However, it is not possible to predict just how much force is needed to cause muscle damage. Keep in mind that warm muscles are more pliable (that is, more easily stretched and less likely to tear) than cold muscles. Therefore, before lifting a heavy object or engaging in any activity that requires quick, jerking movements, go through a thorough warm-up. Even

acute muscle soreness A pain that develops during or immediately following physical activities that were too long or too intense.

delayed-onset muscle soreness (DOMS) Pain that develops 24 to 48 hours after physical activity that is excessive in duration or intensity.

strain Damage to a muscle that ranges from a minor separation of fibres to a complete tearing of the muscle.

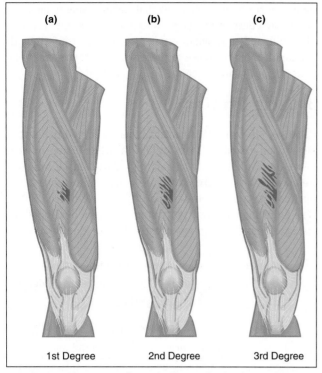

(a)   (b)   (c)

1st Degree   2nd Degree   3rd Degree

FIGURE 13.3 The extent of muscle damage in the three categories of muscle strains. (a) First-degree strain with minimal disruption of muscle fibres. (b) Second-degree strain with significant tearing and hemorrhage. (c) Third-degree strain with complete tear and loss of function.

though a good warm-up should prevent muscle strains, muscle contractions that are more strenuous than normal may result in DOMS.

Tendonitis

Cause **Tendons** are the tissue that connects muscles to bone. **Tendonitis**, which is the inflammation or swelling of a tendon, is one of the most common physical activity–related injuries (Prentice, 2004). As muscles shorten and pull on tendons, the tendons move across other tendons, muscles, and soft tissue. This movement, if unaccustomed, can cause irritation and swelling in the tendon. Once tendonitis develops, pain associated with movement is the first symptom. Swelling, redness, and warmth generally follow. Tendonitis can occur in a number of areas, such as the elbow and shoulder, and is a common injury for runners, tennis players, and weight lifters.

tendons   Tissue that connects muscles to bone.

tendonitis   Inflammation or swelling of a tendon.

sprain   Damage to a ligament that occurs if excessive force is applied to a joint.

ligaments   Connective tissue that connects bones, provides joint support, and determines the direction and range of joint motion.

Prevention   Tendonitis is generally caused by strenuous, prolonged muscle contractions. Therefore, the best prevention of tendonitis is to avoid overuse. If you feel tendon pain or discomfort during a workout, stop the activity. This will prevent further irritation and reduce the severity of tendon damage. If you cannot stop using the muscle and tendon causing the pain, follow the measures for the management of injuries discussed at the end of this chapter.

Ligament Sprains

Cause   A **sprain** is caused by damage to a ligament (Prentice, 2004). **Ligaments** are tough, inelastic bands of connective tissue that connect the bones, provide joint support, and determine the direction and range of motion of joints. Ligament damage can occur if excessive force is applied to a joint. One of the most common sites of ligament damage is the ankle. When walking or running on an uneven surface it is easy to "turn" an ankle, which means that the ankle joint was rotated so that the body weight was placed on the side of the foot. Because the ankle joint is not designed to rotate to that degree, this kind of stress on the joint causes the ligaments to be damaged. Like muscle strains, ligament damage is classified into three degrees as follows:

1st-Degree: Stretching and separation of a limited number of ligament fibres, resulting in minor instability of the joint (Figure 13.4a). Minor pain and swelling likely result.

2nd-Degree: Tearing and separation of a significant number of ligament fibres (Figure 13.4b). Moderate instability of the joint with definite pain, swelling, and stiffness occur.

3rd-Degree: Total tearing or separation of the ligament, causing major instability of the joint (Figure 13.4c). Nerves may be damaged and pain may subside quickly. Considerable swelling generally occurs.

Prevention   To prevent ligament strains, you are advised to develop adequate strength in all joints and in the muscles surrounding the joints. This should be accomplished by an overall strength and endurance training program (discussed in Chapter 5). However, if you have a particular joint that has been injured previously or is weak, it is important to try to maintain maximum strength in the muscles surrounding the joint, because strong muscles provide additional support.

The development of lightweight metal alloys has made it possible to construct braces that provide added support to joints and therefore offer some protection from ligament damage. These braces should not be used as a replacement for developing adequate strength in the muscles and joints. These braces are commonly used in football and basketball, sports recognized for inducing knee damage. Without these

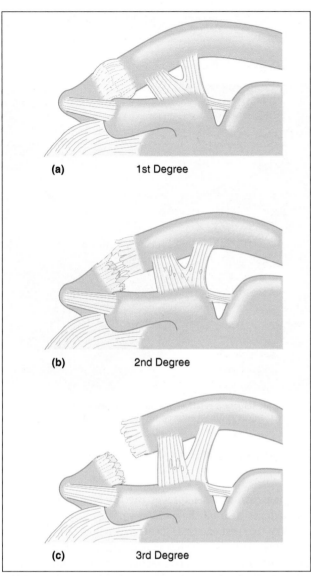

(a)   1st Degree

(b)   2nd Degree

(c)   3rd Degree

FIGURE 13.4 The extent of damage in the three categories of sprains, which involve damage to the ligaments that support joints. (a) First-degree sprain with minimal disruption of tendons in the shoulder. (b) Second-degree sprain with significant tearing. (c) Third-degree sprain with complete tearing and loss of joint stability.

expensive, high-tech devices, the best protection against torn ligaments is to refrain from activities that may subject a joint to high stress, including tennis, soccer, racquetball, football, and basketball.

Torn Cartilage

Cause   **Cartilage** is a tough connective tissue that forms a pad on the end of bones in certain joints, such as the elbow, knee, and ankle. Cartilage acts as a shock absorber to cushion the weight of one bone on another and to provide protection from the friction due to joint movement. Although this pad is made of the toughest of connective tissue, it can

be damaged and torn (Prentice, 2004). Unusually high forces or unusual movements cause tearing of cartilage, which results in joint pain. This type of injury, and severe ligament damage as well, normally requires surgical correction. A Closer Look on page 298 describes one procedure used to repair damage in joints.

Prevention   The only preventive measure for torn cartilage is eliminating those activities that are likely to cause the problem. Again, activities that may result in torn cartilage include any that produce excessive stress on the joint or forceful movements that take the joint outside its normal range of motion.

Common Injuries to the Lower Extremities

We have discussed the cause and prevention of several general activity-related injuries. Since many physical fitness and sport programs involve weight-bearing activities such as running, walking, and aerobic fitness classes, it is important to examine specific injuries involving the legs.

In general, walking does not result in a large number of injuries. Walking is likely the most prescribed physical activity for people of all ages because of the low risk for injury and the ease with which it can be done. As a result, it is the number one physical activity participated in by most Canadians (Cameron, Craig, Stephens, & Ready, 2002). As reported previously, one-quarter to three-quarters of all runners develop one or more leg injuries as a result of overtraining. Further, recent studies report that approximately 50 percent of all participants in aerobic fitness classes develop leg injuries. Most of these injuries occur in the foot and the knee as a result of the stress placed on the legs and feet. The force of the foot landing on the running surface (or aerobics floor) is approximately 2.5 times greater than the body weight of the person. Thus, in the case of a 65 kg runner, the amount of force generated when the foot strikes the pavement is 162 kg! It is easy to see how injuries might occur with this level of stress.

Patella–Femoral Pain Syndrome

Cause   **Patella–femoral pain syndrome (PFPS)** is a common injury manifested as pain behind the patella, or kneecap (Prentice, 2004). Also known as "runner's knee" or *chondromalacia*, PFPS may account for almost 10 percent of all

> **cartilage**   Connective tissue that forms a pad on the end of bone in certain joints including the knee, elbow, and ankle.
>
> **patella-femoral pain syndrome (PFPS)**   A common injury, sometimes called "runner's knee," that is manifested as pain behind the kneecap (patella).

Arthroscopic Surgery: A High-Tech Approach to Joint Repair

Whenever severe ligament or cartilage damage occurs around a joint, as commonly happens to the knee in individuals who play football, soccer, and basketball, the usual remedy is surgery. Traditional surgical techniques require the surgeon to cut the joint open in order to repair it, causing additional trauma to the joint and resulting in prolonged recuperation and rehabilitation. Now, however, a commonly used surgical technique called **arthroscopic surgery** allows surgeons to repair joint injuries without causing further trauma to the joint.

In arthroscopic surgery, surgeons use only two or three small incisions to gain entry into the damaged joint. Through these incisions they insert small micro-optic devices to allow them to see inside the joint, as well as a microsurgery tube that enables them to cut and remove small pieces of damaged tissue and to sew the remaining tissue together. Because the surgeons need make only a few minor incisions, less surgical damage occurs—which translates into less pain and shorter recovery and rehabilitation times than with conventional surgical techniques.

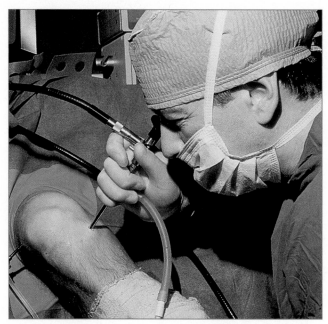

arthroscopic surgery A surgical procedure that uses only two or three small incisions to gain entry to the damaged joint.

Arthroscopic surgery is relatively painless and requires much less recovery time than conventional surgery, which requires opening the joint capsule.

---

visits to sports injury clinics, or 20 to 40 percent of all knee problems (Adirim & Cheng, 2003). Although the precise causes of PFPS remain unclear, the condition results when the patella gets "off track" (Figure 13.5), which causes excessive wear of the patella and pain. Among the factors that predispose an individual to PFPS are misalignment of the quadriceps (thigh muscles) that extend the knee, overuse or prolonged immobilization of the muscles, acute trauma, obesity, and genetics.

When these factors are present, the increased forces and repetitive movements of physical activity cause pain and may result in cracking and popping sounds during movement. Over time and with increased use, the articular (joint) cartilage may begin to degenerate, which eventually may lead to osteoarthritis.

Prevention PFPS can be prevented by limiting stress on the knee. Remember to limit unnecessary stresses on the knee such as squatting and excessive running, jumping, step aerobics, and stair climbing. Further, the chances of developing PFPS can be reduced by strengthening the quadri-

ceps muscles, which improves the tracking of the patella and reduces wear on the patellar surface.

The two best exercises for strengthening the quadriceps are knee extension exercises over the last 20 degrees of extension, and isometric contractions of the quadriceps muscles with the leg fully extended (try to press the back of the knee to the floor while lying on your back) (Prentice, 2004).

Finally, proper athletic footwear may reduce the chances of developing PFPS. If you develop any of the symptoms of PFPS, see your physician or a podiatrist (foot specialist) to discuss the possibility that footwear may be contributing to the problem.

Treatment An aggressive rehabilitation program that includes quadriceps strengthening, rest, and anti-inflammatory drugs has proved beneficial for more than 70 percent of PFPS patients. Although ice neither prevents PFPS nor rehabilitates the joint, it (like anti-inflammatory agents) may provide some relief from the pain and inflammation.

Shin Splints

Cause **Shin splints** (medial tibial stress) is a generic term referring to pain associated with injuries to the front of the lower leg (Prentice, 2004). Three of the most common injuries that cause shin splints are strain and irritation of one or sev-

shin splints Pain in the front of the lower leg.

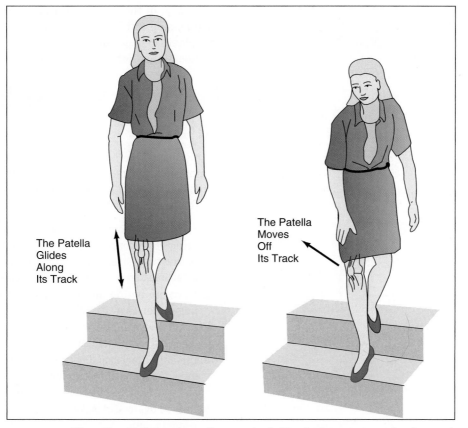

FIGURE 13.5 When the thigh muscles pull correctly (left), the kneecap stays in place and glides easily in its track. With PFPS (right), the thigh muscles pull unevenly and the kneecap gets "off track." This results in uneven pressure on the back of the kneecap, which causes excessive wear and pain.

The Patella Glides Along Its Track

The Patella Moves Off Its Track

eral muscles and tendons located in the lower leg (Figure 13.6); inflammation of tissue connecting the two bones of the lower leg, the tibia and the fibula; and microscopic breaks (called *stress fractures;* discussed next) in either the tibia or the fibula. Other reasons for shin splints include poor biomechanical structure in the feet and the use of improper footwear when walking, jogging, or running.

Prevention   Shin splints can be avoided by running on softer surfaces; by wearing well-padded, shock-absorbing shoes; and by progressively increasing the intensity from walking to running. If shin pain develops, it could be due to a fracture or break of bones and therefore should not be regarded lightly. High-impact activities such as running should be stopped; substitute low-impact activities such as cycling or swimming. Stretching muscles located in the front and back of the lower leg may help prevent the problem as well.

Stress Fractures

Cause   **Stress fractures** are tiny cracks or breaks in bone. Although stress fractures can occur in any leg bone, the long bones of the foot extending from the bones in the heel to the toes (the metatarsal bones) are especially susceptible

(Figure 13.7). Indeed, these are the most common sites of stress fractures in the body. Stress fractures result from excessive force applied to the leg and foot during running or other types of weight-bearing activities (Boden, Osbahr, & Jimenez, 2001). The most likely candidates for this injury are individuals with high arches or poor flexibility of the lower body, and people who increase training intensity or duration too rapidly.

Prevention   People with high arches should seek advice from their physicians or podiatrists, who might prescribe arch supports, which aid in preventing stress-related problems. Again, a key factor in preventing stress fractures is to avoid overtraining by increasing your training load gradually. Remember, increase the intensity or duration no more than 10 to 15 percent per week. Often, a lack of flexibility in the hips and the back of the legs will cause the body's weight to shift so that some bones become chronically overloaded and fracture. Thus, maintaining flexibility in the hips and the back of the legs will reduce your chances of developing a stress fracture.

stress fractures   Tiny cracks or breaks in the bone.

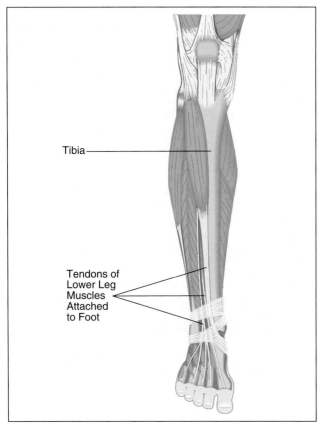

FIGURE 13.6 Locations of the muscles and tendons that are often irritated in shin splints.

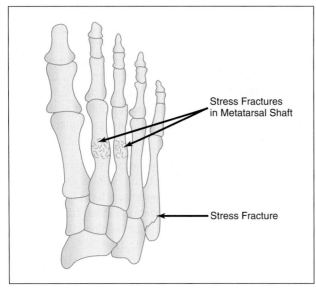

FIGURE 13.7 Stress fractures in the metatarsals.

R.I.C.E. **R**est, **I**ce, **C**ompression, and **E**levation. An acronym representing a treatment protocol for physical activity–related injuries.

If pain in the foot or leg makes you suspect a stress fracture, stop activities that involve the injured area. See your physician to get an X-ray of the area. If a stress fracture is present, only rest can assist the healing process.

Reducing Your Risk of Injury

In this chapter we have discussed the causes and prevention of some general and specific activity-related injuries. Listed below are six key ways to reduce your risk of injury due to physical activity.

1. Engage in a program of muscle-strengthening exercises using all major muscle groups. Maintaining a balance of muscular strength around joints will prevent muscular imbalance and reduce the incidence of injury.
2. Warm up before and cool down after all workouts. Remember that stretching during the warm-up may help prevent injuries, and stretching during the cool-down will help maintain flexibility.
3. Use proper footwear. Good shoes are obviously important for activities such as running and aerobic fitness classes and can reduce your chance of injury.
4. Do not overtrain! A key factor in physical activity–related injuries is improper training techniques. Gradual progression of intensity and duration is essential in preventing injuries.
5. Ensure adequate recovery time is part of your training routine. Rest is an important part of any successful training program.
6. Consider alternatives to high-impact activities such as speedwalking, cycling, or swimming.

To assess your training program with respect to the risks of injury it may pose, see Laboratory 13.1.

Management of Injuries

As mentioned previously, most people who engage in regular physical activity will experience some type of injury at some point in time. The following sections discuss injury treatments and provide an overview of the rehabilitation process.

Any injury that results in extreme pain or the possibility of a broken bone should be examined by a physician. Often an X-ray is taken to determine if there are any broken bones. The following treatment regimen should be followed for less severe injuries (strains, sprains, tendonitis, and so on).

Initial Treatment of Injuries

The objectives of the initial treatment of physical activity–related injuries are to decrease pain, limit swelling, and prevent further injury (Prentice, 2004). These objectives can be met by a combination of rest, ice, compression, and elevation. The acronym **R.I.C.E.** (R-rest, I-ice, C-compression, E-elevation) is an easy way to remember this treatment protocol. The elements of R.I.C.E. should be applied as soon as possible after the injury.

Rest is required to prevent further injury. Movement of injured tissues will aggravate the injury and result in further damage. Any movement that causes pain should be avoided.

Application of *ice* to an injury reduces swelling by reducing blood flow. Minimizing swelling around an injury will reduce the pain and lead to more rapid healing. Ice should be placed in a cloth wrap to prevent frostbite. Ice should be applied for 20- to 30-minute periods, 3 to 4 times a day for 2 days after the injury.

Compression of the injured area also reduces swelling. The amount of compression applied is important. It should be enough to reduce fluid collection around the damaged area but not severe enough to inhibit blood flow. Snugly wrapping the injured area with an elastic bandage is usually sufficient to control swelling. Placing a bag of ice in the last two or three wraps of the elastic bandage incorporates pressure and reduces swelling at the same time.

Finally, while resting it is beneficial to elevate the injured area, above the level of the heart if possible. *Elevation* reduces blood pressure and may therefore reduce swelling. Approximately 3 days following the injury, start a rehabilitation program, as outlined in the next section. If you have any doubts about whether the injury is ready for rehabilitation, delay another 24 to 48 hours.

Rehabilitation

The rehabilitation of minor injuries occurs naturally. That is, after an injury has healed and swelling has subsided, most people will begin to move the injured area at a comfortable rate dependent upon the pain involved. As the pain subsides, more movement can occur, until a normal range of motion is restored. However, this rehabilitation regimen has several drawbacks. First, it is very slow. Depending on the injury, the natural rehabilitation process may take five to ten times as long as an aggressive rehabilitation program. Second, the damaged area may be reinjured because many people attempt to return to full use of the injured area too quickly. A secondary injury often results in much greater damage than the first and can weaken the tissue and lead to recurring injuries for life. Third, for many types of injury, the lack of an aggressive rehabilitation program can prevent the return of full function because the scar tissue that develops limits normal range of motion. Fortunately, these problems may be overcome by an active rehabilitation process.

A relatively new rehabilitation technique that is implemented after the R.I.C.E. procedures have been followed is called **cryokinetics** (Bleakley, McDonough, & MacAuley, 2004). It uses approximately 12 minutes of ice application followed by 3 minutes of light exercise followed by another 3 minutes of cold. The 3 minutes of exercise and 3 minutes of ice should be repeated for five cycles. Activity of the injured limb during this treatment must be guided by the pain associated with its use. Start with an intensity that provides little or no pain. Intensity can be increased gradually as long as pain does not increase. If pain increases during the cryokinetic therapy, stop the treatment and resume the R.I.C.E. procedures until the pain subsides (Figure 13.8).

The initial management of an injury is critical and determines the time required for completion of the rehabilitation process. For example, a regimen of cryokinetics initiated after a third-degree ankle sprain (2 to 3 days post-injury) results in complete recovery within 2 weeks. In contrast, if the cryokinetic treatment starts late (5 to 7 days post-injury), the recovery may take 4 to 5 weeks.

cryokinetics A relatively new rehabilitation technique implemented after healing has been completed. It incorporates alternating periods of treatment using ice, exercise, and rest.

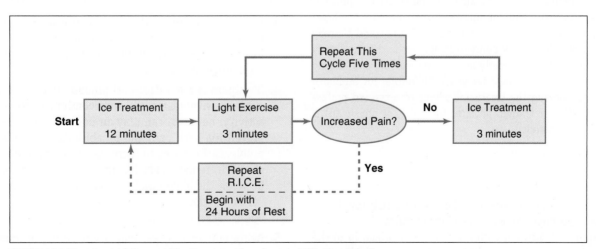

FIGURE 13.8 The steps of the cryokinetics procedure for rehabilitating injuries.

Can Deep-Water Running Help Your Recovery?

With an injury that prevents you from being physically active, the benefits of training are quickly reversed. Your cardiovascular endurance decreases measurably after 2 to 3 weeks without training. However, it is now well accepted that, with reduced training, you can maintain your fitness at a high level for several months. The intensity and specificity of cross-training workouts are most important in determining how much fitness you lose when you take time off from training. Of course, you need to find a method of cross training that will allow your injury to heal. Depending on the injury, you may be able to perform various types of cross training such as cycling, rowing, or using a cross-country skiing simulator to maintain your fitness while your injury heals. Since these methods provide some load on your muscles, you should use them for optimal effect. Unfortunately, some leg injuries are aggravated by these exercises.

An alternative is to run in the water. Deep-water running with a flotation vest provides an excellent training stimulus and more closely simulates land running than many of the other cross-training options. Running in the water is a total body activity that works your legs, trunk, and arms, and stresses your cardiovascular system.

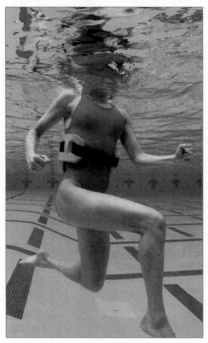

Aerobic performance is maintained with deep-water running for up to 6 weeks in trained endurance athletes, and sedentary individuals can actually improve their fitness level. In addition, there is some evidence of improvement in anaerobic measures and in upper-body strength in individuals engaging in deep-water running. A reduction in spinal loading also constitutes a role for deep-water running in the prevention of injury. The specific benefits you can derive from deep-water running include

- maintenance of or improvement in running performance.
- simulation of any type of running workout with the support of the water.
- ease of simulating interval training since the water adds resistance to your limbs.
- reduced muscle soreness with strenuous workouts because you eliminate eccentric contractions.
- effective maintenance of body composition since you can maintain high levels of energy expenditure.
- provides a workout to upper body musculature.
- strengthens hip adductors/abductors, lower leg musculature, feet, and abdominal muscles.
- improves flexibility when a stretching routine is included.

As pain subsides and the range of motion returns, full recovery may be accelerated if a program of strength training and flexibility exercises is added to the treatment process. This is especially true for muscle injuries, because the healing process may cause the muscle to shorten and thereby limit flexibility. A key point to remember is that an injury that does not heal properly may cause recurring pain during activity and may persist for years. Therefore, for stubborn injuries, seeking the treatment advice of a trained professional (athletic trainer, physical therapist, or physician) is often recommended.

Summary

1. Overtraining constitutes the greatest risk for developing a physical activity–related injury.
2. Injuries associated with running occur primarily in the foot and knee because of the stress placed on the legs and feet. The factors most closely associated with running injuries are improper training techniques, inadequate shoes, and alignment problems in the legs and feet.
3. Factors associated with injuries in fitness classes include participating in more than three sessions per week, wearing improper shoes, and exercising on nonresilient surfaces.
4. Back pain is a multifactoral problem that usually subsides without medical intervention. Physical activity, however, can play an important role in preventing back pain and rehabilitating some back problems. Exercises to increase flexibility and strength, reduce body fat, improve muscle balance between the abdominal and back muscles, and prevent osteoporosis can decrease your risk of developing back problems.
5. Acute muscle soreness may occur during or immediately after physical activity. This type of injury

may be due to muscle damage, accumulation of fluid within the muscle, and/or chemical imbalances within the muscle itself.

6. Delayed-onset muscle soreness (DOMS) sometimes occurs 24 to 48 hours after activity. Eccentric exercise increases the chance that DOMS will occur.

7. When a muscle is forced to contract against excessive resistance, fibres are damaged. This damage is referred to as a strain and can range from a minor separation of fibres to a complete tear.

8. Tendonitis is one of the most common overuse problems associated with physical activity. The term literally means inflammation of a tendon.

9. A sprain is caused by damage to a ligament, a type of connective tissue that provides support for joints. In contrast, torn cartilage refers to damage to the tough, connective tissue that serves as a cushioning pad between the ends of bones.

10. Common injuries to the lower extremities include PFPS, in which the particular cartilage on the back of the kneecap (patella) may be damaged by chronic use; shin splints, a condition that encompasses several different injuries to the front of the lower leg; and stress fractures, which are microscopic breaks in the bone.

11. The following guidelines can help you reduce your risk of developing a physical activity–related injury:

   - Engage in a program of muscle-strengthening to keep a balance in strength around joints.
   - Warm up before and cool down after each workout.
   - Use the proper equipment (especially footwear).
   - Increase exercise intensity and duration slowly throughout your training program.
   - Maintain the proper rest-to-exercise ratio. Do not overtrain!
   - Consider alternatives to high-impact activities.

12. For treating injuries, remember the R.I.C.E. protocol: rest, ice, compression, and elevation.

13. Recently, an effective new technique for injury rehabilitation called cryokinetics has come into use. This treatment calls for alternating periods of cold applications, exercise, and rest.

Study Questions

1. What is *overtraining*? How does it occur?

2. What are considered the primary causes of running injuries?

3. Discuss the injuries that may result from running.

4. Discuss the risks of injury associated with fitness classes and the factors thought to cause the injuries.

5. Differentiate between acute muscle soreness and delayed-onset muscle soreness.

6. Compare and contrast a strain and a sprain.

7. Define tendonitis and describe the best method of prevention/treatment.

8. What is the cause of PFPS, and how should it be treated?

9. What causes shin splints, and how can they be prevented?

10. List the guidelines that should be followed to minimize the risk of injury from increased physical activity.

11. Define the R.I.C.E. protocol and discuss its use.

12. Discuss the use of cryokinetics as a rehabilitation technique.

13. Define the following terms:

arthroscopic surgery	overtraining syndrome
cartilage	tendons
ligament	shin splints
stress fracture	tendonitis

Suggested Reading

Dufek, J. S. (2002). Exercise variability: A prescription for overuse injury prevention. *ACSM's Health & Fitness Journal, 6(4)*, 18–23.

Weblinks

Canadian Physical Medicine and Rehabilitation Services
www.canadianwellness.com/physical/physical.asp
Provides information on physical medicine, rehabilitation, and sports medicine services applicable for professional practitioners in the field of physical therapy, sports medicine, physiotherapy, and rehabilitation.

St. John Ambulance, Canada
www.sja.ca
A website dedicated to enabling Canadians to improve their health, safety, and quality of life through training and community service.

Canadian Society for Exercise Physiology
www.csep.ca
Promotes the generation, synthesis, transfer, and application of knowledge and research related to exercise physiology (encompassing physical activity, fitness, health, and human performance).

References

Adirim, T. A., & Cheng, T. L. (2003). Overview of injuries in the young athlete. *Sports Medicine, 33(1),* 75–81.

Bleakley, C., McDonough, S., & MacAuley, D. (2004). The use of ice in the treatment of actue soft-tissue injury: A systematic review of randomized controlled trials. *American Journal of Sports Medicine, 32(1),* 251–261.

Boden, B. P., Osbahr, D. C., & Jimenez, C. (2001). Low-risk stress fractures. *American Journal of Sports Medicine, 29(1),* 100–111.

Cameron, C., Craig, C. A., Stephens, T., & Ready, T. A. (2002). *Increasing physical activity: Supporting an active workforce.* Ottawa: Canadian Fitness and Lifestyle Research Institute.

Connolly, D. A., Sayers, S. P., & McHugh, M. P. (2003). Treatment and prevention of delayed onset muscle soreness. *Journal of Strength and Conditioning Research, 17(1),* 197–208.

Devereaux, M. W. (2004). Low back pain. *Primary Care, 31(1),* 33–51.

Dufek, J. S. (2002). Exercise variability: A prescription for overuse injury prevention. *ACSM's Health & Fitness Journal, 6(4),* 18–23.

Duffey, M. J., Martin, D. F., Cannon, D. W., Craven, T., & Messier, S. P. (2000). Etiologic factors associated with anterior knee pain in distance runners. *Medicine and Science in Sports and Exercise, 32(11),* 1825–1832.

Francis, L. L., Francis, P. R., & Welshone-Smith, K. (1985). Aerobic dance injuries: A survey of instructors. *The Physician and Sports Medicine, 13(2),* 105–111.

Hreljac, A., Marshall, R. N., & Hume, P. A. (2000). Evaluation of lower extremity overuse injury potential in runners. *Medicine and Science in Sports and Exercise, 32(9),* 1635–1641.

Lac, G., & Maso, F. (2004). Biological markers for the follow-up of athletes throughout the training season. *Pathologie Biologie, 52,* 43–49.

Macintyre, J., & Joy, E. (2000). Foot and ankle injuries in dance. *Clinics in Sports Medicine, 19(2),* 351–368.

Maher, C. G. (2004). Effective physical treatment for chronic low back pain. *Orthopedic Clinics of North America, 35(1),* 57–64.

Murphy, D. F., Connolly, D. A., & Beynnon, B. D. (2003). Risk factors for lower extremity injury: A review of the literature. *British Journal of Sports Medicine, 37(1),* 13–29.

Powers, S., & Howley, E. (2004). *Exercise physiology: Theory and application to fitness and performance* (5th ed.). Dubuque, IA: McGraw-Hill.

Prentice, W. E. (2004). *Rehabilitation techniques for sports medicine and athletic training* (4th ed.). Dubuque, IA: McGraw-Hill.

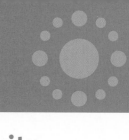

LABORATORY 13.1

Prevention of Injuries During Physical Activity

Name_____ Age _____ Sex _____ Date _____

The following lab is designed to help you identify and eliminate ways in which your physical activity may cause injuries.

DIRECTIONS

For the following measures associated with the prevention of injury, place a check by those you have incorporated into your physical activity (and, in some cases, into your life in general). For any measure not checked, write in the space provided exactly what changes you plan to implement to reduce or eliminate the risks associated with that measure.

PREVENTIVE MEASURE	CHANGES TO IMPLEMENT
_____ Proper shoes worn for the activity	_____
_____ Proper warm-up included	_____
_____ All muscle groups involved in the activity stretched	_____
_____ Over-stretching of the neck and back avoided	_____
_____ Extension and rotation of the spine avoided	_____
_____ Lifting of extremely heavy objects avoided	_____
_____ Quick, jerking movements avoided	_____
_____ All muscle groups involved in the activity strengthened and balanced	_____
_____ Training program properly designed	_____
_____ Appropriate frequency of physical activity used	_____
_____ Appropriate intensity of physical activity used	_____
_____ Appropriate time of physical activity used	_____
_____ Proper techniques used	_____
_____ (For running) firm, level surface used	_____
_____ Proper cool-down included	_____
_____ Device for supporting muscle or joint used (if training cannot be suspended)	_____

CHAPTER 14

Prevention of Cardiovascular Disease

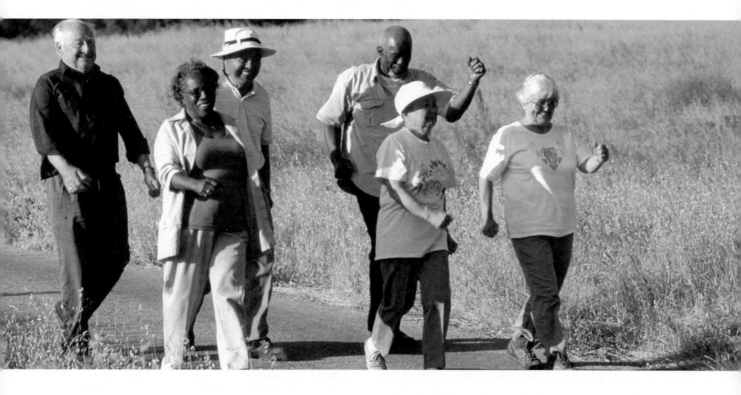

After studying this chapter, you should be able to

1. Identify the number one cause of death in Canada.

2. Identify four common cardiovascular diseases.

3. Outline the primary and secondary risk factors associated with the development of coronary heart disease.

4. Identify the coronary heart disease risk factors that can be modified by lifestyle changes.

5. Outline how physical activity is effective at directly and indirectly preventing heart disease.

6. List the steps involved in reducing your risk of coronary heart disease.

7. Outline the link between dietary sodium and hypertension.

8. Identify the total blood cholesterol levels associated with low, moderate, and high risk of developing coronary heart disease. Identify the cutoff values for blood fats indicative of risk for coronary heart disease.

9. Outline the relationship between diet and elevated blood cholesterol.

10. Outline the potential role of antioxidants in preventing atherosclerosis.

Cardiovascular diseases are a major health problem around the world and account for millions of deaths each year. Cardiovascular disease is the leading cause of death for men and women in Canada (Statistics Canada, 1997). Numerous factors increase your risk for developing cardiovascular disease. Some factors are not within your control (age, sex, and ethnicity). Other factors, such as lifestyle (smoking, physical activity, dietary intake) are within your control and may need to be modified to ensure you have the lowest risk possible for developing cardiovascular disease. In this chapter the incidence and impact of cardiovascular disease in Canada as well as the risk factors for developing cardiovascular disease are discussed. The chapter closes with a section on how to reduce your risk for developing cardiovascular disease.

Cardiovascular Disease in Canada

Although public awareness is often more focused on cancer and AIDS, **cardiovascular disease**—any disease that affects the heart or blood vessels—remains the number one cause of death in Canada.

In 1995, cardiovascular disease accounted for 36 percent of all male deaths and 39 percent of all female deaths in Canada (Statistics Canada, 1998a). Not everyone is affected by cardiovascular diseases at the same rate. Older people, men, and some ethnicities are at greater risk. (See Fitness and Wellness for All, opposite, for a brief discussion of the segments of the population at greatest risk of cardiovascular diseases.) Cardiovascular disease is also a major cause of disability and accounts for more hospitalizations than any other disease (Heart and Stroke Foundation of Canada, 1995). Although it is impossible to place a value on human life, the economic impact of cardiovascular disease is prohibitive, with an annual estimated cost in 1998 of $18 billion. Figure 14.1 illustrates the most recent values derived for the direct and indirect costs of cardiovascular diseases. Direct costs, in 1998 dollars, for hospital care, other institutional care, physician services, other health professional services, drugs, research, and so on were $6818 million. Indirect costs calculated for lost productivity due to premature mortality or disability were $11 654 million.

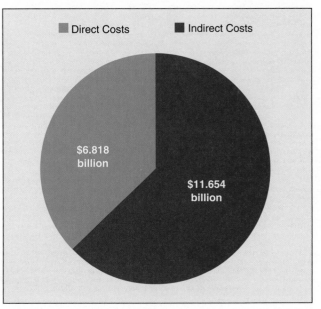

FIGURE 14.1 Annual direct and indirect costs (1998 dollars) of cardiovascular disease in Canada. Total cost = $18 billion.

Source: Economic Burden of Illness in Canada, 1998, Public Health Agency of Canada. Reproduced with the permission of the Minister of Public Works and Government Services Canada, 2005.

Cardiovascular Diseases

Although literally hundreds of diseases impair normal cardiovascular function, the four most common cardiovascular diseases are arteriosclerosis, coronary heart disease, stroke, and hypertension.

Arteriosclerosis

Arteriosclerosis is not a single disease but rather a group of diseases characterized by a narrowing or "hardening" of the arteries. The end result of any form of arteriosclerosis is that blood flow to vital organs may be impaired due to progressive blockage of the artery. **Atherosclerosis** is a special type of arteriosclerosis that results in arterial blockage due

cardiovascular disease   Any disease that affects the heart or blood vessels.

arteriosclerosis   A group of diseases characterized by a narrowing or "hardening" of the arteries.

atherosclerosis   A special type of arteriosclerosis that results in arterial blockage due to buildup of a fatty deposit inside the blood vessel.

Who Is at Greatest Risk of Cardiovascular Disease?

Ethnicity, sex, age, family history, and socioeconomic status affect an individual's risk of developing cardiovascular disease. These factors also explain why cardiovascular disease is more prevalent in certain segments of the Canadian population. Individuals of African, South Asian, and First Nations descent are at greater risk of developing cardiovascular disease compared to the Canadian population as a whole. A possible reason for the increased risk may be related to higher rates of hypertension in these populations. Between the ages of 20 and 65, men are at greater risk than women for developing cardiovascular disease. Risk for cardiovascular disease increases with age for men and women over the ages of 45 and 55 years, respectively. A positive family history also increases risk of cardiovascular disease. If there is history of heart attack or stroke prior to the age of 65 years, angina, or the tendency to develop high blood cholesterol or blood pressure, you are at a greater risk for developing cardiovascular diseases. Finally, individuals who earn low incomes experience higher incidences of heart disease and obesity (a secondary risk factor for heart disease).

Source: Heart and Stroke Foundation of Canada. Risk Factors—Coronary Heart Disease Risk Factor. Retrieved June 2, 2004, from http://ww1.heartandstroke.ca/Page.asp?PageID=110&ArticleID=589&Src=heart.

---

to buildup of a fatty deposit (called *atherosclerotic plaque*) inside the blood vessel. This plaque deposit is typically composed of cholesterol, cellular debris, fibrin (a clotting material in the blood), and calcium. Atherosclerosis is a progressive disease that begins in childhood, and symptoms appear later in life. Figure 14.2 illustrates the progression of arterial blockage caused by atherosclerosis. Note that atherosclerosis is not an "all or none" disease but occurs in varying degrees, with some arteries exhibiting little blockage and others exhibiting major obstruction. Development of severe atherosclerosis within arteries supplying blood to the heart is the major contributor to almost all heart attacks. When a coronary artery is severely occluded (90 to 95 percent), complete blockage (heart attack) occurs in that artery when a blood clot cannot pass through.

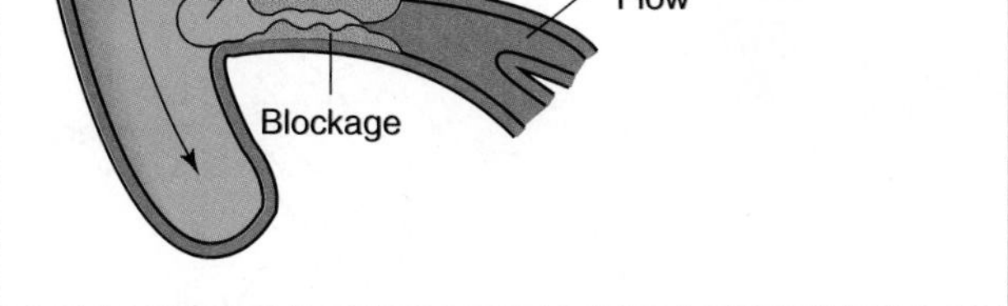

FIGURE 14.2 Progressive stages of atherosclerosis. The three cross-sections show (from left to right) a "normal" artery that has no blockage, and two arteries that have 30 and 95 percent blockages, due to the progressive buildup of plaque.

Coronary Heart Disease

Coronary heart disease is the major disease of the cardiovascular system. **Coronary heart disease (CHD)**, also called *coronary artery disease,* is the result of atherosclerotic plaque forming a blockage in one or more coronary arteries (the blood vessels supplying the heart with oxygen; Figure 14.3). When the degree of blockage of a major coronary artery reaches 75 percent, the resulting lack of blood flow to the working heart muscle causes chest pain. This chest pain is called *angina pectoris* and occurs most frequently during physical activity or emotional stress (Barrow, 1992).

When blood clots form around the atherosclerotic plaque of coronary arteries, severe blockage or restriction of blood flow occurs. Complete blockage of coronary blood flow results in a **heart attack** (also called a **myocardial infarction**). Figure 14.4 illustrates what happens during a heart attack when there is complete blockage in the left coronary artery. The end result is the death of heart muscle cells in the left ventricle; the severity of the heart attack is judged by how many heart muscle cells are damaged. A "mild" heart attack may damage only a small portion of the heart, whereas a "major" heart attack may destroy a large number of heart muscle cells. Because the number of heart muscle cells destroyed during a heart attack determines the patient's chances of recovery, recognizing the symptoms of a heart attack and getting prompt medical attention are crucial. In fact, it is suggested that medical attention within 2 hours of

coronary heart disease (CHD) CHD is the result of atherosclerotic plaque forming a blockage in one or more coronary arteries.

heart attack (myocardial infarction) Complete blockage of coronary arteries resulting in the death of heart cells.

Heart and Coronary Arteries

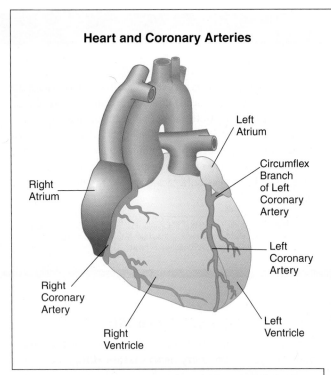

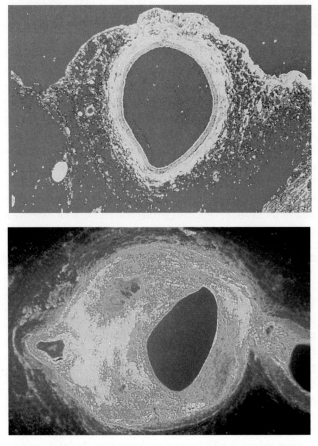

FIGURE 14.3 Locations of the coronary arteries. The photographs on the right show a normal coronary artery (top) and an atherosclerotic coronary artery (bottom).

Source: From Melvin H. Williams, *Lifetime Fitness and Wellness*, 3rd ed. Copyright © 1993 Wm. C. Brown Communications, Inc. Reprinted by permission of Times Mirror Higher Education Group, Inc., Dubuque, Iowa. All rights reserved.

the first symptom increases survival rates (Heart and Stroke Foundation of Canada and ACTI-MENU, 1999). Approximately 12 percent of Canadians who experience a heart attack die within 30 days (Canadian Institute for Health Information, 2003). The long-term (1-year) survival rate after 30 days is 91 to 93 percent (A Closer Look, p. 312).

Stroke

A **stroke** occurs when the blood supply to the brain is reduced for a prolonged period of time. A common cause of stroke is blockage (due to atherosclerosis) of arteries in the head or neck leading to the brain (Figure 14.5). Strokes can also occur when a cerebral (brain) blood vessel ruptures and disturbs normal blood flow to that region of the brain.

Similar to a heart attack, which results in death of heart cells, a stroke results in the death of brain cells. The severity of the stroke may range from slight to severe, depending

stroke When the blood supply to the brain is reduced for a prolonged period of time, usually as a result of blockage of arteries in the head or neck.

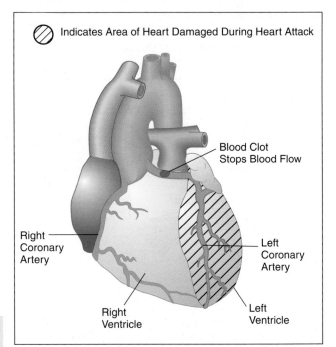

FIGURE 14.4 Effect of a myocardial infarction (heart attack). The cross-hatched area of the heart is damaged due to a stoppage of blood flow during the heart attack.

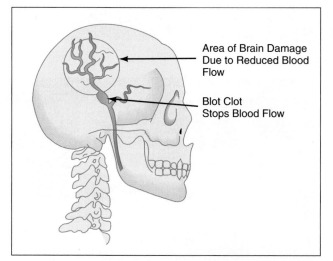

Area of Brain Damage Due to Reduced Blood Flow

Blot Clot Stops Blood Flow

FIGURE 14.5 How blockage of an artery in the brain causes a stroke. Cessation of blood flow through an artery supplying the brain produces damage to the portion of the brain supplied by that artery (indicated by the circle).

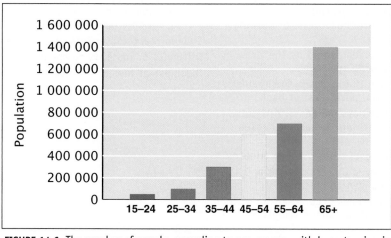

FIGURE 14.6 The number of people, according to age groups, with hypertension in Canada.

Source: Adapted from Statistics Canada CANSIM database, Table 105-0010.

Hypertension

Hypertension refers to chronic high blood pressure. High blood pressure occurs when the force exerted by the heart is greater than normal *(systolic blood pressure)* or when the pressure of blood on the arterial wall is greater than normal *(diastolic blood pressure)*. Clinically, hypertension is generally defined as a resting blood pressure over 140 mm Hg systolic or 90 mm Hg diastolic (Barrow, 1992). The force of the blood against the arterial walls when the heart contracts and pumps blood to the body is called systolic blood pressure (Greenberg, Dintiman, Myers Oakes, Irwin, & Morrow, 2004). The force of blood on the arterial walls when the heart is relaxed is called diastolic blood pressure (Greenberg et al., 2004). A systolic blood pressure of 120 to 139 mm Hg or a diastolic blood pressure of 80 to 89 mm Hg are considered prehypertensive (Chobanian et al., 2003). In 90 percent of hypertension cases, the exact cause of the high blood pressure is unknown; this type of hypertension is called *essential hypertension*. Approximately 10 percent of hypertension cases are caused by a specific disease (such as kidney disease). This type of hypertension is called *secondary hypertension,* because the hypertension is secondary to a primary disease.

The prevalence of hypertension in Canada is remarkably high (Figure 14.6). Factors that increase your risk of hypertension include lack of physical activity, a high-salt diet, obesity, chronic stress, family history of hypertension, sex (men have a greater risk than women), and ethnicity (blacks have a greater risk than whites).

Hypertension is a health problem for several reasons. First, high blood pressure increases the workload on the heart; this may eventually damage the heart muscle's ability to pump blood effectively throughout the body (Barrow, 1992). Second, high blood pressure may damage the lining of arteries, resulting in the development of atherosclerosis and therefore increasing the risk of CHD and stroke (Barrow, 1992). Third, high blood pressure increases the risk of death from kidney failure (Statistics Canada, 1998a).

Although physical activity causes acute increases in systolic blood pressure, this type of blood pressure elevation is transient and is not considered hypertension (i.e., hypertension is chronically elevated blood pressure). Further, the increase in blood pressure during physical activity does not damage the heart or blood vessels.

on the location and the number of brain cells damaged. Minor strokes may involve a loss of memory, speech problems, disturbed vision, or mild paralysis in the extremities. By contrast, severe strokes may result in major paralysis or death. Approximately 7.1 percent of all deaths in Canada each year are a result of stroke (Canadian Institute for Health Information, 2003). Approximately 19 percent of individuals who have a stroke die within the first 30 days (Canadian Institute for Health Information, 2003). Survival rates after 30 days are strongest, with 85 to 88 percent likely to still be living 6 months later. Similar to surviving a heart attack, the key to surviving a stroke is to obtain medical treatment within 2 hours following the appearance of the first symptoms (Heart and Stroke Foundation of Canada and ACTI-MENU, 1999) (A Closer Look, p. 312).

hypertension High blood pressure, generally defined as a blood pressure of 140 mm Hg systolic or 90 mm Hg diastolic or greater.

A CLOSER LOOK

The Warning Signs of Cardiovascular Disease

Recognizing the warning signs of a heart attack or stroke and knowledge of the appropriate emergency action could save your life or that of someone else. Special attention is given to the warning signs, or lack thereof, in women.

What to Do in the Event of a Heart Attack or Stroke

If you or someone near you experiences any of the symptoms listed below for 2 minutes or longer, call 911 or get to the nearest hospital that offers emergency cardiac care. If you are trained in cardiopulmonary resuscitation (CPR) and the patient is not breathing or does not have a pulse, call 911 and start CPR immediately. In any cardiac emergency, rapid action may mean the difference between life and death.

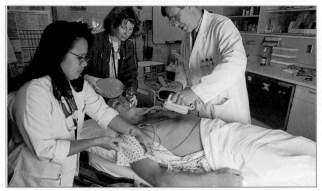

The chances of surviving a heart attack or stroke are greatest when medical attention is obtained within 2 hours of initial symptoms.

Angina

Different types of chest pain

With or without pain in the arm, neck, or jaw

Pain lasts from a few seconds to a few minutes

Occurs most often with effort or strong emotions

Generally relieved by rest or nitroglycerin under the tongue or by spray within 5 or 10 minutes

Heart Attack

Severe chest pain, in different forms (a feeling of tightening, pressure, heaviness, or burning, etc.)

May be accompanied by the following symptoms:

- pain that spreads to shoulders, arms, neck, jaw, or back
- dizziness, paleness, difficulty breathing, sweating, nausea, vomiting, or anxiety

Usually lasts more than 10 minutes

Not relieved by rest or by 2 or 3 doses of nitroglycerin

Can sometimes occur silently, with none of the above symptoms

Stroke

Sudden weakness or loss of sensation in the mouth, arm or leg, on only one side of the body

Sudden reduction or loss of vision

Difficulty or inability to speak

Dizziness or loss of balance

Women:

For many women, angina may happen while at rest. Some may feel more pain in the neck or lower jaw, or they may feel out of breath, nauseated, or tired instead of or in addition to chest pain.

Women:

An estimated 50% of heart attacks in women cause no severe pain. For many women, the classic list of symptoms is replaced by vaguer symptoms:

- pain in the neck, jaw, or arms
- heaviness in the shoulder blades, back, or the pit of the stomach
- feeling out of breath, tired, sweating, nausea, vomiting

Note:

These symptoms can sometimes be vaguer, particularly among the elderly. Watch for a sudden change in behaviour, like unusual slowness, indifference, or an inability to dress or feed oneself.

Source: Adapted from ACTI-MENU, *Do You Have a Healthy Heart?* ACTI-MENU, 2004. www.actimenu.ca

It is estimated that 25 percent of Canadian men and 18 percent of Canadian women have high blood pressure. The percentage of the population with hypertension increases with age (Figures 14.6 and 14.7). Prior to the age of 45 years, the number of men living with hypertension is greater than the number of women (Figure 14.7). However, given the fact that men most often die younger than women, the percentage of the population living with hypertension is greater in women.

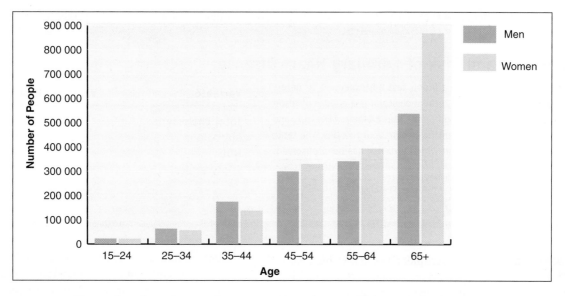

FIGURE 14.7 The number of people, according to sex and age groups, with hypertension in Canada.

Source: Adapted from Statistics Canada CANSIM database table 105-0010.

Hypertension is often called *the silent killer*. Because the condition lacks symptoms, many people are not aware that they are hypertensive. Although severe hypertension may result in headaches and dizziness, these symptoms are often absent. Therefore, without annual medical checkups or blood pressure screenings, hypertension may not be detected for many years.

Risk Factors Associated with Coronary Heart Disease

In an effort to understand the causes and reduce the occurrence of CHD, researchers have identified a number of primary and secondary risk factors that increase the chances of developing CHD and stroke. *Primary risk factors* are factors directly related to the development of CHD and stroke. In contrast, *secondary risk factors* are those that increase the risk of CHD, but their direct contribution to the disease process has not been precisely determined.

Primary Risk Factors

The Heart and Stroke Foundation of Canada and its provincial associates regularly publish new information concerning the *primary and secondary risk factors* associated with the development of CHD and stroke. Figure 14.8 illustrates how these risk factors are divided into those that are controllable and those that you cannot do anything about (Heart and Stroke Foundation of Canada, 2004). Uncontrollable risk factors for heart disease include age and sex, ethnic descent, and family history. Controllable factors include the primary risk factors hypertension, hyperlipidemia, smoking, and

physical inactivity. Controllable factors also include the secondary risk factors type 2 diabetes, obesity, and stress. The greater the number of CHD risk factors an individual has, the greater the likelihood that he or she will develop CHD (Figure 14.8).

Hypertension   Hypertension is a unique risk factor because it is a disease and a risk factor for stroke and CHD. As mentioned earlier, hypertension is considered a disease because it forces the heart to work harder than normal, which can eventually damage the heart muscle. As a CHD risk factor, it contributes to the development of CHD by accelerating the rate of atherosclerosis development (Bouchard, Shepard, Stephens, Sutton, & McPherson, 1990; Heart and Stroke Foundation of Canada, 2004).

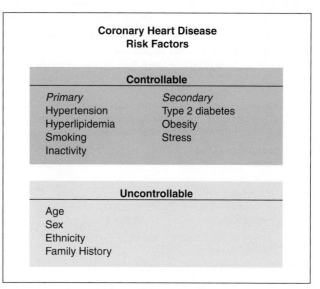

FIGURE 14.8 Coronary heart disease risk factors.

Blood Fats and Risk of Coronary Heart Disease

A variety of components of a blood test are examined to determine risk for CHD. Although total cholesterol is a good indication of risk for CHD, a more thorough profile that examines LDL, HDL, and triglycerides more clearly identifies where your risk lies. The table at the right lists the values at which CHD risk has been observed.

Source: Connelly, P. W., MacLean, D. R., Horlick, L., O'Connor, B., Petrasovityz, A., Little, J. A.: Canadian Heart Health Surveys Research Group. (1992). Plasma lipids and lipoproteins and the prevalence of risk for coronary heart disease in Canadian adults. *Canadian Medical Association Journal, 146(11)*, 1977–1987.

Variable	Value (millimoles/litre)
Total cholesterol	≥ 5.2
LDL	≥ 3.4
HDL	< 0.9
Triglycerides	≥ 2.3

Hyperlipidemia   **Hyperlipidemia** refers to high blood cholesterol levels. As discussed in Chapter 7, cholesterol is a type of fat that can be consumed in the diet or synthesized in the body. The risk of CHD increases as blood cholesterol increases.

Because cholesterol is not soluble in blood, it is combined with proteins in the liver so it can be transported in the bloodstream. The combination of cholesterol, triglycerides, and protein results in two major forms of cholesterol: **low-density lipoproteins (LDL)** and **high-density lipoproteins (HDL)**. LDL are composed of relatively small amounts of protein and large amounts of cholesterol. LDL promotes fatty plaque accumulation in the coronary arteries (atherosclerosis) that contributes to heart disease (Heart and Stroke Foundation of Canada and ACTI-MENU, 1999). HDL are composed of relatively large amounts of protein and small amounts of cholesterol. HDL protect against the fatty plaque accumulation in the coronary arteries by taking this plaque to the liver to be processed (Heart and Stroke Foundation of Canada and ACTI-MENU, 1999). **Triglycerides** are another type of fat found in the blood. These fats also increase risk for CHD (Heart and Stroke Foundation of Canada and ACTI-MENU, 1999). Thus, the association between blood cholesterol and CHD involves LDL, HDL (Barrow, 1992; Third Report of the National Cholesterol Education Program Expert Panel on Detection, Evaluation, and Treatment of High Blood

Cholesterol in Adults, 2001; Thomas & LaFontaine, 2001) and triglycerides (Heart and Stroke Foundation of Canada and ACTI-MENU, 1999). Specifically CHD risk is related to elevated levels of LDL and triglycerides with or without low levels of HDL. CHD risk is lowest, then, in individuals with lower levels of LDL and triglycerides combined with elevated HDL. Because of these relationships, LDL has been called "bad cholesterol" while HDL has been called "good cholesterol."

Even though the risk of developing CHD is best predicted from LDL and HDL levels in the blood, measurement of total blood cholesterol (the sum of all types of cholesterol) also provides a good indication of CHD risk (Barrow, 1992; Canadian Institute for Health Information, 2003). As shown in Figure 14.9, a total blood cholesterol concentration less than 5.2 mmol/L or 200 mg/dL (milligrams per decilitre) indicates a low risk of developing CHD, whereas a concentration 5.2 mmol/L or greater than 240 mg/dL indicates a high CHD risk (Barrow, 1992; Thomas & LaFontaine, 2001). Values between 200 and 239 mg/dL indicate moderate risk.

Guidelines for assessing CHD risks using blood levels of total cholesterol, LDL, HDL, and triglycerides are presented in A Closer Look, above.

Smoking   It is estimated that 21.5 percent of Canadians smoke (Statistics Canada, 2004). Cigarette smoking is most likely the single greatest cause of disease and premature

hyperlipidemia   High blood cholesterol levels; generally a total blood cholesterol concentration greater than 240 mg/dl.

low-density lipoproteins (LDL)   A combination of protein, triglycerides, and cholesterol in the blood, composed of relatively large amounts of cholesterol.

high-density lipoproteins (HDL)   A combination of protein, triglycerides, and cholesterol in the blood, composed of relatively large amounts of protein.

triglycerides   A type of fat consumed and manufactured in the body.

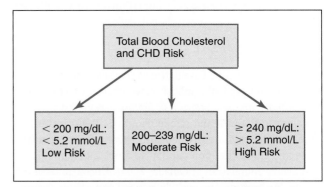

FIGURE 14.9 Total blood cholesterol levels and CHD risks.

death in Canada. It has been linked to more than 30 health problems, including cancer, lung disease, and cardiovascular disease. In regard to smoking and cardiovascular disease, a smoker's risk of developing CHD is far greater than that of a nonsmoker (Figure 14.10). Furthermore, your risk of heart disease increases with the number of cigarettes you smoke. Smoking is also considered the greatest risk factor for sudden cardiac death (sudden death due to cardiac arrest, a heart attack, or irregular heartbeats). In addition, smoking promotes the development of atherosclerosis in peripheral blood vessels (arterial blockage in the arms or legs). Finally, smokers who have a heart attack are more likely to die within an hour after the attack than non-smokers.

Is the risk of cardiovascular disease increased for nonsmokers who breathe secondhand cigarette smoke? Unfortunately, the answer is yes. Passive inhalation of cigarette smoke increases the risk for cardiovascular and lung disease (Canadian Institute for Health Information, 2003). This prompted the banning of smoking in many public places, including airplanes, restaurants, universities and colleges, hospitals, and shopping malls.

Cigarette smoking influences your risk of cardiovascular disease in at least four ways (Greenberg et al., 2004). First, cigarette smoke contains the drug nicotine, which increases heart rate and blood pressure. Second, smoking increases your blood's ability to clot, which raises your risk of heart attack. Third, nicotine influences the way your heart functions, leading to irregular heartbeats (called *arrhythmias*). These arrhythmias can lead to sudden cardiac death. Finally, cigarette smoking increases your chance of developing atherosclerosis by elevating the amount of cholesterol in the blood and encouraging fat deposits in arterial walls.

When people stop smoking, the benefits are immediate and long lasting (Heart and Stroke Foundation of Canada and ACTI-MENU, 1999). In fact, your risk of a heart attack decreases dramatically within only one year of not smoking (Negri, LaVecchia, D'Avanzo, Nobili, & LaMalfa, 1994). Furthermore, your risk for developing heart disease is comparable to a non-smoker 10 years after smoking cessation (Negri et al., 1994).

Physical Inactivity

In 1992, the American Heart Association added physical inactivity (defined as a lack of regular exercise) to the list of major risk factors for the development of CHD. Around the same time the Heart and Stroke Foundation of Canada, Health Canada, and the Canadian Society for Exercise Physiology also recognized the role of a sedentary lifestyle in increasing risk of CHD. The addition of physical inactivity to the list of primary risk factors for CHD is based on a large volume of research that suggests the incidence of CHD is much greater in people who do not engage in regular physical activity (Blair et al., 1989; Bouchard et al., 1990; Kohl, 2001; Paffenbarger, Hyde, Wing, & Hsieh, 1986; Thomas & LaFontaine, 2001).

How does physical activity reduce the risk for CHD? First, physical activity, engaged in regularly and of suffi-

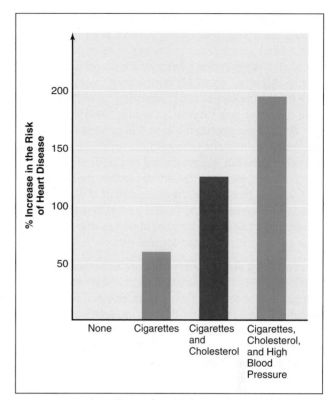

FIGURE 14.10 The effects of multiple risk factors for coronary heart disease.

cient intensity, results in positive changes in peripheral and central circulation, skeletal muscle and myocardium, and lipid and carbohydrate metabolism (Kavanagh, 2001). Physical activity and exercise training also help to prevent atherosclerotic CHD (Thompson et al., 2003). Furthermore, physical activity plays an important role in managing other CHD risk factors including hypertension, low HDL, elevated triglyceride levels, obesity, and possibly cigarette use (Thompson et al., 2003). Thus, physical activity has a primary and secondary role in reducing risk of CHD.

Family History It is firmly established that inherited traits can increase your risk of CHD and stroke (Barrow, 1992; Heart and Stroke Foundation of Canada and ACTI-MENU, 1999). This means that children of parents with CHD are more likely to develop CHD than children of parents who do not have CHD. Current evidence suggests that the familial risk for CHD may be linked to factors such as high blood cholesterol, high blood pressure, diabetes, and obesity (Barrow, 1992).

Ethnicity is also a consideration, because African, Asian, and First Nations populations are at greater risk for CHD than whites. One reason for the greater risk is the high rate of hypertension in these ethnicities, although the cause of that is unknown.

Sex Men have a greater risk of developing CHD and stroke than women. In fact, men have more heart attacks than women, particularly at younger ages (Statistics Canada,

1998b). Figure 14.11 illustrates the number of men and women according to age group who've been hospitalized with a heart attack. Prior to the age of 75 years, the number of men experiencing a heart attack far outstrips that of women. After the age of 80, more women than men experience heart attacks; this is not surprising, given that women tend to outlive men (Statistics Canada, 1998a).

Much of the protection against CHD in women is linked to the female sex hormone estrogen. Estrogen increases HDL cholesterol, reduces LDL cholesterol, and may be involved in maintaining the suppleness of the arteries so that the blood vessel walls are less receptive to the accumulation of plaque (Heart and Stroke Foundation of Canada and ACTI-MENU, 1999). Although the risk of CHD increases in women after menopause, it never becomes as great as for men (Barrow, 1992).

Increasing Age Advancing age increases the risk of developing CHD. The explanation for this observation is that the buildup of arterial plaque is an ongoing process; the longer one lives, the greater the buildup. Another related factor is that people tend to be less physically active as they get older. The increased prevalence of CHD with age is illustrated by the statistic that more than 50 percent of all heart attack victims are 65 or older (Statistics Canada, 1998).

Secondary Risk Factors

Secondary risk factors are those that increase the risk of CHD, but their direct contribution to the disease process is unclear. You can think of secondary risk factors as those that increase your risk of developing a *major* risk factor. At present, the Heart and Stroke Foundation of Canada recognizes type 2 diabetes, obesity, and stress as secondary risk factors.

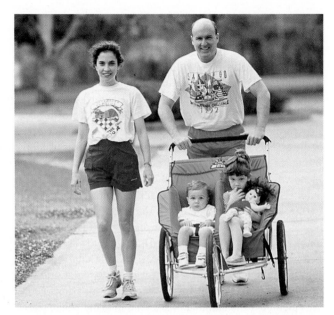

Even modest physical activity (walking for 20 to 30 minutes per day 3 to 5 times per week) can reduce your risk of developing cardiovascular disease.

Type 2 Diabetes As noted in Chapter 1, type 2 diabetes is a disease that results in elevated blood sugar levels because the body is unable to use blood sugar properly. Type 2 diabetes occurs most often in middle age and is common in people who are overweight. In addition to increasing your risk of kidney disease, blindness, and nerve damage, diabetes increases your risk of CHD and stroke. The link between diabetes and CHD is well established; more than 80 percent of all people with diabetes die from some form of

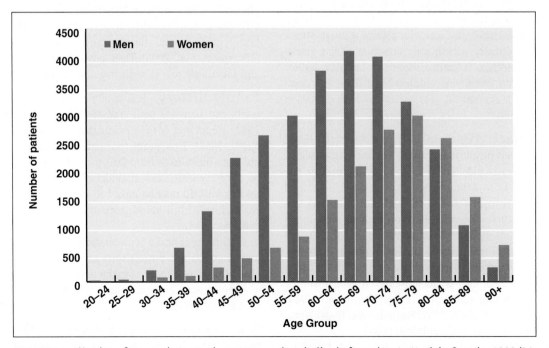

FIGURE 14.11 Number of men and women, by age group, hospitalized after a heart attack in Canada, 1993/94.

Source: Adapted from the Statistics Canada publication *Health Reports*, Catalogue 82-003,1998, Vol. 10, No. 2, October 29, 1998.

cardiovascular disease. The role of diabetes in increasing your risk of CHD may be tied to the fact that individuals with diabetes often have elevated blood cholesterol levels, are hypertensive, and are inactive (Bouchard et al., 1990).

Obesity   Compared with individuals who maintain their ideal percentage body fat, individuals who are obese are more likely to develop CHD, even if they have no other major risk factors (Bouchard et al., 1990). Further, obesity is often associated with elevated blood cholesterol levels and may contribute to hypertension (Bouchard et al., 1990).

Of particular interest is the fact that a person's fat distribution pattern affects the risk of CHD. As discussed in Chapter 2, a waist girth greater than 102 cm for men and 88 cm for women indicates a significant risk for CHD. The physiological reason for the link between CHD and regional fat distribution is related to the research findings that abdominal obesity was significantly related to elevated triglyceride levels, low HDL concentrations, and hypertension (Reeder et al., 1997).

The fact that obesity is associated with a high incidence of hypertension is well established; however, the exact physiological link between obesity and hypertension is less clear. Possible causes of hypertension in individuals who are obese include a high-salt diet, which elevates blood pressure, and increased vascular resistance, which results in the need for higher pressure to pump blood to the tissues (Barrow, 1992). The role of sodium in promoting hypertension is discussed in Nutritional Links to Health and Fitness, page 318.

Stress   Stress increases the risk of CHD; however, the exact link between stress and CHD is unclear and continues to be studied. Nonetheless, it seems likely that stress contributes to the development of several major CHD risk factors. For example, stress may be linked to lifestyle habits. People under stress may start smoking in an effort to relax, or stress could influence smokers to smoke more than they normally would. Under stress, people may eat poorly and neglect physical activity (Heart and Stroke Foundation of Canada and ACTI-MENU, 1999). Further, stress increases the risk of developing hypertension and elevated blood cholesterol. The physiological connection between stress and hypertension appears to be the release of stress hormones, which elevate blood pressure. Currently, it is unclear how stress is linked to high blood cholesterol.

Reducing Your Risk of Heart Disease

Although cardiovascular disease remains the number one killer in Canada, incidence of the disease has declined over the past 30 years. This drop is due primarily to people reducing their risk factors for CHD. Table 14.1 contains a list of the primary and secondary CHD risk factors discussed earlier in the chapter. Note that four of the seven major risk factors and all three of the contributory factors can be modified by behaviour. Therefore, 70 percent of the 10 risk factors presented in Table 14.1 can be modified to reduce your risk of developing cardiovascular disease.

How does one implement a CHD risk reduction program? The first step is the identification of your risk status. This can be done by completing Laboratory 14.1 on page 323 and by carefully examining Table 14.1. The next step is to implement a positive, healthy lifestyle to modify the CHD risk factors that can be altered.

Modification of Primary Risk Factors

The four primary CHD risk factors that can be modified are hypertension, hyperlipidemia, smoking, and physical inactivity.

Hypertension can be reduced in several ways. Individuals who are prehypertensive should also follow these health-promoting lifestyle changes (Chobanian et al., 2003). The

Risk Factor	Risk Factor Classification	Is Behaviour Modification Possible?	Behaviour Modification to Reduce Risk
Smoking	Primary	Yes	Smoking cessation
Hypertension	Primary	Yes	Physical activity and dietary intake
High blood cholesterol	Primary	Yes	Physical activity and dietary intake
Physical inactivity	Primary	Yes	Physical activity
Heredity	Primary	No	
Sex	Primary	No	
Increasing age	Primary	No	
Diabetes	Secondary	Yes	Dietary intake, physical activity
Obesity	Secondary	Yes	Weight loss, dietary intake, physical activity
Stress	Secondary	Yes	Stress management, physical activity

TABLE 14.1 Primary and Secondary Risk Factors for the Development of Coronary Heart Disease

Data from Heart Facts, American Heart Association, 1993.

High Sodium Intake Increases the Risk of Hypertension

A key factor in regulating blood pressure is dietary sodium. High sodium intake results in an elevated blood volume, which promotes higher blood pressure. Therefore, monitoring sodium intake is an important factor in preventing or controlling hypertension.

As mentioned in Chapter 7, sodium (contained in table salt) is a required micronutrient, but the daily requirement for most people is small (less than 400 mg, or one-quarter teaspoon). Even athletes or labourers who lose large amounts of water and electrolytes through sweat rarely require more than 3000 mg (1.5 tsp) of salt per day. Many Canadians consume far too much salt.

What is the maximum amount of dietary sodium that the body can tolerate without developing hypertension? Even though a definitive answer to this question is not available, hypertension is rare in countries where sodium intake is less than 2000 mg (1 tsp) per day.

The key to lowering your sodium intake is avoiding foods that are high in salt (see the table below). Take the time to learn which foods contain a lot of sodium and limit your intake to less than 2000 mg (1 tsp) per day (Durstine & Thompson, 2000).

Food	Serving Size	Sodium Content (mg)
Bologna	56 g	700
Cheese		
Processed	28 g	305
Cheddar	28 g	165
Parmesan	28 g	525
Devilled crab	1	2085
Hamburger patty	1 small	550
Pickles (dill)	1 medium	900
Pizza (cheese)	1 slice (36 cm diameter)	600
Potato chips	20	300
Pretzels	28 g	890
Salami	84 g	1047
Soup		
Chicken noodle	250 mL	1010
Vegetable beef	250 mL	1046
Soy sauce	25 mL	1320
Wiener	1	495

recommendations from the Canadian Hypertension Education Program are for people to modify their lifestyles in the following ways (Touyz et al., 2004):

- Do 30 to 45 minutes of physical activity most (4 to 5) days of the week.
- Maintain an ideal body weight (a BMI of 18.5 to 24.9).
- Limit alcohol consumption to two or fewer standard drinks per day with weekly intake not exceeding 14 drinks for men and 9 drinks for women.
- Eat a reduced-fat, low-cholesterol diet that emphasizes fruits, vegetables, and low-fat dairy products, and maintains adequate intakes of potassium, magnesium, and calcium.
- Restrict salt intake to less than 2000 mg (1 tsp) per day.
- Employ strategies to manage stress.

For more complete details on these recommendations see Touyz et al. (2004) in the Suggested Reading list. In some instances, medication may be required to control high blood pressure.

Hyperlipidemia may be lowered by altering your dietary intake, physical activity, and drug treatment (Barrow, 1992; Durnstine & Thompson, 2000). One of the simplest ways of reducing cholesterol is through diet. Decreasing your intake of saturated fats and cholesterol may significantly reduce your blood cholesterol levels (Nutritional Links to Health and Fitness, p. 320).

A vegetarian diet, defined as one that does not include meat, fish, or fowl, is low in saturated fat and cholesterol and higher in antioxidants such as vitamins C and E and phytochemicals (American Dietetic Association; Dietitians of Canada, 2003). As a result, a vegetarian diet is associated with lower body mass, a reduced mortality rate from heart disease, lower blood cholesterol levels, lower blood pressure, and lower rates of hypertension and type 2 diabetes (American Dietetic Association; Dietitians of Canada, 2003). Controversy exists concerning the effectiveness of a nutritional intake high in antioxidants in preventing CHD. See the Nutritional Links to Health and Fitness box below.

As noted previously, the risk of CHD for smokers decreases as soon as they quit. Clearly, smoking cessation is an important way of reducing CHD risk. Fitness and wellness expert Dr. Melvin Williams offers the following advice on smoking (Kohl, 2001): "If you don't smoke, don't start! If you smoke, quit!" Unfortunately, for most people smoking is a difficult habit to break.

Adding physical activity to your daily routine is another simple way to improve your CHD profile. Even modest levels of physical activity (e.g., 20 to 30 minutes of walking 3 to 5 times per week) reduces the risk of CHD development due to physical inactivity (Blair et al., 1989; Bouchard et al., 1990; Kavanagh, 2001; Paffenbarger et al., 1986; Thompson et al., 2003, Touyz et al., 2004). In addition, regular aerobic exercise modifies other CHD risk factors by positively influencing blood pressure, body composition, and blood cholesterol levels.

Modification of Secondary Risk Factors

The three secondary CHD risk factors that can be modified are obesity, type 2 diabetes, and stress. Body weight loss can be achieved through a combination of diet modification and physical activity (Chapter 8). For example, a nutritional intake reduced in calories and fat coupled with an increase in physical activity will help reduce excess body fat. Regular physical activity can reduce the risk of developing type 2 diabetes. Relaxation techniques (discussed in Chapter 9) can help in counteracting the effects of a stressful lifestyle and therefore reduce the risk for development of CHD.

Reducing Your Risk of Coronary Heart Disease: A Final Word

Regardless of your family history, you can reduce your risk of disease by positively modifying your CHD risk factors. The more changes you make to lower your CHD risk, the better your chances are of preventing cardiovascular disease. Be prepared for occasional backsliding (e.g., eating a high-fat meal or missing opportunities to be physically active); however, when this occurs, quickly regain your focus and return to a healthy lifestyle. CHD risk factor management can add quality and years to your life. Take action today and lower your CHD risk. See A Closer Look (p. 320) for answers to some frequently asked questions about heart disease, nutritional intake, and physical activity.

NUTRITIONAL LINKS TO HEALTH AND FITNESS

Can Antioxidant Vitamins Reduce Your Risk of Coronary Heart Disease?

Free radicals are molecules with an unpaired electron in their outer orbital. While understanding the chemistry of these molecules is not essential, it is important to know that formation of free radicals can result in "oxidative injury" to cells. This free radical–mediated oxidative injury has been linked to many diseases, including CHD. In this regard, research indicates that oxidative injury inside blood vessels is a major contributor to the development of atherosclerosis and CHD. The mechanism that explains this observation relates to the role of oxidative stress in the pathogeneses of atherosclerosis (Antoniades, Tousoulis, Tentolouris, Totuouzas, & Stefanadis, 2003). Extensive research clearly shows that free radicals, particularly reactive oxygen species, play a critical role in the oxidative damage to arterial walls. Antioxidants are believed to reduce the effect of free radicals and improve endothelial function (Antoniades et al., 2003; Hasnaian & Mooradian, 2004). Since antioxidant vitamins (e.g., vitamins E and C and beta carotene) can prevent radical-mediated oxidative injury, it has been reasoned that dietary supplementation with antioxidant vitamins may reduce your risk of CHD (Leeds, 1998). Although some studies reported that antioxidant supplementation reduced the risk of arteriosclerosis, many studies failed to find that antioxidant supplementation protected against atherosclerosis (Hasnain & Mooradian, 2004; Kinlay et al., 2004). Further, one research study found an increased risk for heart failure with long-term vitamin E supplementation in individuals with vascular disease or type 2 diabetes (Lonn et al., 2005). Moreover, most studies showing protective effects of antioxidants used vitamin supplements at doses above the Dietary Reference Intakes (DRI). This has raised concern among many dietitians, who argue that high doses of these vitamins may result in toxic side effects. Until additional research is performed, the best advice is to eat plenty of fresh fruits and vegetables to obtain as many antioxidants as possible from your nutritional intake (Leeds, 1998).

Diet and Blood Cholesterol Levels

One of the easiest dietary means of reducing your blood cholesterol is to reduce your intake of saturated fat and cholesterol. Saturated fats stimulate cholesterol synthesis in the liver and therefore contribute to elevated blood cholesterol. Saturated fats are found mostly in meats and dairy products; avoiding high intake of these foods can reduce your blood cholesterol levels. The table in this box lists the cholesterol content of selected foods. See the Appendices for a more complete listing.

Food	Serving Size	Cholesterol (mg)	Saturated Fat (g)
Bacon	2 slices	30	0.7
Beef (lean)	224 g	150	12
Butter	25 mL	32	0.4
Cheese			
Processed	28 g	27	5.4
Cheddar	28 g	30	5.9
Egg	1 (boiled)	113	2.8
Hamburger			
patty	1 small	68	5.9
Milk (whole)	250 mL	33	5
Milkshake	300 mL	54	8.2
Pizza (meat)	1 slice (36 cm diameter)	31	8
Sausage	84 g	42	8.6
Wiener	1	30	5.2

Frequently Asked Questions about Heart Disease, Nutritional Intake, and Physical Activity

Can dietary modifications or regular physical activity slow the progression of atherosclerosis?
Several studies have concluded that a nutritional intake low in saturated fat can retard the development of atherosclerotic plaques in blood vessels, and regular physical activity prevents the progression of atherosclerosis (Touyz et al., 2004). Clearly, then, a lifestyle that includes a low-fat dietary intake and regular physical activity is a good strategy for slowing the buildup of atherosclerotic plaques.

Some physicians are recommending patients take Aspirin daily to reduce the risk of heart attack. How does Aspirin provide this benefit?
A heart attack occurs when part of the heart muscle is damaged by a stoppage of blood flow through arteries that supply that region of the heart. This often occurs when a blood clot forms and blocks an artery that has been narrowed by the buildup of atherosclerotic plaque. Extensive research indicates that daily doses of Aspirin can prevent heart attacks by reducing the likelihood that blood platelets will stick together and precipitate a blood clot.

Consult your physician before beginning a daily regimen of Aspirin, since Aspirin may not be appropriate for people with bleeding disorders, liver disease, kidney disease, or peptic ulcers, or for individuals allergic to Aspirin.

I've read newspaper accounts of several cases of sudden cardiac death in young athletes. How great is the risk?
Each year only a few cases of sudden cardiac death are reported. Given that millions of young people participate in regular physical activity or sports, the likelihood that a healthy young person will die from sudden cardiac death is extremely small.

Can a medical exam identify people at risk for sudden cardiac death during exercise?
Yes. The combination of a medical history and a physical exam by a qualified physician can usually identify individuals with undetected heart disease that would place them at risk of sudden cardiac death during strenuous physical activities (Rowland, 1999).

Summary

1. Heart disease is the number one cause of death in Canada and the United States. In Canada, 36 percent of all male and 39 percent of all female deaths annually are attributed to cardiovascular diseases.

2. Cardiovascular disease refers to any disease that affects the heart and blood vessels. Common cardiovascular diseases include arteriosclerosis, coronary artery disease, stroke, and hypertension.

3. Coronary risk factors are those that increase your chance for developing coronary heart disease.

4. Coronary risk factors are classified as primary or secondary. Primary risk factors are those that directly increase the risk of coronary heart disease. Secondary risk factors may increase your chance of developing coronary heart disease by promoting the development of a primary risk factor.
5. Primary risk factors for the development of coronary heart disease include hypertension, hyperlipidemia, smoking, and physical inactivity.
6. Secondary risk factors for the development of coronary heart disease include type 2 diabetes, obesity, and stress.
7. Your risk of developing coronary heart disease can be reduced by modification of the following risk factors: hypertension, hyperlipidemia, smoking, physical inactivity, obesity, and stress.
8. A nutritional intake low in saturated fats and cholesterol with plenty of fruits and vegetables may also reduce risk for developing coronary artery disease.

Study Questions

1. Identify the number one cause of death in Canada.
2. Define the following terms:

   cardiovascular disease   atherosclerosis
   coronary heart disease   systolic blood pressure
   coronary artery disease   diastolic blood pressure
   hypertension   HDL, LDL

3. List the primary and secondary risk factors for the development of coronary heart disease.
4. Discuss the difference between *primary* and *secondary* risk factors for the development of coronary heart disease.
5. High-density and low-density lipoproteins have been labelled "good" and "bad" cholesterol, respectively. Explain.
6. Which primary coronary heart disease risk factors can be modified?
7. Which secondary coronary heart disease risk factors can be modified?
8. How does a high-salt diet contribute to hypertension?
9. What is the link between diet and blood cholesterol?
10. How does smoking increase your risk of developing cardiovascular disease?
11. How are arteriosclerosis and atherosclerosis related?
12. How does physical activity prevent cardiovascular diseases?

Suggested Reading

Peterson, J. A. (2000). Take ten: 10 ways to protect your heart. *ACSM's Health and Fitness Journal, 4(2)*, 48.

Thomas, T., & LaFontaine, T. (2001). Exercise, nutritional strategies, and lipoproteins. In J. Roitman (Ed.), *ACSM's Resource Manual for Guidelines for Exercise Testing and Prescription* (4th ed.). Philadelphia: Lippincott, Williams & Wilkins.

Thompson, P. D., Buchner, D., Piña, I. L., Balady, G. J., Williams, M. A., Marcus, B. H., Berra, K., Blair, S. N., Costa, F., Franklin, B., Fletcher, G. F., Gordon, N. F., Pate, R. R., Rodriguez, B. L., Yancey, A. K., & Wenger, N. K. (2003). Exercise and physical activity in the prevention and treatment of atherosclerotic cardiovascular disease. *Circulation, 107*, 3109–3116.

Touyz, R. M., Campbell, N., Logan, A., Gledhill, N., Petrella, R., & Padwal, R. (2004). Canadian Hypertension Education Program. The 2004 Canadian recommendations for the management of hypertension: Part III—Lifestyle modifications to prevent and control hypertension. *Canadian Journal of Cardiology, 20(1)*, 55–59.

Weblinks

Statistics Canada

www.statcan.ca

Contains the most recent statistics on rates of morbidity and mortality for diseases of the heart, cerebrovascular diseases, diabetes, and diseases of the arteries, arterioles, and capillaries.

Heart and Stroke Foundation of Canada

www.heartandstroke.ca

Community-driven and -oriented foundation that strives to provide the most reliable information on heart disease and stroke in Canada.

Canadian Diabetes Association

www.diabetes.ca

An online resource for people with, and affected by, diabetes and for health care professionals treating those affected by the disease.

***Canadian Medical Association Journal* (CMAJ)**

www.cmaj.ca

Open and free access to the leading health sciences journal in Canada. CMAJ is a general medical journal that publishes original research, review articles, commentaries and editorials, practice updates, and health news.

Canadian Society for Exercise Physiology

www.csep.ca

Promotes the generation, synthesis, transfer and application of knowledge and research related to exercise physiology (encompassing physical activity, fitness, health, and human performance).

References

American Dietetic Association; Dieticians of Canada. (2003). Position of the American Dietetics Association and

Dieticians of Canada: Dieticians of Canada. *Canadian Journal of Dietetic Practice and Research, 64(2),* 62–81.

Antoniades, C., Tousoulis, D., Tentolouris, C., Totuouzas, P., & Stefanadis, C. (2003). Oxidative stress, antioxidant vitamins, and atherosclerosis. From basic research to clinical practice. *Herz, 28(7),* 628–638.

Barrow, M. (1992). *Heart talk: Understanding cardiovascular diseases.* Gainesville, FL: Cor-Ed Publishing.

Blair, S. N., Kohl, H. W., Paffenbarger, R. S., Clark, D. G., Cooper, K. H., & Gibbons, L. W. (1989). Physical fitness and all-cause mortality: A prospective study of healthy men and women. *Journal of the American Medical Association, 262,* 2395–2401.

Bouchard, C., Shephard, R., Stephens, T., Sutton, J., & McPherson, B. (1990). *Exercise, fitness, and health: A consensus of current knowledge.* Champaign, IL: Human Kinetics.

Canadian Institute for Health Information. (2003). *Health care in Canada, 2003.* Ottawa: Author.

Chobanian, A. V., Bakris, G. L., Black, H. R., Cushman, W. C., Green, L. A., Izzo, J. L., Jr., Jones, D. W., Materson, B. J., Oparil, S., & Roccella, E. J. (2003). Seventh report of the Joint National Committee on Prevention, Detection, Evaluation, and Treatment of High Blood Pressure: The JNC-7 report. *Journal of the American Medical Association, 289(19),* 2560–2572. Erratum 2003: *290(2),* 197.

Durstine, J. L., & Thompson, R. (2000). Exercise modulates blood lipids and exercise plan. *ACSM's Health and Fitness Journal, 4(4),* 44–46.

Greenberg, J. S., Dintiman, G. B., Myers Oakes, B., Irwin, J. D., & Morrow, D. (2004). *Physical fitness and wellness Canadian edition* (2nd ed.). Toronto: Pearson.

Hasnaian, B. I., & Mooradian, B. A. (2004). Recent trials of antioxidant therapy: What should we be telling our patients? *Cleveland Clinical Journal of Medicine, 71(4),* 327–334.

Heart and Stroke Foundation of Canada. (1995). *Heart disease and stroke in Canada.* Ottawa: Author.

Heart and Stroke Foundation of Canada. (2004). *Risk factors—Coronary heart disease risk factor.* Retrieved June 2, 2004, from ww1.heartandstroke.ca/Page.asp?PageID=110&ArticleID=589&Src=heart.

Heart and Stroke Foundation of Canada and ACTI-MENU. (1999). *Do you have a healthy heart?* Canada: ACTI-MENU.

Kavanagh, T. (2001). Exercise in the primary prevention of coronary heart disease. *Canadian Journal of Cardiology, 17(2),* 155–161.

Kinlay, S., Behrendt, D., Fang, J. C., Delagrange, D., Morrow, J., Witzum, J. L., Rifai, N., Selwyn, A. P., Creager, M. A., & Ganz, P. (2004). Long-term effect of combined vitamin E and C on coronary and peripheral endothelial function. *Journal of American College of Sports Medicine, 18,* 629–634.

Kohl, H. (2001). Physical activity and cardiovascular disease: Evidence for a dose–response. *Medicine and Science in Sports and Exercise, 33(Suppl.),* S472–S483.

Leeds, M. (1998). *Nutrition for healthy living.* Boston: WCB-McGraw-Hill.

Lonn, E., Bosch, J., Yusuf, S., Sheridan, P., Pogue, J., Aarnold, J. M., Ross, C., Arnold, A., Sleight, P., Probstfield, J., & Dagenasi, G. R. (2005). Effects of long-term vitamin E supplementation on cardiovascular events and cancer: A randomized controlled trial. *Journal of the American Medical Association, 293(11),* 2560–2572.

Negri, E., LaVecchia, C., D'Avanzo, B., Nobili, A., & LaMalfa, R. G. (1994). Acute myocardial infarction: Association with time since stopping smoking in Italy. *Journal of Epidemiology and Community Health, 48(2),* 129–133.

Paffenbarger, R. S., Hyde, R. T., Wing, A. L., & Hsieh, C. C. (1986). Physical activity, all-cause mortality of college alumni. *New England Journal of Medicine, 314,* 605–613.

Reeder, B. A., Senthilselvan, A., Després, J-P., Angel, A., Liu, L., Wang, H., & Rabkin, S. W. (1997). The association of cardiovascular disease risk factors with abdominal obesity in Canada. *Canadian Medical Association Journal, 157(1 Suppl),* S39–S45.

Rowland, T. (1999). Screening for risk of cardiac death in young athletes. *Sports Science Exchange, 12(3),* 1–5.

Statistics Canada. (1997). Leading causes of death, 1995. Catalogue No. 84-503-XPB.

Statistics Canada. (1998a) At risk of first or recurring heart disease. Catalogue No. 82-003-XPB.

Statistics Canada. (1998b). Current and future hospitalization after heart attack. Catalogue No. 82-003-XPB.

Statistics Canada. (2003). Canada at a glance, 2003. Catalogue No. 12-581-XPE.

Statistics Canada. (2004). Percentage of smokers in the population. Catalogue No. 82-221-XIE.

Third report of the National Cholesterol Education Program Expert Panel on Detection, Evaluation, and Treatment of High Blood Cholesterol in Adults. (2001). *Journal of the American Medical Association, 285(19),* 1–19.

Thomas, T., & LaFontaine, T. (2001). Exercise, nutritional strategies, and lipoproteins. In J. Roitman (Ed.), *ACSM's Resource Manual for Guidelines for Exercise Testing and Prescription* (4th ed.). Philadelphia: Lippincott, Williams & Wilkins.

Thompson, P. D., Buchner, D., Piña, I. L., Balady, G. J., Williams, M. A., Marcus, B. H., Berra, K., Blair, S. N., Costa, F., Franklin, B., Fletcher, G. F., Gordon, N. F., Pate, R. R., Rodriguez, B. L., Yancey, A. K., & Wenger, N. K. (2003). Exercise and physical activity in the prevention and treatment of atherosclerotic cardiovascular disease. *Circulation, 107,* 3109–3116.

Touyz, R. M., Campbell, N., Logan, A., Gledhill, N., Petrella, R., & Padwal, R. (2004). Canadian Hypertension Education Program. The 2004 Canadian recommendations for the management of hypertension: Part III—Lifestyle modifications to prevent and control hypertension. *Canadian Journal of Cardiology, 20(1),* 55–59.

Understanding Your CVD Risk

Name_____ Age _____ Sex _____ Date _____

Each of us has a unique level of risk for various diseases. Some of these risks are things you can take action to change; others are risks that you need to consider as you plan a lifelong strategy for overall risk reduction. Complete each of the following questions and total your points in each section. If you score between 1 and 5 in any section, consider your risk. The higher the number, the greater your risk. If you answer "don't know" for any question, talk to your parents or other family members as soon as possible to find out if you have any unknown risks.

PART I: ASSESS YOUR FAMILY RISK FOR CVD

1. Do any of your primary relatives (mother, father, grandparents, siblings) have a history of heart disease or stroke?

   Yes ☐ (1 point)　　　No ☐ (0 points)　　　Don't Know ☐

2. Do any of your primary relatives (mother, father, grandparents, siblings) have diabetes?

   Yes ☐ (1 point)　　　No ☐ (0 points)　　　Don't Know ☐

3. Do any of your primary relatives (mother, father, grandparents, siblings) have high blood pressure?

   Yes ☐ (1 point)　　　No ☐ (0 points)　　　Don't Know ☐

4. Do any of your primary relatives (mother, father, grandparents, siblings) have a history of high cholesterol?

   Yes ☐ (1 point)　　　No ☐ (0 points)　　　Don't Know ☐

5. Would you say that your family consumed a high fat diet (lots of red meat, dairy, butter/margarine) during your time spent at home?

   Yes ☐ (1 point)　　　No ☐ (0 points)　　　Don't Know ☐

   Total ☐

PART II: ASSESS YOUR LIFESTYLE RISK FOR CVD

1. Is your total cholesterol level higher than it should be?

   Yes ☐ (1 point)　　　No ☐ (0 points)　　　Don't Know ☐

2. Do you have high blood pressure?

   Yes ☐ (1 point)　　　No ☐ (0 points)　　　Don't Know ☐

3. Have you been diagnosed as prediabetic or diabetic?

   Yes ☐ (1 point)　　　No ☐ (0 points)　　　Don't Know ☐

4. Do you smoke?

   Yes ☐ (1 point)　　　No ☐ (0 points)　　　Don't Know ☐

5. Would you describe your life as highly stressful?

   Yes ☐ (1 point)　　　No ☐ (0 points)　　　Don't Know ☐

   Total ☐

PART III: ASSESS YOUR ADDITIONAL RISKS FOR CVD

1. How would you best describe your current weight?
   a. Lower than what it should be for my height and weight (0 points)
   b. About what it should be for my height and weight
      (1 point)
   c. Higher than it should be for my height and weight
      (1 point)

2. How would you describe the level of exercise that you get each day?
   a. Less than what I should be exercising each day
      (1 point)
   b. About what I should be exercising each day (0 points)
   c. More than what I should be each day (0 points)

3. How would you describe your dietary behaviours?
   a. Eating only the recommended number of calories per day (0 points)
   b. Eating less than the recommended number of calories per day (0 points)
   c. Eating more than the recommended number of calories per day (1 point)

4. Which of the following best describes your typical dietary behaviour?
   a. I eat from the major food groups, trying hard to get the recommended amount of fruits and vegetables
      (0 points)
   b. I eat too much red meat and consume a good deal of saturated fat from meats and dairy products each
      day (1 point)
   c. Whenever possible, I try to substitute olive oil or canola oil for other forms of dietary fat (0 points)

5. Which of the following best describes you?
   a. I watch my sodium intake and try to reduce stress in my life (0 points)
   b. I have a history of chlamydia infection (1 point)
   c. I try to eat 5 to 10 milligrams of soluble fibre each day and to substitute an animal product for a soy
      product in my diet at least once each week (0 points)

Total [   ]

CHAPTER 15

Prevention of Cancer

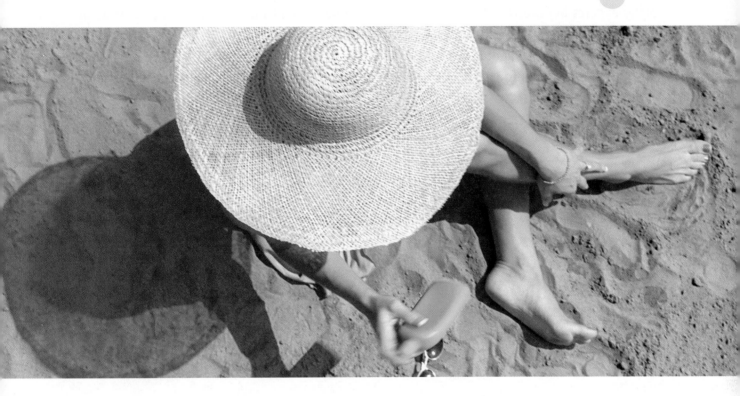

After studying this chapter, you should be able to

1. Define *cancer*.
2. List the seven warning signs of cancer.
3. List the most common types of cancer.
4. Identify factors that influence your risk of developing cancer.
5. Give examples of several types of occupational carcinogens.
6. Outline ways to reduce your risk of skin cancer due to exposure to ultraviolet light.
7. Explain the roles dietary intake and physical activity have in reducing your cancer risk.
8. Explain how regular self-examinations can reduce your risk of cancer.

Cancer is the second leading cause of death in Canada, and death rates continue to climb as the population increases and ages (National Cancer Institute of Canada, 2005). Current predictions are that 38 percent of women and 43 percent of men will develop cancer during their lives. Cancer can strike at any age, although it occurs more frequently in older people. Current statistics forecast that about 41 percent of all Canadians will develop cancer and have a 27-percent chance of dying as a result (Table 15.1).

Although the number of cases is on the rise, the development of new detection and treatment regimens means that cancer need not be a death sentence. According to the Canadian Cancer Society, the number of Canadians successfully surviving cancer continues to increase each year. The key to survival is early detection. If cancers were diagnosed earlier, more than half of cancer deaths could be prevented. The best aids to early detection of cancer are the seven warning signs listed in A Closer Look (p. 329).

Many experts believe that the rise in cancer may be linked to cancer-causing chemicals in water and food supplies as well as diet and lifestyle factors, hormones, infections, genetics, and occupational and environmental factors (Levenson, 2004; National Cancer Institute, 2005). This chapter provides information about the various types of cancers and how to reduce your risk.

	Probability (%) of Developing Cancer in Next 10 Years by Age Group						Lifetime Probability of Developing Cancer		Dying of Cancer	
	30–39	40–49	50–59	60–69	70–79	80–89	%	One in:	%	One in:
Male										
All Cancers	0.6	1.7	6.1	15.5	21.9	20.3	44.0	2.3	28.7	3.5
Prostate	—	0.1	1.7	5.6	6.9	5.3	14.1	7.1	3.9	25.8
Lung	—	0.2	0.9	2.7	4.3	3.7	8.8	11.4	8.1	12.3
Colorectal	—	0.2	0.9	2.1	3.3	3.4	7.3	13.7	3.5	28.4
Lymphoma	0.1	0.2	0.4	0.7	1.1	1.1	2.9	34.3	1.7	59.2
Bladder	—	0.1	0.3	0.7	1.3	1.5	2.7	37.1	1.0	100.0
Kidney	—	0.1	0.3	0.5	0.7	0.6	1.7	57.8	0.7	140.8
Leukemia	—	0.1	0.1	0.4	0.6	0.7	1.5	65.0	1.0	98.0
Oral	—	0.1	0.3	0.4	0.5	0.4	1.4	70.8	0.6	181.8
Stomach	—	—	0.1	0.4	0.6	0.7	1.4	72.4	1.0	103.1
Melanoma	0.1	0.1	0.2	0.3	0.4	0.4	1.3	77.1	0.3	303.0
Pancreas	—	—	0.1	0.3	0.5	0.6	1.2	81.6	1.3	76.9
Female										
All Cancers	1.2	3.0	6.3	10.1	13.6	13.5	38.4	2.6	23.5	4.3
Breast	0.4	1.3	2.4	3.1	3.2	2.5	11.2	8.9	3.7	26.8
Colorectal	—	0.2	0.6	1.3	2.3	2.9	6.4	15.7	3.3	30.6
Lung	—	0.2	0.8	1.7	2.3	1.8	5.9	16.8	5.0	20.0
Lymphoma	0.1	0.1	0.3	0.5	0.8	0.9	2.5	40.1	1.4	69.9
Body of Uterus	—	0.1	0.5	0.7	0.7	0.5	2.3	43.4	0.5	185.2
Ovary	—	0.1	0.3	0.4	0.5	0.4	1.5	66.7	1.1	90.9
Pancreas	—	—	0.1	0.2	0.5	0.6	1.3	78.5	1.3	75.2
Leukemia	—	—	0.1	0.2	0.4	0.5	1.1	89.0	0.7	135.1
Kidney	—	0.1	0.2	0.3	0.4	0.4	1.1	89.9	0.4	227.3
Melanoma	0.1	0.1	0.2	0.2	0.3	0.2	1.1	92.8	0.2	526.3
Bladder	—	—	0.1	0.2	0.3	0.4	0.9	106.6	0.4	256.4
Stomach	—	—	—	0.1	0.3	0.4	0.8	127.7	0.6	175.4
Cervix	0.1	0.1	0.1	0.1	0.1	0.1	0.7	138.2	0.3	384.6
Oral	—	—	0.1	0.2	0.2	0.2	0.7	148.2	0.3	400.0

TABLE 15.1 Probability of Developing Cancer by Age, and Lifetime Probability of Developing and Dying from Cancer

Source: Canadian Cancer Society/National Cancer Institute of Canada: Canadian Cancer Statistics 2005, Toronto, Canada, 2005.

—*Value less than 0.05.*

Note: The probability of developing cancer is calculated based on age- and sex-specific cancer incidence and mortality rates for Canada in 2001 and on life tables based on 1999–2001 all cause mortality rates. The probability of dying from cancer represents the proportion of persons dying from cancer in a cohort subjected to the mortality conditions prevailing in the population at large in 2001.

What Is Cancer?

Cancer, the uncontrolled growth and spread of abnormal cells, is not a single disease but a collection of more than 200 different but related diseases that can occur in almost every tissue and organ in the body (Robbins & Kumar, 1997; Tannock & Hill, 1998). Groups of these abnormal cells result in the growth of new tissue that has no physiologic use, called a *neoplasm*. The neoplastic mass forms a clumping of cells known as a tumour. **Tumours** can be either *benign* or *malignant*. Generally, **benign tumours** are not serious health threats because the cells in them grow and divide relatively slowly and remain localized. In contrast, cells of **malignant tumours** are cancer cells; they grow rapidly and out of control, and they often spread to other locations throughout the body. As cancer cells divide unchecked, the malignant tumour grows in size and invades neighbouring tissue. The growing cancer cells interfere with normal organ function, which may eventually result in potentially fatal organ failure.

The crucial difference between benign-tumour cells and cancer cells is that cancer cells can spread throughout the body—a process called **metastasis**. Thus, for example, cancer cells that arise in the breast may invade breast tissue and eventually spread (metastasize) to other organs (Figure 15.1). Metastasis significantly reduces a cancer patient's chances of survival not only because more organs are affected but also because it is more difficult to treat cancer when it is in more than one location.

When an abnormal growth is discovered in the body, the only way to determine if the growth is a benign or malignant tumour is through biopsy. A biopsy is the surgical removal of a small sample of the tumour for subsequent laboratory analysis.

Types of Cancer

Cancer can develop in almost any organ (Robbins & Kumar, 1997). Skin cancers are more common than cancers of any other organ (National Cancer Institute of Canada, 2005). Other common sites for cancer include the mouth, lung, stomach, colon, kidney, liver, prostate gland, and breast (Table 15.2). There are five broad classifications of cancer made from their microscopic appearance and the body site from which they arise. The name of the cancer is derived from the type of tissue in which it develops. Most human cancers are **carcinomas**, cancers that affect the tissues covering the body surfaces and lining within body cavities. Examples of carcinomas are breast, lung, intestinal, and mouth cancers. They multiply or metastasize through the circulatory or lymphatic system and eventually form solid tumours. **Lymphomas** also develop in the lymphatic system, damaging the infection-fighting regions of the body. Hodgkin's is one form of lymphoma and develops within the lymph nodes (Tortora, 2002).

Sarcomas are any cancer that develops in muscle cells or connective tissues. *Osteogenic sarcoma* is a frequent type

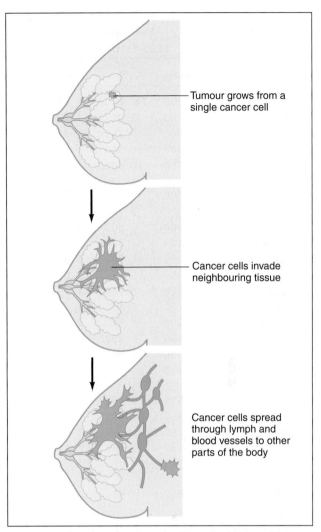

FIGURE 15.1 Growth and metastasis of a malignant breast tumour.

- Tumour grows from a single cancer cell
- Cancer cells invade neighbouring tissue
- Cancer cells spread through lymph and blood vessels to other parts of the body

of childhood sarcoma that destroys normal bone tissue (connective tissue) and eventually metastasizes throughout the body. **Melanomas** are cancerous growths that occur in the skin tissue. Melanomas occur in the part of the skin that

cancer   The uncontrolled growth and spread of abnormal cells.

tumour   A group of abnormal cells. A tumour can be either benign or malignant (cancerous).

benign tumour   Non-cancerous group of cells.

malignant tumour   Cancerous group of cells that grows rapidly; results in deterioration or death.

metastasis   The process of malignant cells spreading through the body.

carcinoma   Malignant tumours that occur in tissue that lines the body.

lymphoma   A cancer that develops in lymphatic tissue.

sarcoma   Any cancer arising from muscle cells or connective tissues.

melanoma   Cancerous growths that develop in the skin cells that create melanin.

	New Cases 2005 Estimates			Deaths 2005 Estimates			Deaths/Cases Ratio 2005 Estimates		
	Total	M	F	Total	M	F	Total	M	F
All Cancers	**149 000**	**76 200**	**72 800**	**69 500**	**36 700**	**32 800**	**0.47**	**0.48**	**0.45**
Lung	22 200	12 000	10 200	19 000	10 700	8 300	0.86	0.89	0.82
Breast	21 800	150	21 600	5 300	45	5 300	0.24	0.30	0.24
Prostate	20 500	20 500	—	4 300	4 300	—	0.21	0.21	—
Colorectal	19 600	10 600	9 000	8 400	4 500	3 900	0.43	0.42	0.43
Non–Hodgkin's Lymphoma	6 400	3 400	3 000	3 000	1 600	1 350	0.46	0.47	0.46
Bladder	5 000	3 700	1 250	1 650	1 150	500	0.34	0.32	0.40
Kidney	4 500	2 800	1 650	1 500	950	570	0.34	0.34	0.34
Melanoma	4 400	2 300	2 000	880	540	340	0.20	0.23	0.17
Leukemia	4 000	2 300	1 700	2 200	1 300	940	0.56	0.56	0.56
Body of Uterus	3 900	—	3 900	710	—	710	0.18	—	0.18
Pancreas	3 400	1 650	1 750	3 300	1 600	1 750	0.99	0.98	0.99
Oral	3 200	2 100	1 050	1 050	710	350	0.33	0.34	0.33
Thyroid	3 100	710	2 400	170	65	100	0.05	0.09	0.04
Stomach	2 800	1 800	1 000	1 900	1 150	730	0.68	0.65	0.72
Brain	2 500	1 350	1 100	1 650	940	720	0.67	0.69	0.65
Ovary	2 400	—	2 400	1 550	—	1 550	0.66	—	0.66
Multiple Myeloma	1 850	1 000	850	1 250	680	590	0.68	0.67	0.69
Esophagus	1 450	1 050	400	1 600	1 200	420	1.13[1]	1.16[1]	1.05[1]
Cervix	1 350	—	1 350	400	—	400	0.30	—	0.30
Larynx	1 150	960	210	510	420	85	0.43	0.44	0.41
Testis	850	850	—	30	30	—	0.04	0.04	—
Hodgkin's Disease	850	460	390	120	70	55	0.14	0.15	0.14
All Other Sites	12 000	6 400	5 600	8 900	4 800	4 100	0.75	0.75	0.74

TABLE 15.2 Cancer Incidence and Death Rates by Site and Sex

Source: Canadian Cancer Society/National Cancer Institute of Canada: Canadian Cancer Statistics 2005, Toronto, Canada, 2005.

—Not applicable.

[1] The high ratio (in excess of 1.0) for cancer of the esophagus may result from incomplete registration of this cancer before death.

Note: Incidence figures exclude an estimated 78 000 new cases of non–melanoma skin cancer (basal and squamous). Total of rounded numbers may not equal rounded total number.

creates melanin or the colour of skin; they often turn that portion of the skin black. Finally, there is **leukemia**, a cancer of the blood-forming organs. It is characterized by rapid growth and distorted development of white blood cells.

After skin cancer, the most common types of cancer are prostate cancer in men and breast cancer in women (National Cancer Institute of Canada, 2005). More than 95

leukemia Cancer of blood-forming organs.

percent of all breast cancers are discovered by women themselves; a routine breast self-examination should be a monthly practice for all women (A Closer Look, p. 329). Although most cancers occur in people over the age of 40, testicular cancer is one of the most common cancers in young men (National Cancer Institute of Canada, 2005). In general, testicular tumours are first noticed as a painless enlargement of the testis. Accordingly, all young men should routinely examine their testicles (A Closer Look, p. 332).

Recently, the largest increase in cancer has been in a deadly form of skin cancer known as *malignant melanoma*

The Seven Warning Signs of Cancer

The best way to survive cancer is to detect it at the earliest possible moment, and early detection can be easier if you know the seven warning signs of cancer. One way to remember them is that each warning sign begins with the first letter of the words in the following sentence:

I **L**oathe **C**ancer, **T**he **B**ig **B**ad **S**courge.

*I*ndigestion or loss of appetite that persists

*L*umps or thickening in the breast or on the lips or tongue

*C*hange in size or colour of a wart or mole

*T*hroat problems: nagging or persistent cough or hoarseness and difficulty in swallowing

*B*leeding that is unexplained from the bowel, nipples, or vagina, or unexplained blood in the urine

*B*owel or bladder habits that change in an obvious way

*S*ores that do not heal or heal only slowly

If you develop any of these signs, see a physician immediately for a cancer screening test.

Breast Self-Examination

The best time to do a breast self-exam is right after your period, when breasts are not tender or swollen. If you do not have regular periods or sometimes skip a month, do it on the same day every month. Use the following procedure to perform your breast self-exam.

1. Lie down and put a pillow under your right shoulder. Place your right arm behind your head (a).
2. Use the finger pads of your three middle fingers on your left hand to feel for lumps or thickening in your right breast. Your finger pads are the top third of each finger.
3. Press firmly enough to know how your breast feels. If you're not sure how hard to press, ask your health care provider. Or try to copy the way your health care provider uses the finger pads during a breast exam. Learn what your breast feels like most of the time. A firm ridge in the lower curve of each breast is normal.
4. Move around the breast in a set way. You can choose either the circle (1), up and down (2), or the wedge (3). Do it the same way every time. It will help you to make sure that you've gone over the entire breast area, and to remember how your breast feels.
5. Now examine your left breast using the right hand finger pads. If you find any changes, see your doctor right away.

You might also want to do a breast self-exam while you're in the shower (b). Your soapy hands will glide over wet skin, making it easy to check how your breasts feel.

For Added Safety: You should also check your breasts while standing in front of a mirror right after you do your breast self-exam each month (c, d). See if there are any changes in the way your breasts look: dimpling of the skin, changes in the nipples, or redness or swelling.

Source: Reprinted by permission of the American Cancer Society, Inc.

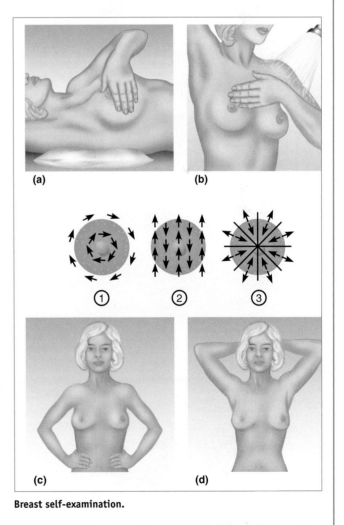

Breast self-examination.

(National Cancer Institute of Canada, 2005). The increase in this type of cancer is likely due to the diminishing layer of ozone in the earth's atmosphere, which protects us from the sun's ultraviolet rays. These rays are the primary cause of skin cancers.

In addition, there has been an increase in lung cancer for women (46 percent) since 1988 (National Cancer Institute,

carcinogens   Cancer-causing agents, which include radiation, chemicals, drugs, and other toxic substances.

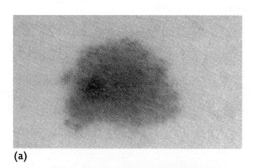

(a)

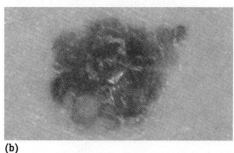

(b)

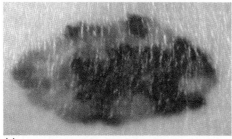

(c)

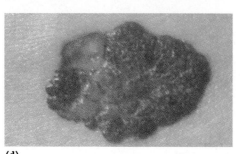

(d)

Malignant melanoma.

2004). The reason for the increased incidence of lung cancer in women is unknown but may be linked to poor air quality (i.e., airborne **carcinogens**) in many cities or being exposed to secondhand smoke.

How Do Normal Cells Become Cancerous?

Cell growth and division is controlled by DNA located within the cell. Normal DNA carefully regulates cell growth and division so that it occurs in a slow and steady fashion. Cancer occurs when DNA is damaged and cell division increases out of control.

DNA damage that results in cancer can occur in response to a number of environmental agents. These cancer-causing agents, called carcinogens, include radiation (including radiation from sunlight), chemicals, hydrocarbons (found in cigarette tar), drugs, and other toxic substances (Robbins & Kumar, 1997; Tortora, 2002). When a carcinogen enters the cell it damages the DNA, which results in a normal cell becoming an abnormal cancer cell (Figure 15.2).

Cancer Risk Factors

The cause of specific cancers is often unknown, but studies reveal that a variety of carcinogens can damage normal cells and start the cancer process. A number of factors play a role in determining your cancer risk (Levenson, 2004; National Cancer Institute of Canada, 2005): heredity, socioeconomic status, radiation exposure, viruses, tobacco use, alcohol use, occupational carcinogens, ultraviolet light, and dietary intake are all considered cancer risk factors (Figure 15.3).

Heredity   If a close blood relation (e.g., father or mother) had cancer, your chances of developing it are three times greater than average (Braakhuis et al., 2004). Although the exact link between heredity and cancer remains unclear, cancers of the breast, stomach, colon, prostate, uterus, ovaries, and lungs appear to run in families. Whether these family patterns of increased cancer risk are due to genetics or the fact that people in the same family experience similar environmental risks remains unclear.

Socioeconomic Status   Past research suggested that there were higher incidences of cancer and cancer deaths among blacks than among whites. The reason for the higher death rate in blacks was unclear, but may have been linked to the fact that cancers in whites are often detected at an earlier, more treatable stage. Current research suggests a weaker link between ethnicity and cancer and a stronger link between lower socioeconomic status and greater incidence of cancer (Baquet, Horm, Gibbs, & Greewald, 1991; Felix-Aaron, Moy, Kang, Chesley, & Clancy, 2005; Mackillop, Zhang-Salomons, Boyd, & Groome, 2000). The incidence of most types of cancer occurs in the lowest socioeconomic strata at twice the average rate in Canada even though it

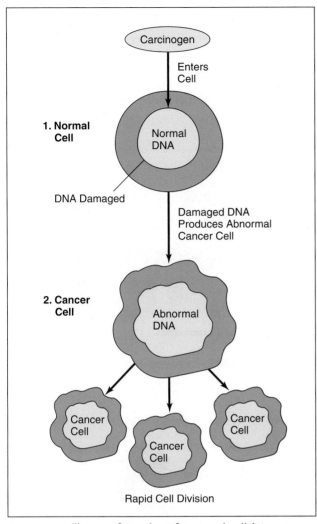

FIGURE 15.2 The transformation of a normal cell into a cancer cell. Entry of a carcinogen into the cell is followed by damage of the DNA.

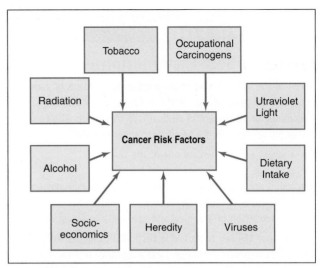

FIGURE 15.3 Cancer risk factors.

has a comprehensive health and social welfare system. The possible reason for this occurrence, as suggested in earlier research, is accessibility. For people who live below the poverty line, consistent access to a doctor is often difficult, whereas those who live within the middle or upper socioeconomic classes may have better access to faster detection and treatment that results in a better prognosis.

Radiation Up to 5 percent of all cancers may be caused by radiation exposure due to medical X-rays, occupational exposure through computer monitors, and environmental radiation (National Radiological Protection Board, 2001; Sasco, 2003). Further, many modern conveniences that emit electromagnetic fields (such as electric blankets) and low-frequency radio waves (such as those associated with cellular telephones) have been implicated in causing cancer.

Viruses It is clear that viruses are linked to many cancers (National Cancer Institute of Canada, 2005). Viruses can cause cancer by invading the cell and damaging DNA. Research has demonstrated that viruses play a role in several blood cancers (leukemia) as well as cancers of the lymphatic system (lymphomas). In addition, evidence suggests that viruses can cause liver, cervical, nose, and pharynx cancer.

Tobacco Tobacco use is the single largest cause of cancer deaths (approximately 25 percent) (Canadian Cancer Statistics, 2005; Single, Rehm, Robson, & Turong, 2000). Heavy smokers are 15 to 25 times more likely to die of cancer than non-smokers (Statistics Canada, 2003). Although the major cancer risk of smoking is the increased chance of developing lung cancer, smoking also increases risk for oral cancers (of the mouth, pharynx, larynx, and esophagus) as well as cancers of the pancreas and bladder (Menvieele, 2004). The average life expectancy for a chronic smoker is 7 years shorter than for a non-smoker.

Even if you don't smoke, evidence shows that second-hand tobacco smoke is also carcinogenic (Canadian Cancer Statistics, 2005). Thus, you should avoid not only active smoking but also inhaling smoke from others. Cigarettes are not the only risk: pipes, cigars, and smokeless tobacco also increase the risk for oral cancers.

Alcohol Heavy use of alcohol increases the risk for oral, esophagus, liver, and breast cancer (*Cancer Weekly*, 2004; Menvieele, 2004; Poschl & Seitz, 2004). Combining drinking and smoking creates an even greater risk for developing cancer. Even moderate drinking has been linked to an increased risk of breast cancer in women.

Occupational Carcinogens Factory workers and people living near factories may have an increased risk of cancer due to specific types of chemicals used or produced by those factories. Industrial chemicals known to be carcinogenic include benzene, nickel, chromate, asbestos, and vinyl chloride (National Cancer Institute, 2004).

Prevention of Cancer **331**

Testicular Self-Examination

Cancer of the testes is one of the most common forms of cancer in men 15 to 34 years of age (National Cancer Institute, 2004), and it accounts for 12 percent of all deaths in this group. The Canadian Cancer Society signals for testicular cancer include

- a slight enlargement of one of the testicles
- a change in the consistency of a testicle
- a dull ache in the lower abdomen or groin (may not occur in all cases of testicular cancer)
- the sensation of dragging and heaviness in a testicle

Because the key to surviving testicular cancer is early detection, all young men should perform a monthly self-examination; this is best done after a warm shower or bath, when the skin of the scrotum (the sac surrounding the testicle) is most relaxed. The examination is performed by rolling each testicle between the thumb and fingers (see the figure in this box). Lumps are generally found on the side or front of the testicle. The presence of a lump does not necessarily indicate cancer, but if you feel any lumps you should call your physician immediately to schedule a medical exam.

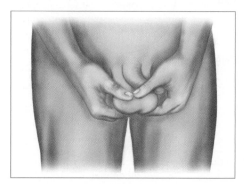

Testicular self-examination.

One of the most common occupational carcinogens is asbestos, a substance formerly used in the building and automobile industries. People who work with radioactive substances may also have increased risk for cancer. Working with coal tars, as in the mining professions, or working near airborne carcinogens, such as in the auto painting business, is also dangerous. Many chemicals used to kill weeds (herbicides) and insects (pesticides) contain potential carcinogens and are found in excessive amounts in some water supplies.

Ultraviolet Light Exposure to the sun or to artificial tanning lights is a major contributor to an increased risk for skin cancer (National Cancer Institute of Canada, 2005). Ultraviolet radiation from these two sources is responsible for more than 700 000 new cases of skin cancer each year. Tanning machines and sun lamps produce ultraviolet rays and present as much risk as the sun's rays. Some tanning salons claim that their equipment emits ultraviolet light at different wavelengths than sunshine and is therefore less dangerous. This is not true! If a sun lamp causes you to tan or burn, it is just as dangerous as the sun.

Nutritional Intake According to the U.S. National Academy of Sciences (2005), nutritional intake is implicated in 60 percent of the cancers in women and 40 percent of the cancers in men (Bianchinni, Kaaks, & Vainio, 2002; Chowdhury, Nishikawa, Blevins, & Rayford, 2000; Levenson, 2004; Millen et al., 2004). A high-fat diet has been linked to breast, colon, and prostate cancer, and it contributes to obesity, which in turn increases the risk for colon, breast, and

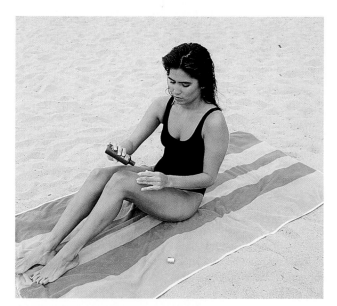

Overexposure to sunlight increases your risk of skin cancer.

uterine cancer. In addition, salt-cured, smoked, and nitrite-cured foods have been linked to cancers of the esophagus and stomach.

Cancer Prevention

Recall from our earlier discussion of coronary heart disease that we can control selected risk factors for heart disease. Many cancers can be prevented in the same way—with lifestyle changes. Indeed, approximately 80 percent of all cancers are related to lifestyle and environmental factors (Levenson, 2004; National Cancer Institute of Canada, 2005). According to the National Cancer Institute, people who lead a healthy lifestyle have only about one-third to one-half the rate of cancer deaths of the general population. Thus, with a change in lifestyle and avoidance of environmental factors that increase your risk, you can prevent many cancers. The first step in reducing your risk of cancer is to identify which cancer risk factors apply to you (see Laboratory 15.1). The next step is to modify those aspects of your environment and lifestyle that increase your chances of developing cancer. Although each individual's heredity is a given, the following cancer risk factors can be modified.

Alcohol Oral cancer and cancers of the larynx, throat, esophagus, and liver occur more frequently among heavy alcohol drinkers (Canadian Cancer Statistics, 2004). Because even moderate alcohol consumption has been implicated as

a cause of some cancers, it is wise to abstain from alcohol consumption or to at least decrease your consumption to a low level. Remember, combining alcohol and tobacco puts you at even greater risk.

Radiation Avoid overexposure to any source of radiation. Medical X-rays, low-frequency radio waves, and other sources of low-level radiation may not be avoidable and are not harmful unless encountered in excess (National Radiological Protection Board, 2001).

Tobacco Cigarette smoking and use of smokeless tobacco increase your risk of cancer. Cigarette smoking is responsible for 87 percent of all lung cancers, and use of chewing tobacco or snuff increases your risk of cancer of the mouth, larynx, throat, and esophagus (Goldenburg et al., 2004; Rodu & Jansson, 2004). Cancer risks can be greatly reduced by abstaining from all tobacco products. If you have never used any tobacco products, don't start. If you are using tobacco

FITNESS AND WELLNESS FOR ALL

Canadian Cancer Society Supports U.S. Initiative to Place Canadian-Style Warnings on Cigarette Packages

The Canadian Cancer Society's director of public issues, Ken Kyle, joined two U.S. Democratic Congressmen in New Jersey in support of legislation that would place Canadian-style warning labels on cigarette packages in the United States.

"Studies in Canada have shown that Canada's new picture-based warnings on cigarette packages are effective at discouraging smoking," said Kyle from a pharmacy in Trenton, NJ, where the news conference was held to generate grassroots support for the legislation.

"The U.S. initiative is further proof that this precedent-setting move is being watched and adopted by the world. Brazil, for example, has already implemented Canadian-style warnings and countries within the European Union are looking into using similar labels," added Kyle.

Introduced in June 2001, the picture-based warnings have gained support from 76 percent of Canadians, according to a recent Environics Research Group national survey. In a different study, among those noticing the new warnings, 43 percent of smokers say they have become more concerned about the health effects of smoking because of them and 44 percent said the new warnings increased their motivation to quit smoking.

"We must break down the image of cool that tobacco companies have manufactured to peddle their poison," said New Jersey Representative Rush Holt. He called on New Jersey pharmacy companies, many of which sell tobacco products in addition to medications, to participate in a local effort to place graphic tobacco

warnings in the storefronts and behind the medicine counters of New Jersey's pharmacies.

"There are few public places more appropriate for combating Big Tobacco's advertising schemes than at the trusted neighborhood pharmacies where New Jersey families get medical advice and buy medications. It is time to give tobacco the image it deserves," said Holt.

The U.S. initiative comes just before the final trial argument in Quebec Superior Court in which Canadian tobacco manufacturers argue that current Tobacco Act restrictions—namely the image-based package warnings and restrictions on tobacco advertising—are in violation of their constitutional right to freedom of expression.

Canada's main tobacco manufacturers, Rothmans, Benson & Hedges, Inc., JTI-Macdonald Corp., and Imperial Tobacco Canada, contend that tobacco advertising and promotion do not increase consumption, and only affect market share among brands.

The federal government and the Canadian Cancer Society—which has intervener status in the trial—argue that there is overwhelming evidence that tobacco advertising does increase smoking and that the restrictions are a "reasonable" limit on the tobacco manufacturers' freedom of expression under section 1 of the Charter of Rights and Freedoms.

Source: Canadian Cancer Society. (2002, July 29). Media release. Retrieved from http://129.33.170.32/ccs/ internet/mediareleaselist/0,3208,3172_15232_ 339341_langid-en,00.html. Reprinted with permission of the Canadian Cancer Society.

products, stop. Many of the detrimental effects of using tobacco products can be reversed if you quit using them.

Occupational Carcinogens

Avoid all industrial pollutants and follow safety procedures in the workplace. In particular, avoid exposure to industrial agents such as radon, dioxins, nickel, chromate, asbestos, and vinyl chloride. If you have questions concerning the carcinogenic risks of chemical exposure in your workplace, contact your provincial Ministry of the Environment. The ministry can provide you with a complete list of cancer-causing chemicals and identify those used in your workplace.

Ultraviolet Light

Prolonged exposure to ultraviolet light from any source increases your risk of developing skin cancer (National Cancer Institute, 2004). Limiting your sun exposure is an obvious way to avoid the carcinogenic effect of ultraviolet light. If you must be exposed to the sun for work or recreation, use a sunscreen to block the effects of ultraviolet rays (A Closer Look, below).

Remember, there is no such thing as a safe tan (Donatelle & Davis, 1991, National Cancer Institute of Canada, 2004). A tan is damaging to your skin, whether you tan quickly or accumulate it slowly over time. Exposure to ultraviolet light is cumulative, and the exposure you get at age 20 may adversely affect you at age 40.

Although skin cancer is the most common cancer, many types of skin cancer are curable if detected and treated early. The key to early detection is self-examination, which should be performed once a month and should include the entire body, particularly those areas exposed to sun. When examining your skin, be alert for the following signs:

1. A sore that doesn't heal. Have it checked if it hasn't healed after 3 weeks and if it bleeds or oozes.
2. A persistent reddish patch of skin that may be painful or itch, or may not bother you at all.
3. A shiny, waxy, scar-like spot that may be yellow or white with irregular borders.
4. A mole that begins to enlarge, thicken, or change colour.
5. A mole that bleeds or ulcerates.
6. A mole that has irregular rather than round borders.
7. A mole with irregular pigmentation; some areas may be light coloured, whereas other areas may be black.

If you have any of these signs, see your health care professional at once (Donatelle & Davis, 1996).

Dietary Intake

Nutrition is probably the most important factor in controlling your risk of cancer (Bianchinni, Kaaks, & Vainio, 2002; Environmental Nutrition, 2004; Levenson, 2004; Millen et al., 2004). Among the primary nutrients in foods that seem to have a protective effect against cancer are vitamins A, E, and C (Kanter, 1995), which appear to protect cells from damage by free radicals (also called *oxygen radicals*). **Free radicals** are normally produced in cells, but when they are produced in large quantities they promote the development of cancer by binding to DNA, altering its structure and function so that the cell divides rapidly and out of control (refer to Figure 15.2). Recent research has shown that vitamins A, E, and C may reduce the risk of cancer because they are antioxidants, substances that remove free radicals from cells and thus prevent DNA damage. These findings have prompted many cancer experts to recommend a dietary plan high in antioxidants (see the Nutritional Links to Health and Fitness box opposite).

Consumption of high-fibre foods lowers your risk of colon and rectal cancers. The apparent advantage of high-fibre foods is that fibre in food increases the frequency of bowel movements, which by decreasing the time the colon and rectum are exposed to dietary carcinogens reduces the risk of cancer.

sun protection factor (SPF)   A sunscreen with an SPF of 15 provides you with 15 times more protection than unprotected skin.

free radicals Promote the development of cancer by binding to DNA, altering its structure and function so that the cell divides rapidly and out of control.

A CLOSER LOOK

Protect Your Skin from Ultraviolet (UV) Rays

Lotions containing a *sunscreen*—a substance that protects the skin from UV radiation—should be applied approximately 30 minutes prior to exposure, because the protective ingredients require several minutes to be absorbed. The sunscreen should have a **sun protection factor (SPF)** of at least 15, which provides you with 15 times greater protection than unprotected skin. The following guidelines can reduce your risk of developing skin cancer from overexposure to ultraviolet rays.

1. Stay out of the sun between 10:00 a.m. and 2:00 p.m., when UV rays are the strongest.
2. If you use any skin preparation containing vitamin A (Retin A), stay out of the sun. Retin A skin lotions increase your susceptibility to UV damage.
3. Avoid sun lamps and tanning booths. If a sun lamp tans you, it damages your skin.
4. When being physically active outdoors use a waterproof sunscreen and apply it often and in adequate quantities.
5. Avoid sunburn by limiting your sun exposure.

Even though dietary fat has been hypothesized to be a risk factor for colon and rectal cancer, recent studies (Chowdhury, Nishikawa, Blevins, & Rayford, 2000; Norat & Roboli, 2001; Sandu, White, & McPherson, 2004; Willett, 2000; Willet, 2001) suggest that fat per se is not a major risk factor in most cancers. These studies indicate instead that consumption of more than 28 grams of red meat or processed meat per day increases your risk of colon and rectal cancers by 12 to 49 percent. The biological link between cancer and the ingestion of red meat remains unclear and is the focus of intensive research. For a list of dietary guidelines for lowering your risk of cancer, see Nutritional Links to Health and Fitness.

Physical Activity Reduces the Risk of Cancer

Some studies (Chakravarthy, Joyner, & Booth, 2002; Hardman, 2001; Slattery & Potter, 2002) provide evidence that regular physical activity may provide some protection against developing, and dying from, cancer. The best evidence comes from studies demonstrating that people who engage in regular physical activity have a lower incidence of colon cancer (Bianchinni, Kaaks, & Vainio, 2002; *Women's Health Weekly*, 2004). In addition, some reports suggest that physical activity reduces the occurrence of breast and uterine cancer in women (Levenson, 2004).

The primary debate about how physical activity protects against cancer centres on the question, "Does physical activity alter the immune system to reduce the formation of cancer cells?" Tumours form normally in everyone from time to time, but the immune system typically destroys the abnormal cells before they increase in number. Therefore, a strong immune system acts to reduce the risk of cancer, whereas a weak immune system may increase your risk of

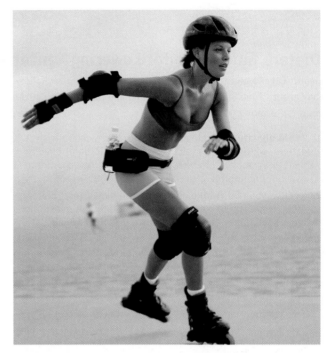

Thirty minutes of physical activity a day pays big dividends in preventing cancer.

cancer. Although numerous studies suggest that physically active individuals have an increased resistance to infection (Lee, 2003) and a decreased incidence of certain forms of cancer (Friedenreich & Orenstein, 2002; Frisch, Wyshak, & Albright, 1985), scientific evidence indicating that physical activity positively alters the immune system is limited (Kiningham, 1998; Malm, 2004). Therefore, it may be that factors other than adaptation of the immune system are responsible for the observation that physical activity is associated with a reduced risk of cancer.

NUTRITIONAL LINKS TO HEALTH AND FITNESS

Foods High in Antioxidants May Reduce Your Risk of Cancer

The antioxidants beta carotene (which the body converts to vitamin A), vitamin C, and vitamin E appear to reduce an individual's risks of cancer (and perhaps of other diseases as well) by neutralizing free radicals (Donatelle & Davis, 1996; Kanter, 1995). Therefore, increasing your dietary intake of antioxidants is an important dietary goal.

Among the best sources of beta carotene are apricots, asparagus, broccoli, carrots, peas, spinach, and tomatoes. Foods that contain substantial amounts of vitamin C include asparagus, broccoli, cauliflower, grapefruit, oranges, peppers, red cabbage, tan-

gerines, and tomatoes. Foods high in vitamin E include vegetable oils, nuts, and seeds; vitamin E is also present in low levels in a variety of other foods.

Dietitians remain divided on whether you should use vitamin supplements to increase your intake of antioxidants. Even though some researchers have suggested that it is safe to supplement your diet with up to 400 units of vitamin E and up to 500 mg of vitamin C (Clarkson, 1991), it remains a good idea to consult a dietitian or health care professional before deciding to use vitamin supplements to raise your dietary intake of antioxidants.

Dietary Guidelines for Lowering Cancer Risk

Health Canada and the Canadian Cancer Society suggest following Canada's Food Guide to Healthy Eating and the following guidelines for lowering your risk of cancer.

1. **Avoid obesity.** Sensible eating habits and regular physical activity will help you avoid excessive weight gain. Obesity increases your risk of colon, breast, gallbladder, prostate, ovarian, and uterine cancers.

2. **Reduce your fat intake.** Reduce the intake of total dietary fat to less than 30 percent of total calories consumed, and reduce the intake of saturated fat to less than 10 percent of total calories. A high-fat diet increases your risk of breast, colon, and prostate cancers.

3. **Eat more high-fibre foods.** Regular consumption of cereals, fresh fruits, and vegetables is recommended. Increasing your fibre intake may reduce your risk of colon cancer.

4. **Include foods rich in vitamins A, C, and E in your daily diet.** These vitamins may reduce your risk of cancer by removing free radicals. See the previous Nutritional Links to Health and Fitness for a list of foods containing these vitamins.

5. **Include cruciferous vegetables in your diet.** Research has shown that broccoli, brussels sprouts, cabbage, cauliflower, and kohlrabi may help reduce the incidence of certain types of cancers. Why these particular vegetables reduce cancer risk is unclear and continues to be the subject of active research.

6. **Eat salt-cured, smoked, and nitrate-cured foods in moderation.** Numerous studies have reported a high incidence of cancer in people who consume large quantities of these foods.

7. **Keep alcohol consumption moderate.** High consumption of alcohol increases the risk of cancers of the mouth, larynx, throat, esophagus, and liver.

Summary

1. The diseases known as cancer are major killers, and the incidence of these diseases is increasing. Currently, cancer is the number two cause of death in Canada.

2. Cancer is the uncontrolled growth and spread of abnormal cells that creates a mass known as a neoplasm. These masses of abnormal cells can form a tumour, which can be classified as either benign (abnormal growth but not life threatening) or malignant (cancerous cells that are life threatening because they will eventually spread to other tissues and disrupt organ function).

3. There are five general classifications of cancer named for their microscopic appearance and the place in the body where they arise: carcinomas, lymphomas, sarcomas, melanomas, leukemia.

4. Carcinogens are cancer-causing agents.

5. Skin cancer is the most common type of cancer. Other common sites of cancer include the mouth, lung, colon, stomach, liver, bone, prostate gland, and breast.

6. Normal cells become cancerous when DNA is damaged, which results in uncontrolled cell division.

7. Heredity, socioeconomic status, radiation, viruses, tobacco, alcohol, occupational carcinogens, ultraviolet light, and a low-fibre, high-fat dietary intake are factors that increase your risk of developing cancer. Cancer risk can be lowered by reducing your exposure to alcohol, radiation, tobacco, occupational carcinogens, and ultraviolet light.

8. Approximately 80 percent of all cancers are related to lifestyle and environmental factors.

9. Dietary intake is probably the most important factor in controlling your risk of cancer. Among the primary nutrients in foods that offer protection from cancer are vitamins A, E, and C, which reduce the risk of cancer by removing free radicals.

10. Engaging in regular physical activity has been shown to reduce the risk of colon, uterine, and breast cancer.

Study Questions

1. Define the following terms:

   cancer
   malignant carcinogen
   benign tumour
   metastasis

2. What is the most common type of cancer?

3. How do normal cells become cancerous?

4. List nine risk factors for cancer.

5. What does SPF stand for, and how is it defined?

6. Physical activity has been shown to reduce the risk of which types of cancer?

7. What is an *antioxidant*? How do antioxidants reduce the risk of cancer?

8. What types of cancer are linked to tobacco use?

9. Name five occupational carcinogens.

10. Discuss the signs of skin cancer.

11. Outline the dietary guidelines for reducing your risk of cancer.

Suggested Reading

Canadian Cancer Society. (2004). *Cancer facts and figures.*

Tannock, I., & Hill, R. P. (Eds.). (1998). *The basic science of oncology.* St. Louis: McGraw-Hill.

Thune, I., & Furberg, A. (2001). Physical activity and cancer risk: Dose–response and cancer, all sites and site specific. *Medicine and Science in Sports and Exercise, 33(Suppl),* S530–S550.

Willett, W. (2001). Diet and cancer: One view at the start of the millennium. *Cancer, Epidemiology, Biomarkers and Prevention, 10,* 3–8.

Weblinks

National Cancer Institute of Canada
www.ncic.cancer.ca
Provides wide-ranging information about cancer and many other health-related issues.

Canadian Medical Association
www.cma.ca
Presents many sources of information about a wealth of medical problems.

WebMD
www.webmd.com
Contains information about a wide variety of diseases and medical problems.

Canadian Cancer Society
www.cancer.ca
Includes up-to-date information, including cancer statistics, risk factors, and current treatments.

References

Baquet, C. R., Horm, J. W., Gibbs, T., & Greewald, P. (1991, April 17). Socioeconomic factors and cancer incidence among blacks and whites. *Journal of National Cancer Institute, 83(8),* 551–557.

Bianchinni, F., Kaaks, R., & Vainio, H. (2002, February). Weight control and physical activity in cancer prevention. *Obesity Review, 3(1),* 5–8.

Braakhuis, B. J., Snijders, P. J., Keune, W. J., Meijer, C. J., Ruijter-Schippers, H. J., Leemans, C. R., & Brakenhoff, R. H. (2004). Genetic patterns in head and neck cancers that contain or lack transcriptionally active human papillomavirus. *Journal of the National Cancer Institute, 96(4).*

Cancer Weekly. (2004, May). Some patterns of alcohol intake are related to the risk of prostate cancer, 177.

Chakravarthy, M. V., Joyner, M. J., & Booth, F. W. (2002, February). An obligation for primary care physicians to prescribe activity to sedentary patients to reduce the risk of chronic health conditions. *Mayo Clinic Proceedings, 77(2),* 1165–1173.

Chowdhury, P., Nishikawa, M., Blevins, G. W., Jr., & Rayford, P. L. (2000, March). Response of rat exocrine pancreas to high-fat and high carbohydrate diet. *Proceedings of the Society of Experimental Biology and Medicine, 223(3),* 310–315.

Clarkson, P. (1991). Vitamins and trace minerals. In D. Lamb & M. Williams (Eds.), *Ergogenics.* Madison, WI: Brown and Benchmark.

Donatelle, R., & Davis, L. (1991). *Access to health* (2nd ed.). Englewood Cliffs, NJ: Prentice Hall.

Environmental Nutrition. (2004, August). Diet guidelines reduce cancer risk and deaths, *27(8),* 1.

Felix-Aaron, K., Moy, E., Kang, M., Chesley, F. D., & Clancy, C. (2005, March 4). Variation in quality of men's health care by race/ethnicity and social class. *Medcare, 3(Suppl),* I72–I81.

Friedenreich, C. M., & Orenstein, M. R. (2002, November). Physical activity and cancer prevention: Etiologic evidence and biological mechanisms. *Journal of Nutrition, 132(11 Suppl),* 3456S–3464S.

Frisch, R. E., Wyshak, G. Albright, N. L., et al. (1985). Lower prevalence of breast cancer and cancers of the reproductive system among former college athletes compared to non-athletes. *British Journal of Cancer, 52,* 885–891.

Goldenberg, D., Lee, J., Koch, W. M., Kim, M. M., Trink, B., Sidransky, D., Moon, C. S. (2004, December). Habitual risk factors for head and neck cancer. *Archives of Otolaryngology, Head and Neck Surgery, 131(6),* 986–993.

Hardman, A. E. (2001, February). Physical activity and cancer risk. *Proceedings of the Nutrition Society, 60(1),* 107–113.

Kanter, M. (1995). Free radicals and exercise: Effects of nutritional antioxidant supplementation. *Exercise and Sport Science Reviews, 23,* 375–397.

Kiningham, R. B. (1998, June 25). Physical activity and the primary prevention of cancer. *Primary Care, 2,* 515–536.

Lee, I. M. (2003, November). Physical activity and cancer prevention—Data from epidemiologic studies. *Medicine and Science in Sports and Exercise, 35(11),* 1823–1827.

Levenson, D. (2004, August 6). Following lifestyle guidelines cuts cancer risk, study shows. *Report on Medical Guidelines Outcomes Resources, 15(15),* 9–10, 12.

Mackillop, W. J., Zhang-Salomons, J., Boyd, C. J., & Groome, P. A. (2000, August 15). Associations between community income and cancer incidence in Canada and the United States. *Cancer, 89(4),* 901–912.

Malm, C. (2004). Exercise immunology: The current state of man and mouse. *Sports Medicine, 34(9),* 555.

Menvieele, G. (2004, June). Smoking, alcohol drinking and cancer risk for various sites of the larynx and hypopharynx: A case control study in France. *European Journal of Cancer Prevention, 13(3),* 165–168.

Millen, A. E., Tucker, M. A., Hartge, P., Halpern, A., Elder, D. E., Guerry, D., IV, Holly, E. A., Sagebiel, R. W., & Potischman, N. (2004, June). Diet and melanoma in a case-control study. *Cancer Epidemiology Biomarkers & Prevention, 13(6)*, 1042–1051.

National Academy of Sciences. (2004). Dietary Reference Intakes. Retrieved on May 15, 2005, from www.nap.edu.

National Cancer Institute of Canada. (2005). *Canadian cancer statistics (2005)*. Retrieved May 15, 2005, from www.ncic.cancer.ca.

National Radiological Protection Board. (2001). X-Rays: How safe are they? Retrieved September 14, 2004, from www.nrpb.org/publications/misc_publications/x-ray_safety_leaflet.pdf.

Norat, T., & Roboli, E. (2001). Meat consumption and colorectal cancer: A review of epidemiological evidence. *Nutritional Reviews, 59*, 37–47.

Poschl, G., & Seitz, H. K. (2004, May/June). Alcohol and cancer. *Alcohol & Alcoholism, 39(3)*, 155.

Robbins, S., & Kumar, V. (1997). *Basic pathology*. Philadelphia: W. B. Saunders.

Rodu, B., & Jansson, C. (2004). Smokeless tobacco and oral cancer: A review of the risks and determinants. *Critical Reviews in Oral Biology and Medicine*, 15(5), 252–263.

Sandu, M., White, I., & McPherson, K. (2001). Systematic review of prospective cohort studies on meat consumption and colorectal cancer risk: A meta-analytical approach. *Cancer Epidemiology Biomarkers & Prevention, 10*, 439–496.

Sasco, A. J. (2003). Breast cancer and the environment. *Hormone Research, 60(3)*, 50.

Single, E., Rehm, J., Robson, L., & Turong, M. V. (2003, June). The relative risks and etiologic fractions of different causes of death and disease attributable to alcohol, tobacco and illicit drug use in Canada. *Canadian Medical Journal, 162(12)*.

Slattery, M. L., & Potter, J. D. (2002, June). Physical activity and colon cancer: Confounding or interaction? *Medical Science Sports Exercise, 34(6)*, 913–919.

Statistics Canada. (2004). Causes of death. Ottawa: Health Statistics Division, Catalogue 84-601-XIE.

Tannock, I., & Hill, R. P. (Eds.). (1998). *The basic science of oncology*. St. Louis: McGraw-Hill, 12.

Tortora, G. (2002). *Principles of human anatomy* (9th ed.). Mississauga, ON: Wiley Canada.

Willett, W. C. (2000). Diet and cancer. *Oncologist, 5*, 393–404.

Willett, W. C. (2001). Diet and cancer: One view at the start of the millennium. *Cancer Epidemiology Biomarkers & Prevention, 10*, 3–8.

Women's Health Weekly. (2004, September). General obesity, not abdominal fat, linked to increased cancer risk in women, 24.

Determining Your Cancer Risk

Name_____ Age _____ Sex _____ Date _____

The purpose of this laboratory is to increase your awareness of your risk of developing all forms of cancer. Complete the following questions by putting a check under either Yes or No.

The more times you put a check under Yes, the more risk factors you have for developing cancer. If you checked Yes even once, you should take steps to modify your lifestyle and reduce your risk for cancer, if it relates to a factor within your control. For some specific information about lowering your cancer risks, see the text.

	Yes	No
1. Do you have a family history of cancer?	_____	_____
2. Do you have a fair complexion?	_____	_____
3. Are you regularly exposed to occupational carcinogens or various types of radiation?	_____	_____
4. Is your skin regularly exposed to excessive sunlight?	_____	_____
5. Do you consume more than 28 g of red meat or of processed meat per day?	_____	_____
6. Do you regularly eat smoked foods?	_____	_____
7. Is your nutritional plan low in fibre?	_____	_____
8. Are you considered clinically obese?	_____	_____
9. Do you consume an excessive amount of alcohol?	_____	_____
10. Do you use tobacco products or breathe secondhand tobacco smoke?	_____	_____

A Lifetime of Physical Activity and Physical Fitness

16

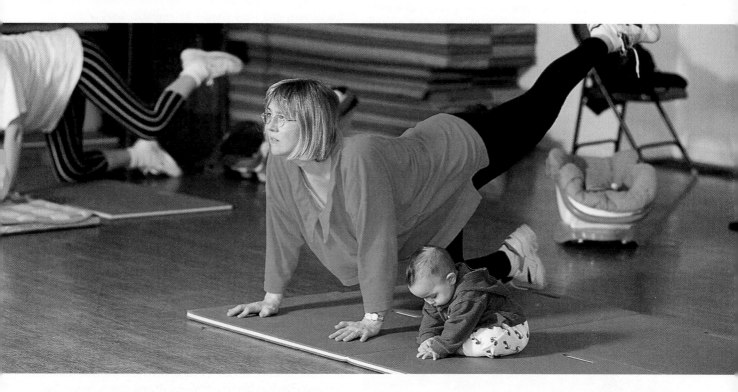

After studying this chapter, you should be able to

1. Identify factors that will assist you in maintaining a physically active lifestyle over your lifetime.
2. Identify the benefits of active living when encountering pregnancy, aging, or disabilities.
3. List several key considerations in choosing a fitness facility.
4. Define the term *fitness expert*.
5. Dispel some common misconceptions about physical fitness.
6. Identify factors to consider when purchasing exercise equipment.
7. List precautions for the use of hot tubs, saunas, and steam baths.

As discussed in Chapter 1, exercise and physical activity must be performed regularly throughout your life to achieve the benefits of physical fitness, wellness, and disease prevention. Fitness cannot be stored! If you stop being physically active, you begin to lose the benefits of physical fitness.

This chapter suggests strategies for maintaining a lifetime physical activity program and the health-related benefits. We also consider key factors in choosing a fitness facility or health club and discuss issues important to being an informed fitness consumer.

Physical Activity Adherence: Lifetime Fitness

Studies have shown that more than 60 percent of adults who start a fitness program quit within the first month (Dishman, 1994; Dishman, 2003). In contrast, people who become physically active and continue with their routine for at least 6 months have an excellent chance of maintaining regular physical activity for years to come (Dishman, 1994). Thus, the first 6 months of your fitness program are critical in determining your lifetime adherence to physical activity. The significance of regular physical activity for several months is probably linked to the fact that 2 to 6 months of training is generally required to bring about significant improvements in physical fitness, including body composition changes (fat loss and muscle development). This positive feedback, once achieved, provides a strong incentive to continue being physically active.

Beginning a lifetime physical activity program requires a strong personal commitment to physical fitness and application of the principles of behaviour modification to change from a sedentary lifestyle to an active lifestyle. In the next sections we discuss several factors that will assist you in maintaining a lifetime commitment to physical activity.

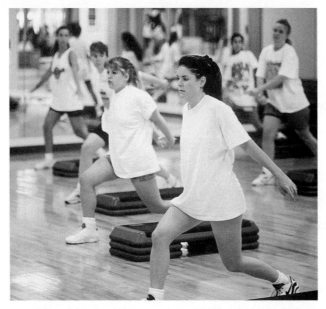

Exercising with friends makes workouts more fun.

Goal Setting for Active Lifestyles

The first step in beginning a successful fitness program is the desire to be physically fit. The second step is establishing short- and long-term fitness goals (goal setting was introduced in Chapter 1 and discussed in detail in Chapter 3). Your goals should be based on your personal needs and desire for fitness, and they should be realistic. Goal setting provides a target to aim for and adds an incentive to maintain regular physical activity. Avoid setting goals that are too stringent. Pushing yourself too hard takes the enjoyment out of physical activity. Table 16.1 provides a few good tips that can help you stick to your goals.

Goals can be designed for either maintenance or improvement. For example, a realistic short-term improvement goal for cardiorespiratory endurance might be to decrease your 2.5-km run time from 15 minutes to 14 minutes during your first 6 months of training. In contrast, a long-term maintenance goal might be to average 30 km of running per week during the first year of training. A key point to remember about fitness goals is that they should be modified from time to time to accommodate changes in your physical fitness needs and to allow you to correct any unrealistic goals you might have set.

Selecting Activities

Physical activity should be fun! Choose physical activities that you enjoy. However, remember that not all enjoyable physical activities will improve the health-related physical fitness components. Which sports or activities provide the best training effect to improve physical fitness components? Table 16.2 evaluates the fitness-building potential of a variety of

Do	Don't
Focus on enjoying the experience.	Push yourself too hard.
Monitor your physical responses.	Let others push you too hard.
Engage in physical activity to reward yourself.	Feel that you have to prove something.

TABLE 16.1 Tips for Establishing a Successful Relationship with Physical Activity.

Source: Adapted from www.uottawa.ca/health/information/nutrition-active.html website, with permission of Health Services, University of Ottawa.

Fitness Ranking

Sport/Activity	Cardiorespiratory Endurance	Upper Body Muscular Strength and Endurance	Lower Body Muscular Strength and Endurance	Flexibility	Caloric Expenditure (calories/min)
Aerobic dance	Good	Good	Good	Fair	5–10
Badminton	Fair	Fair	Good	Fair	5–10
Baseball	Poor	Fair	Fair	Fair	4–6
Basketball	Good	Fair	Good	Fair	10–12
Bowling	Poor	Fair	Poor	Fair	3–4
Canoeing	Fair	Good	Poor	Fair	4–10
Football (flag/touch)	Fair	Fair	Good	Fair	5–10
Golf (walking)	Poor	Fair	Good/fair	Fair	2–4
Gymnastics	Poor	Excellent	Excellent	Excellent	3–4
Handball	Good	Good/fair	Good	Fair	7–12
Karate	Fair	Good	Good	Excellent	7–10
Racquetball	Good/fair	Good/fair	Good	Fair	6–12
Running	Excellent	Fair	Good	Fair	8–15
Skating (ice)	Good/fair	Poor	Good/fair	Good/fair	5–10
Skating (roller)	Good/fair	Poor	Good/fair	Fair	5–10
Skiing (alpine)	Fair	Fair	Good	Fair	5–10
Skiing (nordic)	Excellent/good	Good	Good	Fair	7–15
Soccer	Good	Fair	Good	Good/fair	7–17
Tennis	Good/fair	Good/fair	Good	Fair	5–12
Volleyball	Fair	Fair	Good/fair	Fair	4–8
Waterskiing	Poor	Good	Good	Fair	4–7
Resistance training	Poor	Excellent	Excellent	Fair	4–6

TABLE 16.2 Fitness Evaluation of Various Activities and Sports

Source: From Getchell, B. *Physical fitness: A way of life.* Copyright © 1992. Reprinted by permission of Allyn and Bacon.

popular sports and activities. Note that no one activity is rated as excellent in promoting all aspects of fitness. To achieve total physical fitness, you should participate in several different activities.

Another key consideration is the availability and convenience of the activity. Regardless of how much you enjoy a particular activity, if it is not convenient, your chances of regular participation are greatly reduced. For example, suppose you enjoy swimming—but the pool closest to your home or school is 20 km away, and to make matters worse, the pool hours of operation conflict with your daily schedule. In combination, these two factors decrease your chances of successfully using swimming as your primary type of regular activity. The solution to this problem is simple. Continue to swim when you have the opportunity, but choose another more convenient activity that you enjoy as your regular type of activity. Don't get caught up in the all-or-nothing mentality. Many people believe that if they can't manage to get to the gym for an hour, then they might as well do nothing at all. Engaging in some physical activity, even if it is only for 10 or 20 minutes, is part of a healthy lifestyle.

Planning Physical Activity

Physical activity should be systematic and connected to your goals (Getchell, 1998). This is particularly true during the first several weeks of a fitness program. To achieve your objectives, you must train on a regular basis.

Some suggest that morning physical activity or exercise is better than activity at other times of the day; however, there is no scientific evidence to support the notion that there is an optimal time of day for activity. This is fortunate, because individual preferences vary. Some people prefer to train in the morning hours, whereas others may prefer a noon workout. So try various times throughout the day to find what works best for you. The key to maintaining physical activity is to make it a habit. You would never think to leave the house without showering or brushing your teeth. Similarly, once physical activity is a routine habit there is less inclination to skip it.

Monitoring Progress

Monitoring your progress in achieving or maintaining physical fitness is an important factor in providing feedback and staying motivated. You can monitor your progress in at least two ways. First, maintain a training log to provide feedback concerning the amount of time spent engaging in physical activity. For example, a daily training log can help you monitor the number of kilometres run, the amount of weight lifted, total calories expended during activities, changes in body weight, and so on. A number of commercially available training diaries and computer programs are available.

A second means of monitoring your progress is through periodic physical fitness testing (Chapter 2). Fitness testing provides positive feedback when levels are improving. This type of information can be a useful motivational tool and should be a part of every program.

Social Support

Social support is another key factor in many successful fitness prescriptions. Enjoying interaction with friends or colleagues during activity or in the locker room before or after a workout is an important part of making physical activity fun. See Fitness–Wellness Consumer for some tips on choosing a health club. An excellent way to start being active is to incorporate a buddy system. Physical activity with a friend is an excellent way to start being active on a regular basis, provided that both individuals share the same commitment to improving physical fitness.

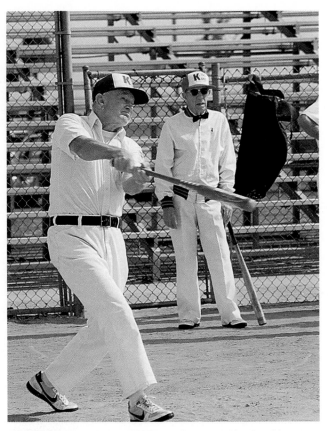

Physical activity can help maintain muscle mass and heart and lung capacity.

FITNESS–WELLNESS CONSUMER

Health Clubs: Choosing a Fitness Facility

While it isn't necessary to join a fitness or health club to become physically fit, many people prefer physical activities in the social environment provided by a club. However, before choosing a facility, consider the following recommendations (Balady, 1998; Industry Canada, 2004):

- Investigate the variety of programs and facilities available in your community before deciding to join any fitness club. Explore not only commercial fitness facilities, but also programs offered by your local YMCA, YWCA, or university.

- Consider the club's location. Is the facility convenient to your home or work?

- Check the club's reputation with the Ministry of Consumer and Business Services or the Canadian Council of Better Business Bureaus. Inquire how long the club has been in business and whether clients have registered complaints.

- Make several trial visits to investigate the cleanliness of the locker rooms, the quality of equipment, and how many people use the facility at your desired workout time.

- Inquire about the qualifications of the program instructors. It is important to ensure that the club's fitness instructors are well trained. See A Closer Look (p. 346) for what a "fitness expert" truly is.

- Consider the club's approach to physical fitness and training. Does it provide routine physical fitness tests and health screening services (e.g., blood pressure measurement)? Do instructors routinely spend time with members, or are members required to seek out instructors to obtain assistance?

- Avoid signing a long-term contract with any fitness or health club. Be wary of contract clauses that waive either the club's liability for injury to you or your right to defend yourself in court.

- Avoid clubs that advertise overnight physical fitness or quick weight loss. After reading this book, you already know that these types of claims are false.

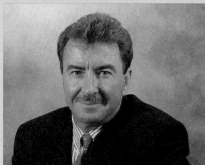

ASK AN EXPERT

Rod Dishman, Ph.D.

Physical Activity Adherence

Dr. Dishman is professor of exercise science and director of the Exercise Psychology Laboratory at the University of Georgia. He is one of the world's leading experts in exercise psychology and issues related to exercise adherence. Dr. Dishman has published numerous scientific papers, books, and book chapters related to exercise adherence. In the following interview, Dr. Dishman addresses several questions related to adherence to regular exercise.

Q: What factors can help me stay motivated to maintain a regular physical activity program?

A: Make regular physical activity your top priority by actions, not just intentions. Schedule a time and pick a place to be active. Many people find engaging in physical activity at lunchtime or at the end of the day invigorating. However, strong intentions often weaken by day's end, when people may feel fatigued and want to rest. If the latter scenario describes you, be physically active earlier rather than later.

If you lack the self-motivation to carry out your physical activity goals, pick other activities or rewards that are important to you and make a commitment not to indulge yourself until daily goals are met. Also, keep a record to ensure that you don't conveniently forget or lie to yourself when you don't meet your desired expectations.

Engineer your environment to make it hard to talk yourself out of physical activity or exercise. Put equipment near your bed at night, so you see it first thing in the morning. Keep a pair of walking shoes in your car or at work to be available whenever opportunities arise.

Contrary to popular belief, there is little evidence that high-intensity physical activity is needed for health benefits. Moderate exertion seems effective too. Pick a type of activity or exercise you most enjoy, a time that best fits your schedule, and an intensity that is pleasurable.

Don't judge the benefits of your activity by fitness gains alone. Research confirms that moderate daily activities such as walking or gardening can have calming and mood-elevating effects and may improve sleep.

Q: How important is goal setting as a motivating factor for getting started in regular physical activity?

A: Specific long-term goals are important to get started. You should also plan a series of short-term, step-by-step goals that are attainable and can bring you closer to your ultimate objective. Distant goals should not change, but immediate daily goals can and often should be flexible. Avoid the abstainer's fallacy that there is only one rigid, unyielding plan that will work for you.

Q: Is it possible to develop a psychological dependence on physical activity or training and, therefore, develop an addiction?

A: In the 1970s, William P. Morgan of the University of Wisconsin described eight cases of running addiction, when a commitment to running exceeded prior commitments to work, family, social relations, and medical advice. Similar cases have been labelled as positive addiction, runner's gluttony, fitness fanaticism, athlete's neurosis, obligatory running, and exercise abuse. Little is understood, however, about the origins, valid diagnosis, or the mental health impact of abusive exercise or training.

Peers as Role Models

Your personal commitment to physical activity and a healthy active lifestyle can be positively influenced by peers who serve as good role models. Most of us know individuals who are regularly active and look and feel terrific. These role models can be motivational to people beginning their own fitness program.

Changing Physical Activity Needs

Chapter 1 discussed the Canadian government's wellness goals for the nation (Health Canada, 2004). The Pan-Canadian Healthy Living Strategy is seeking to improve the overall health of Canadians through all stages of life.

The Active Living Strategy values the integration of all forms of physical activity for all stages of life. You may find that your own physical activity needs change the most during pregnancy, aging, or disability.

Pregnancy Pregnancy causes changes in a woman's physical activity needs and creates some limitations. It does not, however, mean that a woman should stop being physically active. The Canadian Fitness Lifestyle Research Institute outlines the benefits of remaining active while pregnant. In addition, Chapter 12 discusses specific physical activity recommendations. In summary, physical activity can help active moms-to-be experience increased levels of energy, improvement in mood and body image, prevention of gestational

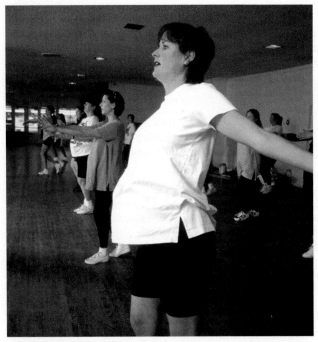
Remaining physically active during pregnancy can shorten labour and recovery times.

Aging The 2000/01 Canadian Community Health Survey indicates that inactivity increases with age, and that a majority of Canadians are at risk of premature death because of lack of physical activity. As we age, some activities become less available. The usual activities we engaged in may be less interesting to us or in some cases harder to perform on a regular basis. We also know there are some natural declines that come with aging. For example, there is a decline in the heart's maximum pumping capacity and heart rate, making strenuous activity difficult. There is also an increase of fatty plaque in blood vessels that causes arteriosclerosis, discussed in Chapter 14.

Aging also takes its toll on the bones and joints, causing a loss of bone strength and density that increases the risk of small fractures and osteoporosis. With increased loss of connective tissue between joints comes inflammation and pain known as arthritis. Chapter 12 covers some of the physiological changes associated with aging and gives some guidelines for healthy active living and physical fitness. It becomes important to find activities that interest you and fit your physical fitness level.

Being physically active is a key element to longevity, independent living, and mental health. Adjustments may have to be made to accommodate flexibility and mobility issues, but accumulating 30 to 60 minutes of moderate-intensity physical activity most days of the week can maintain bone and muscle strength, heart and lung capacity, and flexibility (Health Canada Guide for Older Adults, 2005; Resnick, 2001).

There are a variety of physical activities open to all age groups—from marathon running to swimming, dancing, gardening, or taking the grandchildren for a walk. Regular physical activity has the added benefit of meeting new friends and creating a positive social network. Health Canada's Physical Activity Guide to Healthy Active Living for Older Adults (2005) has some excellent suggestions.

diabetes, easier labour and delivery, and quicker recovery time. The guidelines to achieving these benefits are to

- first discuss your physical activity program with your physician or health care provider.
- engage in activities where the body is supported (e.g., swimming or cycling).
- participate at a comfortable level.
- drink liquids before and after activity.
- take breaks.
- be sensible, take a day off when feeling more tired than usual.

A CLOSER LOOK

What Is a Fitness Expert?

Even though there is currently no standard definition of "fitness expert," anyone who has earned an advanced degree (such as an M.Sc. or a Ph.D.) in exercise science, kinesiology, or exercise physiology from a reputable university can generally be considered a fitness expert or fitness professional. Although individuals with bachelor's degrees in exercise science may have sufficient background to answer many fitness-related questions, the more advanced the degree, the more knowledgeable the individual should be about exercise and physical fitness.

Physical activity and exercise scientists who are actively conducting research in exercise physiology and are active in such professional organizations as the Canadian Society for Exercise Physiology (CSEP) or the Canadian Academy of Sports Medicine (CASM) are generally the best sources of valid information, especially concerning more technical matters. Additionally, physicians or health care professionals with postgraduate training in exercise physiology or a strong personal interest in preventive medicine may be good sources of scientifically based fitness information.

If you having difficulty finding a local fitness expert who can answer your questions, contact the Canadian Society for Exercise Physiology at **www.csep.ca** (185 Somerset St. West, Suite 202, Ottawa, Canada K2P 0J2).

The guidelines given by Health Canada (2005) are to

- build physical activity into your daily routine.
- do the activities you are doing now more often.
- walk wherever and whenever you can.
- start slowly with easy stretching.
- move around frequently.
- take the stairs instead of the elevator.
- carry home the groceries.
- try out an activity at your local community centre.
- accumulate 30 to 60 minutes of moderate activity most days of the week.

As we age, our needs for and interest in physical activity often change. It is thus important to modify your fitness program throughout your life. Many physical activity options exist, so individuals should remain flexible in their habits and be willing to modify their activities as the need arises. Maintaining enthusiasm for physical activity is the foundation of lifetime fitness. See A Closer Look, opposite, for some strategies that can help you adhere to a lifetime of physical activity.

Disabilities According to Health Canada (2005), more than 3.3 million Canadians report some level of disability that presents a limit to their health. When it comes to the physical activity needs of a person with a disability, the challenges may be greater, but disability does not mean inability. It only means that situations may have to be adapted to the person's needs, or a new way of doing things has to be found. For example, those with vision impairment are welcome to bring their guide dogs to the gym with them, while others may request the assistance of a staff member to help with using the equipment.

An inactive lifestyle for individuals with disabilities can create serious side effects, such as weak muscles, weak heart, osteoporosis, and weight gain. Individuals with physical disabilities who manage an active lifestyle benefit in many ways:

- increased strength and flexibility
- reduction of aches and pains
- better circulation
- weight maintenance
- improved physical stamina and self confidence

There are several resources available to Canadians with disabilities who want to get active. Relevant websites are listed at the end of this chapter.

Diet and Fitness Products: Consumer Issues

The fitness boom in Canada has brought an explosion of fitness and diet books, magazines, and a huge number of companies

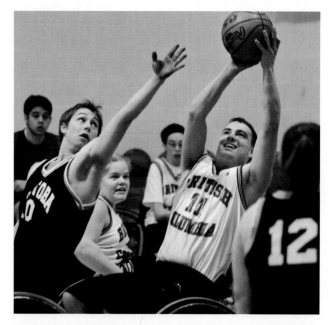

Regular physical activity can increase strength, improve stamina, and help fight depression. Team British Columbia is seen here participating at the Canada Winter Games in 2003.

that produce exercise equipment. Although some fitness books and magazines are written by experts, many are written by individuals with little formal training in exercise physiology. Unfortunately, books and articles written by non-experts often convey misinformation, and some of these writings have created many myths. Further, many exercise products are not useful in promoting physical fitness or weight management. In the next several sections we discuss some key consumer issues related to physical activity, exercise, and weight management.

Common Misconceptions about Physical Fitness

There are numerous misconceptions about physical activity, exercise, physical fitness, and weight management, and to thoroughly discuss them would require hundreds of pages of text. However, we can dispel some common ones.

Yoga Supporters of yoga offer claims that practising it regularly will improve physical fitness, assist in weight loss, and cure a host of diseases. Unfortunately, there is little evidence to support most of these claims (Corbin, 2003). While yoga will improve flexibility and promote relaxation, many yoga positions may cause joint injury, particularly if performed improperly. In short, yoga is not a panacea and should not be the sole contributor to one's fitness prescription.

Hand Weights The popularity of hand-held weights has increased rapidly in the past several years. Some manufacturers claim that using hand weights will greatly increase arm and shoulder strength. Although carrying hand weights will increase the energy expenditure during exercise, 0.5-kg to 1.5-kg hand weights do not promote significant strength gains (particularly in postsecondary-age individuals).

The Keys to Success in Physical Activity Adherence

- Start slowly. For a sedentary or first-time exerciser, any type and amount of physical activity will be a step in the right direction.

- Make only one lifestyle change at a time. Trying for too many major changes at once invites failure. Once you experience success with one change you will be motivated to make other changes.

- Be reasonable. Many people drop out because their expectations are too high or too stringent. Allow sufficient time to reach your goals.

- Find your time to be physically active. Experiment by engaging in physical activities or exercise at different times of the day to learn what works best for you.

- Be active with a friend. Partners can motivate and encourage one another and provide a healthy social experience.

- Make physical activity and exercise a positive habit. Engaging in a desired physical activity routinely will help incorporate it into daily living.

- Mark your progress. An activity journal can be a good motivator. It can include progress in physical condition as well as personal achievements.

Source: Donatelle, R., Davis, L., Munroe, A. J., Munroe, A., & Casselman, M. (2004). *Health: The basics*. Toronto: Pearson Education Canada, 249. Reprinted with permission of Pearson Education Canada Inc.

Further, there are some concerns about the use of hand weights. First, gripping them may increase blood pressure (Graves, Pollock, Montain, Jackson, & O'Keefe, 1987). Individuals with hypertension should seek a physician's advice about the use of hand weights during exercise (Colgan, 2004; Dishman, 1994). Hand weights may also aggravate existing elbow or shoulder arthritis. Finally, some aerobics instructors have banned hand weights in large classes because of the potential danger of hitting someone else with an outstretched hand.

Rubber Waist Belts and Spot Reduction

Recall that spot reduction of body fat is the notion of being able to lose fat from a specific body location. Numerous myths exist concerning the spot reduction effects of such practices as wearing nylon suits or rubber waist bands, as well as exercise focused on a specific body area (e.g., curl-ups). The bottom line is that no method of spot reduction is effective in removing fat from a specific body area (Chapter 8). To lose fat anywhere on your body you need to burn calories through physical activity, exercise, or sport.

Ergogenic Aids

A drug or nutritional product that improves physical fitness and exercise performance is called an **ergogenic aid**. Numerous manufacturers market products that they claim promote strength and cardiovascular endurance. The popularity of these products usually stems from their reported use by champion athletes, but the key concern for the consumer is whether ergogenic aids promote fitness.

Limited scientific evidence supports the notion that nutritional ergogenic aids promote fitness or increase athletic performance. However, anabolic steroids and the drug clenbuterol have increased muscle mass in animals (Picquet, De-Donckner, & Falempin, 2004; Zeman, Peng, Danon, & Etlinger, 2000). Although this may seem to be good news for people who want to increase their muscle mass, the bad news is that these drugs have been shown to be harmful to health. Recent evidence has shown that prolonged use of either drug may result in serious organ damage and, in some cases, death (see Nutrition Links to Health and Fitness,

ergogenic aid A drug or nutritional product that improves physical fitness and exercise performance.

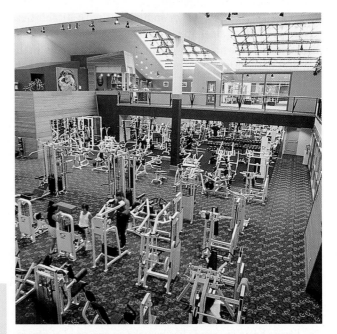

Examine the features of a health club carefully before joining.

Health Canada Requests Recall of Certain Products Containing Ephedra/Ephedrine

Health Canada Notice, January 2002

Health Canada issued a health advisory in June 2001, advising Canadians not to use products containing ephedra/ephedrine with caffeine and other stimulants for purposes of weight loss, body building, or increased energy, concluding that these products pose a serious risk to health. Since the last advisory, a product that combined large doses of ephedrine with caffeine has been reported as a contributing factor in one death.

Stroke, heart attacks, heart rate irregularities, seizures, psychoses, and deaths have also been reported in connection with the use of some products containing ephedra/ephedrine. Health Canada is now removing them from the market.

Ephedra is a botanical source of the alkaloids ephedrine, pseudoephedrine and others. *Ephedra sinica*, whose Chinese name is Ma Huang, has been used in recent years in products marketed for weight loss, body building, and increased energy. Ephedrine is a chemical derivative of the herb *Ephedra sinica* and several other species of ephedra. It stimulates the central nervous and the cardiovascular systems, and causes the lung bronchii to dilate.

Which Groups Are at High Risk? What Are the Side Effects?

Ephedra/ephedrine aggravates conditions such as heart disease, anxiety, and diabetes, and therefore should not be used unless recommended by a health care professional. It should also not be used during pregnancy and lactation.

Adverse effects can include dizziness, decreased appetite, anxiety, gastrointestinal distress, tachycardia, stroke, psychosis, and death. Consumers are advised to check the label for products that combine ephedra/ephedrine with stimulants such as caffeine. Herbs or plants that contain caffeine include coffee, green tea, guarana, maté, and cola nut.

What to Watch Out For

If the product is making a health claim, it should have a drug identification number (DIN). Ephedra/ephedrine products without DINs have not been assessed for safety by Health Canada. This includes all products that are marketed for appetite suppression, weight loss, increased weight tolerance, body-building effects, increased energy or wakefulness, or other stimulant effects. If you are taking a DIN product that contains ephedra and are not sure whether the product meets the recommended standard of 8 mg/dose, 32 mg/day for ephedrine, consult your pharmacist.

STUDY QUESTIONS

1. Are you aware of any friends who use or have used products containing ephedra/ephedrine? What was the product? Why did they decide to take this particular dietary supplement? Did they experience any of the side effects mentioned in this article?

2. What role does the Canadian consumer play in keeping these products off the shelves?

Source: Health Canada Requests Recall of Certain Products Containing Ephedra/Ephedrine, Health Canada, January 9, 2002. Reproduced with the permission of the Minister of Public Works and Government Services Canada, 2005.

---

above) (Colgan, 2004; Lamb & Williams, 1991; Powers & Howley, 2001).

Equipment Many types of fitness-related equipment are available. Every week, magazine and television ads promote "new" devices designed to trim waistlines and build huge muscles overnight. In truth, there are no miracle devices capable of promoting such changes. In fact, there is really no need to buy *any* device to promote fitness. A well-rounded physical fitness program can be designed without equipment. However, if you want to purchase equipment for home use, buy from a reputable and well-established company (Corbin, 2003). Beware of mail-order products, and examine the product before you buy (Corbin, 2003). When in doubt about the usefulness of a product, consult a reputable fitness professional.

Hot Tubs, Saunas, and Steambaths Hot tubs, saunas, and steambaths are popular attractions at many fitness or health clubs. Although they may improve mental attitudes by promoting relaxation, none promotes fat loss or improves physical fitness. While water loss due to perspiration will reduce body weight temporarily, it does not result in fat loss. Further, the lost weight will return as soon as fluids are replenished by eating and drinking.

There are also potential dangers in the use of hot tubs, saunas, and steambaths. One of the major problems concerns the regulation of blood pressure. All of these forms of heat stress increase blood flow to the skin to promote cooling; this reduces blood return to the heart and may reduce blood flow to the brain, resulting in fainting. Therefore, when using a hot tub, sauna, or steambath, note the following precautions (Corbin, 2003):

- Seek a health care professional's advice before use if you suffer from heart disease, hypertension, diabetes, kidney disease, or chronic skin problems, or if you are pregnant.

- Don't use hot bath facilities when you are alone; someone should be present to get emergency help if you develop a health problem, such as fainting.

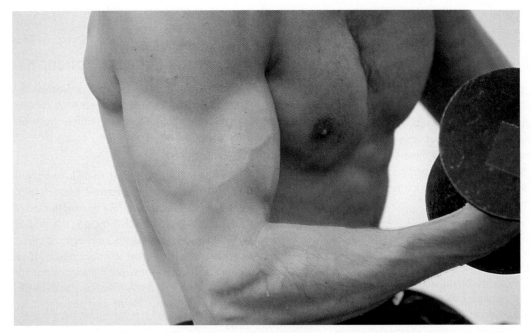

Having a championship physique does not make an individual a fitness expert.

- Don't wear jewellery in hot baths (the metal will absorb heat and may burn your skin).
- Don't drink alcohol prior to or while bathing because alcohol may increase your risk of fainting during heat exposure.
- Don't exercise in a hot tub, sauna, or steambath. The combination of exercise and a hot environment may result in overheating.
- Do not enter a sauna, hot tub, or steambath immediately following vigorous physical activity. Entering a steambath without cooling down after vigorous activity (e.g., snow shovelling) can increase your risk of fainting or pose other more serious health risks.

The duration of stay and recommended temperatures for hot tubs, saunas, and steambaths are as follows:

Hot tub (or whirlpool): Water temperature should not exceed ~38°C (100°F) and the time spent should not exceed 15 minutes.

Sauna: Air temperature should not exceed ~88°C (190°F) and the time spent should not exceed 15 minutes.

Steambath: Air temperature should not exceed ~49°C (120°F) and the time spent should not exceed 10 minutes.

Fitness Books and Magazines   Book stores generally have numerous fitness-related publications on their shelves. Although many fitness books have been written by experts in the field of exercise science, others have been writ-

ten by individuals with little or no formal training in exercise physiology. Dozens of fitness books and magazine articles have been written by models, movie stars, body builders, and even professional or Olympic athletes who have no academic training in exercise science. Clearly, having athletic talent or a good physique does not make an individual a fitness expert.

How do you evaluate the credibility of a physical fitness or weight management book? After reading and studying this book, you should be able to distinguish between fitness facts and fiction. For example, beware of texts that promise overnight results or quick, effortless weight loss. If you have doubts about the validity of a new fitness text contact a reputable fitness professional for advice, for example, by using the Weblinks for this chapter.

Summary

1. Exercise and physical activity must be performed regularly throughout your life to achieve the benefits of physical fitness, wellness, and disease prevention.
2. More than 60 percent of adults who start a regular physical activity program quit within the first month. Evidence suggests that people who start engaging in regular physical activity and continue for 6 months have an excellent chance of maintaining regular physical activity for years.
3. The following are important aspects of maintaining a lifetime commitment to physical activity: goal setting, activity selection, regularity of physical activity, monitoring progress, social support, peers as role models, and modifying your physical activity as a result of aging or other health-related change.

4. The Active Living Strategy values the integration of all forms of physical activity for all stages of life; you may find that your physical activity needs change the most during pregnancy, aging, or disability.

5. Before joining a gym be sure to investigate the facility and its reputation thoroughly.

6. There is no standard definition of a *fitness expert*. However, a fitness expert or professional is, generally, someone who has earned an advanced degree in exercise science, kinesiology, or exercise physiology.

7. Numerous physical fitness misconceptions exist. After studying this book you should be able to distinguish between fact and fiction. If you have doubts about the validity of a new fitness product or textbook, contact a local fitness expert for advice, such as CSEP.

Study Questions

1. Outline the key factors that play a role in maintaining a regular physical activity program.

2. List five points to consider when choosing a health club.

3. Explain what qualifies someone as a *fitness expert*.

4. Discuss the misconceptions associated with yoga, the use of hand weights, the use of rubber weight belts to lose body fat, and dietary ergogenic aids.

5. What factors should be considered when purchasing exercise equipment?

6. List several precautions to consider when using hot tubs, saunas, or steambaths.

7. What percentage of people who start regular physical activity quits within the first month? Discuss the reasons why people do not adhere to physical activity.

8. Discuss the importance of physical activity selection in maintaining physical fitness.

9. List five physical activities or sports considered good or excellent for promoting cardiorespiratory endurance.

10. List five ways to adhere successfully to physical activity.

Suggested Reading

ACSM's guidelines for exercise testing and prescription (6th ed.). (2000). Baltimore: Lippincott, Williams & Wilkins.

Hale, T. (2003). *Exercise physiology: A thematic approach*. Toronto: John Wiley & Sons.

Industry Canada. *Canadian consumer handbook,* (2004 ed.).

Nieman, D. (1999). *Exercise testing and prescription: A health-related approach*. Mountain View, CA: Mayfield.

Powers, S., & Howley, E. (2001). *Exercise physiology: Theory and application to fitness and performance* (4th ed.). St. Louis: McGraw-Hill.

Weblinks

Steadward Centre for Personal & Physical Achievement
www.steadwardcentre.org
Provides fitness and lifestyle programs, instruction, and research for people with physical disabilities.

Canadian Wheelchair Sports Association (CWSA)
www.cwsa.ca
The Canadian Wheelchair Sports Association (CWSA), founded in 1967, is a national sport organization representing wheelchair athletes. It is an incorporated, not-for-profit, organization recognized by Sport Canada.

Active Living Alliance for Canadians with a Disability
www.ala.ca
Provides nationally coordinated leadership, support, encouragement, promotion, and information that facilitates healthy, active living opportunities for Canadians of all abilities across all settings and environments.

Canadian Physical Medicine and Rehabilitation Services
www.canadianwellness.com
Provides information on physical medicine, rehabilitation, and sports medicine services available for professional practitioners in the field.

St. John Ambulance, Canada
www.sja.ca
A website dedicated to enabling Canadians to improve their health, safety, and quality of life through training and community service.

Canadian Society of Exercise Physiology
www.csep.ca
Provides information about the society, conferences, publications, press releases, and offers a physical activity guide.

Canadian Fitness and Lifestyle Research Institute
www.cflri.ca
A national research agency concerned with advising, educating, and informing Canadians and professionals about the importance of leading healthy and active lifestyles.

Ministry of Consumer and Business Services
www.cbs.gov.on.ca
Provides government information about frauds and scams to individuals and businesses to strengthen their knowledge of the marketplace.

Industry Canada Consumer Connection
www.strategis.gc.ca
The Consumer Connection website is published by Industry Canada's Office of Consumer Affairs and offers practical information and tools to help you protect your interest and to spend wisely in the marketplace.

WebMD
www.webmd.com
Includes the latest information on a variety of health-related topics, including diet, exercise, and stress; also contains links to other sites on nutrition, fitness, and wellness topics.

References

Balady, G. (1998, November 6). Health clubs: Are they right for you? *Harvard Men's Health Watch*.

Canadian Fitness and Lifestyle Research Institute. (2004, February 17). *Lifestyle tips: Our relationship with physical activity, CFLRI: The research in active living*. Retrieved from www.uottawa.ca/health/information/nutrition-active.html.

Colgan, M. (2004). *Sports nutrition guide*. Vancouver: Apple Publishing.

Corbin, C. (2003). *Concepts of fitness and wellness: A comprehensive lifestyle approach*. St. Louis: McGraw-Hill.

Dishman, R. K. (1994). *Advances in exercise adherence*. Champaign, IL: Human Kinetics.

Dishman, R. K. (2003). The impact of behavior on quality of life. *Quality Life Resource, 12(Supp. 1)*, 43–9.

Getchell, B. (1998). *Physical fitness: A way of life* (5th ed.). Needham Heights, MA: Allyn and Bacon.

Graves, J., Pollock, M., Montain, S., Jackson, A., & O'Keefe, J. (1987). The effect of hand-held weights on the physiological response to walking exercise. *Medicine and Science in Sports and Exercise, 19*, 260–265.

Health Canada. (2004, February 17). Healthy active living for older adults. Retrieved August 27, 2004, from www.hc-sc.gc.ca.

Industry Canada. (2004, August). *Canada consumer connection*. Retrieved August 2004, from http://strategis.ic.gc.ca.

Lamb, D., & Williams, M. (1991). *Ergogenics: Enhancement of performance in exercise and sport* (vol. 4). Madison, WI: Brown and Benchmark.

Picquet, F., De-Doncker, L., & Falempin, M. (2004, May 1). Enhancement of hybrid-fiber types in rat soleus muscle after clenbuterol administration during hind climbing unloading. *Canadian Journal of Physiology and Pharmacology, 82*, 311–318. Retrieved June 2004, from the National Research Council Canada Research Press website, www.cjpp.nrc.ca.

Powers, S., & Howley, E. (2001). *Exercise physiology: Theory and application to fitness and performance* (4th ed.). St. Louis: McGraw-Hill.

Resnick, B. (2001). Testing a model of exercise behavior in older adults. *Research in Nursing and Health, 24*, 83–89.

Zeman, R. J., Peng, H., Danon, M. J., & Etlinger, J. D. (2000, April). Clenbuterol reduces degeneration of exercised or aged dystrophic muscle. *Muscle Nerve, 23(4)*, 521–528.

Wellness Profile

Name_____ Age _____ Sex _____ Date _____

After reading *Total Fitness and Wellness*, you should be equipped with the knowledge and skills you need to lead a healthy, physically active lifestyle. Take the opportunity now to examine your strengths in six areas of wellness. Write your top three strengths for each factor of wellness below.

PHYSICAL WELLNESS

Maintaining overall physical health and participating in physical activities. Examples of strengths include endurance, balance, and flexibility.

_____

_____

_____

EMOTIONAL WELLNESS

Possessing a positive self-concept and dealing appropriately with your feelings. Strengths may include self-confidence, trust, and optimism.

_____

_____

_____

INTELLECTUAL WELLNESS

Retaining knowledge, thinking critically about issues, making sound decisions, and finding solutions to problems. Examples include inquisitiveness, curiosity, and dedication.

_____

_____

_____

SOCIAL WELLNESS

Developing lasting relationships with family and friends, contributing to the community. Strengths in this area would be compassion and friendliness.

_____

_____

_____

SPIRITUAL WELLNESS

The establishment of personal values and the ability to understand the basic purpose of life. Those experiencing spiritual wellness love life. What aspects of your life bring you spiritual wellness?

_____

_____

_____

ENVIRONMENTAL WELLNESS

Protecting yourself from environmental hazards and minimizing your negative impact on the environment. Behaviours such as recycling and carpooling are strengths in this aspect of wellness.

_____

_____

_____

Is there an aspect of wellness that you need to develop more fully? If so, which one? What can you do now to improve this wellness factor in your life?

_____

_____

_____

LABORATORY 16.2

Evaluating Fitness Products

Name_____ Age _____ Sex _____ Date _____

The benefits of physical activity and exercise are numerous. However, many media sources claim to sell "quick" and "miraculous" products for health and physical fitness. Some advertisements claim that "just a few minutes a day" are needed to lose weight, tone muscles, and trim centimetres. However, we know that true physical fitness requires effort. Complete this activity to practise thinking critically about fitness advertisements.

Find three examples of misleading or false claims on fitness or health products. You can find examples in popular magazines, television or radio ads, or other media sources. Answer the following questions for each of your products.

1. What is misleading or false about the fitness claims?

_____
_____
_____

2. Why is this statement false?

_____
_____
_____

3. Is it written by an expert in the field of exercise and physical fitness?

_____
_____
_____

4. Are the claimed benefits of the product reasonable?

_____
_____
_____

5. Does the claim use gimmick words like "quick," "spot reduce," or "just minutes a day"?

_____
_____
_____

6. Are the advertisers trying to help you or just sell their product?

_____
_____
_____

Keep these ideas in mind to avoid being the victim of fitness ripoffs. If a product sounds too good to be true, it probably is.

Appendix A

Nutritional Content of Common Foods and Beverages

This food composition table has been prepared for Benjamin Cummings and is copyrighted by DINE Systems, Inc., the developer and publisher of the DINE System family of nutrition software for personal computers. The values in this food composition table were derived from the USDA Nutrient Data Base for Standard Reference Release 10 and nutrient composition information from more than 300 companies. Nutrient values used for each food were determined by collapsing similar foods into one food, using the median nutrient values. In the food composition table, foods are listed within eight groups. In order, the eight groups are grains, vegetables, fruits, dairy, protein foods, beverages, alcoholic beverages, and fats/sweets/other.

DINE Systems, Inc.
586 N. French Road
Amherst, NY 14228
(716) 688-2492
FAX (716) 688-2502

APPENDIX A Nutritional Content of Common Foods

NOTE: Carbohydrate value does not include Added Sugar value.

Grains

Amount		Weight	Calories	Protein (g)	Total Fat (g)	Sat. Fat (g)	Carb. (g)	Added Sugar (g)	Fibre (g)	Chol. (mg)	Sodium (mg)	Calcium (mg)	Iron (mg)
Bagel	1 bagel	68 g	175	7	10.22	0.22	32.5	2.25	1.5	0	325	20	1.8
Barley—cooked	125 mL (1/2 cup)	81 g	84	2.25	0.11	0	18.5	0	2.5	0	3	11	0.5
Biscuit	1 biscuit	30 g	100	2	3.78	1.22	13.5	0	0.5	2	262	47	0.7
Bread or roll—wheat	1 slice, 1 roll	27 g	65	2	0.89	0.22	10	2	1.4	0	106	20	0.7
Bread or roll—white	1 slice, 1 roll	28 g	70	2.75	1.11	0.33	11	2	0.5	0	132	20	0.7
Bread—mixed grain	1 slice	25 g	65	2	0.89	0.22	9.75	2.25	1.4	0	106	27	0.8
Bread—oatmeal	1 slice	37 g	90	4	1.78	0.33	10.5	4	1.5	0	140	40	1.1
Bread—pita, wheat	1 pita	57 g	145	5.5	0.89	0.22	28.5	0.5	4.1	0	360	50	1.4
Bread—pita, white	1 pita	57 g	160	6	1	0.22	30	1	1.1	0	300	80	0.7
Bread—raisin	1 slice	26 g	70	2	1	0.33	8.25	3	0.9	0	85	20	0.7
Bread—rye, pumpernickel	1 slice	30 g	80	2.75	0.89	0.11	13	1	1.1	0	185	22	1.1
Bread—wheat	1 slice	28 g	82	3	1	0.33	11.38	2	1.8	0	158.5	22.5	1
Bread—wheat, diet	1 slice	23 g	40	2.5	0.56	0.11	4.25	2	2	0	120	40	0.7
Bread—white	1 slice	27 g	67	2	1	0.22	11	1	0.7	0	135	21	0.7
Bread—white, diet	1 slice	23 g	40	3	0	0	6	1	2	0	110	40	0.7
Bread—whole wheat	1 slice	28 g	69	2.63	1.22	0.17	13	1.38	2	0	127	20	0.9
Breadsticks	1/3 large, 2 small	11 g	36	1.25	0.78	0.22	6	0.5	0.6	0	72	0	0.2
Bulgur	125 mL (1/2 cup)	67 g	113	4.25	0.22	0	23.5	0.5	3	0	3	13	3.7
Cake—non-fat	1 piece	56 g	140	3	0	0	32	15.5	1.2	0	170	0	0
Cereal—bran, fibre	83 mL (1/3 cup)	23 g	62	2	0.78	0.22	7.75	2.75	3.8	0	113	13	3
Cereal—granola	63 mL (1/4 cup)	28 g	130	3	4.89	0.89	13.5	4.5	1.7	0	55	19	0.9
Cereal—granola, fat-free	63 mL (1/4 cup)	28 g	90	2	0	0	21	0.25	2.5	0	20	0	0.4
Cereal—oat flakes	250 mL (1 cup)	46 g	182	5	1.78	0.44	24.75	4.5	3.2	0	115	32	5.8
Cereal—other, cold	250 mL (1 cup)	29 g	110	2	0.22	0.11	19.5	3	0.6	0	226	4	1.8
Cereal—other, hot	167 mL (2/3 cup)	156 g	100	3	0	0	22	0	0.7	0	54	18	1.1
Cereal—sweetened	250 mL (1 cup)	29 g	120	1.25	1	0.44	13	13	0.5	0	210	0	4.5
Cereal—whole grain	188 mL (3/4 cup)	28 g	105	3	0.78	0.22	19	0	2.3	0	160	8	1.4
Cheese ravioli w/sauce	250 mL (1 cup), 6 pieces	263 g	314	13	10.83	6.11	45.13	0.25	3.4	30	733	139	2
Cornbread, hushpuppies	1 square, 3 hushpuppies	51 g	166	3	5.33	1.78	25.75	0	1.6	42	421	87	0.8
Couscous	167 mL (2/3 cup)	108 g	120	4	0	0	26	0	4.3	0	5	0	0.7
Cracker sandwiches	2 large, 5 small	14 g	70	1.75	3.11	1.11	7.75	0.75	0.2	1	135	20	0.4
Crackers	5 crackers	14 g	60	1	2	0.44	8.75	0.75	0.4	0	120	0	0.5
Crackers—butter type	5 large, 10 small	14 g	70	1	3.56	1.11	8	0.25	0.2	1	193	4	0.4
Crackers—crispbread	1 large, 2 small	13 g	40	1	0.89	0.33	8.5	0	1.6	0	112	0	0.5
Crackers—low-fat	2 large, 5 small	14 g	60	2.25	2.33	0.33	10	0	0.6	0	100	0	0.4

Grains, continued

	Amount	Weight	Calories	Protein (g)	Total Fat (g)	Sat. Fat (g)	Carb. (g)	Added Sugar (g)	Fibre (g)	Chol. (mg)	Sodium (mg)	Calcium (mg)	Iron (mg)
Crackers—wheat	4 crackers	18 g	70	1	2.22	0.44	8	0.5	1.5	0	75	0	0.4
Croissants	1 croissant	72 g	310	7	19	11.22	27	6	2	0	240	38	1.8
Croutons	60 mL (4 tablespoons)	10 g	46	1	1.78	0.44	6.25	0.25	0.3	0	124	6	0.3
English muffin	1 muffin	56 g	130	5	0.89	0.33	25	1.5	1.6	0	280	96	1.7
French toast	1 slice	59 g	151	4.25	7.33	1.89	16.25	3.5	0.5	48	277	48	1.1
Fried rice	125 mL (1/2 cup)	99 g	165	4	5.56	1	18.25	0.75	0.6	14	484	14	1.1
Grits	125 mL (1/2 cup)	124 g	73	1.5	0.11	0	16	0	0.3	0	136	0	0.8
Lasagna—meat	1 serving	308 g	350	27.5	23.11	6	31	1.5	2.6	73	1040	275	2.1
Lasagna—vegetable	1 serving	326 g	315	22	12	5.89	27	0.5	4.6	40	970	350	2.3
Macaroni	125 mL (1/2 cup)	66 g	95	3.25	0.33	0.11	19	0	0.9	0	4	5	0.9
Macaroni and cheese	125 mL (1/2 cup)	126 g	191	6	8.56	2.67	22.75	0	1.4	18	434	71	1.2
Macaroni—whole wheat	250 mL (1 cup)	150 g	202	8	1.11	0.22	39	0	7.4	0	10	20	4.5
Matzo or melba toast	1 matzo, 5 melba	19 g	100	3.25	0.56	0.11	22.25	0	0.9	0	6	4	0.9
Meat ravioli with sauce	250 mL (1 cup), 6 pieces	227 g	324	13	8.33	2.89	46.75	0.75	3.1	20	878	54	2.1
Muffins	1 muffin	77 g	240	4.5	8.5	1.67	40	9	2	24.5	310	96.5	1.4
Muffins—fat free	1 muffin	66 g	165	3	0.17		38	10.63	1	0	175	60	0.7
Noodles—chow mein	125 mL (1/2 cup)	25 g	130	3	6.44	1.11	14.5	0	0.5	2	228	4	0.8
Noodles—egg	125 mL (1/2 cup)	160 g	106.5	3.75	1.17	0.22	19.88	0	0.9	26.5	69	9.5	1.3
Noodles—egg, macaroni	250 mL (1 cup)	145 g	190	7	0.56	0.11	37	0	1.1	0	30	14	2.1
Oatmeal—flavored	1 packet	38 g	140	4	2.22	0.44	18	8.25	2.4	0	181	100	4.5
Oatmeal—plain	167 mL (2/3 cup) cooked	176 g	109	4	1.78	0.33	18.25	0	3.3	0	1	15	1.9
Pancakes	1 pancake	38 g	73	2	1.22	0.44	11	1.25	0.5	7	239	50	0.6
Pasta w/parmesan cheese	125 mL (1/2 cup)	134 g	252	6.5	14.67	6.33	22.5	0	1.1	38	479	78	1.5
Rice cake	1 large cake	8 g	35	0.75	0	0	7.5	0	0.3	0	13	0	0
Rice—brown	125 mL (1/2 cup)	97 g	115	2.5	0.67	0.22	25	0	1.8	0	2	12	0.5
Rice—long grain & wild, mix	125 mL (1/2 cup)	88 g	137	3	2	0.56	23	2	0.9	0	579	11	1.1
Rice—seasoned	125 mL (1/2 cup)	107 g	150	3.5	3.78	1.67	23	1	1	5	700	13	1.2
Rice—white	125 mL (1/2 cup)	91 g	92	2	0	0	20.5	0	0.5	0	225	10	0.7
Roll—hamburger/hotdog, wheat	1 roll	43 g	114	4	1.11	0.22	21.25	0.75	2.5	0	242	46	1
Roll—hamburger/hotdog, white	1 roll	43 g	138	3.25	2.44	0.67	22.5	2	1.4	0	271	67	1.3
Roll—hoagie, sub	1 roll	135 g	400	11	7.11	1.78	68.5	4	1.8	0	684	100	3.8
Roll—wheat	1 roll	28 g	77	2.5	1.78	0.44	11.5	1.5	1.1	0	96	50	1
Roll—white	1 roll	34 g	105	3.25	1.67	0.44	16.25	1.75	0.6	0	148	28	1
Salad—pasta	125 mL (1/2 cup)	87 g	250	4	16	3.33	20.75	0	0.7	28	410	40	0.7
Spaghetti	250 mL (1 cup)	128 g	200	7.5	1	0.22	40.5	0	1.1	0	19	14	2
Spaghetti w/meatballs	250 mL (1 cup)	261 g	307	12	10.56	3.89	37	0	2.7	34	1220	53	3.3
Spaghetti—whole wheat	250 mL (1 cup)	144 g	200	9	1.11	0.22	39.5	0	5.8	0	10	20	2.7
Stuffing	125 mL (1/2 cup)	93 g	210	4.5	12.67	3	17.5	2.5	0.5	22	578	40	1.1
Taboule	125 mL (1/2 cup)	80 g	170	3	8.67	1.33	20	0	1.6	0	290	0	0.7
Taco shell	1 shell	11 g	50	0	2	1.11	8	0	0.2	0	5	0	0

Amount	Weight	Calories	Protein (g)	Total Fat (g)	Sat. Fat (g)	Carb. (g)	Added Sugar (g)	Fibre (g)	Chol. (mg)	Sodium (mg)	Calcium (mg)	Iron (mg)
Grains, continued												
Tortilla	1 tortilla	30 g	65	2	1	0.11	12	0	0.9	0	1	42	0.6
Waffles	1 waffle	39 g	110	3	4.33	0.89	13	1.75	0.8	3	279	75	1.8
Vegetables												
Artichokes	125 mL (1/2 cup), 1/2 vegetable	75 g	36	2	0.11	0	7.25	0	2.6	0	42	17	0.8
Asparagus	6 spears, 125 mL (1/2 cup)	90 g	24	1.75	0.33	0.11	3.75	0	1.5	0	4	22	0.6
Asparagus, canned	125 mL (1/2 cup)	122 g	21	1.5	0.33	0.11	2.75	0	1.9	0	425	17	1.5
Bamboo shoots	63 mL (1/4 cup)	30 g	4	0.25	0	0	0.5	0	0.3	0	1	4	0.1
Bamboo shoots—canned	63 mL (1/4 cup)	33 g	6	0.5	0.11	0	1	0	0.6	0	2	1	0.1
Bean sprouts	125 mL (1/2 cup)	59 g	16	1.25	0	0	2.75	0	2.2	0	3	7	0.5
Bean sprouts—canned	125 mL (1/2 cup)	62 g	8	0.75	0	0	1.25	0	2.3	0	149	9	0.3
Beets—canned	125 mL (1/2 cup)	123 g	36	0.75	0	0	8	0	2.9	0	324	17	0.8
Beets—pickled	125 mL (1/2 cup)	119 g	82	0.75	0	0	8.5	11.25	2.8	0	250	13	0.5
Beets—raw, cooked	125 mL (1/2 cup)	99 g	31	0.75	0	0	6.75	0	2.5	0	49	11	0.6
Bok choy—chinese cabbage	125 mL (1/2 cup)	35 g	5	0.25	0	0	0.75	0	0.6	0	23	37	0.3
Broccoli—cooked	125 mL (1/2 cup), 2 spears	85 g	24	1.75	0.11	0	4.25	0	2.5	0	15	68	0.8
Broccoli—raw	125 mL (1/2 cup)	44 g	12	0.75	0.11	0	2	0	1.5	0	12	21	0.4
Brussels sprouts	125 mL (1/2 cup), 4 sprouts	78 g	32	1.5	0.33	0.11	5.75	0	2.4	0	18	24	0.8
Cabbage—raw or cooked	63 mL (1/4 cup) cooked, 125 mL (1/2 cup) raw	36 g	9	0.25	0	0	1.75	0	1	0	7	13	0.2
Carrots—canned	125 mL (1/2 cup)	73 g	17	0.25	0.11	0	3.75	0	2.7	0	176	19	0.5
Carrots—raw or cooked	125 mL (1/2 cup), 6 sticks	69 g	26	0.5	0	0	5.75	0	2.2	0	43	21	0.4
Cauliflower—raw or cooked	125 mL (1/2 cup)	67 g	15	0.75	0.11	0	2.5	0	1.3	0	7	15	0.3
Celery—raw or cooked	125 mL (1/2 cup), 6 sticks	68 g	10	0.25	0	0	2.25	0	1.4	0	51	25	0.2
Chef salad	250 mL (1 cup)	137 g	25	2.5	0.17	0	4	0	2	0	23.5	30.5	0.5
Coleslaw	125 mL (1/2 cup)	92 g	154	0.5	14.44	2.67	4.25	1	1.5	7	287	32	0.4
Corn	1 ear, 125 mL (1/2 cup)	86 g	80	1.75	0.33	0	17.5	0	4.6	0	4	2	0.5
Corn—canned	125 mL (1/2 cup)	120 g	83	1.5	0.44	0.11	13	5.5	4.7	0	324	5	0.4
Cucumber	125 mL (1/2 cup)	52 g	7	0.25	0	0	1.5	0	0.7	0	1	7	0.1
Eggplant	125 mL (1/2 cup)	48 g	13	0.25	0	0	3	0	1	0	2	3	0.2
French fries	1 regular, 313 mL (1-1/4 cups)	85.1 g	241	3	12.72	3.89	29.5	0	2.8	0	129.5	0	1
Fried vegetables/onions	6 onion rings	68 g	180	2	10.78	2.67	15.5	0	1	0	150	12	0.7
Green beans—canned	125 mL (1/2 cup)	68 g	13	0.75	0	0	2.5	0	1.5	0	170	18	0.6
Green beans—raw or cooked	125 mL (1/2 cup)	68 g	20	1	0	0	4	0	1.8	0	3	30	0.7
Greens—collard & mustard	125 mL (1/2 cup)	73 g	16	1.75	0.22	0	3.75	0	1.4	0	15	64	0.7
Greens—mustard, turnip, cooked	125 mL (1/2 cup)	75 g	15	1	0.11	0	2.5	0	1.4	0	16	87	0.7
Greens—mustard, turnip, raw	125 mL (1/2 cup)	28 g	7	0.5	0	0	1.5	0	0.9	0	9	41	0.4
Greens—turnip, canned	125 mL (1/2 cup)	117 g	17	1	0.22	0.11	2.5	0	2.2	0	325	138	1.8
Kale—raw or cooked	125 mL (1/2 cup)	55 g	20	0.75	0.11	0	3	0	1.7	0	15	47	0.6
Lettuce—endive	125 mL (1/2 cup)	25 g	4	0.25	0	0	0.75	0	0.7	0	6	13	0.2
Lettuce—iceberg	250 mL (1 cup)	55 g	7	0.5	0.11	0	1.25	0	0.6	0	5	11	0.3

	Amount	Weight	Calories	Protein (g)	Total Fat (g)	Sat. Fat (g)	Carb. (g)	Added Sugar (g)	Fibre (g)	Chol. (mg)	Sodium (mg)	Calcium (mg)	Iron (mg)
Mixed vegetables—canned	125 mL (1/2 cup)	82 g	39	1.25	0.11	0	8	0	3.5	0	122	22	0.9
Mixed vegetables—frozen	125 mL (1/2 cup)	81 g	22	0.75	0	0	4.5	0	2	0	22	27	0.6
Mushrooms—canned	125 mL (1/2 cup)	78 g	19	1	0.11	0	3.25	0	1.1	0	178	1	0.6
Mushrooms—fresh, cooked	125 mL (1/2 cup)	96 g	25	1.75	0.11	0	4.25	0	1.5	0	1	7	1.7
Mushrooms—raw	125 mL (1/2 cup)	35 g	9	0.5	0	0	1.5	0	0.6	0	1	2	0.4
Okra	125 mL (1/2 cup)	81 g	26	1	0.11	0	5.5	0	2.1	0	5	55	0.5
Onions	125 mL (1/2 cup)	71 g	29	0.5	0.11	0	6.25	0	1.4	0	8	20	0.3
Parsnips	125 mL (1/2 cup), 1/2 vegetable	79 g	64	0.75	0.11	0	14.75	0	3.2	0	8	30	0.5
Peas—green	125 mL (1/2 cup)	85 g	63	3.75	0.11	0	11.5	0	3.5	0	70	19	1.2
Peas—green, canned	125 mL (1/2 cup)	85 g	59	3.25	0.11	0	8	2.75	5.3	0	186	17	0.8
Peas—snowpeas	125 mL (1/2 cup)	79 g	35	2.25	0.11	0	5.75	0	3.4	0	4	37	1.6
Peppers—hot	30 mL (2 tablespoons)	19 g	8	0.25	0	0	1.5	0	0.2	0	1	3	0.2
Peppers—sweet, green	125 mL (1/2 cup), 1/2 vegetable	56 g	12	0.25	0.11	0	2.25	0	0.6	0	2	3	0.6
Peppers—sweet, red	125 mL (1/2 cup)	50 g	12	0.25	0.11	0	2.25	0	0.8	0	2	3	0.6
Potato skins—cheese, bacon	2 halves	96 g	302	11	15.89	7.44	27.5	0	1.4	34	267	225	4.5
Potato—baked/boiled	1/2 baked, 125 mL (1/2 cup)	78 g	73	1.5	0.11	0	16.75	0	1.4	0	4	6	0.3
Potatoes—mashed	125 mL (1/2 cup)	107 g	118	1.5	4.56	1.44	17	0	1.8	4	340	40	0.3
Radishes	2 radishes	9 g	2	0	0	0	0.25	0	0.1	0	2	2	0
Romaine lettuce	250 mL (1 cup)	53 g	9	1	0.11	0	1.25	0	1.3	0	4	19	0.6
Rutabaga	125 mL (1/2 cup)	103 g	35	0.75	0.11	0	7.5	0	2.1	0	19	43	0.5
Salad—potato	125 mL (1/2 cup)	121 g	153	3	7.78	1.89	15	1.5	1.9	47	512	19	0.5
Salad—three bean	125 mL (1/2 cup)	121 g	80	2	0	0	16.25	1.75	5	0	540	20	3.6
Salsa	63 mL (1/4 cup)	57 g	32	0.75	0	0	3	0	0.9	0	680	0	0
Sauerkraut	125 mL (1/2 cup)	118 g	22	0.75	0.11	0	4.5	0	4.1	0	780	36	1.7
Soup—vegetable	250 mL (1 cup)	251 g	81	2	1.56	0.44	11.25	2.25	0.5	2	892	16	1
Spaghetti sauce	125 mL (1/2 cup)	117 g	118	2	5	0.89	12.75	1.5	3.3	0	589	20	1.1
Spaghetti sauce w/meat	125 mL (1/2 cup)	104 g	80	2	3.11	0.67	12.5	2	3.3	0	630	20	1.1
Spinach—canned	125 mL (1/2 cup)	107 g	25	1.75	0.33	0.11	3.25	0	3.9	0	29	135	2.5
Spinach—fresh, cooked	125 mL (1/2 cup)	93 g	24	1.75	0.11	0	3.75	0	3	0	73	131	1.7
Spinach—raw	125 mL (1/2 cup)	28 g	6	0.5	0	0	0.75	0	1.1	0	22	28	0.8
Squash—summer	125 mL (1/2 cup)	96 g	18	0.5	0.11	0	3.75	0	1.5	0	3	22	0.4
Squash—winter	125 mL (1/2 cup)	109 g	41	0.75	0.11	0	9.5	0	3	0	4	23	0.6
Squash—zucchini, fresh, cooked	250 mL (1 cup) raw, 125 mL (1/2 cup) cooked	112 g	18	0.75	0	0	3.5	0	1.4	0	2	19	0.5
Sweet potato	125 mL (1/2 cup)	154 g	98	1.25	0	0	23	0	4	0	11	30	0.5
Sweet potato—candied	125 mL (1/2 cup)	114 g	190	1	0	0	26.5	20	4.4	0	60	20	0.7
Tomatoes—canned or stewed	125 mL (1/2 cup)	121 g	34	0.75	0.11	0	6.5	0.25	2.4	0	305	33	0.7
Tomatoes—raw	125 mL (1/2 cup), 4 slices	86 g	17	0.5	0.11	0	3.5	0	1.3	0	8	6	0.5
Vegetable juice	188 mL (3/4 cup)	182 g	35	1	0	0	8	0	1	0	650	20	0.7
Waterchestnuts—canned	125 mL (1/2 cup)	70 g	34	0.25	0	0	8.25	0	1.5	0	3	3	0.3
Waterchestnuts—raw	125 mL (1/2 cup)	62 g	66	0.75	0	0	15.75	0	1.4	0	9	7	0.4

© 2002, DINE Systems, Inc., 586 N. French Rd., Amherst, NY 14228.

Vegetables, continued

	Amount	Weight	Calories	Protein (g)	Total Fat (g)	Sat. Fat (g)	Carb. (g)	Added Sugar (g)	Fibre (g)	Chol. (mg)	Sodium (mg)	Calcium (mg)	Iron (mg)
Watercress—raw	125 mL (1/2 cup)	17 g	2	0.25	0	0	0.25	0	0.2	0	7	20	0
Wax beans	125 mL (1/2 cup)	68 g	18	1	0.11	0	4.25	0	1.5	0	6	27	0.6
Yams	125 mL (1/2 cup)	70 g	69	1.25	0.11	0	16.75	0	1.8	0	7	8	0.3

Fruits

	Amount	Weight	Calories	Protein (g)	Total Fat (g)	Sat. Fat (g)	Carb. (g)	Added Sugar (g)	Fibre (g)	Chol. (mg)	Sodium (mg)	Calcium (mg)	Iron (mg)
Apple cider	187 mL (3/4 cup)	186 g	94	0	0.11	0	17	6	0.1	0	6	7	0.4
Apples—sweetened	125 mL (1/2 cup)	102 g	68	0	0.11	0	12.5	3.25	2	0	4	4	0.3
Apples—unsweetened	1 fruit, 125 mL (1/2 cup)	133 g	77	0.25	0.44	0.11	20	0	2.1	0	0	8	0.2
Applesauce—sweetened	125 mL (1/2 cup)	128 g	97	0.25	0	0	3.75	10.75	1.1	0	3	8	0.4
Applesauce—unsweetened	125 mL (1/2 cup)	122 g	53	0.25	0	0	12.5	0	2.5	0	2	4	0.2
Apricots—sweetened	1 fruit	80 g	65	0.5	0	0	3.75	10.75	1.1	0	3	8	0.4
Apricots—unsweetened	1 fruit, 2 canned	35 g	17	0.5	0.11	0	4	0	0.8	0	0	5	0.2
Avocados	1/2 fruit, 125 mL (1/2 cup)	113 g	166	2	14.22	2.56	7.25	0	2.7	0	10	12	1
Banana	1 fruit, 125 mL (1/2 cup)	114 g	105	1	0.33	0.22	24	0	2.3	0	1	7	0.4
Blueberries—sweetened	125 mL (1/2 cup)	122 g	103	0.5	0.11	0	8.5	16.25	2.3	0	3	7	0.4
Blueberries—unsweetened	125 mL (1/2 cup)	75 g	41	0.5	0.22	0	9	0	1.7	0	2	5	0.2
Cherries—sweetened	125 mL (1/2 cup)	128 g	106	0.75	0	0	12.25	13	0.9	0	4	13	0.4
Cherries—unsweetened	10 fruits, 125 mL (1/4 cup)	93 g	44	0.75	0	0	10	0	0.9	0	2	12	0.4
Dates	5 fruits, 63 mL (1/4 cup)	43 g	118	0.75	0.22	0.11	28.5	0	3.7	0	1	14	0.5
Dried fruit	63 mL (1/4 cup), 8 pieces	32 g	92	1	0	0	21.75	0	2.4	0	9	11	0.7
Figs, sweetened	2 fruit	57 g	45	0.25	0	0	7	3.75	1.3	0	1	15	0.2
Figs—unsweetened	4 fruit, 125 mL (1/2 cup)	67 g	144	1.63	0.61	0.11	37	0	6.4	0	4	74.5	1
Fruit cocktail	125 mL (1/2 cup)	125 g	56	0.5	0.11	0	14.5	2.5	1.4	0	6.5	8	0.4
Fruit cocktail—sweetened	125 mL (1/2 cup)	127 g	83	0.5	0	0	8.75	11	1.4	0	8	8	0.3
Fruit cocktail—unsweetened	125 mL (1/2 cup)	123 g	50	0.5	0	0	11.5	0	1.4	0	4	6	0.3
Grapefruit—sweetened	125 mL (1/2 cup)	127 g	76	0.5	0	0	10	8	0.5	0	2	18	0.5
Grapefruit—unsweetened	1/2 fruit, 125 mL (1/2 cup)	120 g	39	0.5	0	0	9	0	0.7	0	0	14	0.2
Grapes—sweetened	125 mL (1/2 cup)	128 g	94	0.5	0	0	10.5	12	0.5	0	7	12	1.2
Grapes—unsweetened	20 fruits, 125 mL (1/2 cup)	84 g	48	0.5	0	0	11.5	0	0.5	0	2	8	0.2
Guava	1 fruit	90 g	45	0.5	0.33	0.11	9.5	0	5	0	2	18	0.3
Juice—unsweetened	188 mL (3/4 cup)	186 g	90	0.5	0	0	22.5	0	0.2	0	8	16	0.5
Kiwi fruit	1 fruit	76 g	46	0.75	0	0	10	0	2.1	0	4	20	0.3
Mango	1/2 fruit, 125 mL (1/2 cup)	93 g	61	0.5	0.33	0.11	14.25	0	1.8	0	2	9	0.2
Melon	125 mL (1/2 cup)	97 g	30	0.5	0.11	0	7	0	0.7	0	9	8	0.2
Nectarines	1 fruit	137 g	68	1	0.56	0.11	14.5	0	3.3	0	0	6	0.2
Olives	3 olives	12 g	15	0.25	1.56	0.22	0.25	0	0.3	0	234	8	0.2
Orange	1 fruit, 125 mL (1/2 cup)	134 g	63	1	0	0	14	0	3.9	0	1	53	0.2
Papaya	1/2 fruit, 125 mL (1/2 cup)	146 g	56	0.75	0	0	12.75	0	1.8	0	4	35	0.2
Peaches—sweetened	125 mL (1/2 cup)	125 g	94	0.5	0	0	5.25	17	1.2	0	8	3	0.4
Peaches—unsweetened	1 fruit, 125 mL (1/2 cup)	113 g	44	0.5	0	0	10.75	0	1.3	0	3	5	0.1
Pears—sweetened	2 halves	158 g	103	0.5	0	0	6	18.5	3.2	0	8	8	0.4

Fruits, continued

Amount		Weight	Calories	Protein (g)	Total Fat (g)	Sat. Fat (g)	Carb. (g)	Added Sugar (g)	Fibre (g)	Chol. (mg)	Sodium (mg)	Calcium (mg)	Iron (mg)
Pears—unsweetened	1 fruit, 125 mL (1/2 cup)	136 g	98	0.75	0.67	0	25	0	4.3	0	0	18	0.4
Pineapple—sweetened	2 slices, 125 mL (1/2 cup)	120 g	93	0.5	0	0	7.5	15	0.9	0	2	15	0.4
Pineapple—unsweetened	2 slices, 125 mL (1/2 cup)	108 g	70	0.25	0	0	17.5	0	0.9	0	2	6	0.4
Plums—sweetened	2 plums	89 g	67	0.5	0.11	0	8	7.75	0.7	0	17	9	0.7
Plums—unsweetened	1 raw, 2 canned	69 g	37	0.5	0	0	8.25	0	0.9	0	1	5	0.2
Prunes—cooked	125 mL (1/2 cup), 7 fruits	123 g	136	1.25	0.33	0	32	0	4.9	0	3	29	1.4
Prunes—dried	125 mL (1/2 cup)	74 g	209	2	0.44	0	49.25	0	6.8	0	4	45	2.1
Pumpkin—canned	125 mL (1/2 cup)	122 g	41	0.75	0.11	0.11	8.75	0	3.5	0	6	32	1.7
Raisins	63 mL (1/4 cup)	38 g	109	1	0	0	26	0	2.5	0	5	19	0.8
Raspberries—sweetened	125 mL (1/2 cup)	132 g	117	0.75	0.11	0	12	18.25	4.2	0	0	19	0.5
Raspberries—unsweetened	125 mL (1/2 cup)	62 g	30	0.5	0.22	0	6.5	0	3	0	0	14	0.3
Strawberries—sweetened	125 mL (1/2 cup)	133 g	100	0.5	0.11	0	9	15	2	0	4	14	0.6
Strawberries—unsweetened	125 mL (1/2 cup)	74 g	24	0.5	0.22	0	5.5	0	1.6	0	2	11	0.5
Tangerines—sweetened	125 mL (1/2 cup)	126 g	76	0.5	0	0	10	8.5	0.9	0	8	9	0.4
Tangerines—unsweetened	1 fruit, 125 mL (1/2 cup)	102 g	43	0.5	0	0	9.75	0	0.9	0	2	14	0.1
Watermelon	125 mL (1/2 cup)	80 g	25	0.5	0.22	0.22	5	0	0.3	0	2	6	0.2

Dairy

Amount		Weight	Calories	Protein (g)	Total Fat (g)	Sat. Fat (g)	Carb. (g)	Added Sugar (g)	Fibre (g)	Chol. (mg)	Sodium (mg)	Calcium (mg)	Iron (mg)
Buttermilk	250 mL (1 cup)	245 g	99	8.75	2	1.33	11.25	0	0	9	257	285	0.1
Cheese spread	30 mL (2 tablespoons)	28 g	81	3.5	6.56	4.33	2	0	1	89	293	95	1
Cheese—American	28 g (1 ounce), 1 slice	28 g	106	6.75	8.22	5.44	0.5	0	0	27	406	174	0.1
Cheese—cheddar	28 g (1 ounce), 1 slice	28 g	113	7.5	8.67	5.89	0.5	0	0	30	177	203	0.2
Cheese—cottage	125 mL (1/2 cup)	109 g	113	14.5	4.78	3.11	3	0	0	17	440	65	0.2
Cheese—cottage, non-fat	125 mL (1/2 cup)	113 g	90	14	0	0	7	0	0	10	400	60	0
Cheese—cottage, low-fat	125 mL (1/2 cup)	113 g	96	15	1.22	0.78	4	0	0	5	440	74	0.2
Cheese—mozzarella	28 g (1 ounce), 1 slice	28 g	80	6	5.67	3.67	0.5	0	0	22	106	147	0.1
Cheese—mozzarella, light	28 g (1 ounce)	28 g	72	7.25	4.11	2.78	0.75	0	0	16	150	183	0.1
Cheese—non-fat	28 g (1 ounce), 1 slice	28 g	40	8	0	0	1	0	0	5	290	210	0
Cheese—parmesan/romano	15 mL (1 tablespoon)	5 g	20	2	1.33	0.89	0.25	0	0	4	82	61	0
Cheese—provolone	28 g (1 ounce), 1 slice	28 g	100	7.75	7	4.78	0.5	0	0	20	248	214	0.2
Cheese—reduced fat	28 g (1 ounce), 1 slice	28 g	80	8	5	3	1	0	0	20	220	350	0
Cheese—ricotta	125 mL (1/2 cup)	124 g	216	15	14.89	10	3.75	0	0	63	104	257	0.5
Cheese—ricotta, part skim	125 mL (1/2 cup)	119 g	166	14.5	8.67	5.67	6.25	0	0	37	143	369	0.3
Cheese—Swiss	28 g (1 ounce)	28 g	101	8	6.89	4.67	0.75	0	0	25	231	246	0.1
Hot cocoa prepared w/milk	250 mL (1 cup)	250 g	218	8	9	5.67	13.5	11.25	3	33	123	298	0.8
Ice cream	125 mL (1/2 cup)	70 g	148	2.5	7.44	4.67	4.5	11.75	0.2	30	58	88	0.3
Ice milk	125 mL (1/2 cup)	66 g	110	3	2.78	1.89	10	8	0.3	8	75	100	1
Lowfat chocolate milk	250 mL (1 cup)	258 g	175	8.5	3.78	2.33	12.25	16	1.3	12	150	294	0.7
Meal replacement drinks	250 mL (1 cup)	314 g	200	14	1	0.44	36	17	4	5	230	500	6.3
Milk—chocolate	250 mL (1 cup)	250 g	208	8.5	7.89	5.11	10.5	14.5	1.1	30	149	280	0.6
Milk—low-fat	250 mL (1 cup)	244 g	112	8.75	3.56	2.22	11.25	0	0	14	123	299	0.1

© 2002, DINE Systems, Inc., 586 N. French Rd., Amherst, NY 14228.

Dairy, continued

	Amount	Weight	Calories	Protein (g)	Total Fat (g)	Sat. Fat (g)	Carb. (g)	Added Sugar (g)	Fibre (g)	Chol. (mg)	Sodium (mg)	Calcium (mg)	Iron (mg)
Milk—skim	250 mL (1 cup)	245 g	86	9	0.44	0.33	11.5	0	0	4	126	302	0.1
Milk—whole	250 mL (1 cup)	244 g	150	8.5	7.67	5	11	0	0	33	120	291	0.1
Tofutti	125 mL (1/2 cup)	66 g	150	2.5	6.67	1.11	9	11	1.5	0	105	1	0.6
Yogurt—frozen	125 mL (1/2 cup)	96 g	100	3	1.78	1.11	8	10.25	0.1	7	59	100	1
Yogurt—low-fat w/fruit	1 container	227 g	240	9	3	2	27	16	0.3	10	120	330	1
Yogurt—non-fat w/fruit	1 container	96 g	95	3.5	0	0	8	12	0	0	70	150	1
Yogurt—plain, low-fat	1 container	227 g	142	11.25	3.67	2.44	15.75	0	0	15	160	422	0.6
Yogurt—plain, non-fat	1 container	227 g	110	11	0.22	0.22	16	0	0	4	160	430	1
Yogurt—plain, whole milk	1 container	198 g	145	8.75	6.89	4.56	11.5	0	0	32	123	312	0.6
Yogurt—w/fruit, artificial sweetener	1 container	184 g	90	7	0.67	0.44	14	0	0.5	5	110	250	1

Protein Foods

	Amount	Weight	Calories	Protein (g)	Total Fat (g)	Sat. Fat (g)	Carb. (g)	Added Sugar (g)	Fibre (g)	Chol. (mg)	Sodium (mg)	Calcium (mg)	Iron (mg)
Bacon substitute	1 strip	12 g	52	3	4.11	1.56	0	0	0	13	207	1	0.2
Beans—baked	125 mL (1/2 cup)	121 g	140	6	1.67	0.67	15	7.5	6	8	423	60	2.1
Beans—black	125 mL (1/2 cup)	86 g	113	6.5	0.33	0.11	20.75	0	4.4	0	1	24	1.8
Beans—kidney, pinto	125 mL (1/2 cup)	86 g	115	6.5	0.33	0.11	22.25	0	4.5	0	2	33	2.4
Beans—kidney, pinto, canned	125 mL (1/2 cup)	125 g	104	5.75	0.22	0	19.5	0	6.1	0	445	35	1.6
Beans—lima	125 mL (1/2 cup)	90 g	94	5.5	0.22	0.11	17.5	0	4.6	0	26	25	1.8
Beans—lima, canned	125 mL (1/2 cup)	124 g	93	4.75	0.22	0.11	17.5	0	5.8	0	309	35	2
Beans—navy, chickpeas	125 mL (1/2 cup)	87 g	132	6.75	1	0.22	23.75	0	4.8	0	4	52	2.4
Beans—navy, chickpeas, canned	125 mL (1/2 cup)	126 g	146	7	0.78	0.11	27.5	0	5	0	473	51	2
Beans—white, canned	125 mL (1/2 cup)	131 g	153	8.25	0.22	0.11	29.25	0	5	0	7	96	3.9
Beans—white, split peas	125 mL (1/2 cup)	93 g	125	7	0.22	0.11	23	0	5.3	0	2	66	2.6
Beef stew	250 mL (1 cup)	247 g	207	9	9	4.22	16.5	0.5	2.5	53	616	29	2.6
Beef—corned	85 g (3 ounces)	85 g	182	15.25	12.11	5.22	0	0.25	0	65	768	11	1.5
Beef—mixed dish	250 mL (1 cup)	186 g	310	18.25	13.56	5.89	23.5	1.25	2.1	68	840	52	3.5
Biscuit w/egg, meat, cheese	1 biscuit	168 g	489	19.25	31.22	9.67	29	4	0.8	347	1240	151	2.9
Bologna sandwich	1 sandwich	106 g	311	18.75	18	6.56	22	3.75	1.7	32	845	60	2.5
Broadbeans—fava	125 mL (1/2 cup)	85 g	93	11	0.22	0	17	0	4.4	0	4	31	1.3
Broadbeans—fava, canned	125 mL (1/2 cup)	128 g	91	5.5	0.11	0	16.25	0	4.5	0	580	34	1.3
Burrito	1 burrito	230 g	213	6	7.22	3.56	29	0	3.2	33	558	53	2.3
Caviar	15 mL (1 tablespoon)	16 g	40	8	2.11	0.78	0.5	0	0.4	94	240	44	1.8
Cheeseburger (large) & roll	1 sandwich	280 g	711	4.25	43.33	16.78	33	4	1	113	1164	295	5
Cheeseburger (low-fat) & roll	1 sandwich	219 g	370	32	14	5	35	3.5	1.6	75	890	200	3.6
Cheeseburger (small) & roll	1 sandwich	172 g	461	24	27.56	13.67	25.25	3	0.8	95	906	245	3.3
Chicken breast sandwich	1 sandwich	195 g	509	29	26.89	4.78	34.75	1.75	1.7	83	1082	80	2.7
Chicken fingers/nuggets	4 fingers, 6 nuggets	98.5 g	275	26	14	3.11	15.25	0	0.4	49	558	7	0.8
Chicken salad	125 mL (1/2 cup)	84 g	179	15.75	12.22	2.89	0.75	0.75	0.3	118	329	21	0.9
Chicken wings	10 wings	257 g	617	14.75	46.56	13.56	15	1	0.4	198	1581	36	1.8
Chicken w/skin	85 g (3 ounces)	85 g	189	39	9.22	2.56	0	0	0	70	60	12	1

© 2002, DINE Systems, Inc., 586 N. French Rd., Amherst, NY 14228.

Protein Foods, continued

	Amount	Weight	Calories	Protein (g)	Total Fat (g)	Sat. Fat (g)	Carb. (g)	Added Sugar (g)	Fibre (g)	Chol. (mg)	Sodium (mg)	Calcium (mg)	Iron (mg)
Chicken w/out skin	85 g (3 ounces)	85 g	147	24.5	3.89	1.11	0	0	0	72	63	12	0.9
Chicken—fried, no skin	4 ounces	113 g	107	19.25	4.22	1.33	0.25	0	0	50	46	9	0.8
Chicken—fried, w/skin	85 g (3 ounces)	85 g	155	15.75	8.44	2.44	4.75	0	0.2	52	149	11	0.8
Chicken—mixed dish	250 mL (1 cup)	216 g	365	15.25	17.78	5.56	13.5	0	1	103	600	30	2.2
Chickpeas	125 mL (1/2 cup)	101 g	138	6.5	1.67	0.11	24.75	0	4.8	9	183	39	2
Chili con carne	250 mL (1 cup)	247 g	286	15.75	12.44	5.78	28.5	0	6.5	43	964	86	3
Chili—vegetarian	250 mL (1 cup)	226 g	240	18	12	1.78	13	2	16.4	0	860	6	3.2
Chimichanga	1 chimichanga	182 g	425	18.5	17.11	8.33	41.25	0	5.2	30	933	145	4
Chop suey	250 mL (1 cup)	250 g	300	26	16	4.33	13	0	1.5	68	1053	60	4.8
Chow mein—beef or chicken	187 mL (3/4 cup)	165 g	65	6.5	1.44	0.56	5.25	0.75	1.4	26	845	80	1.3
Clams, oyster, shrimp-fried	4 pieces	43 g	103	5.25	6.11	1.11	6	0	0.1	23	183	20	0.6
Clams, oysters, shrimp	125 mL (1/2 cup)	90 g	71	12.25	1.22	0.33	2.5	2	0	62	108	41	6
Coconut—shredded	30 mL (2 tablespoons)	10 g	44	0.25	3	2.67	2.25	2.25	0.4	0	24	1	0.2
Crabmeat	85 g (3 ounces)	85 g	86	12.5	1	0.22	4.5	0	0	26	713	25	0.4
Egg salad	125 mL (1/2 cup)	103 g	267	11	22.89	5.78	1	3	0.3	418	513	43	1.8
Egg—boiled, poached	1 egg	50 g	79	6.5	5.56	2.11	0.5	0	0	274	69	28	1
Egg—fried, scrambled	1 egg	55 g	89	6.25	6.78	3	1	0	0	281	150	37	0.9
Egg—omelet	1 omelet (3 eggs)	228 g	382.5	24.13	25.17	7.33	6	0	0.4	675	625	171.5	2.6
Egg—substitute	63 mL (1/4 cup)	56 g	43	5.5	1.56	0.22	1.5	0	0	0	115	30	0.8
Eggroll	1 eggroll	85 g	173	6.75	4.56	0.89	25	3	0.8	7	471	20	1.1
Enchilada	1 enchilada	178 g	322	10.5	16.89	9.67	30	0	5.8	42	1052	276	2.2
Fish casserole	250 mL (1 cup)	259 g	407	18.5	23.78	7.56	26.25	0.75	1.8	70	1314	182	2.3
Fish sandwich	1 sandwich	177 g	488	19	26.56	5.89	39.25	3.75	1.5	70	928	46	2
Fish sticks	3 pieces	57 g	150	6.75	8.22	2.22	12	0.75	0.7	15	280	0	0.5
Fish—fried	85 g (3 ounces)	85 g	209	8.75	11.56	2.67	16.25	1.25	0.7	39	350	0	0.5
Fish—not fried	85 g (3 ounces)	85 g	81	17	1	0.33	7.5	0	0	45	57	13	0.4
Fish—smoked, pickled	28 g (1 ounce)	28 g	56	6.25	2.33	0.67	0	0	0	14	235	5	0.3
Grilled cheese sandwich	1 sandwich	120 g	442	17	30.67	13.78	23	2.25	1.7	53	1200	402	1.8
Ground beef—lean	187 mL (3/4 cup)	85 g	228	22.5	13.94	5.44	0	0	0	76.5	62.5	8	2.1
Ground beef—regular	187 mL (3/4 cup)	85 g	246	20.75	17.56	6.89	0	0	0	80	71	9	2.1
Ham	85 g (3 ounces)	85 g	124	15.75	6.56	2.33	0	0	0	41	1064	6	0.8
Ham sandwich	1 sandwich	140 g	343	23.5	15.89	7.67	23	2	1.7	60	1577	229	2.5
Hamburger (large) & roll	1 sandwich	228 g	594	27.5	33	12.67	33.25	2	0.9	101	688	87	4.8
Hamburger (low-fat) & roll	1 sandwich	206 g	320	22	10	4	35	3.5	1.6	60	670	150	3.6
Hamburger (small) & roll	1 sandwich	137 g	355	22	19.33	8.22	22.25	3	1.7	95	556	71	3.2
Hot dog	1 hot dog	50 g	144	5.75	12.89	5.22	0.25	1.25	0	30	547	20	0.7
Hot dog and roll	1 sandwich	105 g	298	9.25	17.56	6.67	20	2.5	0.7	29	880	60	2.2
Julienne salad	500 mL (2 cups)	483 g	489	47.5	29	13.89	7.5	0	3.5	281	1340	360	3.4
Lamb	85 g (3 ounces)	85 g	169	19.75	11.11	5.33	0	0	0	68	49	8	1.5
Lentils	125 mL (1/2 cup)	99 g	115	7.75	0.22	0	20.25	0	2.8	0	2	19	3.3
Liver	85 g (3 ounces)	85 g	127	17.75	4.56	2	2.5	0	0	258	52	8	5.8
Luncheon meat—beef, pork	2 slices	56 g	152	8.5	12.22	5.11	0	1	0	36	696	6	0.8

Protein Foods, continued

	Amount	Weight	Calories	Protein (g)	Total Fat (g)	Sat. Fat (g)	Carb. (g)	Added Sugar (g)	Fibre (g)	Chol. (mg)	Sodium (mg)	Calcium (mg)	Iron (mg)
Luncheon meat—chicken, turkey	2 slices	56 g	64	11.5	1.33	0.44	0	0	0	24	716	6	0.6
Luncheon meat—lean	2 slices	56 g	90	8	4	3.11	3	1.5	0	30	586	0	0.8
Meatloaf	85 g (3 ounces)	85 g	204	16	12	4.44	7	0.25	0.7	104	303	18	2
Miso	125 mL (1/2 cup)	138 g	284	14.25	7.33	1.11	39.25	0	7.4	0	5032	92	3.8
Nuts—mixed	45 mL (3 tablespoons), 26 nuts	28 g	170	4.25	13.56	2.22	6.25	0	1.6	0	170	20	1.1
Pâté	15 mL (1 tablespoon)	13 g	41	2	3.67	1.44	0	0	0	51	91	9	0.7
Peanut butter	30 mL (2 tablespoons)	32 g	190	9	14.56	2.78	4.5	2	2.4	0	150	11	0.6
Peanut butter & jelly sandwich	1 sandwich	101 g	371	12.25	17.89	3.56	26.5	17.75	3.8	0	426	66	2.2
Peanuts	45mL (3 tablespoons), 32 nuts	28 g	164	6.25	12.33	1.78	5.25	0	2.5	0	110	7	0.5
Peas—black-eyed	125 mL (1/2 cup)	86 g	100	5.75	0.33	0.11	18.25	0	8.3	0	3	21	2.2
Peas—black-eyed, canned	125 mL (1/2 cup)	120 g	92	5	0.33	0.11	16.5	0	8.2	0	359	24	1.2
Pepperoni	85 g (3 ounces)	85 g	440	16.5	41.56	14.56	2.25	2	0	72	1589	5	0.6
Pizza—cheese & vegetable	1 slice	130 g	249	12.5	9.22	5.11	30	0.5	4	15	518	195	2.3
Pizza—cheese topping	1 slice	65 g	199	11.5	8.44	4.44	28.25	0.5	2	17	456	250	1.2
Pizza—cheese, meat & vegetable	1 slice	120 g	270	16	12.44	6	26.5	0.5	3.5	27	682	230	2.5
Pizza—French bread	1 slice	164 g	410	17.5	19.22	8	39	2	2	35	1030	200	2.7
Pizza—meat topping	1 slice	106 g	271	11.5	13	5.33	27	0.5	1.2	20	733	132	1.8
Pork and beans	125 mL (1/2 cup)	126 g	134	6.5	1.89	0.67	17	8	6.6	9	521	71	2.1
Pork chop	85 g (3 ounces)	85 g	217	23.5	12.89	4.89	0	0	0	70	48	21	0.8
Pork chop—lean cut	85 g (3 ounces)	85 g	177	23	8	0	0	0	0	0	0	0	0
Pork feet	227 g (8 ounces)	227 g	138	14.5	8.78	3.22	0	0	0	71	597	32	1.1
Pork rinds	85 g (3 ounces)	113 g	458	51.75	26	10	0	0	0	80	2275	19	0.5
Pork roast	85 g (3 ounces)	85 g	232	23	15	5.56	0	0	0	78	53	16	1
Pork roast—lean cut	85 g (3 ounces)	85 g	180	24	8.33	3.11	0	0	0	78	55	14	1.2
Pork spareribs	113 g (4 ounces)	113 g	132	10.25	9.89	3.89	0	0	0	41	31	16	0.6
Pork—fresh, fried	113 g (4 ounces)	114 g	144	11	11.22	4.22	0	0	0	41	25	4	0.4
Pork—fresh, roasted	113 g (4 ounces)	114 g	164	15.75	10.22	3.89	0	0	0	54	37	4	0.6
Refried beans	125 mL (1/2 cup)	113 g	135	6	1.33	0.56	18	0	6	0	400	40	2.2
Roast beef sandwich	1 sandwich	164 g	353	27.25	14.89	7.33	30.25	2.25	1.7	49	766	87	4.1
Roast beef—lean cut	85 g (3 ounces)	85 g	156	24.75	5.67	1.89	0	0	0	69	54	4	2.7
Roast beef—regular	85 g (3 ounces)	85 g	222.5	22.75	13.5	5.11	0	0	0	69.5	53	5	2.4
Sausage	85 g (3 ounces)	85 g	264	12	22.33	8.67	0	1.5	0	42	774	12	1.2
Seafood or fish salad	125 mL (1/2 cup)	104 g	160	13.5	9.78	2.33	1.75	0.25	0.4	142	250	31	0.9
Sloppy Joe sandwich	1 sandwich	146 g	302	18.5	13.78	6	23.75	2.5	1.4	63	509	31	0.9
Soybeans—roasted	63 mL (1/4 cup)	44 g	205	14.25	10.22	1.56	13.5	0	1.9	0	1	89	2
Steak	85 g (3 ounces)	85 g	191	24	9.33	3.44	0	0	0	71	54	7	2.7
Steak—lean cut	85 g (3 ounces)	85 g	176	24.5	7.89	3	0	0	0	69	56	5	2.4
Submarine/hoagy	1 submarine	401 g	934	34.5	51.22	12.67	73.25	3.75	3.1	87	1538	294	5.7
Sweet & sour chicken, pork	250 mL (1 cup)	258 g	426	17.5	13.89	3.33	23.5	31.75	1.3	83	1209	27	1.9

© 2002, DINE Systems, Inc., 586 N. French Rd., Amherst, NY 14228.

	Amount	Weight	Calories	Protein (g)	Total Fat (g)	Sat. Fat (g)	Carb. (g)	Added Sugar (g)	Fibre (g)	Chol. (mg)	Sodium (mg)	Calcium (mg)	Iron (mg)
Taco	1 taco	171 g	370	21	18.44	11.11	26.5	0	3.4	57	802	221	2.4
Taco salad	375 mL (1—1/2 cup)	198 g	279	13.5	13.33	6.67	24	0	4.3	44	763	192	2.3
Tahini	15 mL (1 tablespoon)	16 g	92	2.5	7.33	1.11	3.75	0	1.5	0	10	109	2.2
Tofu	85 g (3 ounces)	85 g	65	6.75	2.33	0.33	2.25	0	1	0	8	68	1.1
Tostada	1 tostada	198 g	325	13.75	13.89	9.67	28	0	7.5	40	834	214	2.2
Tripe	113 g (4 ounces)	113 g	61	12.5	1.11	0.67	0	0	0	58	44	77	0.3
Tuna casserole	250 mL (1 cup), 18 chips	231 g	248	16	10.44	3.33	26.75	0	0.7	36	1072	120	1.4
Tuna in oil	125 mL (1/2 cup)	74 g	142	22	5.44	1.11	0	0	0	18	275	7	0.8
Tuna in water	125 mL (1/2 cup)	74 g	90	19.25	1.44	0.44	0	0	0	28	400	0	0.7
Tuna salad	125 mL (1/2 cup)	102 g	183	14	9.44	1.89	2.25	0	0.4	13	412	23	0.8
Tuna sandwich	1 sandwich	120 g	364.5	16.25	23	4.11	24.13	2.25	1.7	25	599	53	2
Turkey hot dog	1 hot dog	45.4 g	102	6.5	8	3.11	0.25	1.5	0	51	641	51	0.9
Turkey sandwich	1 sandwich	194 g	355	30.25	14.67	2.67	23.5	2.25	1.7	76	385	75	3.3
Turkey w/skin	85 g (3 ounces)	85 g	168	24	7.89	2.11	0	0	0	70	57	20	1.5
Turkey w/out skin	85 g (3 ounces)	85 g	137	25.5	3.22	1	0	0	0	72	64	19	1.5
Veal	85 g (3 ounces)	85 g	195	25.63	10.17	4	0	0	0	95.5	69.5	16.5	1
Veal—lean cut	85 g (3 ounces)	85 g	167	27	5.33	1.67	0	0	0	98	76	20	1
Veal—mixed dish	1 serving	168 g	327	28.25	17.78	9.78	9.5	0.75	1.7	137	634	138	3.7
Venison	85 g (3 ounces)	85 g	147	25.75	3.11	1.22	0	0	0	95	280	6	3.8
Beverages													
Beer—non-alcoholic	375 mL	359 g	55	0.75	0	0	11	0	0	0	19	25	0.1
Coffee	250 mL (1 cup)	237 g	5	0.25	0	0	1	0	0	0	7	6	0.6
Coffee—decaffeinated	250 mL (1 cup)	239 g	3	0.25	0	0	0.75	0	0	0	8	8	0.1
Cola	375 mL	366 g	150	0	0	0	0	37	0	0	70	0	0
Cola—diet	375 mL	360 g	2	0.25	0	0	0.25	0	0	0	70	0	0
Cola—diet, no caffeine		358 g	2	0	0	0	0	0	0	0	70	0	0
Cola—no caffeine	375 mL	363 g	155	0	0	0	0	38.75	0	0	73	0	0
Juice drink	187 mL (3/4 cup), 1 juice box	190 g	106	0	0	0	6.5	19.5	0	0	7	1	1
Mellow Yellow, Mountain Dew	375 mL	371 g	177	0	0	0	0	44	0	0	30	0	0
Non-cola—diet, no caffeine	375 mL	342 g	4	0	0	0	0.5	0	0	0	42	0	0
Non-cola—no caffeine	375 mL	364 g	157	0	0	0	0	37.75	0	0	46	2	0.1
Postum	5 mL (1 teaspoon)	3 g	12	0	0	0	3	0	1.3	0	0	0	0
Tea—herbal, no caffeine	250 mL (1 cup)	240 g	4	0	0	0	0.75	0	0	0	3	5	0.2
Tea—plain	250 mL (1 cup)	239 g	3	0	0	0	0.5	0	0	0	0	0	0
Wine—non-alcoholic	156 mL	136 g	42	0.5	0	0	9.75	0	0	0	7	12	0.6
Beverages—Alcoholic													
Beer	375 mL	360 g	145	1	0	0	13.25	0	0	0	8	12	0
Beer—light	355 mL	355 g	110	1	0	0	7	0	0	0	8	15	0
Chianti	156 mL	148 g	106	0.25	0	0	2.5	0	0	0	8	12	0.6
Cocktail—mixed drink	1 cocktail	134 g	139	0	0	0	1	1.5	0	0	6	4	0.1

© 2002, DINE Systems, Inc., 586 N. French Rd., Amherst, NY 14228.

Beverages—Alcoholic, continued

Food	Amount	Weight	Calories	Protein (g)	Total Fat (g)	Sat. Fat (g)	Carb. (g)	Added Sugar (g)	Fibre (g)	Chol. (mg)	Sodium (mg)	Calcium (mg)	Iron (mg)
Liqueur	47 mL	50 g	167	0	0.11	0	8.5	9.5	0	0	4	1	0
Liquor	47 mL, 1 jigger, 23 mL (1-1/2 tablespoons)	42 g	110	0	0	0	0	0	0	0	0	0	0
Vermouth	156 mL	148 g	100	0.25	0	0	1	0	0	0	8	12	0.4
Wine	156 mL	148 g	104	0.25	0	0	2.5	0	0	0	12	12	0.4
Wine cooler	375 mL	360 g	173	0.75	0	0	7.75	9.75	0	0	25	32	1.4
Wine—light	156 mL	148 g	73	0.5	0	0	1	0	0	0	10	13	0.6

Fats/Sweets/Other

Food	Amount	Weight	Calories	Protein (g)	Total Fat (g)	Sat. Fat (g)	Carb. (g)	Added Sugar (g)	Fibre (g)	Chol. (mg)	Sodium (mg)	Calcium (mg)	Iron (mg)
Bacon	1 slice	9.25 g	37	2.35	3.11	1.16	0.09	0.05	0	8	160.5	0.88	0.2
Bacon bits	23 mL (1-1/2 tablespoons)	7 g	21	2.5	1.11	0.33	0	0	0	6	181	0.1	0.1
Breakfast milk powder	1 packet	36 g	130	6	0	0	0	26.25	0.4	0	185	80	4.5
Brownie	1 square	38 g	150	2	6.22	1.67	6.5	15	0.9	10	105	1	0.7
Butter	5 mL (1 teaspoon), 1 pat	5 g	34.7	0	3.81	2.41	0	0	0	10.7	39.7	0.7	0.3
Cake	1 piece	98 g	280	4	11.33	3	15.25	22.25	0.5	56	285	57	1
Candy—chewy	28 g (1 ounce)	28 g	109	0	1	0.56	1.5	20.5	0	0	32	1	0
Candy—chocolate & peanut butter	47 g (1-1/2 ounces)	47 g	237	6	13.78	5.89	4	22	2.5	3	90	34	0.7
Candy—chocolate	28 g (1 ounce)	28 g	150	2	8.22	4.78	2.25	15	0.8	6	24	50	0.3
Candy—chocolate covered	28 g (1 ounce)	28 g	132	1.25	5.56	2.11	3	13.25	1.5	3	43	33	0.4
Candy—fudge	1 cube	28.4 g	119	1	4.06	1.06	1.7	17.93	0.4	2.7	54.1	27	0.3
Candy—hard	5 pieces	28 g	110	0	0	0	2.75	27.5	0	0	7	1	0.1
Catsup	15 mL (1 tablespoon)	15 g	17	0	0	0	2.75	1.5	0.2	0	168	3	0.1
Cheese puffs	250 mL (1 cup)	28 g	160	2	9.78	1.78	16	0	0.3	0	330	0	0.4
Cheese sauce	63 mL (1/4 cup)	70 g	71	3.5	3.56	1.89	6.5	0	0	10	412	139	0.1
Chili sauce	15 mL (1 tablespoon)	15 g	17	0.25	0	0	2.75	1.25	0.9	0	196	2	0.1
Chip dip	63 mL (1/4 cup)	60 g	120	2	10	6	4	0.5	0	40	360	80	0
Coffee whitener	15 mL (1 tablespoon)	11 g	22	0	2.11	1.33	0	1	0	0	12	1	1
Cookies—fig bars	2 bars	28 g	100	1	1.78	0.44	10.5	10.5	1.2	1	90	20	0.7
Cookies—non-fat	2 cookies	23 g	75	1	0	0	17.5	6.5	0.6	0	115	0	0.2
Cookies—oatmeal raisin	3 cookies	40 g	195	2.25	8.11	1.89	13.5	13.5	1.4	1	150	0	0.8
Cookies—others	3 cookies	42 g	180	1.5	8.11	2.89	10	15	0.3	3	131	1	0.7
Corn chips	250 mL (1 cup)	28 g	152	2	9.44	1.33	16	0	1.3	0	205	36	0.2
Cream cheese	30 mL (2 tablespoons)	30 g	106	2.5	10.22	6.67	1	0	0	34	90	24	0.4
Cream cheese—light	30 mL (2 tablespoons)	28 g	80	3	7	4	1	0	0	25	115	20	1
Cream—coffee, half & half	15 mL (1 tablespoon)	15 g	25	0.5	2.22	1.44	0.5	0	0	8	6	15	0
Cream—whipped	15 mL (1 tablespoon)	5 g	15	0.25	1.33	1.11	0.25	0.25	0	2	4	3	1
Cupcakes	250 mL (1 cup)cake	39 g	140	1.25	4.56	1.89	8.5	15	0.7	12	121	24	0.6
Danish	1 danish	71 g	252	4.5	11.67	3.67	10.25	19	0.7	14	249	36	1.1
Danish—non-fat	1 danish	33 g	90	2	0	0	20	9.75	0.2	0	85	20	0
Dessert topping—no sugar	15 mL (1 tablespoon)	5 g	5	0	0.56	0.44	0	0	1	4	5	2	1

© 2002. DINE Systems, Inc., 586 N. French Rd., Amherst, NY 14228.

Amount	Weight	Calories	Protein (g)	Total Fat (g)	Sat. Fat (g)	Carb. (g)	Added Sugar (g)	Fibre (g)	Chol. (mg)	Sodium (mg)	Calcium (mg)	Iron (mg)
Diet bar	1 bar	31 g	120	2	4	1.44	19	9.5	3	1	30	150	2.7
Doughnut or sweet roll	1 doughnut, 1 sweet roll	60 g	220	3.75	9.89	3.33	29.5	18	1	5	230	22	1.1
Frozen desserts—non-fat	125 mL (1/2 cup)	68 g	100	2	0.22	0.11	23.5	9.5	0.4	1	48	100	0
Frozen yogurt cone—low-fat	1 serving	85 g	105	4	1	0.56	22	13	0.1	3	80	112	0.2
Frozen yogurt sundae—low-fat	1 sundae	171 g	240	6	3	2.33	50.5	43	0.8	6	170	190	0.1
Gelatin	125 mL (1/2 cup)	127 g	105	2	1	1	23	22	0	0	57	0	0
Gelatin—sugar free	125 mL (1/2 cup)	121 g	8	1.5	0	0	0	0	0	0	31	0	0
Granola bars	1 bar	28 g	133	2	6	2	18.25	13	0.6	0	70	20	0.5
Gravy	63 mL (1/4 cup)	60 g	30	1	1.44	0.56	2.25	0.5	0.1	1	260	3	0.4
Hollandaise sauce	63 mL (1/4 cup)	64 g	230	2.25	23.44	8.44	2.5	0	0	140	316	50	1
Honey	10 mL (2 teaspoons)	14 g	42	0	0	0	0	10.5	0	0	1	1	0.1
Hot cocoa mix	1 envelope	26 g	110	1.5	2.78	1.56	3.5	16	1.1	2	165	40	0.7
Ice cream bar	1 bar	57 g	172	2	11.78	7.11	6	11.5	0.3	17	50	80	0
Jam or jelly	10 mL (2 teaspoons)	13 g	35	0	0	0	1	7.5	0.1	0	1	1	1
Lard	15 mL (1 tablespoon)	13 g	115	0	12.22	5	0	0	0	12	0	0	0
Margarine—stick	5 mL (1 teaspoon), 1 pat	5 g	33.7	0	3.52	0.67	0	0	0	0	44.3	1.3	0
Margarine—stick, light	5 mL (1 teaspoon), 1 pat	5 g	20	0	2.22	0.33	0	0	0	0	36.7	0.33	0.3
Margarine—tub	15 mL (1 tablespoon)	14 g	101	0	8.89	2	0	0	0	0	152	4	0
Margarine—tub, light	15 mL (1 tablespoon)	14 g	50	0	5.89	1	0	0	0	0	110	1	1
Marshmallows	2 pieces	14 g	47	0.25	0	0	1	11.75	0	0	7	2	0.1
Mayonnaise	15 mL (1 tablespoon)	14 g	100	0.25	11	1.89	0.25	0.25	0	8	74	1	1
Mayonnaise—light	15 mL (1 tablespoon)	14 g	48	0.25	4.56	1	0.75	1	0	5	95	1	1
Mayonnaise—non-fat	15 mL (1 tablespoon)	16 g	12	0	0	0	3	3	0	0	190	0	0
Meal replacement bar	1 serving	48 g	270	11	14	5	24	22.5	0	0	330	250	4.5
Milkshake	313 mL (1-1/4 cups)	290 g	368	10	12.78	8.22	26.5	19.25	0.5	54	243	375	0.5
Milkshake—low-fat	1 serving	293 g	320	10.75	1.33	0.56	66	44.75	0	10	170	327	0.1
Miracle Whip	15 mL (1 tablespoon)	14 g	64	0	5.89	0.89	2.5	0.5	0	5	95	2	1
Miracle Whip—non-fat	15 mL (1 tablespoon)	16 g	20	0	0	0	5	5	0	0	210	0	0
Molasses	15 mL (1 tablespoon)	20 g	55	0	0	0	0	14.5	0	0	11	75	1.8
Mustard	5 mL (1 teaspoon)	5 g	6	0.25	0.33	0	0.25	0	0	0	60	0	0
Non-cola—diet	375 mL 1-1/2 cups)	369 g	2	0	0	0	0.5	0	0	0	8	0	0
Nutrasweet—Equal	1 packet	1 g	4	0.5	0	0	0	0.5	0	0	0	0	0
Oil	15 mL (1 tablespoon)	14 g	120	0	12.78	1.89	0	0	0	0	0	0	0.1
Pickles—dill	2 spears	61 g	7	0	0.11	0	1	0.75	0.9	0	584	9	0.4
Pickles—sweet	1 pickle, 3 slices	18 g	18	0	0	0	0.5	4	0.3	0	107	2	0.2
Pie—custard or cream	1 slice	152 g	346	6.75	13.11	6.22	20.75	25.75	1	125	375	122	0.8
Pie—fruit	1 slice	158 g	405	4	16.22	5.33	34.75	25.25	4	6	423	17	1.6
Pie—pecan	1/6 of 23 cm pie	138 g	575	7	29.67	5.67	33	37.25	2.2	100	305	65	4.6
Popcorn	250 mL (1 cup)	11 g	32	0.75	1.44	0.44	5.5	0.75	0.8	0	68	0	0.2
Popsicle	1 popsicle	69 g	50	0	0	0	0	13	0	0	10	0	0
Potato chips	250 mL (1 cup), 20 chips	28 g	150	2	9.67	2	15	0	1.4	0	190	0	0.4
Pretzels	167 mL (2/3 cup)	28 g	110	2.75	0.89	0.22	21.75	1	0.9	0	610	9	1.4

Fats/Sweets/Other, continued

	Amount	Weight	Calories	Protein (g)	Total Fat (g)	Sat. Fat (g)	Carb. (g)	Added Sugar (g)	Fibre (g)	Chol. (mg)	Sodium (mg)	Calcium (mg)	Iron (mg)
Pudding	125 mL (1/2 cup)	147 g	150	4.5	2.22	1.44	10	18	0	9	443	152	0
Pudding—diet	125 mL (1/2 cup)	132 g	90	4	2.44	1.57	13	0	0.4	9	423	152	0.1
Relish	30 mL (2 tablespoon)	28 g	35	0	0	0	1.25	7.5	0.2	0	243	6	0.2
Saccharin	1 packet	1 g	2	0	0	0	0	0	0	0	2	0	0
Salad dressing	15 mL (1 tablespoon)	16 g	80	0	8.22	1.33	0.25	0.25	1	0	146	2	1
Salad dressing—light	15 mL (1 tablespoon)	15 g	16	0.25	0.33	0.11	0.75	0.5	0.3	0	137	1	1
Salad dressing—no oil	15 mL (1 tablespoon)	17 g	12	0	0	0	2.5	0	0.7	0	0	1	1
Salad dressing—non-fat	15 mL (1 tablespoon)	15 g	16	0	0	0	3	3	0	0	143	0	0
Salt	4 shakes	0 g	0	0	0	0	0	0	0	0	64	0	0
Sherbet	125 mL (1/2 cup)	97 g	136	1	1.89	1.22	6	23.5	0	7	44	52	0.2
Soft drinks	375 mL (1-1/2 cups)	369 g	156	0	0	0	0	39.5	0	0	22	0	0
Soup—beef or chicken	250 mL (1 cup)	266 g	74	4.25	2.22	0.67	8.5	0	1	7	910	17	0.9
Soup—bouillon, broth	1 cube, packet(s), 250 mL (1 cup)	5 g	9	0.75	0.22	0.11	0.25	1	0	1	965	1	0.1
Soup—broth based, no salt	250 mL (1 cup)	241 g	135	5.75	3.89	0.78	16.5	0	2.8	0	115	47	1.8
Soup—cream, chowder	250 mL (1 cup)	246 g	140	5.5	6.11	2.89	14	0	0.9	22	1010	150	0.6
Soup—low salt	250 mL (1 cup)	246 g	110	4	3	1	12	0	0.5	2	100	17	1.3
Soup—miso	250 mL (1 cup)	199 g	152	4.5	6.44	0.89	19	0	3	0	490	20	1.3
Sour cream	30 mL (2 tablespoons)	24 g	52	0.5	5.11	3.11	1	0	0	10	34	28	0
Sour cream—imitation	30 mL (2 tablespoons)	26 g	50	1.5	4.67	4	1.5	0	0	2	20	14	0
Sour cream—non-fat	30 mL (2 tablespoons)	28 g	16	2	0	0	2	0	0	0	20	40	0
Soy sauce	15 mL (1 tablespoon)	18 g	10	1.25	0	0	1.25	0	0	0	1015	3	0.4
Steak/Worcestershire sauce	15 mL (1 tablespoon)	15 g	11	0	0	0	1	1.75	0	0	143	0	0
Sugar	5 mL (1 teaspoon)	4 g	15	0	0	0	0	3.75	0	0	0	0	0
Sunflower seeds	30 mL (2 tablespoons)	19 g	116	3.75	10.78	1.11	4	0	1.7	0	1	11	1.3
Syrup—pancake, table	30 mL (2 tablespoons)	40 g	110	0	0	0	0	27.5	0	0	21	1	1
Tortilla chips	250 mL (1 cup), 10 chips	19 g	95	1.25	4.67	1.33	12	0	0.9	0	123	23	0.3
White sauce	63 mL (1/4 cup)	63 g	99	2.5	5.67	2.22	6	0	0.1	8	222	73	0.2

Appendix B

Nutritional Content of Fast Foods*

Arby's
Burger King
Jack in the Box
KFC
McDonald's
Pizza Hut
Taco Bell

APPENDIX B Nutritional Content of Fast Foods

Name	Serving Size	Gram weight	Calories	Protein (g)	Carb. (g)	Total Fat (g)	Sat. Fat (g)	% Calories from Fat	Chol. (mg)	Sodium (mg)	Fibre (g)	Sugar (g)	Calcium (mg)	Iron (mg)	Vit. A (IU)	Vit. C (mg)
Arby's																
Arby's – Breakfast																
Egg, Scrambled	1 egg	50	70	6	0	5	2	65.22	220	70	0	0	20	0.72	*	0
French Toastix w/o Powdered Sugar or Syrup (5 oz)	3 hotcakes	124	370	7	48	17	4	41.02	0	440	4	*	70	1.80	*	0
Sausage Patty	39 g	39.70	200	7	1	19	7	84.24	60	290	0	0	0	0.72	*	0
Arby's – Sides																
French Fries, Cheddar, Curly	regular	170	450	7.50	52	25	6	48.60	5	1420	0	*	80	2.70	*	12
French Fries, Curly, Medium	regular	128	380	5	49	19	4.50	44.19	0	1100	0	*	0	1.80	*	12
French Fries, Homestyle, Medium	regular	142	420	5	57	19	3	40.81	0	830	4	*	0	1.44	*	21
Jalapeno Bites	regular	110	330	7	29	21	9	56.76	40	670	2	*	40	0.72	*	1.20
Mozzarella Sticks	regular	137	470	18	34	29	14	55.65	60	1330	2	*	400		*	1.20
Onion Petals	regular	113.40	410	4	43	24	3	53.47	0	300	2	*	20	0.72	*	0
Potato Cakes	2 cakes	85.10	220	2	21	14	3	57.80	0	460	3	*	0	1.08	*	6
Potato, Baked Broccoli 'n Cheddar	1 potatoe	384	550	14	71	25	13	39.82	50	730	7	*	250	3.96	*	63.60
Arby's – Poultry and Seafood																
Chicken Finger Meal	1 meal	303	880	35	81	47	8	47.69	60	2240	0	*	0	1.80	*	9
Chicken Finger Snack	1 snack	208	610	20	62	32	6	46.75	30	1610	0	*	0	1.80	*	9
Fish Fillet Sandwich	1 sandwich	223	540	23	51	27	7	45.08	40	880	2	*	80	3.60	*	1.20
Roast Turkey Deluxe, Low-fat	1 sandwich	196	230	19	33	5	1.50	17.79	25	870	4	*	60	2.70	*	9
Arby's – Sandwiches																
Barbecue Sandwich, Arby-Q	1 sandwich	186	380	19	42	15	5	35.62	30	990	3	*	100	3.60	*	4.80
Chicken Bacon 'N Swiss Sandwich	1 sandwich	222	610	37	52	30	9	43.13	75	1620	5	*	200	2.70	*	2.40
Chicken Breast Fillet Sandwich	1 sandwich	216	560	30	49	28	6	44.37	55	1080	6	*	80	2.70	*	1.20
French Dip Sub	1 sub	200	490	30	43	22	8	40.41	56	1440	3	*	120	6.30	*	1.20
Grilled Chicken Deluxe Sandwich	1 sandwich	247	420	30	42	16	4	33.33	60	930	3	*	80	2.70	*	12
Grilled Chicken Sandwich, Low-fat	1 sandwich	179	280	30	33	5	1.50	15.15	50	920	4	*	50	2.52	*	4.80
Italian Sub	1 sub	291	800	28	49	54	16	61.21	85	2610	2	*	350	4.50	*	9

* Values unavailable.

Name	serving Size	Gram weight	Calories	Protein (g)	Carb. (g)	Total Fat (g)	Sat. Fat. (g)	% Calories from Fat	Chol. (mg)	Sodium (mg)	Fibre (g)	Sugar (g)	Calcium (mg)	Iron (mg)	Vit. A (IU)	Vit. C (mg)
Arby's, continued																
Roast Beef Sandwich, Regular	1 sandwich	158	400	23	36	20	7	43.27	40	1030	3	*	50	4.50	*	0
Roast Chicken Club	1 sandwich	239	540	37	39	29	8	46.19	70	1590	3	*	200	2.70	*	2.40
Roast Chicken Deluxe, Low-fat	1 sandwich	196	260	23	32	5	1.50	16.98	40	950	4	*	60	2.70	*	9
Turkey Sub	1 sub	303	670	29	49	39	10	52.94	60	2130	2	*	350	4.50	*	9
Arby's – Beverages and Shakes																
Milk	250 mL	227	120	8	12	5	3	36	20	120	0	*	300	0.36	*	2.40
Orange Juice	313 mL	283	140	1	34	0	0	0	0	0	0	*	0	0	*	78
Shake, Chocolate	313 mL	292	390	8	69	9	6	20.82	10	270	0	*	250	0.90	*	*
Shake, Jamocha	313 mL	292	380	8	66	9	6	21.49	10	300	0	*	250	0.90	*	*
Shake, Strawberry	313 mL	292	380	8	67	9	6	21.26	10	270	0	*	250	0.90	*	*
Shake, Vanilla	313 mL	292	380	8	67	9	6	21.26	12	270	0	*	250	0.90	*	0
Arby's – Salads																
Salad, Garden, w/ 1 Crouton Packet and 2 Saltine Crackers	1 salad	290	110	9	16	3	0	21.26	0	150	1	*	200	0.36	*	72
Salad, Grilled Chicken, Low-fat	1 salad	401	190	25	16	4	0.50	18	40	530	1	*	200	0.36	*	75
Salad, Roast Chicken, Low-fat	1 salad	401	200	25	16	5	0.50	21.53	40	800	1	*	200	0.36	*	75
Arby's – Breads																
Biscuit w/Margarine	1 bisquit	78.50	270	5	26	16	3	53.73	0	750	0	*	0	0	*	0
Croissant	1 croissant	62	260	6	28	16	10	51.43	20	300	0	*	0	2.70	*	0
Arby's – Dessert and Snacks																
Turnover, Iced Apple	1 turnover	96.10	360	4	54	14	3	35.20	0	180	6	*	0	1.44	*	1.20
Turnover, Iced Cherry	1 turnover	97.80	350	4	53	14	3	35.59	0	190	0	*	0	1.44	*	4.80

* Values unavailable.

*Source: CyberSoft, Inc. Copyright 2001 by CyberSoft, Inc.

Burger King

Name	Serving Size	Gram weight	Calories	Protein (g)	Carb. (g)	Total Fat (g)	Sat. Fat. (g)	% Calories from Fat	Chol. (mg)	Sodium (mg)	Fibre (g)	Sugar (g)	Calcium (mg)	Iron (mg)	Vit. A (IU)	Vit. C (mg)
Burger King – Breakfast																
Biscuit w/Egg	1 sandwich	132	380	11	37	21	5	49.61	140	1010	1	3	60	2.70	200	0
Biscuit w/Sausage	1 sandwich	130	490	13	36	33	10	60.24	35	1240	1	3	40	2.70	0	0
Biscuit w/Sausage, Egg, & Cheese	1 sandwich	188	620	20	37	43	14	62.93	185	1650	1	4	150	2.70	500	0
French Toast Sticks	5 sticks	113	440	7	51	23	5	47.15	2	490	3	12	60	1.80	0	0
Burger King – Sides																
French Fries, Medium, Salted	1 serving	116	400	3	50	21	8	47.13	0	820	4	0	0	0.72	0	0
French Fries, Unsalted, Medium	1 serving	116	400	3	50	21	8	47.13	0	760	4	0	0	0.72	0	0
Hash Brown Rounds, Large	1 serving	128	410	3	42	26	10	56.52	0	750	4	0	0	1.08	0	0
Onion Rings, Medium	1 serving	94	380	5	46	19	4	45.60	2	550	4	4	100	0.72	0	0
Cini-Minis, w/o Vanilla Icing	4 rolls	108	440	6	51	23	6	47.59	25	710	1	20	60	2.70	1000	1.20
Burger King – Chicken																
Chicken Tenders, 5 Pieces	5 pieces	77	230	14	11	14	4	55.75	40	590	0	0	0	0.36	0	0
Patty, BK Broiler Chicken Breast	1 serving	99	140	21	4	4	1	26.47	90	570	*	*	*	*	*	*
Burger King – Burgers																
Cheeseburger	1 serving	133	360	21	27	19	9	47.11	60	760	1	4	150	2.70	300	0
Cheeseburger, Bacon	1 serving	140	400	24	27	22	10	49.25	70	940	1	4	150	2.70	300	0
Cheeseburger, Double Patty	1 serving	198	580	38	27	36	17	55.48	120	1060	1	5	250	4.50	400	0
Cheeseburger, Double Whopper	1 serving	374	1010	55	47	67	26	59.64	180	1460	3	8	300	7.20	750	9
Cheeseburger, Whopper	1 serving	295	760	35	47	48	17	56.84	110	1380	3	8	250	4.50	750	9
Hamburger	1 serving	120	320	19	27	15	6	42.32	50	520	1	4	80	2.70	100	0
Hamburger, Double Whopper	1 serving	349	920	49	47	59	21	58.03	155	980	3	8	150	7.20	500	9
Hamburger, Whopper	1 serving	270	660	29	47	40	12	54.22	85	900	3	8	100	4.50	500	9
Burger King – Sandwiches																
Chick 'n Crisp Sandwich	1 sandwich	139	460	16	37	27	6	53.41	35	890	3	3	40	1.80	0	0
Chicken Sandwich	1 sandwich	229	710	26	54	43	9	54.74	60	1400	2	4	100	3.60	0	0
Croissan'wich w/ Sausage & Cheese	1 sandwich	106	450	13	21	35	12	69.84	45	940	1	3	100	1.80	200	0
Fish Sandwich, BK Big	1 sandwich	252	720	23	59	43	9	54.13	80	1180	3	4	80	3.60	100	0

* Values unavailable.

Name	Serving Size	Gram weight	Calories	Protein (g)	Carb. (g)	Total Fat (g)	Sat. Fat. (g)	% Calories from Fat	Chol. (mg)	Sodium (mg)	Fibre (g)	Sugar (g)	Calcium (mg)	Iron (mg)	Vit. A (IU)	Vit. C (mg)
Burger King – Beverages and Shakes																
Chocolate Shake, Medium	1 serving	397	440	12	75	10	6	20.55	30	330	4	67	300	2.70	400	0
Coca Cola Classic®, Medium	687 mL	660	280	0	70	0	0	0	0		0	70	0	0	0	0
Diet Coke®, Medium	687 mL	660	1	0	0	0	0	0	0		0	0	0	0	0	0
Sprite®, Medium	687 mL	682	260	0	66	0	0	0	0		0	66	0	0	0	0
Vanilla Shake, Medium	1 medium	397	430	13	73	9	5	19.06	30	330	2	66	400	0	400	6
Burger King – Dessert																
Pie, Dutch Apple	1 serving	113	300	3	39	15	3	44.55	0	230	2	22	0	1.44	0	6

*Source: CyberSoft, Inc. Copyright 2001 by CyberSoft, Inc.

Name	Serving Size	Gram weight	Calories	Protein (g)	Carb. (g)	Total Fat (g)	Sat. Fat (g)	% Calories from Fat	Chol. (mg)	Sodium (mg)	Fibre (g)	Sugar (g)	Calcium (mg)	Iron (mg)	Vit. A (IU)	Vit. C (mg)
Jack in the box – Breakfast																
Breakfast Jack Sandwich	1 sandwich	126	280	17	28	12	5	37.50	190	750	1	3	150	3.60	400	3.60
Breakfast Sandwich, Ultimate	1 sandwich	243	600	34	39	34	10	51.17	400	1470	2	7	300	3.60	750	6
French Toast Sticks w/Bacon	1 serving	131	470	12	53	23	4	44.33	30	700	2	10	100	0.72	0	0
Pancake w/Bacon	1 serving	157	370	12	59	9	2	22.19	30	1020	3	14	80	2.70	0	0
Jack in the box – Sides																
Egg Rolls	3 egg rolls	170	440	15	40	24	6	49.54	35	1020	4	5	80	4.50	750	12
French Fries, Curly, Chili Cheese	1 serving	230	650	14	60	41	12	55.49	25	1760	4	3	150	2.70	750	0
French Fries, Curly, Seasoned	1 serving	125	410	6	45	23	5	50.36	0	1010	4	0	40	1.80	300	0
French Fries, Regular	1 serving	113	350	4	46	16	4	41.86	0	710	3	0	10	0.72	0	6
Hash Browns	1 serving	57	170	1	14	12	2	64.29	0	250	1	0	10	0.18	0	0
Stuffed Jalapenos	7 jalapenos	168	530	14	46	31	12	53.76	60	1730	3	5	300	1.44	1000	21
Onion Rings	1 serving	125	410	6	45	23	5	50.36	0	1010	4	0	40	2.70	200	18
Potato, Bacon-Cheddar Wedges	1 serving	265	800	20	49	58	16	65.41	55	1470	4	2	350	1.44	500	9
Jack in the box – Chicken and Seafood																
Chicken Breast Pieces	5 pieces	150	360	27	24	17	3	42.86	80	970	1	0	20	1.80	200	1.20
Chicken Teriyaki Bowl	1 serving	502	670	26	128	4	1	5.52	15	1730	3	27	100	4.50	6500	24
Fish & Chips	1 serving	281	780	19	86	39	9	45.53	45	1740	6	2	20	2.70	100	15
Jack in the box – Burgers																
Cheeseburger	1 burger	115	320	14	30	16	6	45	40	720	2	5	150	3.60	300	1.20
Cheeseburger, Bacon Ultimate	1 burger	302	1020	58	37	71	26	62.71	210	1740	1	7	300	7.20	750	0.60
Cheeseburger, Double Patty	1 burger	165	460	24	32	27	12	52.03	80	1090	2	5	200	4.50	500	2.40
Cheeseburger, Jumbo Jack	1 burger	282	680	31	39	45	16	59.12	115	1130	2	9	250	4.50	1000	9
Hamburger	1 burger	103	280	12	30	12	4	39.13	30	490	2	5	100	3.60	100	1.20
Hamburger, Jumbo Jack	1 burger	267	590	27	39	37	11	55.78	90	670	2	10	150	4.50	500	9
Hamburger, Sourdough Jack	1 burger	233	690	34	37	45	15	58.78	105	1180	2	3	200	4.50	750	9

*Source: CyberSoft, Inc. Copyright 2001 by CyberSoft, Inc.

Name	Serving Size	Gram weight	Calories	Protein (g)	Carb. (g)	Total Fat (g)	Sat. Fat. (g)	% Calories from Fat	Chol. (mg)	Sodium (mg)	Fibre (g)	Sugar (g)	Calcium (mg)	Iron (mg)	Vit. A (IU)	Vit. C (mg)
Jack in the box – Sandwiches																
Chicken Fajita Pita Sandwich	1 sandwich	187	280	24	25	9	4	29.24	75	840	3	5	150	2.70	1250	0
Chicken Sandwich	1 sandwich	184	420	16	39	23	4	48.48	40	950	2	4	100	2.70	200	4.80
Croissant, Sausage	1 sandwich	187	700	21	38	51	20	66.04	240	1000	0	6	100	1.80	400	0.60
Grilled Chicken Fillet Sandwich	1 sandwich	242	480	27	39	24	6	45	65	1110	4	6	200	4.50	400	9
Philly Cheesesteak Sandwich	1 sandwich	234	580	33	56	16	8	28.80	80	1860	1	3	200	2.70	400	3.60
Jack in the box – Beverages and Shakes																
Iced Tea, Regular	625 mL	600	0	0	0	0	0	0	0	0	0	0	0	0	0	0
Minute Maid® Lemonade, Regular,	625 mL	560	190	0	65	0	0	0	0	100	0	65	0	0	0	0
Barq's® Root Beer, Regular,	625 mL	627	180	0	50	0	0	0	0	40	0	50	0	0	0	0
Strawberry Ice Cream, Regular	500 mL	473	640	10	85	28	15	39.87	85	300	0	67	350	0	750	0
Jack in the box – Mexican																
Taco	1 serving	82	170	7	12	10	4	54.22	20	460	2	1	100	1.08	300	1.20
Taco, Monster	1 serving	125	270	12	19	17	6	55.23	30	670	4	2	200	1.44	400	1.20
Jack in the box – Salads																
Salad, Chicken Garden	1 salad	253	200	23	8	9	4	39.51	65	420	3	4	200	0.72	3500	12
Jack in the box – Desserts and Snacks																
Cake, Carrot	1 serving	99	370	3	54	16	3	38.71	40	340	2	28	20	1.44	5350	0.60
Cake, Double Fudge	1 serving	85	300	3	50	10	2	29.80	50	320	1	25	40	1.98	300	0.60
Cheesecake	1 serving	103	320	7	32	18	10	50.94	65	220	1	22	50	0.18	700	3
Turnover, Hot Apple	1 serving	107	340	4	41	18	4	47.37	0	510	2	12	10	1.80	100	10.20

KFC

KFC – Sides

Name	Serving Size	Gram weight	Calories	Protein (g)	Carb. (g)	Total Fat (g)	Sat. Fat. (g)	% Calories from Fat	Chol. (mg)	Sodium (mg)	Fibre (g)	Sugar (g)	Calcium (mg)	Iron (mg)	Vit. A (IU)	Vit. C (mg)
Barbecue Baked Beans	1 regular	156	190	6	33	3	1	14.75	5	760	6	13	80	1.80	400	**
Cole Slaw	1 regular	142	232	2	26	13.50	2	52.03	8	284	3	20	30	**	450	34.20
Corn on the cob	1 regular	162	150	5	35	1.50	0	7.78	0	20	2	8	**	**	100	3.60
Macaroni & Cheese	1 regular	153	180	7	21	8	3	39.13	10	860	2	2	150	**	1000	**
Potato Salad	1 regular	160	230	4	23	14	2	53.85	15	540	3	9	20	2.70	500	**
Potato Wedges	1 regular	135	280	5	28	13	4	46.99	5	750	5	1	20	1.80	**	1.20
Potato, Mashed w/Gravy	1 regular	136	120	1	17	6	1	42.86	1	440	2	0	**	0.36	**	**

KFC – Chicken

Name	Serving Size	Gram weight	Calories	Protein (g)	Carb. (g)	Total Fat (g)	Sat. Fat. (g)	% Calories from Fat	Chol. (mg)	Sodium (mg)	Fibre (g)	Sugar (g)	Calcium (mg)	Iron (mg)	Vit. A (IU)	Vit. C (mg)
Chicken Wing, Honey-Barbecue	6 pieces	189	607	33	33	38	10	56.44	193	1145	1	18	40	1.44	400	4.80
Chicken Wing, Hot	6 pieces	135	471	27	18	33	8	62.26	150	1230	2	0	40	1.44	**	**
Chicken, Breast, Extra Crispy	1 breast	168	470	39	17	28	8	52.94	160	874	1	0	20	1.08	**	**
Chicken, Breast, Original Recipe	1 breast	153	400	29	16	24	6	54.55	135	1116	1	0	40	1.08	**	**
Chicken, Drumstick, Extra Crispy	1 drumstick	67	195	15	7	12	3	55.10	77	375	1	0	**	0.72	**	**
Chicken, Drumstick, Original Recipe	1 drumstick	61	140	13	4	9	2	54.36	75	422	0	0	**	0.72	**	**
Chicken, Popcorn, Larger	1 regular	170	620	30	36	40	10	57.69	73	1046	0	0	20	0.72	0	0
Chicken, Thigh, Extra Crispy	1 thigh	118	380	21	14	27	7	63.45	118	625	1	0	20	1.08	**	**
Chicken, Thigh, Original Recipe	1 thigh	91	250	16	6	18	4.50	64.80	95	747	1	0	20	0.72	**	**
Chicken, Whole Wing, Extra Crispy	1 wing	55	220	10	10	15	4	62.79	55	415	1	0	**	0.36	**	**
Chicken, Whole Wing, Original	1 wing	47	140	9	5	10	2.50	61.64	55	414	0	0	**	0.36	**	**
Crispy Chicken Strips	3 strips	115	300	26	18	16	4	45	56	1165	1	1	**	1.08	100	**
Pot Pie, Chunky Chicken	1 pot pie	368	770	29	69	42	13	49.09	70	2160	5	8	100	1.80	4000	1.20

KFC – Sandwiches

Name	Serving Size	Gram weight	Calories	Protein (g)	Carb. (g)	Total Fat (g)	Sat. Fat. (g)	% Calories from Fat	Chol. (mg)	Sodium (mg)	Fibre (g)	Sugar (g)	Calcium (mg)	Iron (mg)	Vit. A (IU)	Vit. C (mg)
Chicken Sandwich, Tender Roast w/o Sauce	1 sandwich	177	270	31	26	5	1.50	16.48	65	690	1	1	40	1.80	**	**
Chicken Sandwich, Triple Crunch w/o Sauce	1 sandwich	176	390	25	39	15	4.50	34.53	50	650	2	0	40	2.70	**	**

** Contains less than 2% of the daily value of these nutrients.

*Source: CyberSoft, Inc. Copyright 2001 by CyberSoft, Inc.

Name	Serving Size	Gram weight	Calories	Protein (g)	Carb. (g)	Total Fat (g)	Sat. Fat. (g)	% Calories from Fat	Chol. (mg)	Sodium (mg)	Fibre (g)	Sugar (g)	Calcium (mg)	Iron (mg)	Vit. A (IU)	Vit. C (mg)
KFC – Bread																
Biscuit	1 biscuit	56	180	4	20	10	2.50	48.39	0	560	0	2	20	1.08	**	**
KFC – Desserts and Snacks																
Cake, Double Chocolate-Chip	1 serving	76	320	4	41	16	4	44.44	55	230	1	28	40	1.80	0	0
Little Bucket Parfait, Chocolate Creme	1 serving	113	290	3	37	15	11	45.76	15	330	2	25	40	1.08	**	0
Little Bucket Parfait, Fudge Brownie	1 serving	99	280	3	44	10	3.50	32.37	145	190	1	35	20	1.08	100	0
Little Bucket Parfait, Lemon Creme	1 serving	127	410	7	62	14	8	31.34	20	290	4	50	200	0.72	100	2.40
Pie, Apple	1 slice	113	310	2	44	14	3	40.65	0	280	0	23	0	1.08	0	0
Pie, Pecan	1 slice	113	490	5	66	23	5	42.16	65	510	2	31	20	1.44	200	0
Pie, Strawberry Creme	1 slice	78	280	4	32	15	8	48.39	15	130	2	22	0	0.72	100	2.40

** Contains less than 2% of the daily value of these nutrients.

*Source: CyberSoft, Inc. Copyright 2001 by CyberSoft, Inc.

McDonald's

Name	Serving Size	Gram weight	Calories	Protein (g)	Carb. (g)	Total Fat (g)	Sat. Fat. (g)	% Calories from Fat	Chol. (mg)	Sodium (mg)	Fibre (g)	Sugar (g)	Calcium (mg)	Iron (mg)	Vit. A (IU)	Vit. C (mg)
McDonald's – Breakfast																
Biscuit, Bacon, Egg, & Cheese	1 sandwich	168	540	21	36	34	10	57.30	250	1550	1	4	200	2.70	500	*
Biscuit, Sausage w/Egg	1 sandwich	178	550	18	35	37	10	61.10	245	1160	1	3	100	2.70	300	*
Burrito, Breakfast	1 serving	117	320	13	21	20	7	56.96	195	660	1	2	150	1.80	500	9
Egg McMuffin	1 sandwich	136	290	17	27	12	4.50	38.03	235	790	1	3	200	2.70	500	1.20
Hotcakes w/ Margarine & Syrup	1 serving	228	600	9	104	17	3	25.29	20	770	3	40	100	4.50	400	*
Hotcakes, Plain	1 serving	156	340	9	58	8	1.50	21.18	20	630	3	9	100	4.50	*	*
Hash Browns	1 serving	53	130	1	14	8	1.50	54.55	0	330	1	0		0.36	*	2.40
Sausage w/Egg McMuffin®	1 sandwich	162	440	19	27	28	10	57.80	255	890	1	3	250	2.70	500	*
Spanish Omelette Bagel	1 sandwich	258	690	27	59	38	14	49.85	275	1560	10	10	250	4.50	750	15
Ham, Egg, & Cheese Bagel	1 sandwich	218	550	26	58	23	8	38.12	255	1490	9	10	200	4.50	750	*
Steak, Egg, & Cheese Bagel	1 sandwich	245	660	36	57	31	11	42.86	285	1300	9	9	200	5.40	750	*
McDonald's – Chicken																
Chicken McNuggets®	6 pieces	108	290	15	20	17	3.50	52.22	55	540	2	0	20	0.72	*	*
McDonald's – Burgers																
Cheeseburger	1 burger	121	320	16	35	13	6	36.45	40	830	2	7	250	2.70	300	2.40
Cheeseburger, Quarter Pounder	1 burger	200	530	28	38	30	13	50.56	95	1310	2	9	350	4.50	500	2.40
Hamburger	1 burger	107	270	13	35	8	3.50	27.27	30	600	2	7	200	2.70	200	2.40
Hamburger, Big Mac	1 burger	216	570	26	45	32	10	50.35	85	1100	3	8	250	4.50	300	3.60
Hamburger, Quarter Pounder	1 burger	172	430	23	37	21	8	44.06	70	840	2	8	200	4.50	100	2.40
French Fries, Medium	1 serving	147	450	6	57	22	4	44	0	290	5	0	20	1.08	*	18
McDonald's – Sandwiches																
Crispy Chicken Sandwich	1 sandwich	234	550	23	54	27	4.50	44.10	50	1180	2	7	200	3.60	300	6
Filet-o-Fish Sandwich	1 sandwich	156	470	15	45	26	5	49.37	50	890	1	5	200	1.80	200	*
McDonald's – Beverages and Shakes																
McFlurry, Oreo®	1 serving	337	570	15	82	20	12	31.69	70	280	0	69	450	1.08	1250	2.40
Milkshake, Chocolate, Large	687 mL	458	582	15.57	93.89	16.95	10.59	25.64	59.54	444	3.66	81	518	1.42	425.94	1.83
Milkshake, Vanilla, Large	687 mL	458	508	16.03	81.98	13.74	8.51	23.78	50.38	375	1.83	80	558	0.41	595.40	3.66

* Values unavailable.

*Source: CyberSoft, Inc. Copyright 2001 by CyberSoft, Inc.

Name	Serving Size	Gram weight	Calories	Protein (g)	Carb. (g)	Total Fat (g)	Sat. Fat. (g)	% Calories from Fat	Chol. (mg)	Sodium (mg)	Fibre (g)	Sugar (g)	Calcium (mg)	Iron (mg)	Vit. A (IU)	Vit. C (mg)
McDonald's – Salads																
Salad, Shaker, Chef	1 salad	206	150	17	5	8	3.50	45	95	740	2	2	150	1.44	1500	15
Salad, Shaker, Garden	1 salad	149	100	7	4	6	3	55.10	75	120	2	1	150	1.08	1500	15
Salad, Shaker, Grilled-Chicken Caesar	1 salad	163	100	17	3	2.50	1.50	21.95	40	240	2	1	100	1.08	1250	12
McDonald's – Desserts and Snacks																
Cinnamon Roll	1 serving	95	390	6	50	18	5	41.97	65	310	2	24	60	1.44	400	*
Cookie, Chocolate-Chip	1 serving	35	170	2	22	10	6	48.39	20	120	1	13	20	1.08	200	*
Danish, Cheese	1 serving	105	400	7	45	21	5	47.61	40	400	2	16	80	1.44	300	*
Ice Cream Cone, Vanilla, Lower-Fat	1 serving	90	150	4	23	4.50	3	27.27	20	75	0	17	100	0.36	300	1.20
Pie, Baked Apple	1 serving	77	260	3	34	13	3.50	44.15	0	200	0	13	20	1.08	*	24
Sundae, Hot Fudge	1 serving	179	340	8	52	12	9	31.03	30	170	1	47	250	0.72	500	1.20
Sundae, Strawberry	1 serving	178	290	7	50	7	5	21.65	30	95	0	46	200	0.36	500	1.20

* Values unavailable.

*Source: CyberSoft, Inc. Copyright 2001 by CyberSoft, Inc.

Pizza Hut

Name	Serving Size	Gram weight	Calories	Protein (g)	Carb. (g)	Total Fat (g)	Sat. Fat. (g)	% Calories from Fat	Chol. (mg)	Sodium (mg)	Fibre (g)	Sugar (g)	Calcium (mg)	Iron (mg)	Vit. A (IU)	Vit. C (mg)
Pizza Hut – Pasta																
Cavatini Pasta	1 serving	357	480	21	66	14	6	26.58	8	1170	9	12	150	3.60	1250	*
Cavatini Supreme Pasta	1 serving	396	560	24	73	19	8	30.59	10	1400	10	11	150	4.50	1500	*
Spaghetti w/ Marinara Sauce	1 serving	473	490	18	91	6	1	11.02	0	730	8	10	150	3.60	1000	*
Spaghetti w/ Meat Sauce	1 serving	467	600	23	98	13	5	19.47	8	910	9	10	100	3.60	1750	*
Pizza Hut – Pizza																
Cheese, Hand-Tossed, Med.	1 slice	103	309	14	43	9	4.80	26.21	11	848	3.40	8	190	1.26	450	2.40
Cheese, Pan, Med.	1 slice	111	361	13	44	15	5.70	37.19	11	678	3.30	1	200	2.52	500	2.40
Cheese, Thin & Crispy, Med.	1 slice	79	243	11	27	10	4.90	37.19	11	653	2.40	1	190	1.26	450	2.40
Chicken Supreme, Hand-Tossed, Med.	1 slice	116	291	15	44	6	3	18.62	17	841	3.50	9	120	1.26	400	6
Chicken Supreme, Pan, Med.	1 slice	125	343	15	45	12	3.90	31.03	16	671	3.40	2	150	2.70	400	6
Chicken Supreme, Thin & Crispy, Med.	1 slice	102	232	13	29	7	3.20	27.27	19	681	2.50	2	120	1.44	400	7.20
Meat Lover's, Thin & Crispy, Med.	1 slice	107	339	15	28	19	7.80	49.85	35	970	2.60	1	140	1.80	450	2.40
Meat Lover's, Hand-Tossed, Med.	1 slice	121	376	17	44	15	6.40	35.62	30	1077	3.60	8	140	1.62	400	2.40
Meat Lover's, Pan, Med.	1 slice	129	428	16	45	21	7.30	43.65	29	607	3.40	1	140	2.88	450	2.40
Pepperoni, Hand-Tossed, Med.	1 slice	100	301	13	43	8	4	24.32	15	867	3.20	8	120	1.26	350	2.40
Pepperoni, Pan, Med.	1 slice	106	353	12	44	14	4.80	36	14	697	3.10	1	130	2.52	350	2.40
Pepperoni, Thin & Crispy, Med.	1 slice	74	235	10	27	10	4.10	37.82	14	672	2.10	1	120	1.26	350	2.40
Supreme, Hand-Tossed, Med.	1 slice	123	333	15	44	11	4.90	29.55	18	927	3.70	9	130	1.62	400	6
Supreme, Pan, Med.	1 slice	130	385	14	45	17	5.70	39.33	18	757	3.60	1	140	2.88	400	6
Supreme Pizza, Thin & Crispy, Med.	1 slice	110	284	13	29	13	5.50	41.05	20	784	2.80	2	130	1.62	400	16.80
Veggie Lover's, Hand-Tossed, Med.	1 slice	120	281	12	45	6	3	19.15	7	771	3.80	9	130	1.44	450	9.60
Veggie Lover's, Pan, Med.	1 slice	125	333	11	46	12	3.90	32.14	7	601	3.60	2	130	2.88	450	9.60
Pizza Hut – Desserts and Snacks																
Apple-Dessert Pizza	1 slice	81	250	3	48	4.50	1	16.56	0	230	2	25	*	1.08	*	*
Cherry-Dessert Pizza	1 slice	81	250	3	47	4.50	1	16.84	0	220	3	24	*	1.44	450	*
Pizza Hut – Breads																
Bread Stick	1 serving	38	130	3	20	4	1	28.13	0	170	1	1	*	1.08	*	*
Bread, Garlic	1 slice	37	150	3	16	8	1.50	48.65	0	240	1	1	40	1.44	500	*

* Values unavailable.

Taco Bell

Taco Bell – Mexican

Name	Serving Size	Gram weight	Calories	Protein (g)	Carb. (g)	Total Fat (g)	Sat. Fat. (g)	% Calories from Fat	Chol. (mg)	Sodium (mg)	Fibre (g)	Sugar (g)	Calcium (mg)	Iron (mg)	Vit. A (IU)	Vit. C (mg)
Bean Burrito, 7 Oz	1 burrito	198	370	13	54	12	3.50	28.72	10	1080	12	3	150	2.70	2250	0
Burrito Supreme, Beef, 8.75 Oz	1 burrito	248	430	17	50	18	7	37.67	40	1210	9	4	150	2.70	2500	4.80
Burrito Supreme, Chicken, 8.75 Oz	1 burrito	248	410	20	49	16	6	34.29	45	1120	8	4	150	1.80	2250	4.80
Burrito Supreme, Steak, 8.75 Oz	1 burrito	248	420	21	48	16	6	34.29	35	1140	8	4	150	2.70	2250	3.60
Chalupa Supreme, Beef, 5.5 Oz	1 chalupa	156	380	14	29	23	8	54.62	40	580	3	3	150	1.80	300	4.80
Chalupa Supreme, Chicken, 5.5 Oz	1 chalupa	156	360	17	28	20	7	50	45	490	2	3	100	1.80	200	4.80
Chalupa Supreme, Steak, 5.5 Oz	1 chalupa	156	360	17	27	20	7	50.56	35	500	2	3	150	2.70	100	3.60
Enchirito, Beef, 7.5 Oz	1 enchirito	213	370	18	33	19	9	45.60	50	1300	9	2	300	1.80	5000	1.20
Enchirito, Chicken, 7.5 Oz	1 enchirito	213	350	21	32	16	8	40.45	55	1210	7	2	250	1.80	5000	1.20
Enchirito, Steak, 7.5 Oz	1 enchirito	213	350	22	31	16	8	40.45	45	1220	7	2	250	2.70	4500	0
Gordita Supreme, Beef, 5.5 Oz	1 gordita	156	300	17	27	14	5	41.72	35	550	3	4	150	1.80	100	3.60
Gordita Supreme, Chicken, 5.5 Oz	1 gordita	156	300	16	28	13	5	39.93	45	530	3	4	150	1.44	200	3.60
Gordita Supreme, Steak, 5.5 Oz	1 gordita	156	300	17	27	14	5	41.72	35	550	3	4	150	1.80	100	3.60
Grilled Stuft Burrito, Beef, 10.3 Oz	1 burrito	292	730	27	75	35	11	43.57	65	2090	11	4	350	5.40	1500	9
Grilled Stuft Burrito, Chicken, 10.3 Oz	1 burrito	292	690	33	73	29	8	38.10	70	1900	8	4	300	5.40	1250	9
Grilled Stuft Burrito, Steak, 10.4 Oz	1 burrito	295	690	30	72	30	8	39.82	60	1970	8	4	300	6.30	1250	6
Mexican Pizza, 6.75 Oz	1 pizza	191	390	18	28	25	8	55.01	45	930	8	2	250	2.70	1750	6
Mexican Rice, 4.75 Oz	1 order	135	190	5	23	9	3.50	41.97	15	750	1	1	150	1.44	5000	1.20
Nachos, 3.5 Oz	1 order	99	320	5	34	18	4	50.94	5	560	3	2	100	0.72	300	0
Nachos Bellgrande, 11 Oz	1 order	312	760	20	83	39	11	46	35	1300	17	4	200	3.60	500	4.80
Nachos Mucho Grande, 18 Oz	1 order	510	1320	31	116	82	25	55.66	75	2670	18	6	250	5.40	1000	12
Nachos Supreme, 7 Oz	1 order	198	440	14	44	24	7	48.21	35	800	9	3	150	2.70	0	3.60

Taco Bell, continued

Taco Bell – Dessert and Snacks

Name	Serving Size	Gram weight	Calories	Protein (g)	Carb. (g)	Total Fat (g)	Sat. Fat. (g)	% Calories from Fat	Chol. (mg)	Sodium (mg)	Fibre (g)	Sugar (g)	Calcium (mg)	Iron (mg)	Vit. A (IU)	Vit. C (mg)
Pintos 'n Cheese, 4.5 Oz	1 order	128	180	9	18	8	4	40	15	640	10	1	150	1.80	2250	0
Quesadilla, Cheese, 4.25 Oz	1 quesadilla	170	350	16	31	18	9	46.29	50	860	3	2	350	0.72	400	0
Quesadilla, Chicken, 6 Oz	1 quesadilla	170	400	25	33	19	9	42.43	75	1050	3	2	350	0.72	500	1.20
Seven-Layer Burrito, 10 Oz	1 burrito	283	520	16	65	22	7	37.93	25	1270	13	4	200	3.60	1500	6
Soft Taco Supreme, Beef, 5 Oz	1 taco	142	260	11	22	13	6	46.99	40	590	3	3	100	1.08	400	3.60
Soft Taco Supreme, Chicken, 4.75 Oz	1 taco	135	240	14	21	11	5	41.42	45	490	2	3	100	0.72	300	3.60
Soft Taco Supreme, Steak, 4.75 Oz	1 taco	135	240	15	20	11	5	41.42	35	510	2	2	100	1.08	200	3.60
Soft Taco, Beef, 3.5 Oz	1 taco	99	210	11	20	10	4	42.06	30	570	3	1	80	1.08	400	0
Soft Taco, Chicken, 3.5 Oz	1 taco	99	190	13	19	7	2.50	32.98	35	480	2	1	80	0.72	200	1.20
Soft Taco, Steak, 3.5 Oz	1 taco	99	190	14	18	7	3	32.98	25	490	1	1	100	1.08	200	0
Double-Decker Taco, 7 Oz	1 taco	198	330	14	37	15	5	39.82	30	740	9	2	100	1.80	400	0
Double-Decker Taco Supreme, 7 Oz	1 taco	200	380	15	39	18	7	42.86	40	760	9	3	150	1.80	400	3.60
Taco Supreme, 4 Oz	1 taco	113	210	9	14	14	6	57.80	40	350	3	2	100	1.08	400	3.60
Taco Salad w/Salsa, 19 Oz	1 salad	539	850	30	69	52	14	54.17	70	2250	16	12	300	6.30	1450	30
Taco, 2.75 Oz	1 taco	78	170	9	12	10	4	51.72	30	330	3	1	80	0.72	400	0
Tostada, 6.25 Oz	1 tostada	177	250	10	27	12	4.50	42.19	15	640	11	2	150	1.80	2500	1.20
Cinnamon Twists, 1.25 Oz	1 order	35	150	1	27	4.50	1	26.56	0	190	1	13	0	0.36	0	0

Glossary

1-mile walk test A field test designed to evaluate cardiorespiratory endurance. The objective of the test is to complete a 1-mile walk in the shortest possible time.

1.5-mile run test A field test designed to evaluate cardiorespiratory endurance. The objective of the test is to run/walk a 1.5-mile distance in the shortest possible time.

10-percent rule Intensity or time of activity should not be increased more than 10 percent per week.

acclimatization The physiological adaptations that occur to assist the body in adjusting to environmental extremes.

acute muscle soreness A pain that develops during or immediately following physical activities that were too long or too intense.

adaptation An attempt to cope with any given stressor.

adenosine triphosphate (ATP) A high-energy compound synthesized and stored in small quantities in muscle and other cells. The breakdown of ATP results in a release of energy that can be used to fuel muscular contraction.

aerobic Means "with oxygen"; in cells pertains to energy-producing biochemical pathways that use oxygen to produce energy.

aerobics A common term that describes all forms of exercise designed to improve cardiorespiratory fitness (e.g., jogging, walking, cycling, and swimming).

agonist The muscle doing the majority of the movement, also known as the *primary mover*.

AIDS Acquired Immune Deficiency Syndrome: a fatal disease that develops from infection by the human immunodeficiency virus (HIV).

air displacemnt plethysmography (ADP) A method of determining body composition in which body volume is measured in an enclosed chamber.

amino acids The basic structural unit of proteins.

anabolic steroids Synthetic hormones (usually testosterone) that cause the body to produce muscle and prevent muscle breakdown.

anaerobic threshold The level of intensity above which the aerobic system cannot supply enough energy and the body fatigues quickly. Specifically, the work intensity during graded, incremental exercise at which there is a rapid accumulation of blood lactic acid.

anaerobic Means "without oxygen"; in cells pertains to energy-producing biochemical pathways that do not require oxygen to produce energy.

androgenic steroids Weaker anabolic steroids.

anorexia nervosa An eating disorder characterized by a dramatic weight loss achieved through strict dieting.

antagonist One or more muscles assisting primary muscles in a particular movement, also known as the *secondary movers* or *stabilizers*.

antioxidants Chemicals that prevent a damaging form of oxygen (called *oxygen free radicals*) from causing destruction to cells.

arteries The blood vessels that transport blood away from the heart.

arteriosclerosis A group of diseases characterized by a narrowing or "hardening" of the arteries.

arthroscopic surgery A surgical procedure that uses only two or three small incisions to gain entry to the damaged joint.

asthma A condition that reduces the size of the airways leading to the lungs; it can result in a sudden difficulty in breathing.

atherosclerosis A special type of arteriosclerosis that results in arterial blockage due to buildup of a fatty deposit inside the blood vessel.

behaviour modification A technique used in psychological therapy to promote desirable changes in behaviour.

benign tumour Non-cancerous group of cells.

binge eating disorder An eating disorder that involves frequent sessions of consuming large amounts of food without attempting to avoid calorie absorption.

bioelectrical impedance analysis (BIA) A convenient, rapid, non-invasive technique used to provide an estimate of body composition.

body composition The relative amount of fat and lean body tissue (muscle, organs, bone) found in the body.

body mass index (BMI) The ratio of body weight (kg) divided by height squared (m^2).

breathing exercises A simple way of achieving relaxation by regulating the speed and depth of breathing.

bulimia nervosa An eating disorder characterized by a strong desire to be thin interrupted by binge eating followed by efforts to avoid calorie absorption and feelings of guilt and lack of control.

calorie The amount of energy necessary to raise the temperature of 1 gram of water 1°C; the unit of measure used to quantify food energy or the energy expended by the body.

cancer The uncontrolled growth and spread of abnormal cells.

capillaries Thin-walled vessels that permit the exchange of oxygen and carbon dioxide and nutrients between the blood and tissues.

carbohydrates A key energy source for muscular contraction. Dietary sources of carbohydrates are breads, grains, fruits, and vegetables.

carbon monoxide A gas produced during the burning of fossil fuels such as gasoline and coal; also present in cigarette smoke.

carcinogens Cancer-causing agents, which include radiation, chemicals, drugs, and other toxic substances.

carcinoma Malignant tumours that occur in tissue that lines the body.

cardiorespiratory system Refers to the cooperative work of the circulatory (heart, blood, vascular system) and respiratory (lungs) systems.

cardiovascular disease Any disease that affects the heart or blood vessels.

cartilage A tough, connective tissue that forms a pad on the end of bones in certain joints, such as the elbow, knee, and ankle.

cellulite The "lumpy," hard fat that often gives skin a dimpled look.

chlamydia A sexually transmitted infection caused by a bacterial infection within the reproductive organs and spread through vaginal, anal, and oral sex.

cholesterol A type of derived fat in the body that is necessary for cell and hormone synthesis.

cocaine A powerful stimulant derived from the leaves of the South American coca shrub, which grows primarily in the Andes Mountains.

complete proteins Contain all the essential amino acids and are found only in foods of animal origin (meats and dairy products).

complex carbohydrates Carbohydrates that provide micronutrients and the glucose necessary for producing energy. They are contained in starches and fibre.

concentric contractions Dynamic contractions that result in muscle shortening.

convection Heat loss by the movement of air (or water) over the surface of the body.

cool-down A 5- to 15-minute period of low-intensity activity that immediately follows the primary conditioning period.

coronary heart disease (CHD) CHD is the result of atherosclerotic plaque forming a blockage in one or more coronary arteries.

coronary heart disease The result of plaque forming a blockage in one or more coronary arteries.

creeping obesity A slow increase in body fat over several years.

cross training The use of a variety of physical activities for improving cardiorespiratory endurance.

cycle ergometer test A field test performed on a cycle ergometer designed to evaluate cardiorespiratory endurance.

delayed-onset muscle soreness (DOMS) Pain that develops 24 to 48 hours after physical activity that is excessive in duration or intensity.

derived fats A class of fats that do not contain fatty acids and are not soluble in water.

diabetes A metabolic disorder characterized by high blood glucose levels.

diastolic blood pressure The pressure of the blood in the arteries at the level of the heart during the resting phase of the heart (diastole).

distress Stress that may negatively affect health.

drug abuse Excessive use of a drug leading to negative personal, family, social, or professional consequences.

drug misuse Taking a drug for a purpose other than for which it was intended.

drug use Consuming a drug in the way it was intended to be used.

dual-energy X-ray absorptiometry (DXA) A method used to estimate fat, lean, and bone mineral content.

dynamic contractions Muscle contractions in which there is movement of a body part.

dynamic stretching A technique that develops an active range of motion through the process of slow and controlled movements.

eating disorders A range of unhealthy eating and body weight issues.

eccentric contractions Dynamic contractions that result in the muscle lengthening.

ergogenic aid A drug or nutritional product that improves physical fitness and exercise performance.

essential amino acids Amino acids that cannot be manufactured by the body and therefore must be consumed in the diet.

eustress Good stress.

evaporation The conversion of water (or sweat) to a gas (water vapour); the most important means of removing heat from the body during physical activity.

exercise metabolic rate (EMR) The energy expenditure during physical activity.

exercise prescription guidelines Guidelines that incorporate regular exercise in accordance with the FITT principles that can be tailored to individual needs. It incorporates fitness goals, type of exercise, warm-up, workout (primary conditioning), and cool-down.

exercise stress test A diagnostic test designed to determine if a subject's cardiovascular system responds normally to exercise.

exercise A specific physical activity (often called *training*) that causes the exertion of the muscles, heart, and lungs through various movements.

fartlek training Fartlek is a Swedish word meaning "speed play," and refers to an interval-type training in which sprints are inserted into long, slow runs.

fast-twitch fibres Muscle fibres that contract rapidly and fatigue quickly.

fat An efficient storage form for energy, because of the energy content.

fatty acids The basic structural unit of triglycerides.

fibre A stringy, nondigestible carbohydrate found in whole grains, vegetables, and fruits in its primary form, cellulose.

flexibility The ability to move joints freely through their full range of motion.

free radicals Promote the development of cancer by binding to DNA, altering its structure and function so that the cell divides rapidly and out of control.

frequency of exercise The number of times per week that one intends to be active.

fructose Also called *fruit sugar;* a naturally occurring sugar found in fruits and in honey.

galactose A simple sugar found in the breast milk of humans and other mammals.

general adaptation syndrome A pattern of responses to stress that consists of an alarm stage, a resistance stage, and an exhaustion stage.

genital herpes A general term for a family of diseases caused by viral infections; highly contagious and transmitted through hand-to-genital contact, oral, anal, or vaginal sex.

glucose A sugar molecule that can be used by the body in its natural form for energy.

glycogen The storage form of glucose in the liver and skeletal muscles.

glycolysis Metabolic process in which carbohydrates are broken down to ATP.

gonorrhoea A common sexually transmitted infection, transmitted through vaginal, anal, and oral contact.

healthy active lifestyle A lifestyle that values and incorporates physical activity into everyday living.

heart attack (myocardial infarction) Complete blockage of coronary arteries resulting in the death of heart cells.

heart rate Number of heartbeats per minute.

heat injury Bodily injury that can occur when the heat load exceeds the body's ability to regulate body temperature.

high-density lipoproteins (HDL) A combination of protein, triglycerides, and cholesterol in the blood, composed of relatively large amounts of protein.

homeotherms Animals that regulate their body temperatures to remain close to a set point. Humans regulate their body temperatures around the set point of 37°C (98.6°F).

humidity The amount of water vapour in the air.

hydrocarbons Chemical compounds that contain carbon and hydrogen.

hydrostatic weighing A method of determining body composition that involves weighing an individual on land and in water.

hyperlipidemia High blood cholesterol levels; generally a total blood cholesterol concentration greater than 240 mg/dl.

hyperplasia An increase in the number of muscle fibres.

hypertension (high blood pressure) Usually considered to be a blood pressure of greater than 140 for systolic or 90 for diastolic.

hypertrophy An increase in muscle fibre size.

incomplete proteins Proteins that are missing one or more of the essential amino acids; can be found in numerous vegetable sources.

intensity of exercise The amount of physiological stress or overload placed on the body during exercise.

intermediate fibres Muscle fibres that possess a combination of the characteristics of fast- and slow-twitch fibres.

interval training Repeated sessions or intervals of relatively intense exercise.

isocaloric balance When energy intake equals energy expenditure.

isokinetic contractions Concentric or eccentric dynamic contractions performed at a constant speed.

lactic acid A byproduct of glucose metabolism, produced primarily during intense exercise.

lactose Also called *milk sugar;* a simple sugar found in milk products; it is composed of galactose and glucose.

leukemia Cancer of blood-forming organs.

ligaments Connective tissue within the joint capsule that holds bones together.

lipoproteins Combinations of protein, triglycerides, and cholesterol in the blood.

long, slow distance training Continuous exercise that requires a steady, submaximal exercise intensity, generally around 70 percent HRmax.

low-density lipoproteins (LDL) A combination of protein, triglycerides, and cholesterol in the blood, composed of relatively large amounts of cholesterol.

lymphoma A cancer that develops in lymphatic tissue.

macronutrients Carbohydrates, fats, and proteins, which are necessary for building and maintaining body tissues and providing energy for daily activities.

malignant tumour Cancerous group of cells that grows rapidly; results in deterioration or death.

maltose Also called *malt sugar;* a simple sugar found in grain products; it is composed of two glucose molecules linked together.

marijuana A plant mixture (stems, leaves, or seeds) containing the active chemical tetrahydrocannabinol.

meditation An ancient method that aims to produce relaxation and achieve inner peace.

melanoma Cancerous growths that develop in the skin cells that create melanin.

metastasis The process of malignant cells spreading through the body.

micronutrients Nutrients in food, such as vitamins and minerals, that regulate the functions of the cells.

minerals Chemical elements (e.g., sodium and calcium) required by the body for normal functioning.

momentum stretching Uses momentum to force a joint or limb beyond a normal range of motion.

motor unit A motor nerve and the muscle fibres it controls.

muscular endurance The ability of a muscle or muscle group to generate force over and over again or to sustain muscular contractions.

muscular strength The maximum amount of force that can be produced during one contraction.

myocardial infarction (MI) (also called a heart attack) Damage to the heart due to a reduction in blood flow, resulting in the death of heart muscle cells.

negative caloric balance When more calories are expended than consumed.

nitrogen dioxide An amber-coloured gas found in smog.

nonessential amino acids Eleven amino acids that the body can make and therefore are not necessary in the diet.

nutrients Substances in food that are necessary for good health.

obesity An excessive accumulation of body fat to the extent that it puts one's health at risk.

omega-3 fatty acid A type of unsaturated fatty acid that lowers blood cholesterol and triglycerides and is found primarily in fresh or frozen mackerel, herring, tuna, and salmon.

one-repetition maximum (1 RM) test Measurement of the maximum amount of weight that can be lifted one time.

organic Refers to foods that are grown without pesticides.

osteoporosis The loss of bone mass and strength, which increases the risk of bone fractures.

overeating The consumption of excessive calories that leads to a positive caloric balance.

overload principle Stressing the body or a specific muscle beyond what it is used to, in order to improve physical strength.

overtraining Results from exercising too hard, too fast, or too frequently with an inadequate amount of rest between sessions.

overweight Refers to a body weight greater than expected for a specific height.

ozone A gas produced by a chemical reaction between sunlight and the hydrocarbons emitted from car exhausts.

particulates Tiny solid particles or liquid droplets that are suspended in the air.

patella-femoral pain syndrome (PFPS) A common injury, sometimes called "runner's knee," that is manifested as pain behind the kneecap (patella).

photochemical smog The brownish-yellow haze resulting from the combination of hydrocarbons and nitrogen oxides.

physical activity Any bodily movement produced by the skeletal muscles that expends energy.

physical fitness The ability of the body to function at optimal efficiency with an improved physiological state that can lead to improved health and longevity.

positive caloric balance When more calories are consumed than expended.

progression principle Placing gradual and increasing stress on the body, producing positive changes.

progressive resistance exercise (PRE) The application of the overload principle to strength and endurance training programs.

proprioceptive neuromuscular facilitation (PNF) A technique that combines stretching with alternating contraction and relaxation of muscles to improve flexibility.

psychosocial stressors The many events in daily life that can cause good or bad stress.

pulmonary circuit The blood vascular system that circulates deoxygenated blood from the right side of the heart, through the lungs, and back to the left side of the heart.

R.I.C.E. cryokinetics A relatively new rehabilitation technique implemented after healing has been completed. It incorporates alternating periods of treatment using ice, exercise, and rest.

recruitment The process of involving more muscle fibres to increase muscular force.

recuperation principle The body requires recovery periods between exercise training sessions in order to adapt to the stress of exercise. Therefore, a period of rest is essential for achieving maximal benefit from exercise.

repetition maximum (RM) The maximal load that a muscle group can lift a specified number of times before tiring.

resting metabolic rate (RMR) The amount of energy the body requires to perform all necessary functions associated with maintaining life.

reversibility principle Fitness gains made through training will be lost when training is stopped for long periods of time or permanently.

sarcoma Any cancer arising from muscle cells or connective tissues.

saturated fatty acid A type of fatty acid that comes primarily from animal sources (meat and dairy products) and is solid at room temperature.

self-efficacy The belief in one's ability to accomplish the task at hand.

self-esteem A sense of satisfaction with oneself.

set The number of repetitions performed consecutively without resting.

sexually transmitted infections (STIs) A group of more than 20 diseases generally spread through sexual contact.

shin splints Pain in the front of the lower leg.

sit and reach test A field test that measures the flexibility of the muscles in the lower back and in the back of the thigh.

skinfold measurements A field test in which measurement of representative samples of subcutaneous fat provides a means of estimating overall body fatness.

slow-twitch fibres Muscle fibres that contract slowly and are highly resistant to fatigue.

specificity of training The development of muscular strength and endurance is specific to the muscle group exercised and the training intensity.

specificity principle The effect of training is specific to those muscles involved in the activity.

spot reduction The false notion that exercise applied to a specific region of the body will result in fat loss in that region.

sprain Damage to a ligament that occurs if excessive force is applied to a joint.

starches Long chains of sugars commonly found in foods such as corn, grains, potatoes, peas, and beans.

static contractions Muscle contractions in which muscular tension is developed but no movement of body parts takes place.

static stretching Stretching that slowly lengthens a muscle to a point where further movement is limited.

step test A field test that involves bench stepping designed to evaluate cardiorespiratory endurance.

strain Wear and tear on the mind and body while trying to adapt to a stressor.

strain Damage to a muscle that ranges from a minor separation of fibres to a complete tearing of the muscle.

stress fractures Tiny cracks or breaks in the bone.

stress The way your mind and body react when you are forced to adapt to the persons and/or situations around you.

stressor A factor that produces distress or eustress.

stretch reflex Involuntary contraction of a muscle that occurs due to rapid stretching of that muscle.

stroke volume The amount of blood pumped per heartbeat.

stroke When the blood supply to the brain is reduced for a prolonged period of time, usually as a result of blockage of arteries in the head or neck.

sucrose Also called *table sugar;* a molecule composed of glucose and fructose.

sulphur dioxide A yellowish-brown gas that is a byproduct of burning fossil fuels.

sun protection factor (SPF) A sunscreen with an SPF of 15 provides you with 15 times more protection than unprotected skin.

syphilis A sexually transmitted infection transmitted through direct sexual contact; caused by a bacterial infection and cured by antibiotics.

systemic circuit The blood vascular system that circulates oxygenated blood from the left side of the heart, throughout the body, and back to the right side of the heart.

systolic blood pressure The pressure of the blood in the arteries at the level of the heart during the contraction phase of the heart (systole).

target heart rate (THR) zone The range of heart rates that corresponds to an exercise intensity of approximately 50 to 85 percent VO_2max and results in improvements in aerobic capacity.

temperature inversion A weather condition occurring when a layer of cool air is trapped under a layer of warmer air.

tendonitis Inflammation or swelling of a tendon.

tendons Connective tissue that connects muscles to bones.

threshold for health benefits The minimum level of physical activity required to achieve the health benefits of exercise.

time (duration) of physical activity The amount of time invested in performing the primary workout.

training threshold A training intensity above 50 percent of VO_2max where there is an improvement in cardiorespiratory fitness.

trans fatty acid A type of fatty acid that increases cholesterol in the blood and is a major contributor to heart disease.

triglycerides The form of fat broken down and used to produce energy to power muscle contractions.

triglycerides A type of fat consumed and manufactured in the body.

tumour A group of abnormal cells. A tumour can be either benign or malignant (cancerous).

type 1 diabetes Also called *insulin-dependent diabetes;* a result of abnormally low levels of insulin.

type 2 diabetes Also called *non–insulin-dependent diabetes* or *adult-onset diabetes;* a result of a reduced ability of insulin to transport glucose from the blood to the cells.

type of exercise The specific type of exercise to be performed.

unsaturated fatty acid A type of fatty acid that comes primarily from plant sources and is liquid at room temperature.

valsalva manoeuvre Breath holding during an intense muscle contraction; can reduce blood flow to the brain and cause dizziness and fainting.

variety principle Training blocks that alternate between low, medium, and high intensity to challenge the body and facilitate improvements.

veins Blood vessels that transport blood toward the heart.

venereal warts Warts caused by a small group of viruses called human papilloma viruses; spread through sexual contact.

visualization A relaxation technique that uses appealing mental images to promote relaxation and reduce stress; also called *imagery.*

vitamins Small molecules that play a key role in many bodily functions.

VO_2max Maximum aerobic power is an indication of the fitness of the cardiorespiratory system. Specifically, it refers to the highest oxygen consumption achieved during an exercise test.

waist girth The measurement taken at the smallest point of the waist, usually at the level of the umbillicus (navel).

warm-up A brief period of activity that precedes a workout so that muscle temperature and blood flow increase.

wellness A state of healthy living that includes physical, emotional, intellectual, spiritual, social, environmental, and occupational health.

Index

Photo Credits